Congenital Anomalies of the Brain, Spine, and Neck

Guest Editors

HEMANT A. PARMAR, MD
MOHANNAD IBRAHIM, MD

NEUROIMAGING CLINICS OF NORTH AMERICA

www.neuroimaging.theclinics.com

Consulting Editor
SURESH K. MUKHERJI, MD

August 2011 • Volume 21 • Number 3

SAUNDERS an imprint of ELSEVIER, Inc.

W.B. SAUNDERS COMPANY
A Division of Elsevier Inc.

1600 John F. Kennedy Boulevard • Suite 1800 • Philadelphia, Pennsylvania 19103-2899

http://www.theclinics.com

NEUROIMAGING CLINICS OF NORTH AMERICA Volume 21, Number 3
August 2011 ISSN 1052-5149, ISBN 13: 978-1-4557-1110-9

Editor: Joanne Husovski
Developmental Editor: Donald Mumford

Neuroimaging Clinics of North America (ISSN 1052-5149) is published quarterly by Elsevier Inc., 360 Park Avenue South, New York, NY 10010-1710. Months of issue are February, May, August, and November. Business and editorial offices: 1600 John F. Kennedy Blvd., Suite 1800, Philadelphia, PA 19103-2899. Business and editorial offices: 6277 Sea Harbor Drive, Orlando, FL 32887-4800. Periodicals postage paid at New York, NY, and additional mailing offices. Subscription prices are USD 314 per year for US individuals, USD 436 per year for US institutions, USD 158 per year for US students and residents, USD 363 per year for Canadian individuals, USD 546 per year for Canadian institutions, USD 461 per year for international individuals, USD 546 per year for international institutions and USD 226 per year for Canadian and foreign students and residents. To receive student/resident rate, orders must be accompanied by name of affiliated institution, date of term, and the *signature* of program/residency coordinator on institution letterhead. Orders will be billed at individual rate until proof of status is received. Foreign air speed delivery is included in all *Clinics* subscription prices. All prices are subject to change without notice. POSTMASTER: Send address changes to *Neuroimaging Clinics of North America*, Elsevier Health Sciences Division, Subscription Customer Service, 3251 Riverport Lane, Maryland Heights, MO 63043. Telephone: 1-800-654-2452 (U.S. and Canada); 314-447-8871 (outside U.S. and Canada). Fax: 314-447-8029. E-mail: journalscustomerservice-usa@elsevier.com (for print support); journalsonlinesupport-usa@elsevier.com (for online support).

Reprints. For copies of 100 or more of articles in this publication, please contact the Commercial Reprints Department, Elsevier Inc., 360 Park Avenue South, New York, NY 10010-1710. Tel.: 212-633-3812; Fax: 212-462-1935; E-mail: reprints@elsevier.com.

Neuroimaging Clinics of North America is covered by *Excerpta Medical/EMBASE,* the RSNA Index of Imaging Literature, *MEDLINE/PubMed (Index Medicus),* MEDLINE/MEDLARS, SciSearch, Research Alert, and Neuroscience Citation Index.

Printed and bound by CPI Group (UK) Ltd, Croydon, CR0 4YY

Transferred to Digital Print 2011

GOAL STATEMENT

The goal of *Neuroimaging Clinics of North America* is to keep practicing radiologists and radiology residents up to date with current clinical practice in radiology by providing timely articles reviewing the state of the art in patient care.

ACCREDITATION

The *Neuroimaging Clinics of North America* is planned and implemented in accordance with the Essential Areas and Policies of the Accreditation Council for Continuing Medical Education (ACCME) through the joint sponsorship of the University of Virginia School of Medicine and Elsevier. The University of Virginia School of Medicine is accredited by the ACCME to provide continuing medical education for physicians.

The University of Virginia School of Medicine designates this enduring material activity for a maximum of 15 *AMA PRA Category 1 Credit*(s)™ for each issue, 60 credits per year. Physicians should claim only the credit commensurate with the extent of their participation in the activity.

The American Medical Association has determined that physicians not licensed in the US who participate in this CME activity are eligible for a maximum of ***15*** AMA PRA Category 1 Credit(s)™ for each issue, 60 credits per year.

Credit can be earned by reading the text material, taking the CME examination online at http://www.theclinics.com/home/cme, and completing the evaluation. After taking the test, you will be required to review any and all incorrect answers. Following completion of the test and evaluation, your credit will be awarded and you may print your certificate.

FACULTY DISCLOSURE/CONFLICT OF INTEREST

The University of Virginia School of Medicine, as an ACCME accredited provider, endorses and strives to comply with the Accreditation Council for Continuing Medical Education (ACCME) Standards of Commercial Support, Commonwealth of Virginia statutes, University of Virginia policies and procedures, and associated federal and private regulations and guidelines on the need for disclosure and monitoring of proprietary and financial interests that may affect the scientific integrity and balance of content delivered in continuing medical education activities under our auspices.

The University of Virginia School of Medicine requires that all CME activities accredited through this institution be developed independently and be scientifically rigorous, balanced and objective in the presentation/discussion of its content, theories and practices.

All authors/editors participating in an accredited CME activity are expected to disclose to the readers relevant financial relationships with commercial entities occurring within the past 12 months (such as grants or research support, employee, consultant, stock holder, member of speakers bureau, etc.). The University of Virginia School of Medicine will employ appropriate mechanisms to resolve potential conflicts of interest to maintain the standards of fair and balanced education to the reader. Questions about specific strategies can be directed to the Office of Continuing Medical Education, University of Virginia School of Medicine, Charlottesville, Virginia.

The faculty and staff of the University of Virginia Office of Continuing Medical Education have no financial affiliations to disclose.

The authors/editors listed below have identified no professional/financial affiliations for themselves or their spouse/partner:

Aaron H. Baer, MD; Daniel JG Baxter, MD, CM, FRCPC; Sonia Bermúdez, MD; James Chen, BS; Aaron A. Cohen-Gadol, MD, MSc; Michael A. DiPietro, MD; Tamara Feygin, MD; Hugh JL Garton, MD; Lydia Gregg, MA, CMI; Sachin K. Gujar, MBBS, MD; Khaled Hammoud, MD; Shawn L. Hervey-Jumper, MD; Joanne Husovski, (Acquisitions Editor); Mohannad Ibrahim, MD (Guest Editor); Steven J Kasten, MD; Sudhir Kathuria, MD; Cormac O. Maher, MD; Mohit Maheshwari, MD; Maria T. Mantilla, MD; Shraddha S. Mukerji, MD; Sara Nuñez, MD; Amit Pandya, MD; Hemant A. Parmar, MD (Guest Editor); Charles Raybaud, MD; Stephanie Rufener, MD; Lubdha M. Shah, MD (Test Author); Karuna Shekdar, MD; Manohar Shroff, MD, FRCPC; Nicholas M. Wetjen, MD; and Elysa Widjaja, MD.

The authors listed below have identified the following professional/financial affiliations for themselves or their spouse/partner:

Dheeraj Gandhi, MD, MBBS is a consultant for Covidian/EV3 Merlin, and is an industry funded research/investigator for AOD Inc.

Suresh K. Mukherji, MD (Consulting Editor) is a consultant for Philips.

Disclosure of Discussion of Non-FDA Approved Uses for Pharmaceutical Products and/or Medical Devices

The University of Virginia School of Medicine, as an ACCME provider, requires that all faculty presenters identify and disclose any off-label uses for pharmaceutical and medical device products. The University of Virginia School of Medicine recommends that each physician fully review all the available data on new products or procedures prior to clinical use.

TO ENROLL

To enroll in the Neuroimaging Clinics of North America Continuing Medical Education program, call customer service at 1-800-654-2452 or sign up online at http://www.theclinics.com/home/cme. The CME program is available to subscribers for an additional annual fee of USD 196.

Neuroimaging Clinics of North America

FORTHCOMING ISSUES

Tropical Neuroradiology
Rakesh Gupta, MD, *Guest Editor*

Intracranial Infections
Guarang Shah, MD, *Guest Editor*

Neuroradiology Applications of High-Field MR Imaging
Winfried Willinek, MD, *Guest Editor*

RECENT ISSUES

May 2011

Stroke Imaging
Pamela W. Schaefer, MD, *Guest Editor*

February 2011

Clinical Applications of Diffusion Imaging of the Brain
L. Celso Hygino da Cruz Jr, MD, *Guest Editor*

November 2010

Neuroradiology Emergencies
Alisa D. Gean, MD, *Guest Editor*

August 2010

State of the Art Brain Tumor Diagnostics, Imaging, and Therapeutics
Meng Law, MD, *Guest Editor*

RELATED INTEREST

Neurologic Clinics, February 2009 (pages 285–301)
Pediatric Neuroimaging by authors Ahmed Abdelhalim and Ronald Alberico
Laszlo Mechtler, MD, *Guest Editor*
www.neurologic.theclinics.com

Contributors

CONSULTING EDITOR

SURESH K. MUKHERJI, MD, FACR
Professor and Chief of Neuroradiology and Head, and Neck Radiology; Professor of Radiology, Otolaryngology Head and Neck Surgery, Radiation Oncology, Periodontics and Oral Medicine, University of Michigan Health System, Ann Arbor, Michigan

GUEST EDITORS

HEMANT A. PARMAR, MD
Associate Professor, Department of Radiology, University of Michigan Health System, Ann Arbor, Michigan

MOHANNAD IBRAHIM, MD
Assistant Professor, Department of Radiology, University of Michigan Health System, Ann Arbor, Michigan

AUTHORS

AARON H. BAER, MD
Department of Radiology, University of Michigan Health System, Ann Arbor, Michigan

DANIEL J.G. BAXTER, MD CM, FRCPC
Neuroradiologist, Diagnostic Imaging, University of Toronto, Toronto, Ontario, Canada

SONIA BERMÚDEZ, MD
Associate Professor of Medicine, University El Bosque, Bogotá, Colombia; Chief, Neuroradiology Section, Department of Diagnostic Imaging, Fundacion Santa Fe de Bogotá University Hospital, Bogotá DC, Colombia

JAMES CHEN, BS
Department of Radiology, Johns Hopkins Hospital, Baltimore, Maryland

AARON A. COHEN-GADOL, MD, MSc
Assistant Professor, Department of Neurological Surgery, Indiana University, Indianapolis, Indiana

MICHAEL A. DIPIETRO, MD
John F. Holt Collegiate Professor, Department of Radiology, University of Michigan Health System, Ann Arbor, Michigan

TAMARA FEYGIN, MD
Assistant Professor of Radiology, Neuro-radiology Division, Department of Radiology, The Children's Hospital of Philadelphia, University of Pennsylvania, Philadelphia, Pennsylvania

DHEERAJ GANDHI, MBBS, MD
Director, Endovascular Surgical Neuroradiology Program. Johns Hopkins University Hospital and Johns Hopkins Bayview; Associate Professor of Radiology, Neurology and Neurosurgery, Johns Hopkins University Hospital and Johns Hopkins Bayview, Baltimore, Maryland

HUGH J.L. GARTON, MD
Associate Professor, Department of Neurosurgery, University of Michigan, Ann Arbor, Michigan

LYDIA GREGG, MA, CMI
Illustrator, Department of Radiology, Johns Hopkins Hospital, Baltimore, Maryland

SACHIN K. GUJAR, MBBS, MD
Assistant Professor of Radiology, Division of Neuroradiology, Johns Hopkins University School of Medicine, Baltimore, Maryland

KHALED HAMMOUD, MS
College of Human Medicine, Michigan State University, Lansing, Michigan

SHAWN L. HERVEY-JUMPER, MD
Resident, Department of Neurosurgery, University of Michigan, Ann Arbor, Michigan

MOHANNAD IBRAHIM, MD
Assistant Professor, Department of Radiology, University of Michigan Health System, Ann Arbor, Michigan

STEVEN J. KASTEN, MD
Assistant Professor, Department of Plastic Surgery, University of Michigan Health System, Ann Arbor, Michigan

SUDHIR KATHURIA, MD
Departments of Radiology and Neurosurgery, Johns Hopkins Hospital, Baltimore, Maryland

CORMAC O. MAHER, MD
Assistant Professor, Department of Neurosurgery, University of Michigan, Ann Arbor, Michigan

MOHIT MAHESHWARI, MD
Department of Radiology, Medical College of Wisconsin, Milwaukee, Wisconsin

MARIA T. MANTILLA, MD
Associate Professor of Neuroradiology Section, Department of Diagnostic Imaging, Reina Sofia Clinic, International Sanitas Organization, Colsanitas University Clinic "Reina Sofía," Bogotá, Colombia

SHRADDHA S. MUKERJI, MD
Department of Pediatric Otolaryngology, University of Texas Medical Branch, Galveston, Texas; Department of Radiology, University of Michigan, Ann Arbor, Michigan

SURESH K. MUKHERJI, MD, FACR
Professor and Chief of Neuroradiology and Head, and Neck Radiology; Professor of Radiology, Otolaryngology Head and Neck Surgery, Radiation Oncology, Periodontics and Oral Medicine, University of Michigan Health System, Ann Arbor, Michigan

SARA NUÑEZ, MD
Associate Professor of Medicine and Neuroradiology Section, Colombia University Clinic, International Sanitas Organization; Neuroradiology Section, Country Clinic, Bogotá, Colombia

AMIT PANDYA, MD
Department of Radiology, University of Michigan Health System, Ann Arbor, Michigan

HEMANT A. PARMAR, MD
Associate Professor, Department of Radiology, University of Michigan Health System, Ann Arbor, Michigan

CHARLES RAYBAUD, MD
Derek Harwood-Nash Chair in Medical Imaging; Professor of Radiology, University of Toronto; Head of Division of Neuroradiology, Hospital for Sick Children, Toronto, Ontario, Canada

STEPHANIE RUFENER, MD
Department of Radiology, University of Michigan Health System, Ann Arbor, Michigan; Mount Scott Diagnostic Imaging Center, Portland, Oregon

KARUNA SHEKDAR, MD
Assistant Professor of Radiology, Neuroradiology Division, Department of Radiology, The Children's Hospital of Philadelphia, University of Pennsylvania, Philadelphia, Pennsylvania

MANOHAR SHROFF, MD, FRCPC
Neuroradiologist; Associate Professor, Diagnostic Imaging, The Hospital for Sick Children, University of Toronto, Toronto, Ontario, Canada

NICHOLAS M. WETJEN, MD
Assistant Professor, Department of Neurologic Surgery, Mayo Clinic, Rochester, Minnesota

ELYSA WIDJAJA, MD
Assistant Professor of Radiology, University of Toronto; Staff Radiologist, Division of Neuroradiology, Hospital for Sick Children, Toronto, Ontario, Canada

Contents

Foreword xi

Suresh K. Mukherji

Demystifying Congenital Malformations for Imaging Specialists xiii

Hemant A. Parmar and Mohannad Ibrahim

Midline Congenital Malformations of the Brain and Skull 429

Sara Nuñez, Maria T. Mantilla, and Sonia Bermúdez

Considering the complexity of congenital midline abnormalities of the brain, it is mandatory to review and summarize the subject, based on embryologic development, developmental biology, clinical approach, neuroimaging, and molecular genetics. There are still several areas of poor knowledge, confusion, and controversy. Pathogenesis in some cases is not clearly understood, and definitions and limits among different diseases are not apparent. This article reviews several malformations of the skull and brain with the aims of making image interpretation easier, enabling an accurate diagnosis, establishing the prognosis, and aiding in genetic counseling.

Development and Dysgenesis of the Cerebral Cortex: Malformations of Cortical Development 483

Charles Raybaud and Elysa Widjaja

The cerebral cortex develops in several stages from a pseudostratified epithelium at 5 weeks to an essentially complete cortex at 47 weeks. Cortical connectivity starts with thalamocortical connections in the 3rd trimester only and continues until well after birth. Vascularity adapts to proliferation and connectivity. Malformations of cortical development are classified into disorders of specification, proliferation/apoptosis, migration, and organization. However, all processes are intermingled, as for example a dysplastic cell may migrate incompletely and not connect appropriately. However, this classification is convenient for didactic purposes as long as the complex interactions between the different processes are kept in mind.

Congenital Arterial and Venous Anomalies of the Brain and Skull Base 545

Sudhir Kathuria, James Chen, Lydia Gregg, Hemant A. Parmar, and Dheeraj Gandhi

Congenital cerebral vascular anomalies include a spectrum of conditions that result from perturbation of normal developmental processes. Although some of these conditions are asymptomatic and well compensated by collateral circulation, others can cause significant morbidity or produce a range of complications for affected patients. Knowledge of the underlying developmental etiologies and the associated imaging characteristics helps fully elucidate the morphologic and hemodynamic details of these lesions and determine the necessity for any intervention.

Congenital Midface Abnormalities 563

Daniel J.G. Baxter and Manohar Shroff

There are a wide variety of congenital midface abnormalities that originate during transformation of the first pair of pharyngeal arches into adult structures. Computed

tomography and magnetic resonance imaging are important components in the comprehensive evaluation of these lesions. A detailed understanding of midface embryogenesis and developmental anatomy is important in directing appropriate patient management.

Congenital Malformations of the Orbit 585

Sachin K. Gujar and Dheeraj Gandhi

This article discusses the embryologic development of the eye and orbital structures. Among the defects presented are anophthalmia and microphthalmia, coloboma, persistent hyperplastic primary vitreous, Coats disease, vascular malformations, encephalocele and nasolacrimal mucocele. Clinical and imaging features of the diseases are presented, along with radiographic images.

Congenital Malformations of the Temporal Bone 603

Shraddha S. Mukerji, Hemant A. Parmar, Mohannad Ibrahim, and Suresh K. Mukherji

Congenital ear or temporal bone malformations are a diagnostic challenge to radiologists and surgeons alike. Newer imaging techniques can detect subtle changes in middle ear and cochlear anatomy. This information is invaluable with increasing use of hearing restoration surgeries and/or cochlear implants in such patients. This article discusses the embryogenesis, classification system, and salient imaging findings of congenital outer, middle ear, and inner ear anomalies in children. Both high-resolution computerized tomography and magnetic resonance imaging scans of the temporal bones are described.

Congenital Cystic Lesions of the Head and Neck 621

Mohannad Ibrahim, Khaled Hammoud, Mohit Maheshwari, and Amit Pandya

This article presents clinical characteristics and radiologic features of congenital cervical cystic masses, among them thyroglossal duct cysts, cystic hygromas, branchial cleft cysts, and the some of the rare congenital cysts, such as thymic and cervical bronchogenic cysts. The imaging options and the value of each for particular masses, as well as present clinical and radiologic images for each, are discussed.

Hemangiomas and Vascular Malformations of the Head and Neck: A Simplified Approach 641

Aaron H. Baer, Hemant A. Parmar, Michael A. DiPietro, Steven J. Kasten, and Suresh K. Mukherji

This article is a review of vascular tumors and malformations that occur in infancy and childhood. It discusses anomalies of arterial, venous, capillary, lymphatic, and mixed vascular endothelium in terms of their varying forms, clinical course, imaging characteristics, complications, and treatment. The comparative utility of various imaging modalities is simplified.

Imaging of Congenital Spine and Spinal Cord Malformations 659

Stephanie Rufener, Mohannad Ibrahim, and Hemant A. Parmar

This article reviews normal embryologic development of the spine and spinal cord and the imaging features of congenital abnormalities of the spine and spinal cord, with particular focus on magnetic resonance imaging. The authors discuss spinal dysraphisms, a heterogeneous group of congenital abnormalities of the spine and spinal cord, and provide information to expand understanding of these complex entities.

Foreword

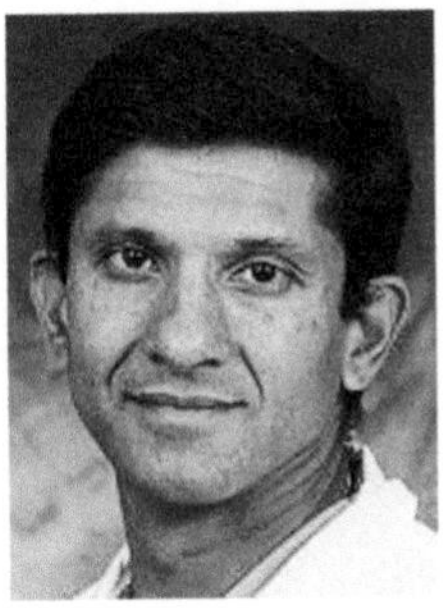

Suresh K. Mukherji, MD
Consulting Editor

One of the most rewarding aspects of academic medicine is having the ability to "make a difference" in the lives of our patients, those we train, and those with whom we work. It is very hard for me to be objective when writing this Foreword since Hemant Parmar, MD and Mohannad Ibrahim, MD are both members of the Neuroradiology Division at the University of Michigan.

I am not sure if words can fully describe how much I admire and respect both of these individuals. There is a saying that in order to be successful, you should always try and hire people who are smarter than you ... and this is certainly the case here! Both Hemant and Mohannad are extraordinary clinical neuroradiologists and are regarded as excellent teachers by our residents and fellows. Both are academically productive and have lectured at numerous national and international meetings. But, most importantly, they are two of the nicest people who I have met and have impeccable character. Both are incredible "team players" and are always willing to help each other and all members of our group.

Hemant and Mohannad both completed dedicated Pediatric Neuroradiology fellowships at Sick Kids Hospital in Toronto. They are very good friends and it has been a pleasure seeing how they interact and always support each other. So, it was a natural choice to invite them to Guest Edit this edition of *Neuroimaging Clinics* on the topic of "Congenital Malformations of Head, Neck, and Spine." They have been able to successfully assemble internationally recognized experts on each subject matter. I think you will find the article content and illustrations of the highest caliber and am confident this issue will become a "classic."

In their Preface, Hemant and Mohannad correctly said that it "was going to be quite a challenging proposition, but the idea of this project was to demystify the embryologic aspect and make the learning of congenital malformations easy and interesting." Well, I think they have fully accomplished all of their objectives and I thank them and their article authors for their extraordinary contributions.

Suresh K. Mukherji, MD
Department of Radiology
University of Michigan Health System
1500 East Medical Center
Ann Arbor, MI 48109-0030, USA

E-mail address:
mukherji@med.umich.edu

Neuroimag Clin N Am 21 (2011) xi
doi:10.1016/j.nic.2011.06.001
1052-5149/11/$ – see front matter

Demystifying Congenital Malformations for Imaging Specialists

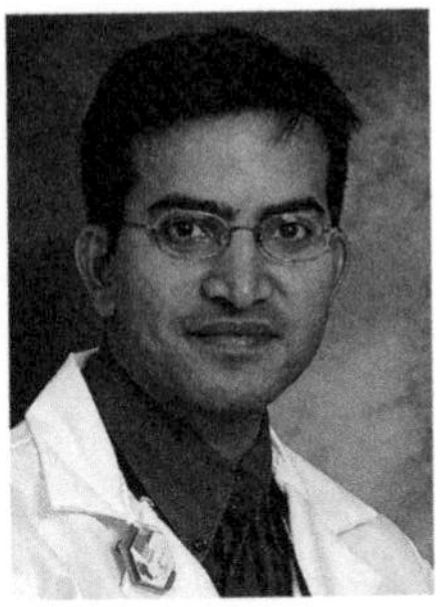

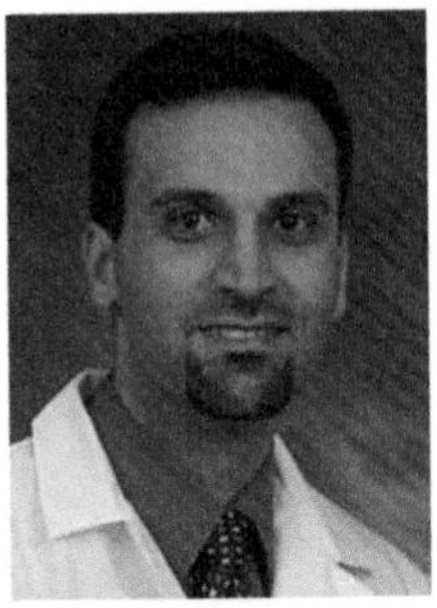

Hemant A. Parmar, MD Mohannad Ibrahim, MD
Guest Editors

Pediatric neuroimaging is generally challenging for radiologists. Like in other areas of pediatric imaging, understanding congenital malformations of the brain, spine, and neck requires detailed knowledge of the basic embryology, something which many of us dread and have long forgotten from our medical school days.

When Suresh approached us to do guest edit an issue of *Neuroimaging Clinics of North America* on "congenital malformations of head, neck and spine," we were humbled and equally honored for the opportunity. We realized it was going to be quite a challenging proposition, but the idea of this project was to demystify the embryologic aspect and make the learning of congenital malformations easy and interesting.

In this publication, we deal with most of the congenital malformations that one can expect to see in pediatric neuroimaging. Each article emphasizes the role of basic embryology in the understanding of imaging manifestation of various malformations. Images are used liberally throughout to help elucidate and graphically exemplify the concepts. We begin with the intracranial congenital malformations and then move to the orbits, temporal bone, neck, and finally, the spinal malformations. We have an article on fetal neuroimaging, emphasizing the role of MRI in diagnosing various malformations in-utero. The final two articles provide a neurosurgeon's perspectives to various intracranial and spinal congenital malformations. Each of the authors is a recognized expert in their field (some have taught and mentored us!) and we would like to express our sincere appreciation and thanks for all their insights and their hard work.

We are grateful to Suresh Mukherji, MD, FACR for extending this invitation to serve as guest editor for *Neuroimaging Clinics*. We would also like to thank Joanne Husovski from Elsevier for all her support, patience, and assistance during the publication of this issue. It is our sincere hope that the readers of the *Neuroimaging Clinics* enjoy this issue and find the information useful in their clinical practice.

Hemant A. Parmar, MD

Mohannad Ibrahim, MD
Department of Radiology
University of Michigan Health System
1500 East Medical Center Drive
Ann Arbor, MI 48109-0302, USA

E-mail addresses:
hparmar@med.umich.edu (H.A. Parmar)
mibrahim@umich.edu (M. Ibrahim)

Neuroimag Clin N Am 21 (2011) xiii
doi:10.1016/j.nic.2011.05.015

Midline Congenital Malformations of the Brain and Skull

Sara Nuñez, MD[a,b,*], Maria T. Mantilla, MD[c], Sonia Bermúdez, MD[d,e]

KEYWORDS

- Congenital, hereditary, and neonatal diseases and abnormalities • Encephalocele • Corpus callosum
- Holoprosencephaly • Central nervous system cysts
- Dandy-Walker syndrome • Rhombencephalon
- Magnetic resonance imaging

Considering the complexity of congenital midline abnormalities of the brain, it is mandatory to review and summarize the subject, based on embryologic development. There are still several areas of poor knowledge, confusion, and controversy. Pathogenesis in some cases is not clearly understood, and definitions and limits among different diseases also unclear. Reviewing these concepts makes image interpretation easier, giving an accurate diagnosis that can help the clinician establish the prognosis and provide genetic counseling. Brain malformations are frequently diagnosed either incidentally or because of patients' overall clinical picture. In some cases the radiologist does not know relevant data from the medical chart, such as the prenatal or family history, which thus can lead to a diagnosis based only on the imaging findings. The latter situation advocates a review of congenital midline abnormalities of the brain in order to clarify concepts and allow a diagnosis that is better oriented. Some investigators believe that a classification system based solely on neuroimaging criteria is not achievable.

MIDLINE CEPHALOCELES

Cephaloceles are an extracranial protrusion of the cerebral tissue and meninges through a congenital defect in the cranial bones. The connection between the protruding tissue and the intracranial cavity remains. Cephaloceles are usually classified according to the location of the skull defect: anterior or posterior in relation to the coronal sutures (**Fig. 1**). Anterior cephaloceles comprise those whereby the swelling is in front of the coronal suture or located in the orbit or nasal cavity; these include interfrontal, frontoethmoidal (nasofrontal, nasoethmoidal, naso-orbital), and nasopharyngeal (transsphenoidal, transethmoidal, sphenoethmoidal, basioccipital) cephaloceles.[1] Posterior cephaloceles are defined as parietal when the defect is between the bregma and the lambda, and occipital when the defect arises between the lambda and the foramen magnum, possibly including one or more of the cervical vertebrae.[2]

Atretic cephaloceles are formes fruste of cephaloceles, which contain a small, noncystic, flat, or

---

The authors have nothing to disclose and there are not conflicts of interest.
[a] Colombia University Clinic, International Sanitas Organization, Avenida de la Esperanza, calle 68 Bogotá, Colombia
[b] Neuroradiology Section, Country Clinic, carrera 16 a No 82-37, Bogotá, Colombia
[c] Department of Diagnostic Imaging, Reina Sofia Clinic, International Sanitas Organization, Colsanitas University Clinic "Reina Sofía", Carrera 31 No. 125ª-23, Bogotá, Colombia
[d] University El Bosque, Carrera 7 B Bis No. 132 - 11 - Bogotá D.C., Bogotá, 110121, Colombia
[e] Neuroradiology Section, Department of Diagnostic Imaging, Fundacion Santa Fe de Bogotá University Hospital, Calle 119 # 7-75 third floor, Bogotá DC, Colombia
* Corresponding author. Radiology and Diagnosis Imaging department, Colsanitas University Clinic Colombia, Calle 23 No. 66-46, Bogotá DC, Colombia.
E-mail address: saranm49@etb.net.co

Neuroimag Clin N Am 21 (2011) 429–482
doi:10.1016/j.nic.2011.05.001
1052-5149/11/$ – see front matter

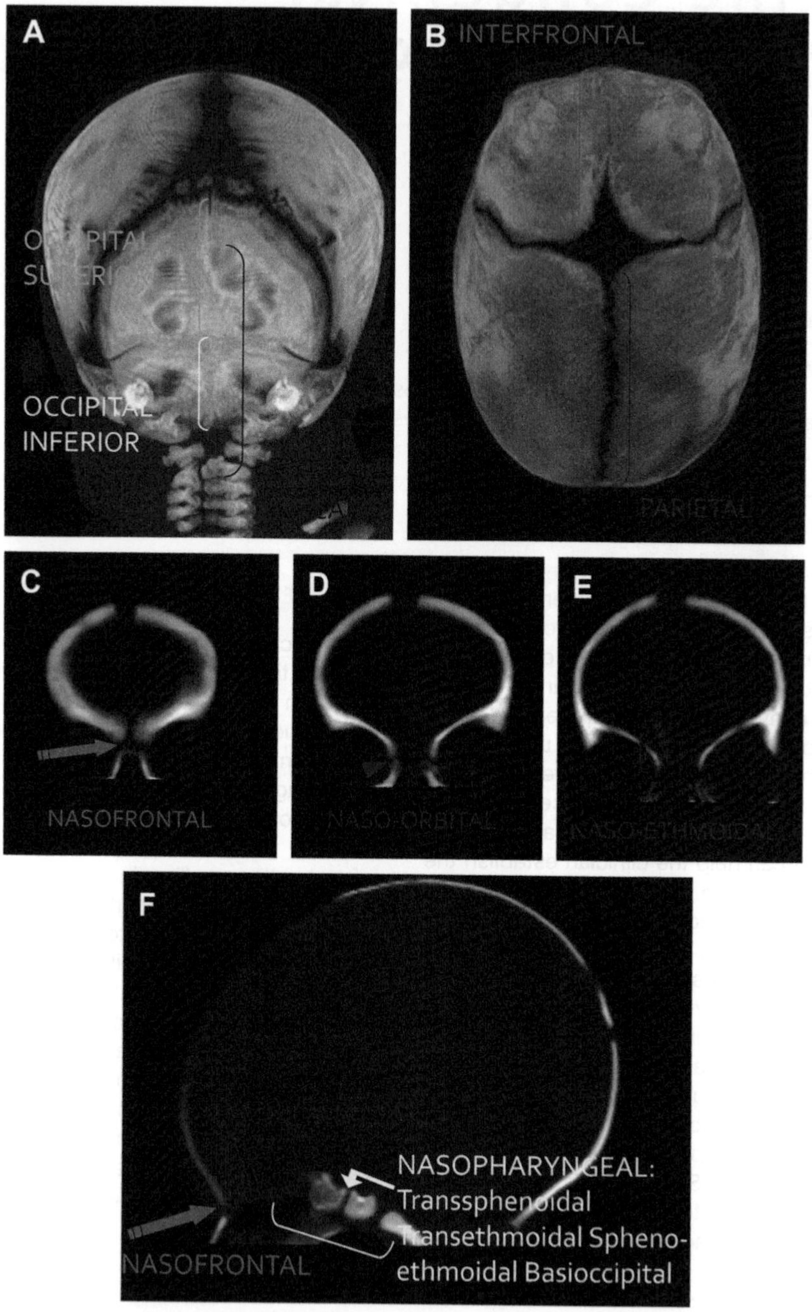

Fig. 1. Classification of cephaloceles according to the skull defect. (*A*) Three-dimensional CT of head. Posterior view of occipital bone demonstrates the location of different occipital cephaloceles: superior, inferior, occipitocervical. (*B*) Three-dimensional CT of head. Superior view of skull illustrates sites of interfrontal and parietal cephaloceles. (*C*) CT coronal image at nasofrontal sutures (*straight arrow*), where nasofrontal cephaloceles occur. (*D*) CT coronal image at the level of the middle third of the medial orbital wall (*arrowhead*), where naso-orbital cephaloceles protrude. (*E*) CT coronal image at frontoethmoidal level (*curved arrow*), where nasoethmoidal cephaloceles are found. (*F*) CT midline sagittal image. Different points of probable nasopharyngeal (transsphenoidal: *angled arrow*) and frontoethmoidal cephaloceles are shown.

nodular lesion. This lesion is situated in the midline of the scalp, either near the vertex (parietal) or just cephalic to the external occipital protuberance (occipital form).[3,4] Other definitions are listed in **Box 1**.

Cephaloceles can also be classified according to the involvement of the cranial vault (interfrontal, parietal, occipital, and lateral) or the skull base (temporal, frontoethmoidal, nasopharyngeal, spheno-orbital, and sphenomaxillary).[3] Nasopharyngeal, temporal and spheno-orbital types are classified as basal cephaloceles by other investigators.[5,6] A detailed histologic examination allows for another classification according to their content: pure meninges (meningocele), meninges and brain (encephalomeningoceles), part of the ventricle (encephalocystocele), or glial-lined cyst containing cerebrospinal fluid (CSF) (gliocele).[7]

The incidence of cephaloceles is approximately 0.8 to 3.0 per 10,000 births.[3,8] Occipital cephaloceles constitute 66% to 89% of the cases,[3] frontoethmoidal 15%, and basal 10%.[5,6] Frontoethmoidal cephaloceles show a relatively high incidence (1:5000 live births) in Southeast Asia.[9,10] There are several factors that influence the incidence of neural tube defects (NTD), such as different genetic alterations, nutrition and the health status of women, frequency of prenatal diagnosis resulting in an elective abortion, and exposure to NTD-inducing toxic agents.[11]

On the fifth day of life, gastrulation starts and establishes 3 germ layers (ectoderm, mesoderm, and endoderm) in the embryo. On days 15 to 16, invagination starts (cells enter Hensen's node and migrate cephalad) to form the notochordal process, which eventually becomes the notochord. The notochord induces the overlying ectoderm to thicken and form the neural plate. Cells of the neural plate form the neuroectoderm, and their induction initiates the neurulation process. The expression of several genes and proteins that participate in the process of gastrulation and neurulation is described in **Box 2**.[12] At about 17 days gestational age (GA), the neural plate thickens laterally and forms the neural folds. These folds contract (due to the underlying actin myofibrils), elevate, and form a depressed medial zone known as the neural groove.[13,14] At about the 20th gestational day, the folds thicken and the surrounding mesenchyme expands simultaneously, leading the edges of the folds to approach one another in the midline, where they fuse at the following levels: the mesencephalic-rhombencephalic boundary, the cervical spine, and the rostral end of the neural groove.[10] As the folding edges of the neural ectoderm join, they are covered by adjacent cutaneous ectoderm. Disjunction of the two ectoderm (cutaneous and neural) types occurs as the edges meet, and the cells at the lateral border or crest of the neuroectoderm begin to dissociate from their neighbors, creating the neural crest (**Fig. 2**).[12] The neural crest cells migrate, and once they reach the prechordal

Box 1
Definitions of skull malformations

- Cranium bifidum occultum: a midline or paired paramedian skull defect, without the prolapsing of meninges or brain (eg, parietal or frontal foramina)
- Exencephaly: acrania with protrusion of the central nervous system (CNS) into the amniotic cavity (in utero) or into the environment (postnatal)
- Anencephaly: acrania with absence of most or all of the brain tissue
- Cutis aplasia congenita: absence of skin in a localized or extended area at birth. Variable depth of the defect (only epidermis or as deep as the dura)

Data from Naidich TP, Altman NR, Braffman BH, et al. Cephaloceles and related malformations. AJNR Am J Neuroradiol 1992;13(2):655–90.

Box 2
Genes and proteins for gastrulation and neurulation

1. Head-forming genes: OTX2, LIM1, HESX1, Secreted factor Cerberus
2. Initiates and maintains integrity of node and primitive streak: gene Nodal (member of Transforming Growth Factor β family)
3. Mesoderm ventralization during gastrulation: BMP-4 (Bone Morphogenetic Protein 4), requires the presence of FGF (Fibroblast Growth Factor secreted by node and primitive streak)
4. Antagonize BMP-4 activity and dorsalize mesoderm to form the notochord and somitomeres in the head region, and induction of neurulation: chordin, noggin, follistatin
5. Proteins of induction (inactivation of BMP-4) of neural plate structures (hindbrain and spinal cord): FGF, WNT3a

Data from Langman J. Second week of development: trilaminar germ disc 65. In: Sadler TW, Langman J, editors. Langman's medical embryology. 9th edition. Philadelphia: Lippincott Williams & Wilkins; 2004. p. 534; and Padmanabhan R. Etiology, pathogenesis and prevention of neural tube defects. Congenit Anom (Kyoto) 2006;46(2):55–67.

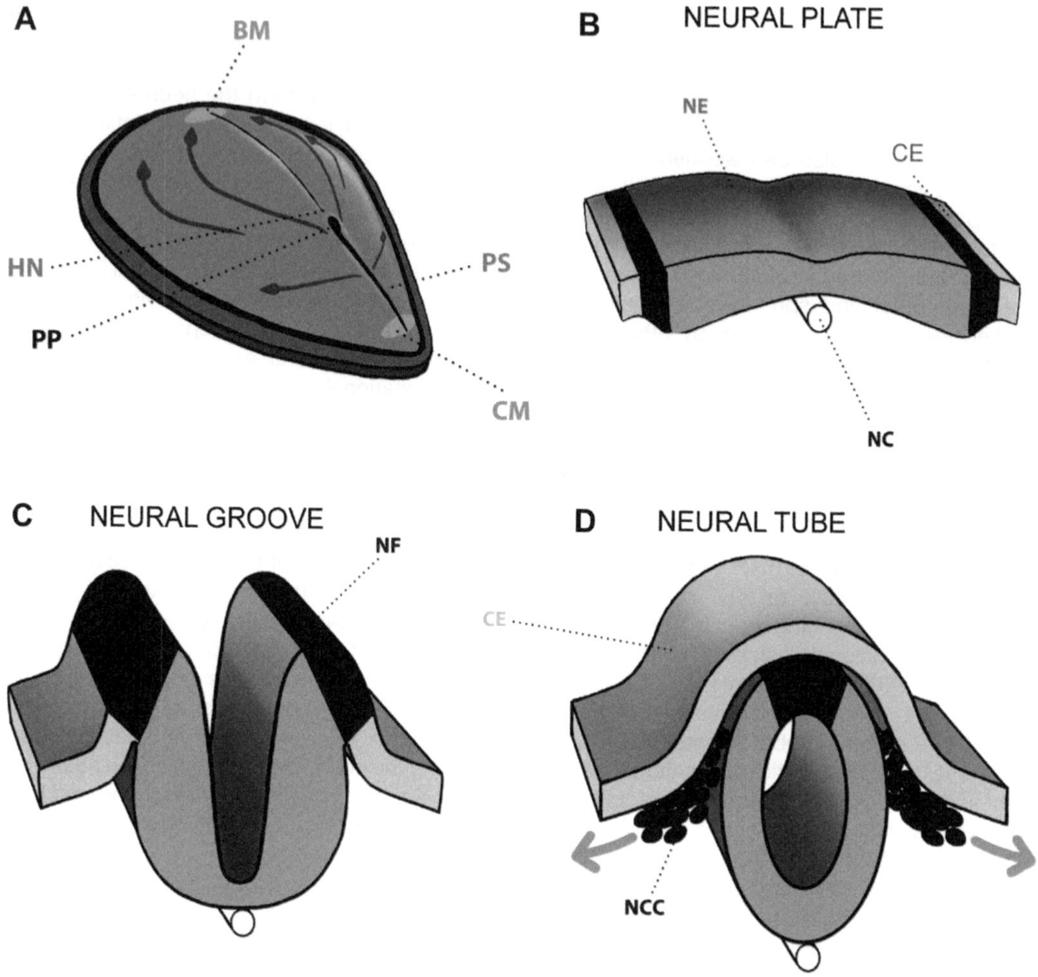

Fig. 2. Summary of neural plate and neural tube formation. Neural plate formation. (*A*) On the fifth day gestational age a group of ectodermal cells proliferate to form the primitive streak along the dorsal surface of the embryo. At the cephalic end of the streak is a rapidly proliferating group of cells, surrounding a primitive pit, known as Hensen's node. On day 15-16 gestational age, cells enter the primitive pit and migrate cephalad to form the notochordal process, which eventually becomes the notochord. The notochord induces the overlying ectoderm to thicken and form the neural plate. Neural tube formation. (*B*) Cells of the neural plate form the neuroectoderm and their induction initiates the neurulation process. Then the neural plate thickens laterally and forms the neural folds. (*C*) These folds contract, elevate and form a depressed medial zone known as the neural groove. (*D*) At about the 20th gestational day, the folds thicken and the surrounding mesenchyme expands simultaneously, leading the edges of the folds to approach one another in the midline. As the folding edges of the neural ectoderm join, they are covered by adjacent cutaneous ectoderm. Disjunction of the two ectoderm (cutaneous and neural) types occurs as the edges meet, and the cells at the lateral border or crest of the neuroectoderm begin to dissociate from their neighbors originating the neural crest cells. BM, bucopharyngeal membrane; CE, cutaneous ectoderm; CM, cloacal membrane; HN, Hensen's node; NC, notochord; NCC, neural crest cells; NE, neuroectoderm; NF, neural folds; PP, primitive pit; PS, primitive streak.

skull base, the overlying neural tube is transformed into prosencephalon, which then differentiates into the diencephalon and telencephalon.[15] Some of the neural crest derivatives include connective tissue and bones of the face and skull, cranial nerve ganglia, and dermis of the face and neck.[12]

The mechanisms leading to the defective closure of the neural tube are still unknown. Recently, Trovato and colleagues[11] proposed that NTD may be due to p53 downregulation or disruption, which diminishes the expression of hepatocyte growth factor/scatter factor (HGF), c-met, and STAT3 genes. Other high-risk factors associated with NTD are listed in **Box 3**.

There are two important embryologic clues in defining the pathogenesis of cephaloceles. First, there is a midline skull defect in congenital nasal cephaloceles, which corresponds with the sites of neural tube closure along the median (implies neurulation disorder). Second, the fact that a skin or an epithelial layer covers the cephaloceles suggests that the neural tube must have closed (implies postneurulation disorder).[10]

There are 4 theories about the pathogenesis of cephaloceles, as follows:

1. Neurulation disorder. Hoving[10] postulated that a disturbance in the disjunction between the cutaneous and the neural ectoderm at the site of final closure of the rostral neuropore, possibly due to a lack of apoptosis, might result in a frontoethmoidal cephalocele. This process can be disturbed at any of the sites of neural tube closure, leading to the various cephaloceles as classified. Examples of these abnormal points of closure and cephaloceles are listed in **Table 1**.[10]
2. Postneurulation. At later stages of embryogenesis isolated focal cranial defects may arise, while the multiple ossification centers coalesce to allow the progressive ossification of the chondrocranium (from 35 days GA until after birth). Certain cephaloceles of the skull base could be secondary to failure of the correct coalescence of the ossification centers, leaving persistent dehiscence between two endochondral ossification centers.[14,16]
3. Defective tissular induction. A defective tissular induction that occurs at early embryogenesis is a plausible explanation of the concurrence of cephaloceles and both cerebral and craniofacial malformations.[15,16] These malformations encounter prosencephaly, agenesis of the corpus callosum, anomalies of the visual and olfactory structures, and midline facial clefts for the anterior cephaloceles, and agenesis of the corpus callosum with dorsal cyst, callosal lipoma, and porencephaly for posterior cephaloceles. These abnormalities could present for anterior cephaloceles, at 28 to 35 days GA, during the induction of the mesoblast (by the notochord and the neural tube) to form the cranial base and facial structures.[16] Blustajn and colleagues[15] explain the association of transsphenoidal cephalocele and both ophthalmologic and endocrine anomalies by this mechanism. If there is no migration of the neural crest cells to the future prechordal skull base region, there is no appropriate induction of the overlying diencephalic neural tube during organogenesis of the optic nerves and the hypothalamic-pituitary axis. In the case of posterior cephaloceles, the defective induction

Box 3
High-risk factors associated with NTD

1. Gene disorders:
   a. Cerebrocostomandibular syndrome
   b. Fraser syndrome
   c. Meckel-Gruber syndrome
   d. Waardenbur syndrome
2. Physical agents:
   a. X-irradiation
   b. Hyperthermia
   c. Stress
3. Drugs:
   a. Thalidomide
   b. Folate antagonists
   c. Androgenic hormones
   d. Valproate
   e. Carbamazepine
   f. Hypervitaminosis A
4. Substance abuse:
   a. Alcohol
5. Chemical agents:
   a. Organic mercury
   b. Lead
6. Maternal infections:
   a. Rubella
   b. Cytomegalovirus
   c. *Toxoplasma gondii*
   d. Syphilis
7. Maternal metabolic conditions:
   a. Phenylketonuria
   b. Diabetes mellitus
   c. Endemic cretinism

Data from Naidich TP, Altman NR, Braffman BH, et al. Cephaloceles and related malformations. AJNR Am J Neuroradiol 1992;13(2):655–90; and Padmanabhan R. Etiology, pathogenesis and prevention of neural tube defects. Congenit Anom (Kyoto) 2006;46(2):55–67.

Table 1
Abnormal points of closure and cephaloceles

Point of Closure	Cephalocele
Foramen cecum (closure of frontal and ethmoid bones)	Frontoethmoid
Between chiasmatic plate and the nasal fields	Basal

Data from Hoving EW. Nasal encephaloceles. Childs Nerv Syst 2000;16(10–11):702–6.

and formation of the membranous cranial roof occur at 38 to 45 days GA. At later stages of embryogenesis, isolated focal cranial defects may arise, while the multiple ossification centers coalesce to allow the progressive ossification of the chondrocranium (from 35 days GA until after birth). Certain cephaloceles of the skull base could be secondary to failure of this process.[16]

4. Intracranial cyst. Diebler and Dulac[16] also proposed another mechanism to explain the association of certain cystic intracranial malformations (such as Dandy-Walker cyst) with cephalocele. Diebler and Dulac mention that an increased intracranial pressure (due to intracranial mass or cyst) may lead to progressive thinning of the neuropil, which evolves into a focal defect in the cranial vault with cephalocele.

Swelling at the level of the cephalocele, bony defect, facial malformations (anterior cephaloceles), and intracranial malformations are certain features shared by patients with cephaloceles (**Table 2**). Magnetic resonance (MR) imaging is the modality of choice for the evaluation of all of these abnormalities; even though computed tomography (CT) is more precise than MR imaging in delineating the margins and extensions of the bony defect.

It is necessary to determine the size, extent, and nature of the contents of the cephalocele. The size of the cephaloceles varies according to their location and type (tissue content within the sac).The dysgenesis of the corpus callosum and hydrocephalus are the most common associated intracranial abnormalities.[9] Encephaloceles are isointense relative to gray matter with most MR imaging sequences, but they may be hyperintense on T2-weighted images because of gliosis.[6,17,18] When cephaloceles contain meninges, they are isointense to CSF. If cephaloceles contain ventricle, in addition to the CSF signal intensity the walls of the ventricles are seen isointense to gray matter.

New techniques such as MR imaging and MR angiography provide precise information about venous sinuses and arteries. Kotil and colleagues[19] have shown that 3-dimensional (3D) Fourier-transformation constructive interference in a steady state (CISS) sequence and T2-weighted reversed (T2R) imaging on 3 Tesla allow a superb demonstration of the intracranial venous anomalies associated with these cephaloceles. These anomalies include an anomalous upward course of the straight sinus ("vertical embryonic positioning of the straight sinus"), elongation of the vein of Galen, and splitting of the superior sagittal sinus. A prominent supracerebellar cistern has also been shown with these techniques.[20,21] This evaluation is crucial for surgical planning, particularly of venous anomalies in occipital, parietal, and atretic parietal cephaloceles.[19,21]

Table 2
Abnormalities associated with cephaloceles

Abnormality	Cephalocele
Dysgenesis corpus callosum (DCC)	TSPH, N-ETH, N-FR, OCC, P, A-P
Arachnoid cyst associated to DCC	P, A-P
Hydrocephalus	I-FR, OCC, P
Optic nerve atrophy	OCC, N-PHR, FR-ETH
Dandy-Walker cyst, Chiari II malformation, microcephaly	OCC, P
Venous anomalies, prominent supracerebellar cistern	OCC, P
Cerebral and cerebellar migration anomalies	OCC
Chiari III	OCC
Interhemispheric lipoma	N-F
Proptosis	N-O

Abbreviations: A-P, atretic parietal; FR-ETH, frontoethmoidal; I-FR, interfrontal; N-ETH, nasoethmoidal; N-FR, nasofrontal; N-O, naso-orbital; N-PHR, nasopharyngeal; OCC, occipital; P, parietal; TSPH, transsphenoidal.
Data from Refs.[3,10,13,16,22]

Occipital Cephalocele

The location of the bony defect in occipital cephaloceles may be infratentorial (**Fig. 3**), supratentorial, or combined.[16] These defects can also involve the posterior arch of C1 and C2 (occipitocervical cephalocele).[2] The occipital cephalocele can be small or large (>50 mm), and is rarely larger in size than the head (giant cephalocele, **Fig. 4**) of the patient.[19] The occipital encephalocele is part of the Chiari III malformation. The features of this malformation are described in detail in the section on posterior fossa malformations. Intracranial malformations and syndromes are associated with occipital cephaloceles, as listed in **Box 4**.

Parietal and Atretic Parietal Cephaloceles

The bony defect in parietal cephaloceles more commonly lies near the posterior or anterior fontanelle. Under this bony defect there is a fenestrated falx or dural dehiscence, leading to the ostium and

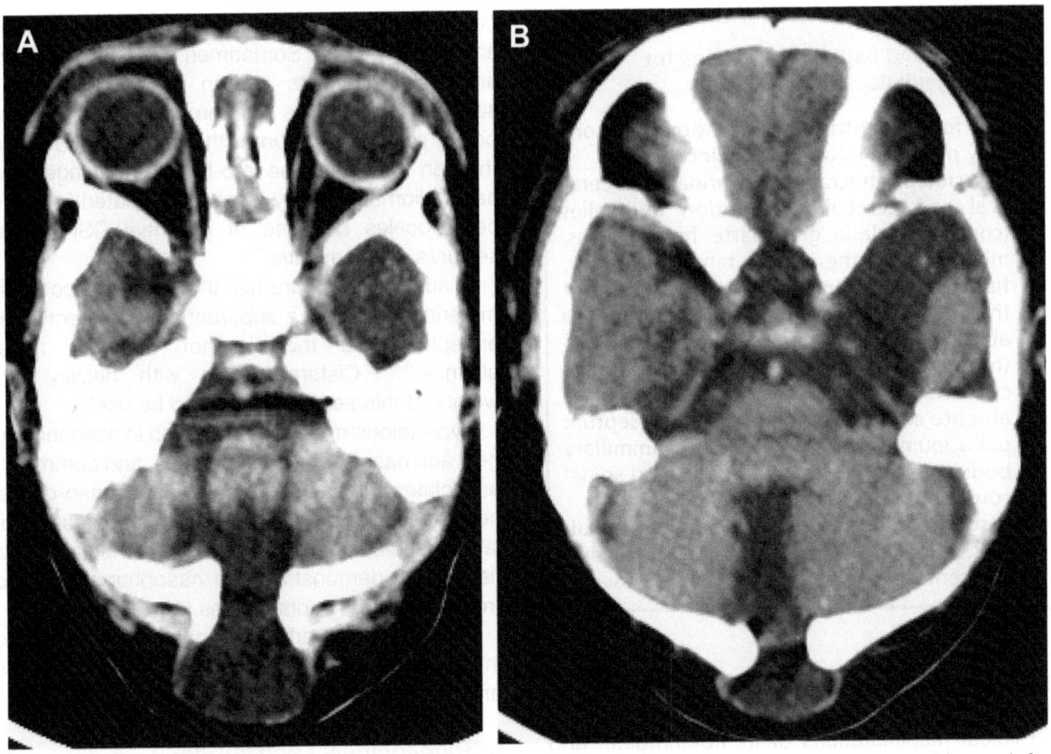

Fig. 3. Occipital inferior cephalocele. Axial CT contiguous images of head (*A* and *B*) show occipital bony defect inferior to the occipital external protuberance (inion) with protrusion of tissue isodense to cerebrospinal fluid (CSF).

the interhemispheric fissure being widened. A tentorial cleft or fenestration is shown as a consequence of the insertion of the separated dural leaves (of the falx), which insert into the ipsilateral tentorial leaf (**Fig. 5**). Some clinical findings of parietal cephaloceles and associated intracranial malformations are mentioned in **Box 5**.

Nowadays, thin-section (1–2 mm) gradient echo (with gradient spoiler) or fast spin echo MR images or thin CT images are available, and are required to visualize the small communication in atretic cephaloceles.[13]

Anterior Cephaloceles

Midline anterior cephaloceles include (a) frontoethmoidal (nasoethmoidal, nasofrontal, and naso-orbital), (b) nasopharyngeal (transethmoidal,

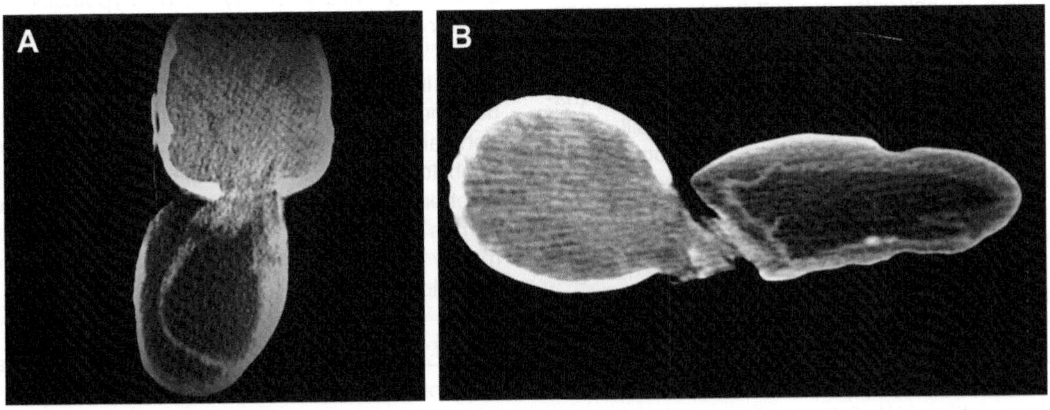

Fig. 4. Giant occipital cephalocele. Coronal (*A*) and axial (*B*) CT images demonstrate the large sac, which contains tissue isodense to both brain parenchyma and CSF.

Box 4
Radiologic and pathologic findings for occipital cephalocele

1. The fourth ventricle and the occipital horn may protrude into the cephalocele
2. Associated intracranial malformations: Cerebral and cerebellar migration anomalies (cortical dysplasia, gray matter heterotopias, microgyria of the medial temporal cortex, faulty convolution, inversion or absence of the dentate fascia and rudimentary to absent amygdala), cystic malformations of the posterior fossa, dorsal interhemispheric cyst, fusion of thalami, partial or complete absence of the anterior commissure, septum pellucidum, fornices, and mammillary bodies. Hydromyelia and a deformed spinal cord, optic nerve atrophy[3,19]
3. Associated syndromes: Chemke, Cryptophthalmos, Knobloch, Meckel, pseudo-Meckel, dyssegmental dwarfism, frontonasal dysplasia[3]

sphenoethmoidal, transsphenoidal, basioccipital), and (c) interfrontal.

Clinical manifestations of frontoethmoidal and nasopharyngeal cephaloceles may consist of nasal stuffiness, rhinorrhea, a broad nasal root, or hypertelorism.[22] These cephaloceles change in size during crying, the Valsalva maneuver, or jugular compression (positive Furstenberg test).[16,23] MR imaging evaluation must involve the specific zone and the entire brain. Associated anomalies with anterior cephaloceles are listed in **Box 6**.

Frontoethmoidal (Sincipital) Cephaloceles

In frontoethmoidal cephaloceles, the internal skull defect is located in the midline, but the external skull defect may vary with the bony surroundings of the defect in the facial skeleton.[7,10] Frontoethmoidal cephaloceles are soft tissue masses connected to the subarachnoid space via an enlarged foramen cecum, and extend to the glabella (nasofrontal) or into the nasal cavity (nasoethmoidal). A bifid or absent crista galli, cribriform plate, or a defect of the frontal bone suggest intracranial extension of the cephalocele, and are fairly well demonstrated with CT. It is important to bear in mind that no bone is seen in the normal neonate at the level of the crista galli and cribriform plate, because the crista galli and midline cribriform plate only start ossifying at 2 months (postnatal) and progress until about 14 months of age.[13]

Nasoethmoidal (intranasal) cephaloceles are usually evident in the pediatric age group, and cause complex deformities in the frontal, orbital, and nasal regions. Sometimes it is a small defect and only manifests late in adulthood. In this setting, misdiagnosis is common as either a nasal polyp, intracerebral tumor that has invaded down through the skull base into the nasal anlage, and nasal gliomas. Biopsy is contraindicated in these cephaloceles because of potential CSF leaks, seizures, or meningitis.[6,17]

In such cases, intrathecal injection of contrast material may show a subarachnoid connection in encephaloceles that is not seen in nasal gliomas.[6,24] Cisternography with heavily T2-weighted thin sections may also be useful.[6]

Hypertelorism is constantly seen in nasopharyngeal and nasofrontal cephaloceles, and commonly associates with nasoethmoidal and naso-orbital cephaloceles. Other facial malformations such as labial fissure, palatine fissure, and median nasal fissure are demonstrated in nasopharyngeal and frontoethmoidal cephaloceles (**Fig. 6**).[13,16]

Because naso-orbital cephaloceles protrude into the orbit, they typically present proptosis and a slightly pulsatile mass.[16]

Nasopharyngeal Cephaloceles

Nasopharyngeal cephaloceles are not obviously seen on clinical examination; because they are occult, they are discovered toward the end of the first postnatal decade. The cephalocele causes obstruction of the nasopharynx, which manifests as a persistent nasal stuffiness or "mouth-breathing." Clinical examination detects a nasal or pharyngeal mass that increases in size with Valsalva maneuver, as mentioned earlier. It must be borne in mind that misdiagnosing nasopharyngeal cephaloceles as a mass might lead to an erroneous biopsy.[13,16] To rule out a nasopharyngeal encephalocele, it is mandatory to perform a neuroradiological evaluation in patients with hypertelorism, diminished visual acuity and hypothalamic-pituitary dysfunction, and/or nasopharyngeal mass.[16] These symptoms are due to the stretching of the inferior portion of the third ventricle, hypothalamus, and optic chiasm into the sac.[13,15] Other ophthalmologic anomalies associated with these cephaloceles include hypoplasia of the optic discs, coloboma, and retinal dysplasia. Agenesis of the corpus callosum is demonstrated in approximately 80% of patients with nasopharyngeal cephaloceles.[13]

Interfrontal Cephaloceles

Interfrontal cephaloceles are frequently located in the inferior part of the metopic suture; nevertheless, they may occupy the entire length of the

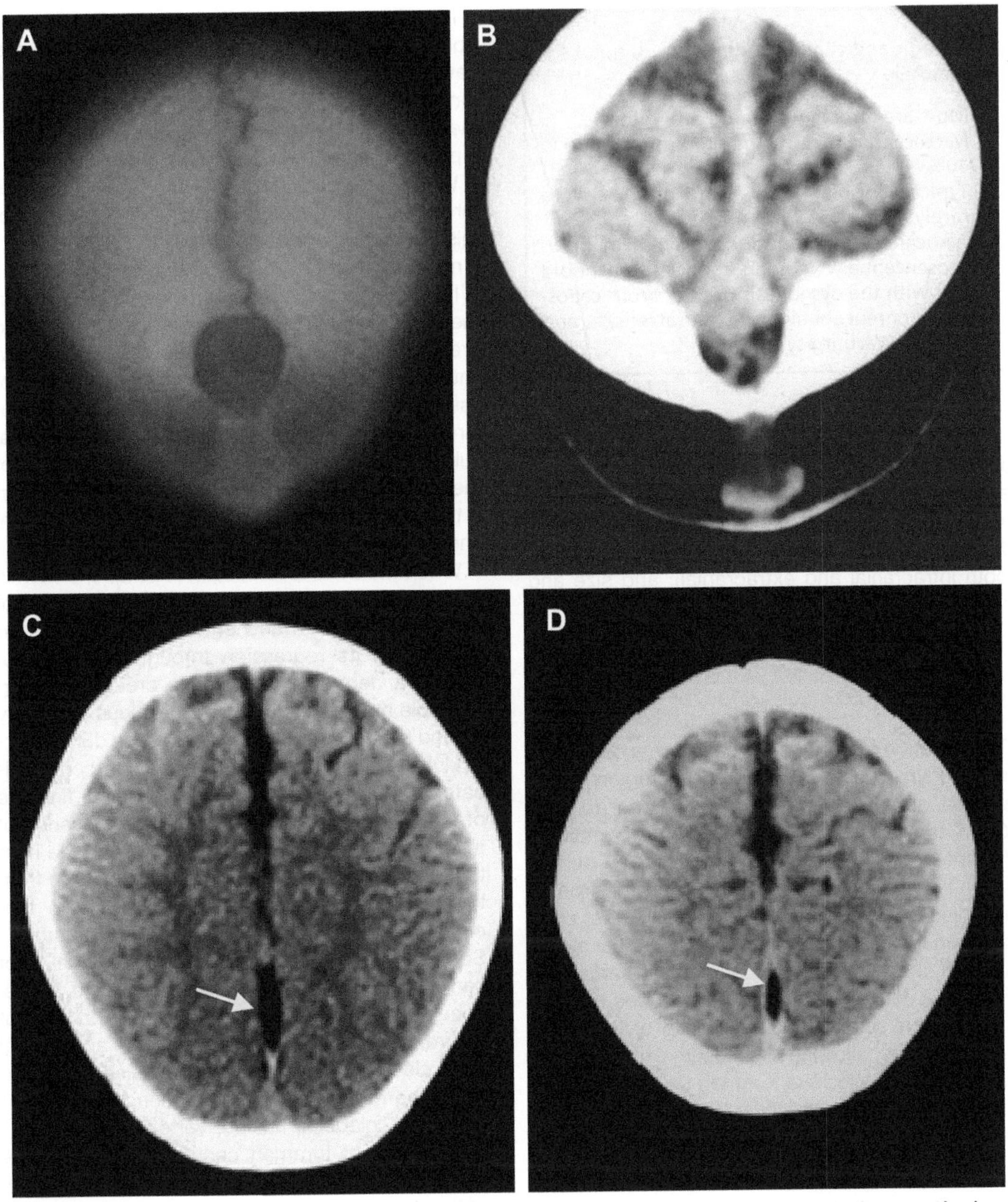

Fig. 5. Atretic parietal cephalocele. Axial CT images (*A*, bone and *B*, soft tissue windows) illustrate the bony defect at a superior parietal level. The widened interhemispheric fissure (*arrow*) secondary to a fenestrated falx (dural dehiscence) is shown at the lower level (*C*, *D*).

suture, which allows the passage to the anterior tips of the frontal lobes or the anterior halves of the cerebral hemispheres. The protrusion of the brain could be asymmetric and extensive, leading to a rotation of the intracranial hemisphere. The associated cerebral malformations such as agyria, holotelencephaly (prosencephaly with arrhinencephaly), and hydrocephalus, and the compression of the herniated brain contribute to the poor prognosis of the interfrontal cephalocele (**Fig. 7**).[16]

The treatment of congenital cephaloceles and CSF leaks includes craniotomies as well as, more recently, endoscopic surgery, and is aimed at performing the resection of the cephalocele and repairing the bony anomalies, particularly hypertelorism.[1] This surgical resection must be

Box 5
Radiologic and clinical findings for parietal cephalocele

1. Most are atretic (5–15 mm) and gliocele
2. Microcephaly in 20%, marked retardation in 40%[3]
3. Typically display hair at the base and are rarely multiple[3]
4. Associated malformations: spectra of holoprosencephaly, vermian agenesis, arachnoid cyst with the dysgenesis of the corpus callosum, porencephalic cysts (atretic), and Walker-Warburg syndrome[3,19]

performed at a very early age to prevent CSF leakage, meningitis, or increase in mass size. The prognosis of the patients with cephaloceles depends on its location, associated anomalies (both intracranial and extracranial), and size and content of the sac.

NASAL DERMOIDS, NASAL GLIOMAS, AND DERMAL SINUS

The migration of neural crest cells forms centers of mesenchymal cells in the frontonasal region. There are spaces between these centers, prior to their fusion and ossification. The fonticulus frontalis is the space between the frontal and nasal bones, which will close postnatally and form the frontonasal suture. The prenasal space is the zone between the nasal bones and the precursor structures of the nasal septum and nasal cartilages. There is a dural diverticulum that extends through the prenasal space, reaches the tip of the nose, and regresses, allowing the closure of this space, which is then called the foramen cecum (situated anterior to the crista galli).[25]

Box 6
Radiologic and pathologic findings for anterior cephalocele

1. Associated anomalies: arrhinencephaly, anophthalmia, microphthalmos, and dysgenesis of the corpus callosum, interhemispheric lipomas, arachnoid cyst, and hydrocephalus.[22] Malformation of cerebral cortical development (schizencephaly)
2. Associated syndrome: aberrant tissue band syndrome[3]
3. Interhemispheric lipoma in nasofrontal cephalocele[6,24]

If brain tissue protrudes through the fonticulus frontalis and communicates with the intracranial cavity, a frontonasal cephalocele is formed. If the fonticulus frontalis closes after the protrusion of the brain tissue, the entrapped tissue constitutes a prenasal cerebral heterotopia (nasal glioma).

When the protrusion of the brain tissue is through the prenasal space without regression of this tissue, and connects to the intracranial cavity, a nasoethmoidal encephalocele arises (**Fig. 8**).[25]

If dysplastic brain tissue remains separated from the intracranial CSF, after its protrusion through the prenasal space an intranasal cerebral heterotopia (intranasal glioma) is formed. There is a stalk of tissue in approximately 15% of cases, without direct fluid-filled tract connection with intracranial subarachnoid spaces.[25] The partial regression of the most superior portion of the dural diverticulum is the postulated explanation for both the prenasal and the intranasal cerebral heterotopia.[13,25]

When the dural diverticulum reaches the dermis and remains attached (incomplete disjunction of the neuroectoderm and cutaneous ectoderm) to the skin in its regression through the prenasal space, a dermal sinus tract is created, leaving a dimple at its orifice. The dermal sinus tract may extend superiorly along the path of the dural diverticulum for variable distance, and can communicate with the intracranial cavity. Clinical findings of the dermal sinus tract include the presence of a dimple or pit (**Fig. 9**) over the nasal bridge near the osteocartilaginous junction (or anywhere from the glabella to the tip of the nose), hairs that emanate from the pit, and sebaceous discharge.[22] Some of the tissue within the sinus dermal tract can create dermoid and/or epidermoid cysts, due to persistent ectodermal elements at sites of suture closure, brain diverticulation, and neural tube closure.[13] These cysts can also be found along the following midline locations: the anterior fontanelle, glabella, nasion, vertex, subocciput,[26] at the level of foramen cecum (adjacent to the crista galli), and adjacent to the anterior margin of the third ventricle.[22]

MR imaging is the best choice to achieve the objective sought in studying these lesions, namely, evaluating the nature (imaging features of the tissue), locating site of origin, and determining the extension of the lesion.

Nasal gliomas are evident near the root of the nose, located paramedian to the bridge of the nose and external to the nasal cavity, while intranasal gliomas are inside the nasal cavity medial to the middle turbinate bone.

MR imaging is the modality of choice for the evaluation of these lesions, which are hypointense to isointense relative to gray matter on T1-weighted

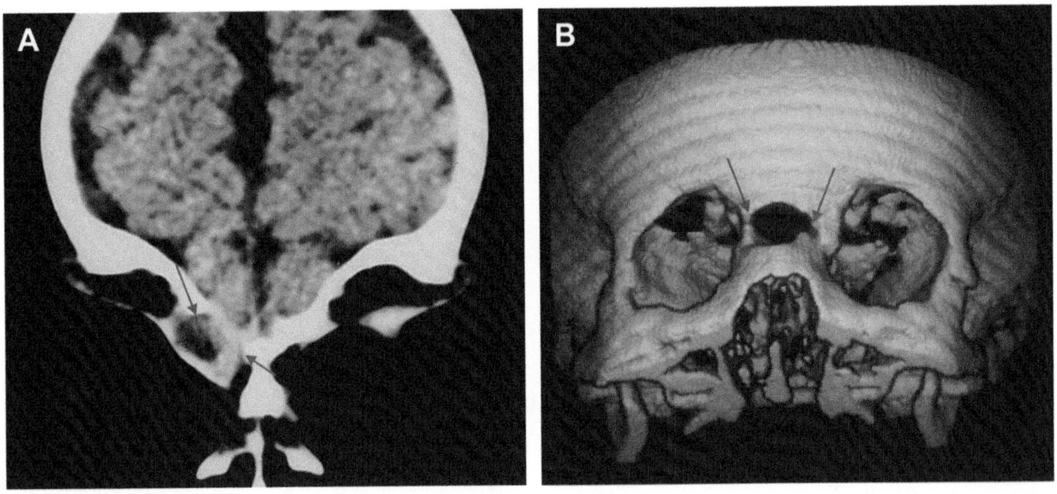

Fig. 6. Nasofrontal cephaloceles. (*A*) Coronal CT (soft tissue window) demonstrates the protrusion (parasagittal toward the right side) of a soft tissue mass through the bony defect (*arrows*) at the frontonasal level. (*B*) Both a nasofrontal bony defect (*arrows*) and hypertelorism are seen on a 3-dimensional frontal view (on bone window).

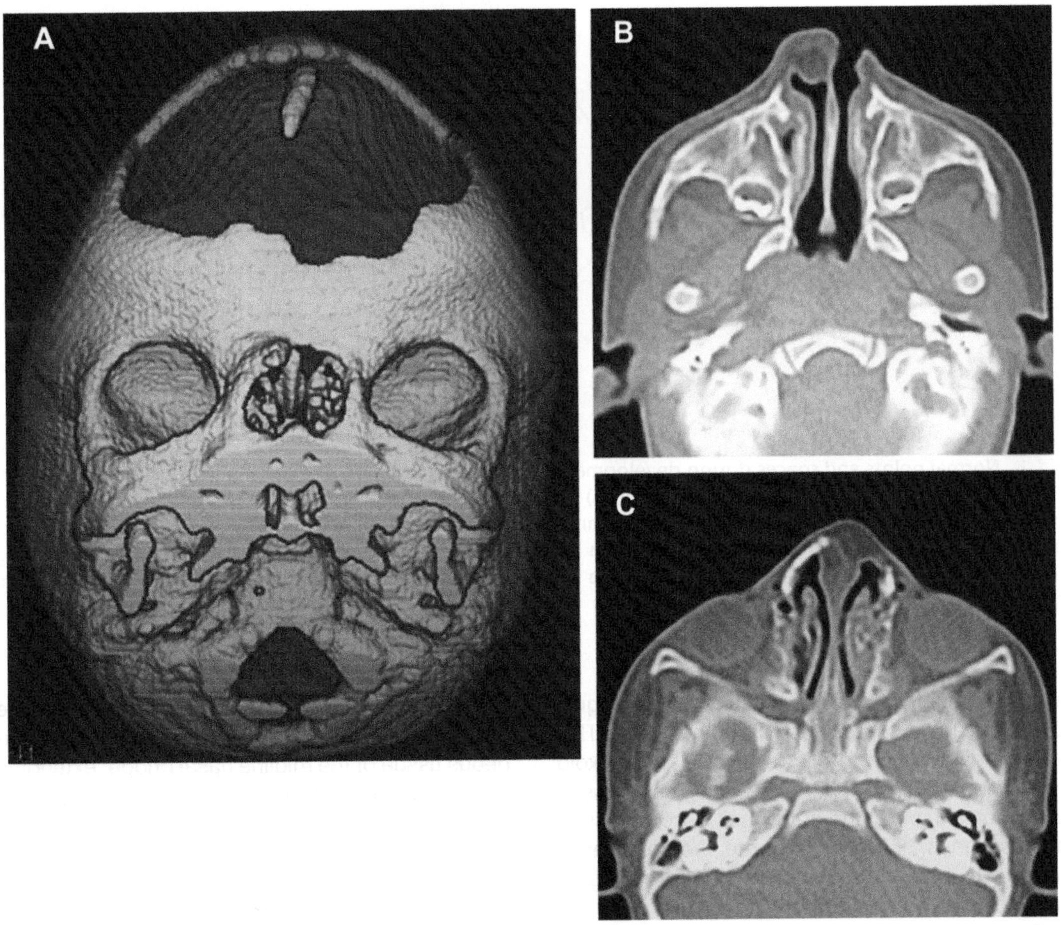

Fig. 7. Interfrontal cephalocele. Bone window images (*A*, 3-dimensional frontal view; *B* and *C*, axial images) demonstrate a large bony defect along the metopic suture, associated with hypertelorism and a craniofacial cleft (left parasagittal).

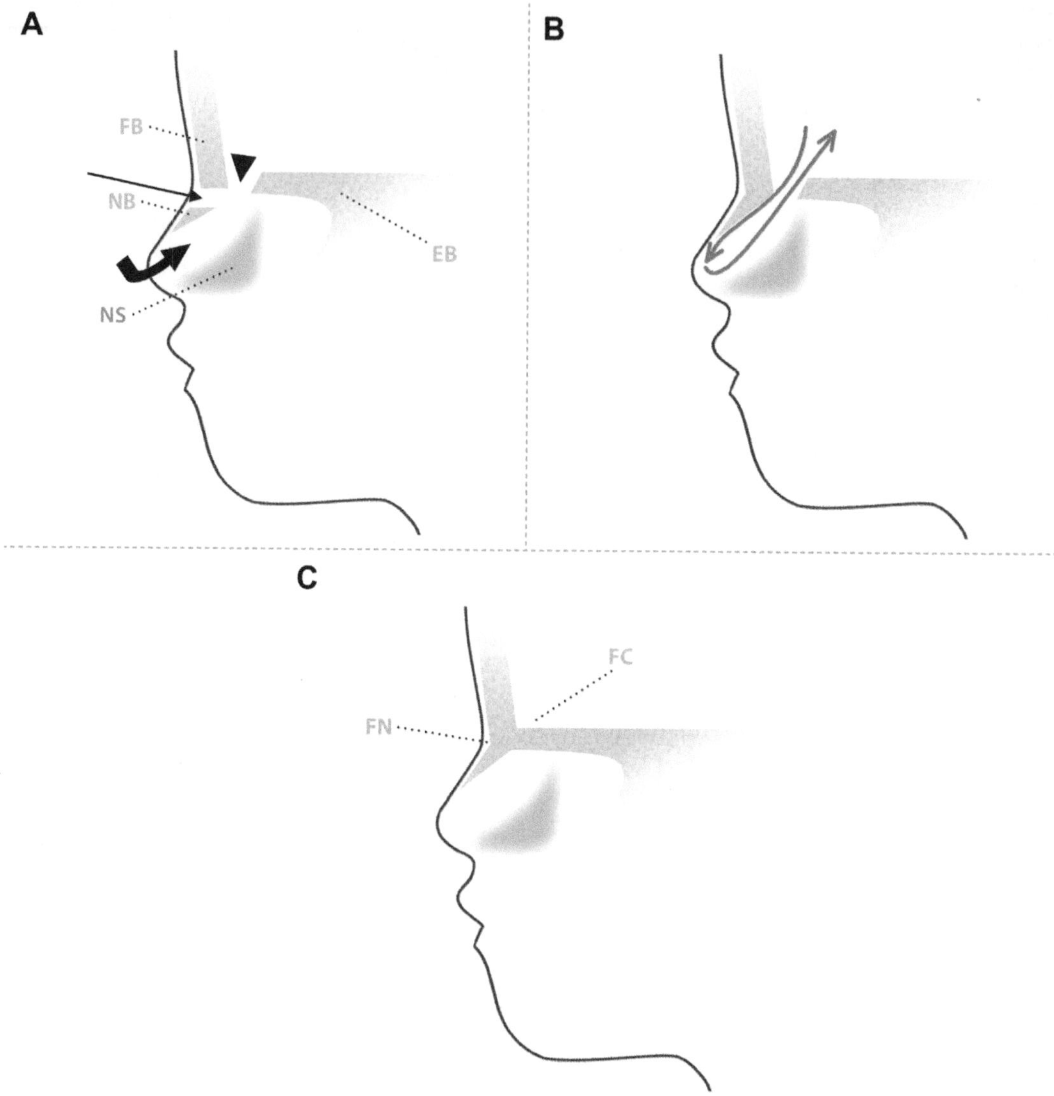

Fig. 8. Normal points and spaces during development of nasofrontal region and anomalies at this level. (*A*) Fonticulus frontalis (between frontal and nasal bones) (*straight arrow*) and prenasal space (between nasal bone and precursor structures of nasal septum and nasal cartilages) (*angled arrow*) are demonstrated. (*B*) Dural diverticulum (*curved* and *long arrows*) extends through the prenasal space, reaches the tip and regresses, allowing the closure of this space, which then is called the foramen cecum (*arrowhead* in *A*). (*C*) Closure and formation of frontonasal suture and foramen cecum.

and T2 -weighted imaging, with a focal high signal on T2-weighted sequences within the lesion. This latter finding is due to gliosis, cysts, and myxoid degeneration. Even though the dysplastic tissue does not enhance, the surrounding compressed mucosa does.[22] To demonstrate the intracranial stalk, a high-resolution surface coil MR imaging method must be applied.[26]

Concerning the dermal sinus tract, not only the features of the sinus tract but also the associated dermoid and epidermoid cysts must be detected. The dermal sinus tract is seen as a hypointense line on T1-weighted images within the subcutaneous tissue of the midline nasal bridge, extending toward the prenasal space.[22]

The epidermoid cysts are isointense to CSF on both T1-weighted (low signal) and T2-weighted (bright signal) images, and show restriction on isotropic diffusion-weighted images.

Because dermoid cysts have fat components, they demonstrate T1 shortening (bright signal) and variable hyperintensity on T2-weighted

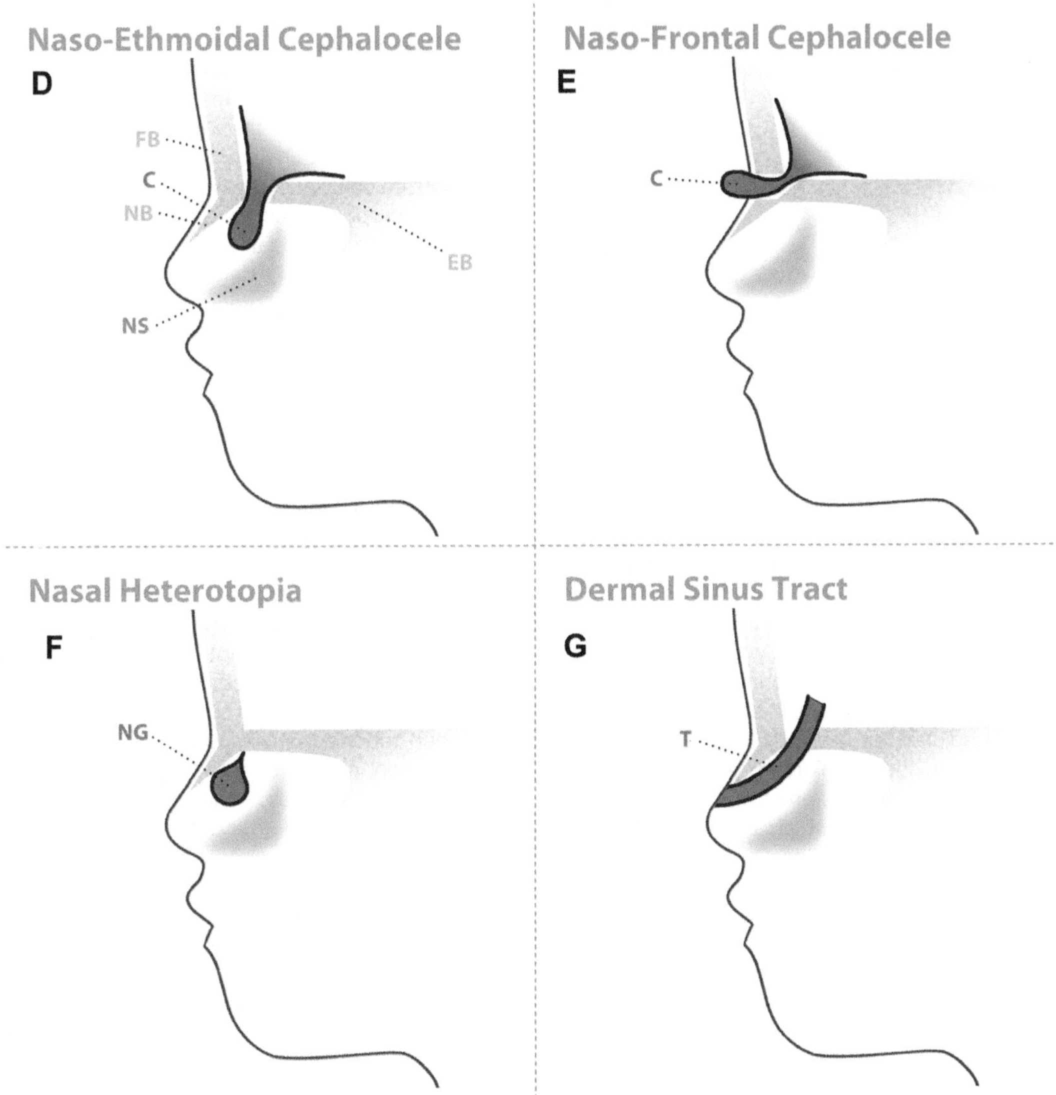

Fig. 8. (*D*) Naso-ethmoidal cephalocele (red sac): protrusion of brain tissue through the prenasal space, without regression of this tissue, and with connection to the intracranial cavity. (*E*) Nasofrontal cephalocele (red sac): protrusion of brain tissue through the fonticulus frontalis with communication with intracranial cavity. (*F*) Nasal cerebral heterotopia (nasal glioma): dysplastic brain tissue remains separated from the intracranial CSF, after its protrusion through the prenasal space. It is shown as a red oval figure, behind the nasal bone. (*G*) Dermal sinus tract is demonstrated as a red tube that slides through the prenasal space and could communicate with intracranial cavity. FB, frontal bone; NB, nasal bone; EB, ethmoid bone; NS, nasal septum and cartilages; FN, frontonasal suture; FC, foramen caecum; C, cephalocele; NG, nasal glioma; T, dermal sinus tract.

images, as well as variable signal intensity on diffusion-weighted images.[22]

A bifid anterior crista galli and an enlarged foramen cecum, plus atypical signal intensity at the foramen cecum, indicate the presence of an intracranial epidermoid or dermoid cyst.[22]

All of the aforementioned lesions can be surgically resected. The nasal dermoid and epidermoid cysts are operated on to avoid potential CNS infection if there is intracranial connection.[26]

ANOMALIES OF THE CORPUS CALLOSUM

The primitive lamina terminalis is part of the rostral wall of the telencephalon, after closure of the anterior neuropore at about 25 days GA. During the

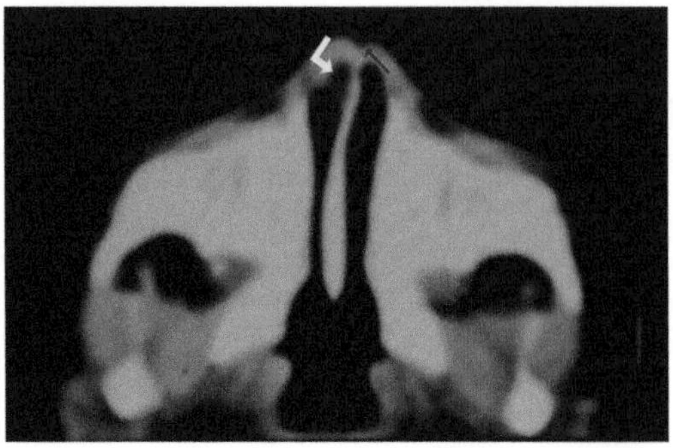

Fig. 9. Dermal sinus tract. CT axial image (soft tissue window) shows a dimple (*straight arrow*) and a dermoid cyst (*angled arrow*) at the tip of the nose.

seventh week GA, the dorsal end (near the paraphysis) of the lamina terminalis thickens and is called the lamina reuniens or commissural plate. The sulcus medianus telencephali medii is a groove developed in the lamina reuniens. The ventral surface of this groove is filled with cellular material from the developing subarachnoid space (meninx primitiva). A bridge or "sling" is formed across the sulcus medianus, probably of this material and of neurons from the developing hemispheres. The cells within this sling express surface molecules and secrete chemicals, which are required to guide the axons across the midline. During the 10th week GA, pioneer axons of different commissures cross the midline in the following order: first the anterior commissure (10th week), second the hippocampal commissure (11th week), and third the corpus callosum. The corpus callosum is sequentially formed, starting with the posterior genu, anterior body, posterior body and anterior genu, the splenium, and finally the rostrum.[13] This knowledge is important in order to differentiate the callosal anomalies, as listed in **Table 3**. Callosal anomalies are associated with anterior and hippocampal commissures anomalies, as mentioned in **Table 4**. According to the injury during embryologic development, Utsunomiya and colleagues[27] summarized callosal anomalies as follows: (a) total defect of corpus callosum, anterior commissure, and psalterium due to failure of lamina reuniens at 6 to 8 weeks GA; (b) total defect of corpus callosum due to failure of callosal precursor at 8 to 10 weeks GA; (c) partial defect of corpus callosum due to partial failure of callosal precursor at 10 to 15 weeks GA; (d) callosal hypoplasia due to failure to association fibers entering massa commissuralis at 11 to 20 weeks GA; (e) atrophy due to failure of commissural fibers in the corpus callosum at 20 weeks GA until after birth.

The development of the corpus callosum is not completed in utero. During the neonatal period and infancy, both postnatal loss and myelination of callosal axons occur.[28] The etiology of corpus callosum dysgenesis is not completely known. Some implicated risk factors are listed in **Box 7**.

Asymptomatic agenesis of the corpus callosum has been reported when found isolated; its incidence is very rare. The more frequent manifestations include seizures, macrocephaly, delayed development, mental retardation, and hypothalamic dysfunction.[13] Dysgenesis of corpus callosum is commonly associated with many syndromes and other cerebral and cerebellar anomalies, such as other telencephalic commissure anomalies, Chiari II malformation, Dandy-Walker malformation, interhemispheric cysts, malformations of cortical development (neuronal migration and organization), cephaloceles, and midline facial anomalies.[13,28]

Table 3
Corpus callosum anomalies

	Corpus Callosum	
Anomaly	**Present**	**Absent or Small**
Agenesis: complete absence	None	All
Hypogenesis: incomplete formation	Posterior genu Anterior body	Anterior/inferior genu Posterior body Splenium, rostrum
Destructive	Splenium, rostrum	Genu, body
Dysgenesis: defective development (holoprosencephaly)	Splenium Genu, splenium Body, splenium	Genu, body, rostrum Body Genu

Data from Barkovich AJ. Congenital malformations of the brain and skull. In: Barkovich AJ, editor. Pediatric neuroimaging. 4th edition. London: Lippincott Williams and Wilkins; 2005. p. 291–405.

Table 4
Commissural anomalies in callosal anomalies

Corpus Callosum	Other Commissures
Agenesis	Anterior: small, absent
—	Hippocampal: small, absent, enlarged
Hypogenesis	Hippocampal: enlarged

Data from Barkovich AJ. Congenital malformations of the brain and skull. In: Barkovich AJ, editor. Pediatric neuroimaging. 4th edition. London: Lippincott Williams and Wilkins; 2005. p. 291–405.

MR imaging is an excellent modality for the assessment of the dysgenesis of the corpus callosum, because it displays not only the features of this anomaly but also other associated ones.

On axial images the following findings are evident: lateral convexity of the frontal horns, parallel lateral ventricles, colpocephaly (disproportionate dilatation of trigones and occipital horns of the lateral ventricles), keyhole dilatation of the temporal horns (deficient cingulate fasciculus), upward extension of the third ventricle into the interhemispheric fissure between lateral ventricles, communication of the third ventricle with the interhemispheric fissure anteriorly, interdigitation of gyri across the midline (due to partial absence of the falx in the interhemispheric fissure), and hypoplasia of the anterior commissure (**Figs. 10** and **11**).[13,28]

Sagittal images are the best sequence for the evaluation of the extent of the dysgenesis of the corpus callosum, which could be absent or incomplete (**Fig. 12**).

On coronal images other features are well shown, such as persistent everted cingulated gyri, medial hemispheric sulci extending into the third ventricle, crescent-shaped lateral ventricles (due to impression on the medial walls of the ventricles by the medially positioned bundles of Probst), incomplete inversion of the hippocampus, and extension of the third ventricle into the interhemispheric fissure. Coronal images also demonstrate that the hippocampal commissure unites the fornices, not the cerebral hemispheres.[13]

The longitudinal callosal bundles of Probst are formed when the axons cannot cross the midline, and are forced to lie laterally to the cingulate gyri and medially to the medial walls of the lateral ventricles, and parallel to the interhemispheric fissure, merging (by its inferomedial borders) with rudimentary fornices.[13] These bundles are brighter on T1 and darker on T2 images than are other white matter fibers. MR imaging findings of corpus callosal dysgenesis are mentioned in **Box 8**.

The lack of formation or destruction of the callosal axons correlate with markedly reduced volume of cerebral white matter. If the callosal anomaly is secondary to an improper guidance of axons across the midline, the volume of the cerebral cortex and the appearance of white matter are normal.[13,29]

Agenesis of corpus callosum presenting interhemispheric cyst (IHC) is classified by Barkovich[13] into two major groups: Type 1, diverticulum of the ventricular system that communicates with the ventricles; and Type 2, multiple cysts, which do not communicate with the ventricles. Type 1 and Type 2 are divided into subgroups depending on the clinical manifestations and associated anomalies. Type 1 IHC is isointense to CSF. Type 2 IHC is slightly hyperintense to CSF on T1-weighted images and isointense to hyperintense on T2-weighted images. Subcortical heterotopia is seen in Type 2.[13]

Box 7
Risk factors of anomalies of corpus callosum

1. Irradiation
2. Deficiencies in riboflavin, folic acid, niacin
3. Maternal infection: rubella, congenital toxoplasmosis
4. Fetal alcohol syndrome
5. Maternal diabetes

Data from Kollias SS, Ball WS Jr, Prenger EC. Cystic malformations of the posterior fossa: differential diagnosis clarified through embryologic analysis. Radiographics 1993;13(6):1211–31.

INTRACRANIAL LIPOMAS

Intracranial lipomas are congenital malformations composed of abnormal collections of fat. Lipomas probably derive from abnormal differentiation of the meninx primitiva, which normally differentiates into the leptomeninges and the subarachnoid space.

The meninx primitiva originates from the mesoderm of the neural crest cells. First, the developing embryo is involved by the meninx primitiva, then (in an established sequence) the inner meninx resorbs, leaving the subarachnoid space. There is an inverse correlation between the pattern of cavitation and dissolution of the meninx with the allotment of intracranial lipomas: the last zone to resorb is the dorsum of the lamina terminalis, and lipomas are more frequent (40%–50%) at the pericallosa area. Other sites for lipomas are the quadrigeminal plate/superior cerebellar cisterns (25%), the suprasellar/interpeduncular cisterns (10%–20%), the cerebellopontine angle cisterns (7%), and the

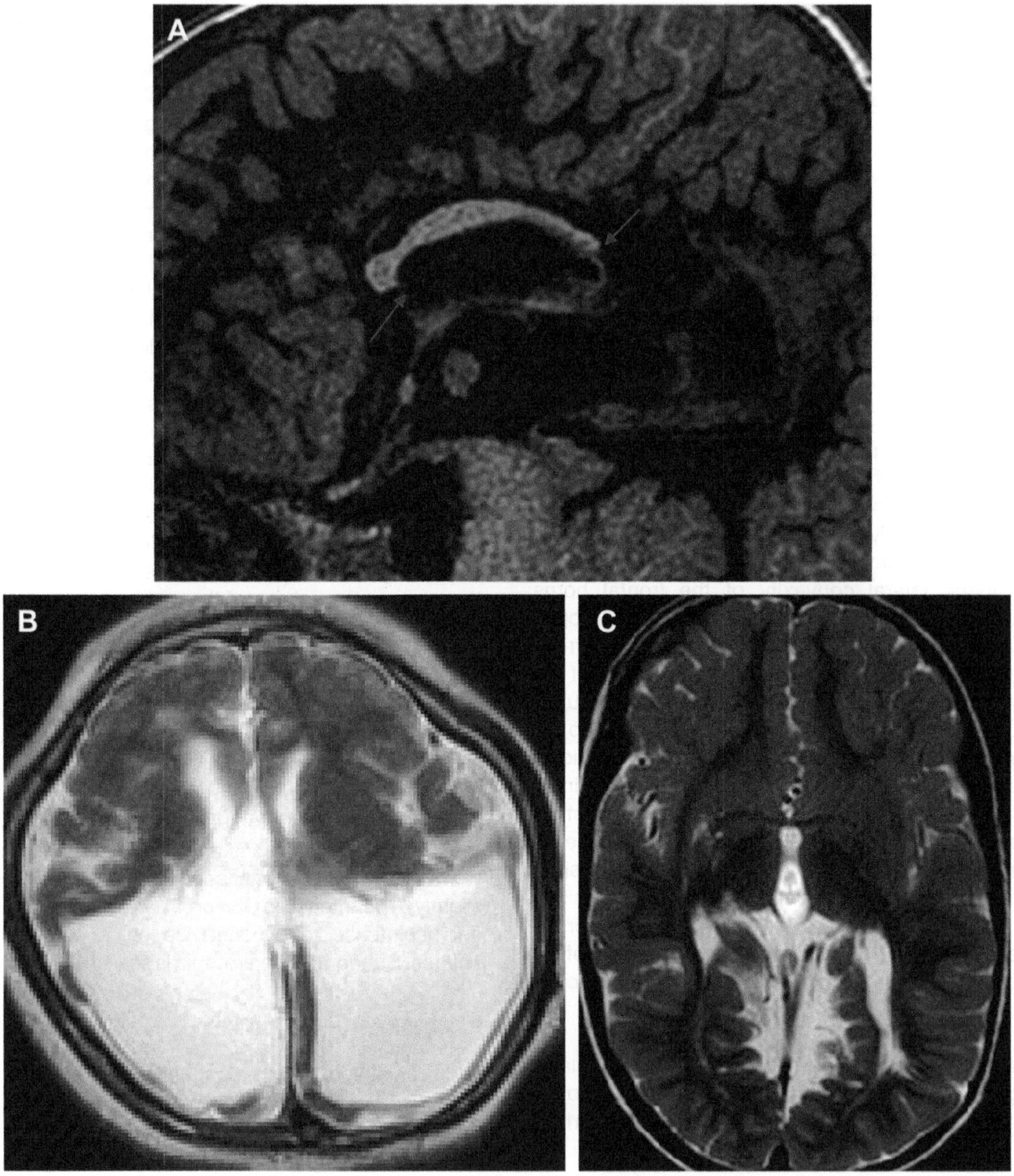

Fig. 10. Dysgenesis of the corpus callosum. (*A*) On sagittal T1-weighted image the absence (*arrow*) of the posterior body and splenium of the corpus callosum are seen. (*B*) Colpocephaly is illustrated on an axial T2-weighted image. (*C*) Hypoplasia of anterior commissure (*arrow*) is shown on axial T2-weighted image.

Sylvian cisterns (5%). Blood vessels and cranial nerves course through these lipomas (within the subarachnoid space).[13,28] Intracranial lipomas are usually asymptomatic and are considered incidental findings, even though some patients present with seizures or cranial neuropathy secondary to involvement of the adjacent neural tissue.[28] Lipomas are habitually juxtaposed to malformed brain, such as callosal lipomas (**Fig. 13**) near callosal hypogenesis, frontal interhemispheric lipomas associated with midline facial clefts, and nasofrontal or nasoethmoidal cephaloceles; even extension of the lipoma into the cephalocele is frequently seen. The term midline craniofacial dysraphism refers to a midline developmental disorder associated with a lipoma of the interhemispheric fissure. Intracranial lipomas are malformations (not tumors) and they increase in bulk only with somatic growth.[13,28]

MR imaging is the best modality for the evaluation of intracranial lesions. Lipomas display a bright

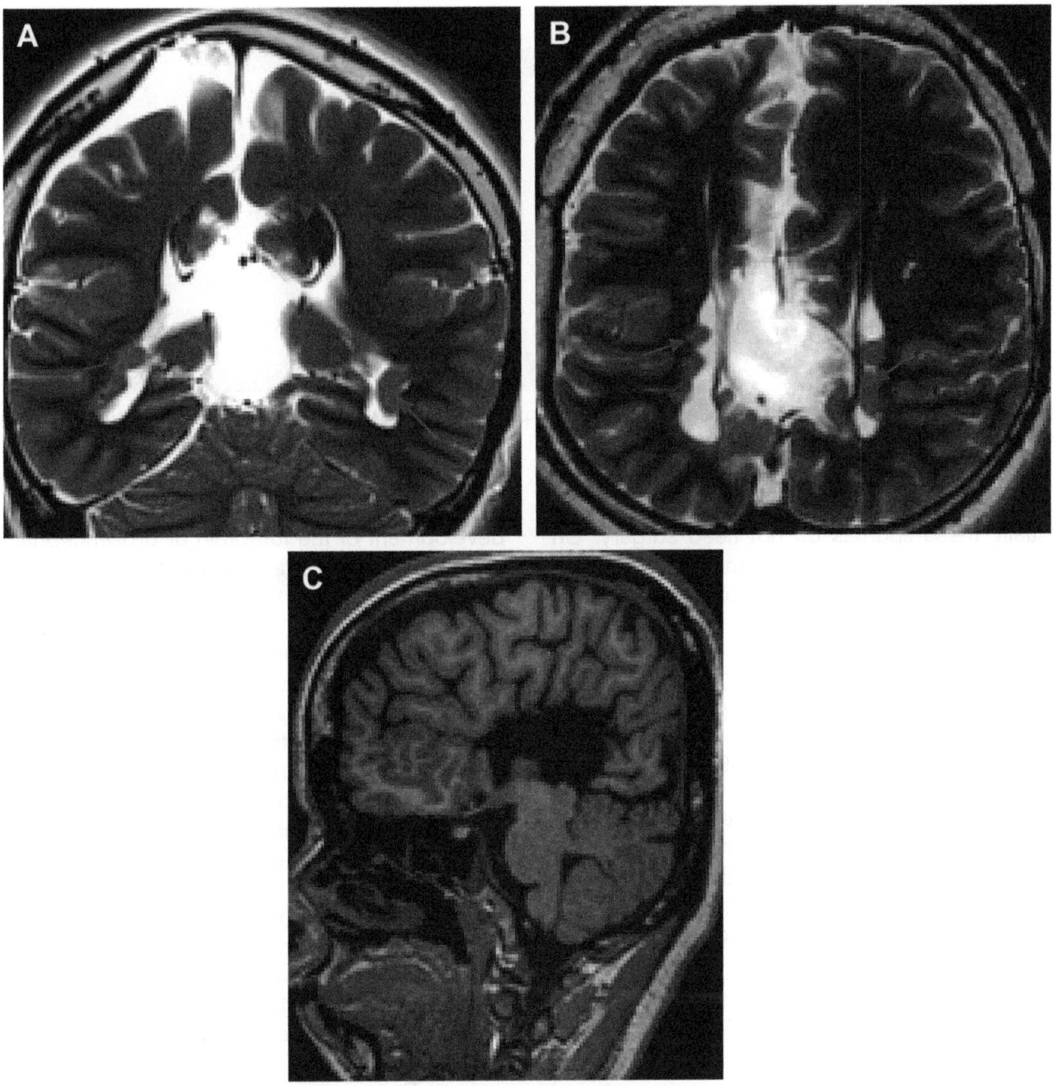

Fig. 11. Agenesis of corpus callosum. (*A*) Hypointense bundles of Probst (*arrowhead*), persistent eversion of the cingulated gyrus, and subependymal heterotopias are demonstrated on a coronal T2-weighted image. (*B*) On an axial T2-weighted image, the ventricles are parallel and subependymal heterotopias are seen. (*C*) Sagittal T1-weighted image shows absence of both the corpus callosum and the cingulated sulcus.

signal on T1-weighted and T2-weighted images, becoming hypointense on fat saturation pulse and on long repetition time images as the echo time increases. Chemical shift is demonstrated in large lipomas, due to the different chemical shifts of water and fat protons, thus helping radiologists differentiate fat from blood.[13] MR imaging findings of intracranial lipomas are listed in **Box 9**.

Intracranial lipomas are divided by the Tart and Quisling classification into curvilinear and tubulonodular types.[30,31] Curvilinear lipomas are frequently posterior, small, and linear, whereas tubulonodular ones are usually anterior, round, or cylindrical. Some lipomas do not fit this pattern, such as the case reported by Chen and colleagues,[30] which is posterior, bulky, and elliptical, without frontal dysraphism.

Interhemispheric lipomas are well delineated, and can prolong inferiorly through the velum interpositum to the choroidal fissure and into the choroid plexus of the ventricles (15%–25%), anteriorly in front of the callosal genu, or posteriorly behind the splenium.[13,30] The flow void caused by the branches of the pericallosal artery traversing pericallosal lipomas can be difficult to differentiate from calcifications on MR imaging.[13]

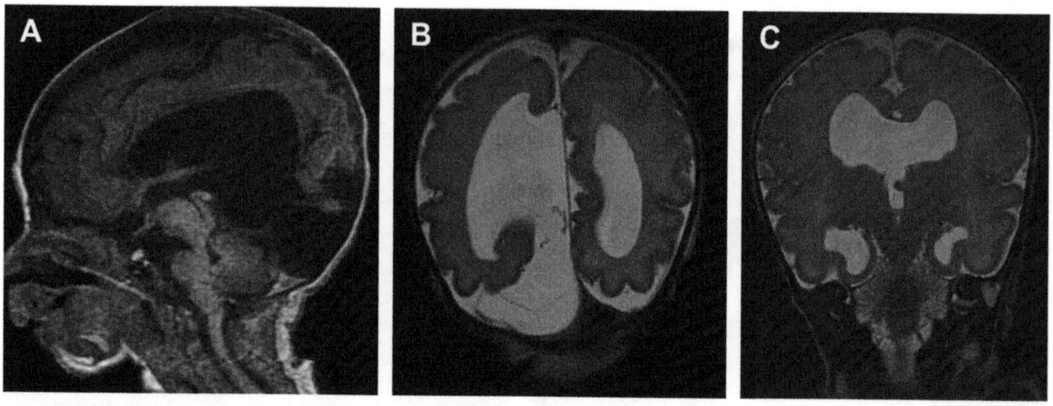

Fig. 12. Hypogenesis of corpus callosum with interhemispheric cyst type I is shown on sagittal T1-weighted image (*A*) and Coronal T2-weighted images (*B, C*).

Usually these lipomas do not need surgery. On rare occasions, shunt placement is required when hydrocephalus is associated with inferior collicular lipomas.[28]

HOLOPROSENCEPHALY, SEPTO-OPTIC DYSPLASIA, AND OTHER VARIANTS

Ventral induction is the third stage of the embryonic period in the development of the CNS. The first and second ones are the formation and separation of the germ layers (neural plate) and dorsal induction with the formation of the neural tube. At the end of the dorsal induction or neurulation the anterior neuropore closes, and the development of the forebrain or prosencephalon begins from the rostral neural tube. The forebrain then divides into the telencephalon and the diencephalon. The telencephalon divides into the anterior pallius that originates the cerebral cortex and the ventral subpallium creates the basal ganglia. The other processes of division of the telencephalon are in the sagittal and rostrocaudal direction, and are named diverticula. The sagittal diverticulation or cleavage creates two dorsolateral vesicles. Failures or defects in the division of the telencephalon are the causes of prosencephalies (**Fig. 14**).[32]

Congenital cleavage anomalies of the middle line, prosencephalies, are a spectrum ranging from the mildest anomaly, the septo-optic dysplasia, to the most severe one, alobar holoprosencephaly. Injuries to the CNS occur as early as 4 to 6weeks GA when prosencephalic cleavage occurs. The compared incidence between fetuses (40/100,000) and live born children (0.48–0.88/100,000) shows a high incidence of fetal loss.[33] Karyotype and genetic anomalies are diverse and are demonstrated in a variable number of cases. The mutation most frequently identified occurs in SHH (sonic hedgehog gene) at 7q36; more often in familial holoprosencephaly (autosomal dominant) SHH has multiple functions in the development of the nervous system, in dorsal-ventral patterning by which the dorsal and ventral regions of the nervous system acquire their distinct anatomic and functional properties. Diverse associations could be present such as maternal diabetes, occupational exposure to metals and herbicides or pesticides, drug abuse, high doses of radiation, eclampsia, and advanced and early maternal age. Concurrent anomalies in patients are variable as well, and include iniencephaly, cephaloceles, cardiac, and osseous anomalies.[34]

Box 8
Anomalies of corpus callosum: imaging findings

1. White matter abnormalities
   a. Probst bundles
   b. Anterior commissure hypoplasia
2. Gyral and sulcal abnormalities
   a. Persistent eversion of cingulated gyrus
   b. Absent cingulated sulcus
   c. Hippocampal hypogenesis
3. Ventricular abnormalities and cysts
   a. Widened third ventricle, superiorly extended into interhemispheric cyst
   b. Colpocephaly, crescentic shape of lateral ventricles on coronal images, parallel or lateral convexity of lateral ventricles on axial images

Data from Caruso P, Robertson R, Setty B, et al. Disorders of brain development. In: Atlas S, editor. Magnetic resonance imaging of the brain and spine, vol. 1. 4th edition. China: Lippincott Willians & Wilkins; 2009.

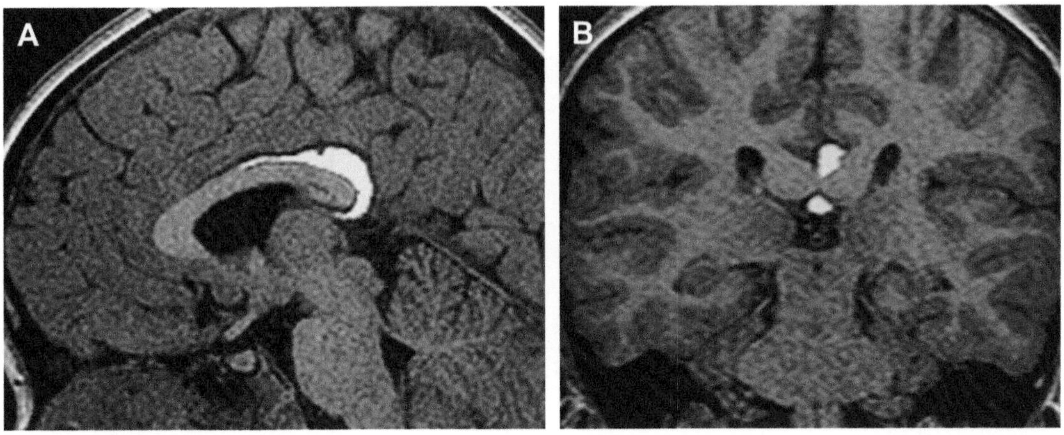

Fig. 13. Callosal lipoma. T1-weighted images (*A*, sagittal; *B*, coronal) demonstrate a curvilinear pericallosal lipoma (high signal), adjacent to the splenium and the posterior body of the corpus callosum. There is slight hypogenesis of the adjacent splenium. The chemical shift artifact is well noticed on sagittal and coronal image.

Cleavage defects mainly affect the prosencephalon and are presented as a unique ventricle with fused frontal lobes, basal nuclei, thalami, and greater association to facial anomalies. These facial anomalies are due to cleavage defects as well, and in the most severe degree there is a unique ocular globe or Cyclops. Ethmocephaly, cebocephaly, premaxillary agenesis, or arhinencephaly with cleft lip are other probable associations.[35] In the other mild forms there are variable degrees of ethmoidohypoplasia, hypotelorism, and orbital anomalies such as ophthalmic hendidura stenosis. All of these anomalies usually have hypothalamic fusion, anterior or posterior pituitary hypoplasia, ectopic posterior pituitary, and a thin or absent pituitary that could either be or not be associated with an endocrinal deficit in correlation with the severity of the anomaly. As the caudate nuclei are the most central structures, these and the central hypothalamic nuclei are the most affected. Also, the abnormal orientation and fusion of the thalami and midbrain is greater in the most severe grades.[36,37]

Box 9
Imaging findings of intracranial lipomas

1. Mass
   a. MR imaging sequences: isointense to fat on T1 and T2, hypointense on saturation fat sequence
   b. Location (cisterns): pericallosal, quadrigeminal, superior cerebellar, suprasellar, interpeduncular, cerebellopontine angle, Sylvian
   c. Extension: choroid plexus of lateral ventricles, areas of lamina terminalis or fornix
   d. Chemical shift artifact: different chemical shift fat and water protons
2. Adjacent structures: hypogenesis corpus callosum, collicular plate
3. Blood vessels and cranial nerves: traverse through the lipoma
4. Calcifications: difficult to differentiate from arterial flow void signals

Data from Barkovich AJ. Congenital malformations of the brain and skull. In: Barkovich AJ, editor. Pediatric neuroimaging. 4th edition. London: Lippincott William and Wilkins; 2005. p. 291–405.

Mental retardation is usually present in the more severe forms and is absent in the milder ones.

Prosencephaly is the unique condition whereby there is absence of the anterior segment, the former in the normal development, if the corpus callosum is partially formed, as in semilobar holoprosencephaly. However, the dorsal "corpus callosum" is composed of axons of the dorsal interhemispheric commissure resembling a true callosal splenium, and has been called pseudocallosum or atypical callosal dysgenesis.[38,39] This condition is related to severe developmental delay. Instead of the normal corpus callosum, a small cortical bridge between the two hemispheres could be present, with a disorganized appearance of the white matter tracts.

There is a relation between the corpus callosum and the typical dorsal cyst in holoprosencephalies. If the dorsal cyst exists there is no development of the corpus callosum. A similar relation exists between the development of the corpus callosum and the dorsal interhemispheric fissure.

The appearances of the ventricle and lobes are some of the main criteria in the differentiation

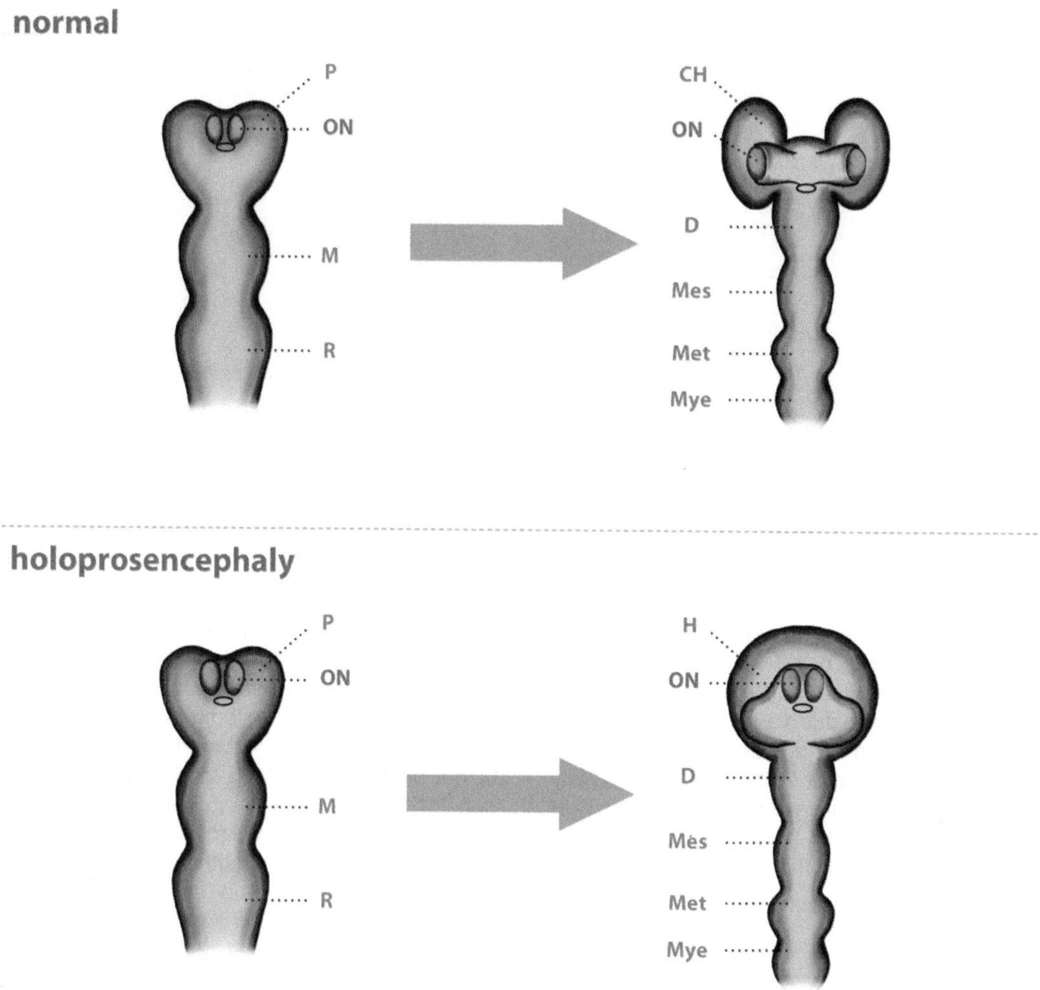

Fig. 14. Normal and abnormal embryology in prosencephalies. P, prosencephalum; ON, optic nerves; M, mesencephalum; R, rhombencephalum; D, diencephalum; Mes, mesencephalum; Met, metencephalum; Mye, myelencephalum.

between alobar, semilobar, or lobar holoprosencephalies. In the alobar form, the temporal lobes and the temporal horns of the ventricle are not depicted. In the semilobar form, the temporal lobes and temporal horns are partially formed with a partially formed interhemispheric fissure, and the frontal horns are not formed (**Figs. 15–17**). In the lobar form both the temporal lobes and horns are normal, and there are hypoplastic or dysplastic frontal horns.

The presence of a posterior cyst that is a posterior extension of the third ventricle is related to the absence of the splenium of the corpus callosum.[38,40]

The Sylvian fissure is relatively abnormal, and in the more severe cases it could be absent. In these cases the M1 segment of the middle cerebral arteries is short, with more branches than usual.[40] The Sylvian angle is formed between the longitudinal axis of the Sylvian fissures. The normal angle is 15° (range 11°–18°). The more horizontal and abnormal is the orientation of these fissures, the bigger is the magnitude of this angle. This angle has greater values in the alobar forms than in the semilobar and lobar ones. In the most severe forms of alobar holoprosencephaly, this angle is as big as $122° \pm 55°$.

Holoprosencephalies can be associated with variable degrees of lobe hypoplasia, cortical dysplasia, zones of cortical flattening, widening of the cortex, and cortical heterotopias (see **Figs. 14–16; Fig. 18**).

MR imaging is the diagnostic technique that displays most of these anomalies. Although

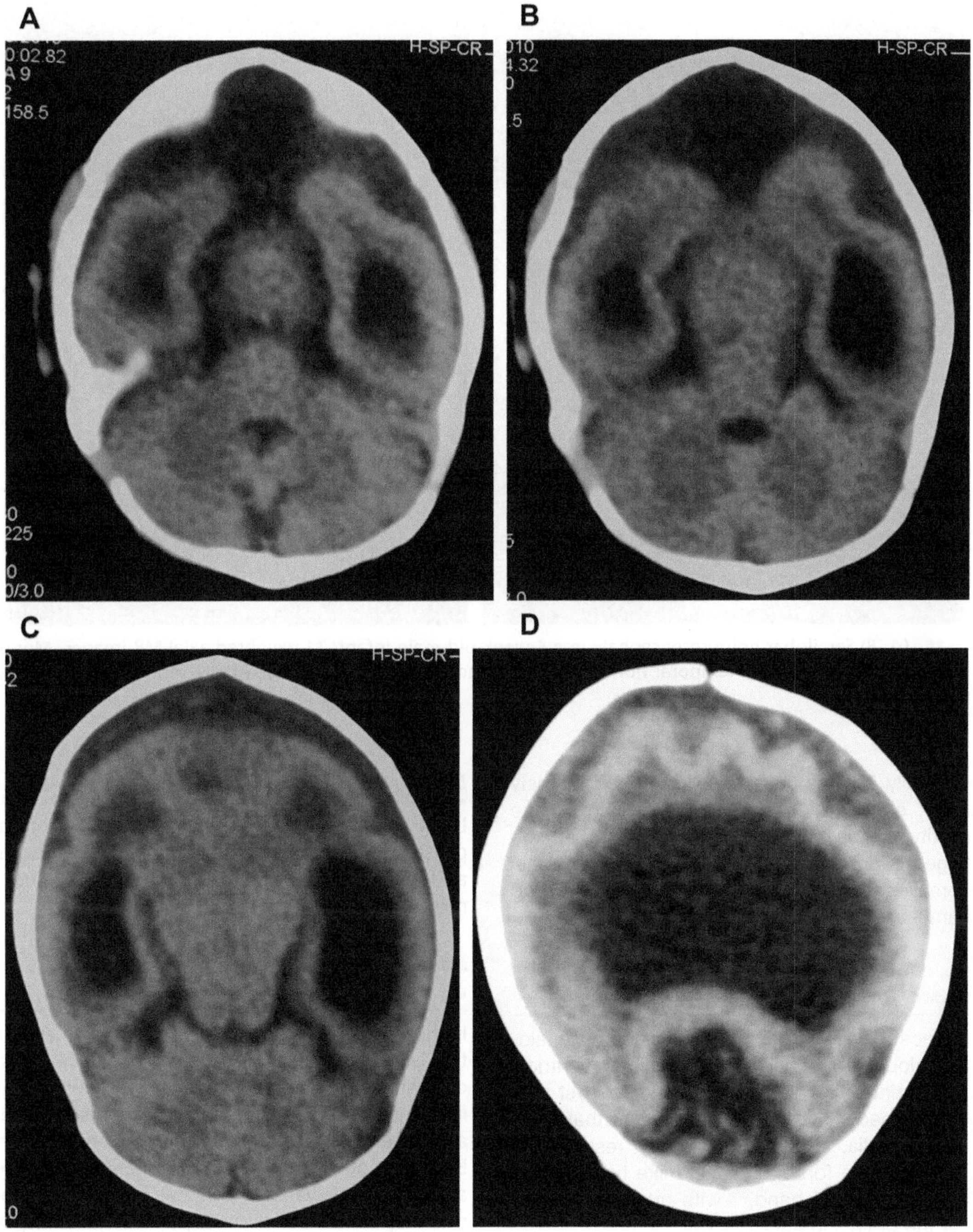

Fig. 15. (*A–D*) Semilobar holoprosencephaly in a 4-week-old male infant: CT axial images. Monoventricle, thalami, and basal ganglia fusion. Frontal lobe hypoplasia, cortical dysplasia. Rudimentary anterior and posterior interhemispheric fissure.

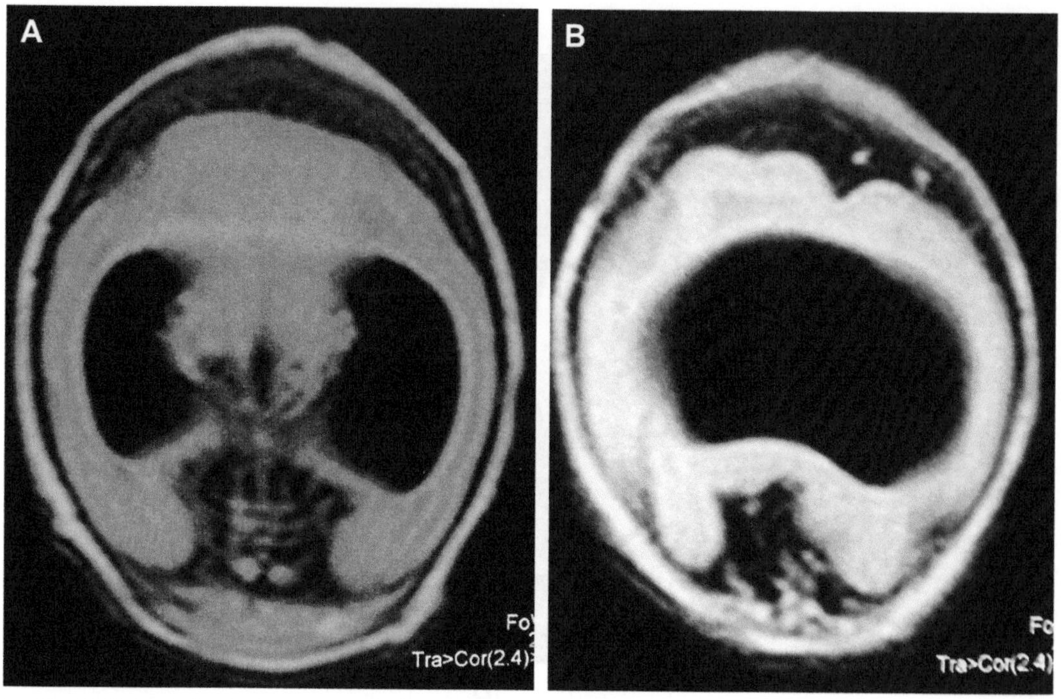

Fig. 16. (*A, B*) Semilobar holoprosencephaly in a 4-week-old male infant: T1-weighted axial MR images. Monoventricle with rudimentary temporal horns, partially fused diencephalum, and partially formed posterior and anterior fissures.

classically 3 types have been described, namely alobar, semilobar, and lobar depending on the severity of the anomaly, often findings on the images overlap because as in other congenital anomalies there is a continuum. The outstanding characteristics are described here.[41]

Alobar Holoprosencephaly

The most severe form of holoprosencephaly, alobar holoprosencephaly, has a unique ventricle that continues with a posterior midline cyst with entirely fused midline structures such as thalamus, basal ganglia, and frontal lobes, resulting in a pancake-like forebrain, shield-like hemisphere, and hippocampal band,[35] with arteries traveling over the brain surface (**Box 10**).

Semilobar Holoprosencephaly

In semilobar holoprosencephaly the midline structures begin to separate and the ventricular structures begin to appear with rudimentary third ventricle, temporal, and occipital horns. The frontal hypoplasia and cortical dysplasia are lesser than in the alobar form and the dorsal cyst is smaller (**Box 11**; see **Figs. 15–18**).

Lobar Holoprosencephaly

Lobar holoprosencephaly, the mildest form of the prosencephalies, presents with better prognosis and with normal or mild facial anomalies, usually mild hypotelorism (**Box 12**; **Figs. 19** and **20**).

Middle Interhemispheric Variant or Syntelencephaly

In the middle interhemispheric variant the fusion of the brain lobes is posterior, which is the main difference compared with the other prosencephalies. The frontal horns of the ventricle are present, and there is a posterior monoventricle.[42,43] Because of the absence of anterior cleavage anomalies, this variant has a low incidence of endocrinopathies, choreiform symptoms, and hypothalamic dysfunction (**Box 13**).[41]

Septo-Optical Dysplasia

This most common condition in females has been classified by Barkovich into two groups.[44] The first one is associated with schizencephaly, usually with partial absence of the septum pellucidum and without anomalies of the optic radiations; the second is associated with complete absence of the septum pellucidum, ventriculomegaly, and

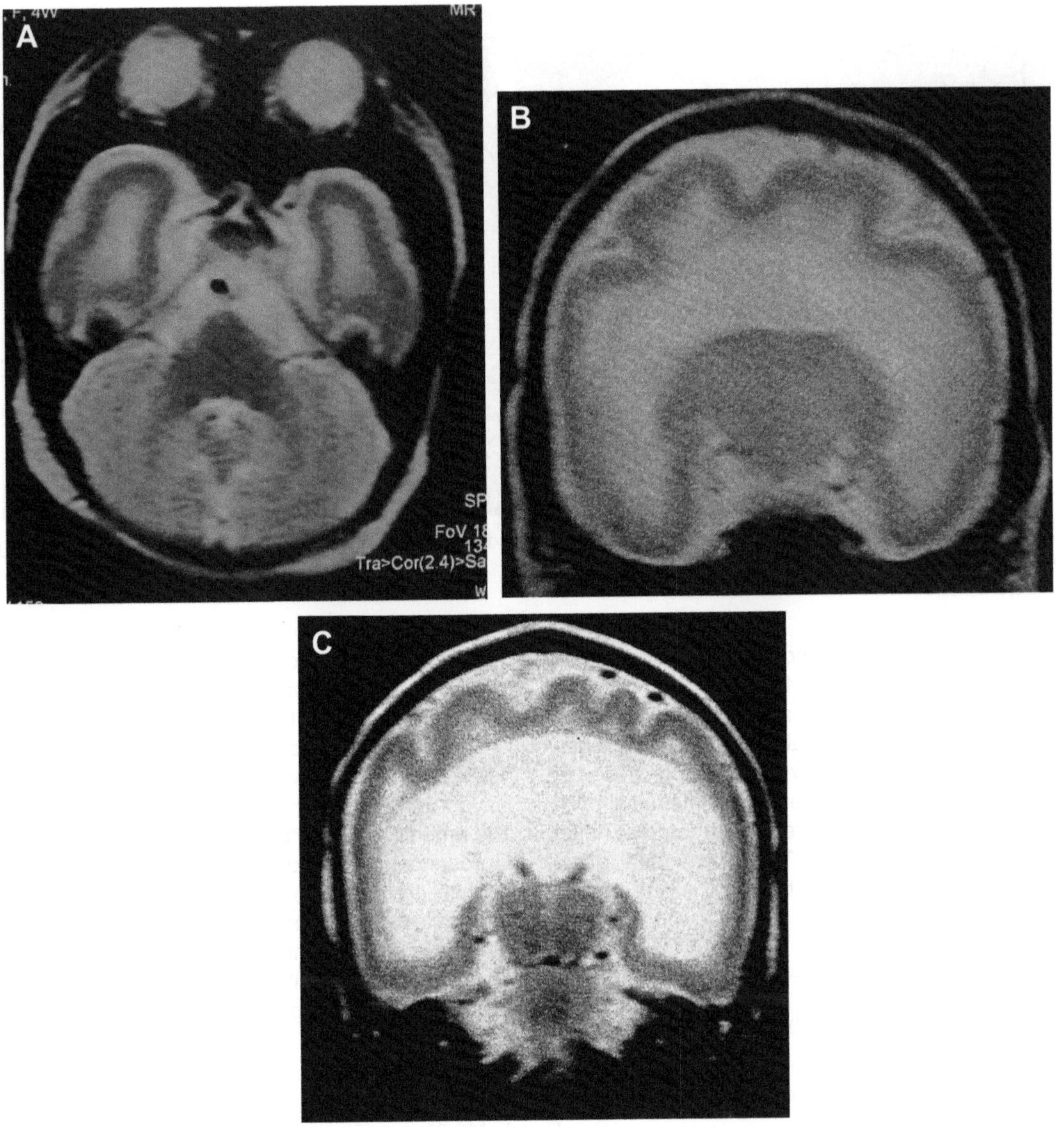

Fig. 17. Semilobar holoprosencephaly in a 4-week-old male infant. Axial (*A*), coronal (*B*), and (*C*) T2-weighted images. Monoventricle with rudimentary temporal horns, diencephalic fusion. Frontal and temporal lobe hypoplasia.

diffuse hypoplasia of the white matter. The association with cortical organization anomalies is classified by some investigators as a third group (**Box 14**; **Figs. 21** and **22**).[45,46]

There is impairment of the hypothalamic-pituitary axis with endocrinopathies.

Unilateral optic nerve hypoplasia and the presence of remnants of the septum pellucidum are associated with a milder phenotype in septo-optical dysplasia, according to the observations of some. On the other hand, abnormalities of the hippocampus and falx are related to severe clinical disease.[47,48]

The isolated absence of the septum pellucidum is a rare anomaly, and its neurologic future is not clear. Some investigators[49] suggest that it could indicate a limbic anomaly; certain symptoms such as psychomotor impairment have been associated with this anomaly (**Fig. 23**).[50]

If some of the bone anomalies, mainly of the facial bones, need to be demonstrated, CT can be used as a complementary diagnosis imaging

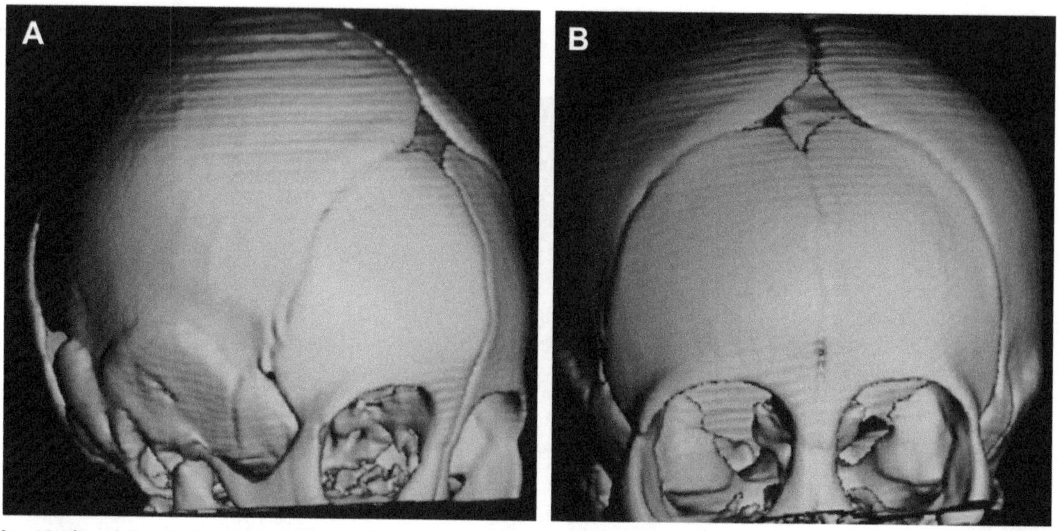

Fig. 18. (*A, B*) Semilobar holoprosencephaly in a 4-week-old male infant: CT 3-dimensional reconstruction. Trigonocephaly and hypotelorism.

that displays a very detailed image of bone anomalies such as a unique frontal bone with the absence of the metopic suture, trigonocephaly (see **Fig. 18**), scaphocephaly, ethmoid hypoplasia, orbital bone anomalies, hypotelorism or hypertelorism, cleft palate, and stenosis of the nasal pyriform aperture due to overgrowth of the nasal process of the maxilla.[51] This is the ideal diagnostic imaging technique to demonstrate one of the variants of holoprosencephaly: the solitary median maxillary central incisor (located exactly in the middle line of the maxilla).

MR angiography or CT angiography are useful for demonstrating vascular anomalies such as azygous A2 anterior cerebral artery, absence of the anterior cerebral artery in cases of alobar holoprosencephaly, and a medial orientation of the middle cerebral arteries. The associated venous anomalies depend on the severity of the anomalies; which are absence or hypoplasia of the superior and inferior longitudinal sinus and, eventually, absence of the straight sinus of higher degree.

Box 10
Alobar holoprosencephaly

1. Monoventricle without a septum pellucidum. Posterior cyst located in the suprapineal recess
2. Corpus callosum absent
3. Hypoplasia and fusion of the frontal lobes
4. Variable degrees of delayed myelin maturation and migration disorders in the frontal lobes cortical, dysplasia, and subcortical heterotopias associated to the absence of corticospinal tracts
5. Unique thalamus associated to basal nuclei and hypothalamic fusion
6. Sylvian fissures displaced anteriorly or absent in correlation with the grade of frontal hypoplasia
7. I (olfactory) and II (optic) cranial nerves could be absent
8. Absence of the anterior falx cerebri and its bone insertion point, the crista galli apophysis
9. Winding network of vessels from the internal carotid arteries

Box 11
Semilobar holoprosencephaly

1. Presence of temporal horns of the lateral ventricles is a distinct feature. Small dorsal cyst
2. Septum pellucidum absent
3. Partially formed third ventricle, without roof.
4. Posterior interhemispheric fissure and falx presence
5. Cortical frontal lobe and hypothalamic fusion
6. Thalami and basal ganglia with incomplete fusion (caudate nuclei)
7. Wide, anteriorly and medially displaced Sylvian fissure
8. Posterior dysplastic corpus callosum (rostrum, genu, and body absent)
9. Azygous anterior cerebral artery

Box 12
Lobar holoprosencephaly

1. Rostral and ventral frontal neocortex fusion
2. Absence of the septum pellucidum
3. Better-formed lateral ventricles, with hypoplasia of the frontal horns. Small or absent dorsal cyst
4. Corpus callosum: absence of rostrum and genu, anterior body variably present, splenium present
5. Anterior interhemispheric fissure could be partially absent
6. Diencephalic fusion (basal ganglia and thalamus) could be mild or absent
7. Azygous anterior cerebral artery

Nowadays, prenatal and newborn diagnosis of holoprosencephaly should be made using ultrasonography or MR imaging.[52,53] Middle-line anomalies such as the absence of the corpus callosum, septum pellucidum, and anomalies of the frontal and third ventricle are very well displayed by ultrasonography[54,55] and fetal MR imaging (**Fig. 24**).[56] Color Doppler is useful for showing vascular anomalies. Fetal MR imaging usually shows more accurate findings than MR imaging.[57]

Diffusion tensor images demonstrate the abnormal white matter tracts present in prosencephalies, such as bilateral absence of corticospinal tracts in alobar type posterior commissural bundle representing the callosal splenium, and posterior limb fibers arching to the motor cortex or coursing dorsally to the (presumably) sensory cortex. The sizes of corticospinal and middle cerebellar peduncle tracts were found to correlate strongly with both holoprosencephaly type and neurodevelopmental score. In septo-optical dysplasia there is a decrease in anisotropy and an increase in mean diffusivity of the optic nerves.[58–61]

PITUITARY AND HYPOTHALAMIC ANOMALIES

The two parts of the pituitary gland, the adenohypophysis (pars glandular, pars intermedia, and pars tubular) and the neurohypophysis (pars nervosa infundibular stalk) have different embryologic origins but they join up as early as 13 weeks GA.

Rathke's pouch originates from the growth of the preinfundibular part of the neural plate and moves caudally to reach the definitive position. It originates the adenohypophysis. At the time the Rathke pouch forms, the oral ectoderm is in direct contact with the neuroectoderm of the ventral forebrain without intervening mesoderm. By stages 20 and 21, the pouch loses its contact with the roof of the mouth.

The neurohypophysis arises from the most rostral part of the secondary prosencephalon, the floor of the rostral forebrain. The portion of

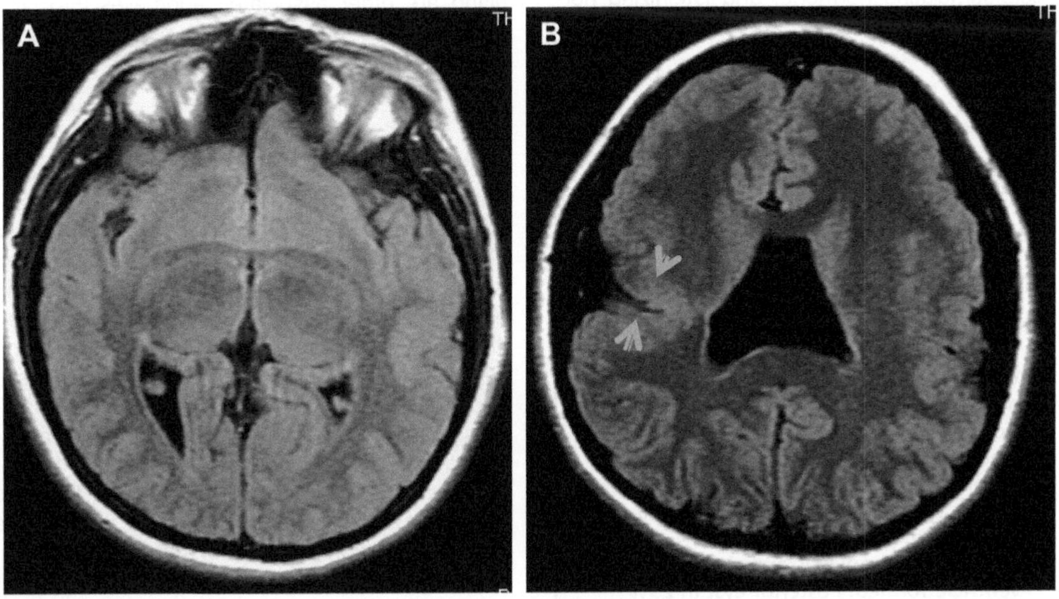

Fig. 19. (*A, B*) Lobar holoprosencephaly in a 16-year-old girl: T2-weighted fluid-attenuated inversion recovery (FLAIR) axial MR images: transversal band anterior to the anterior commissure. Absence of frontal horns of lateral ventricle. Frontal lobe cortical dysplasia with close-lip schizencephaly (*short yellow arrows*).

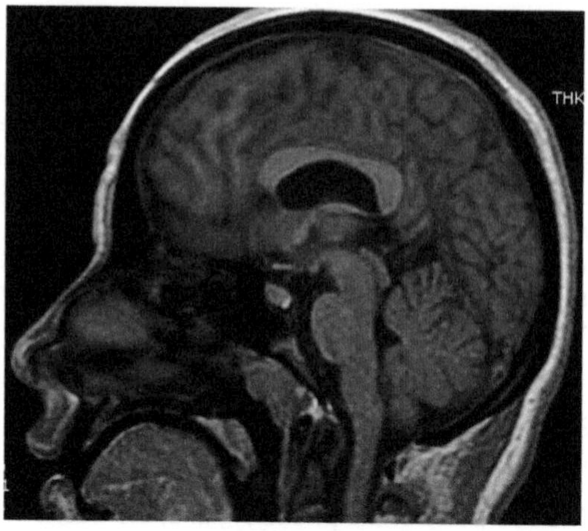

Fig. 20. Lobar holoprosencephaly in a 16-year-old girl: T1-weighted sagittal view. Corpus callosum without the rostrum, and anterior and inferior genu.

the pouch adjacent to the neurohypophyseal evagination forms the pars intermedia. The portion of the adenohypophysis that surrounds the stalk of the neurohypophysis forms the pars tuberalis, and the remaining part forms the pars distalis or glandularis. The oropharyngeal part remains as the pharyngeal hypophysis throughout life. The Rathke pouch migrates together with the pituitary cells, and remnants may be found in the pituitary.

Hormones are produced at a very early developmental stage: adrenocorticotropic and somatotropic at week 8, and prolactin-releasing, follicle-stimulating hormone, and luteinizing hormone at week 12.[33]

Box 13
Middle interhemispheric variant or syntelencephaly

1. Interhemispheric fusion of the Sylvian fissures appearing with abnormal horizontal orientation
2. Posterior frontal and parietal lobes fusion (peri-Rolandic)
3. Very common cortical dysplasia and heterotopias
4. Normal cleavage of the basal ganglia. Thalamus variably fused
5. Separated hypothalamus
6. Corpus callosum: body absence, genu variably present, splenium present
7. Normal or hypoplastic anterior horns. Third ventricle formed. Posterior cyst in 25%
8. Septum pellucidum absent
9. Azygous anterior artery

Box 14
Septo-optical dysplasia

1. Frontal horns: inferiorly pointed and typical square shape in the superior and anterior surface
2. Absent or incomplete anterior septum pellucidum
3. Unilateral or bilateral absence or reduced size of the optic nerves. Hypoplastic chiasm
4. Corpus callosum: mild anterior dysgenesis
5. Nonfusion of midline structures

Posterior Pituitary Ectopia

The hypothesized origins discussed in the literature for this condition are a transection of the pituitary stalk during a traumatic birth, an insult-like hypoxia of the stalk during the perinatal period, or an embryonic abnormality in pituitary gland organogenesis.[62]

The main finding is the absence of the posterior lobe of the pituitary gland with an ectopic posterior pituitary bright spot on the midline in the pituitary stalks, in a thick tuber cinereum or in the hypothalamus. The condition could be associated with the fusion of the tuber cinereum and mammillary bodies, optic chiasma hypoplasia, dysgenesis or agenesis of the septum pellucidum, absence of the internal carotid artery and the carotid canal, platybasia, and basilar impression. Absence of the pituitary stalk and hypoplasia of the pituitary gland are other associated anomalies (**Fig. 25**). Clinically, this anomaly could cause congenital pituitary dwarfism.[63]

Duplicated Pituitary Gland/Stalk

A duplicated pituitary gland or stalk has been classified among the median cleft face syndromes. The pituitary, both the neurohypophysis and adenohypophysis, may have been divided during early development. Midline craniofacial abnormalities are commonly associated: hypertelorism, cleft palate, midline clival defects, choanal atresia, and ectopic adenohypophyseal or hamartomatous pharyngeal masses. The most common associated intracranial anomaly is a midline bar or a mass of soft tissue on the floor of the third ventricle, probably due to arrested cells in the normal migration process of the hypothalamus. Some patients present with associated cerebellar hypoplasia, nonunion of the vertebral arteries, and absence of the massa intermedia between the thalami (**Fig. 26**).[64]

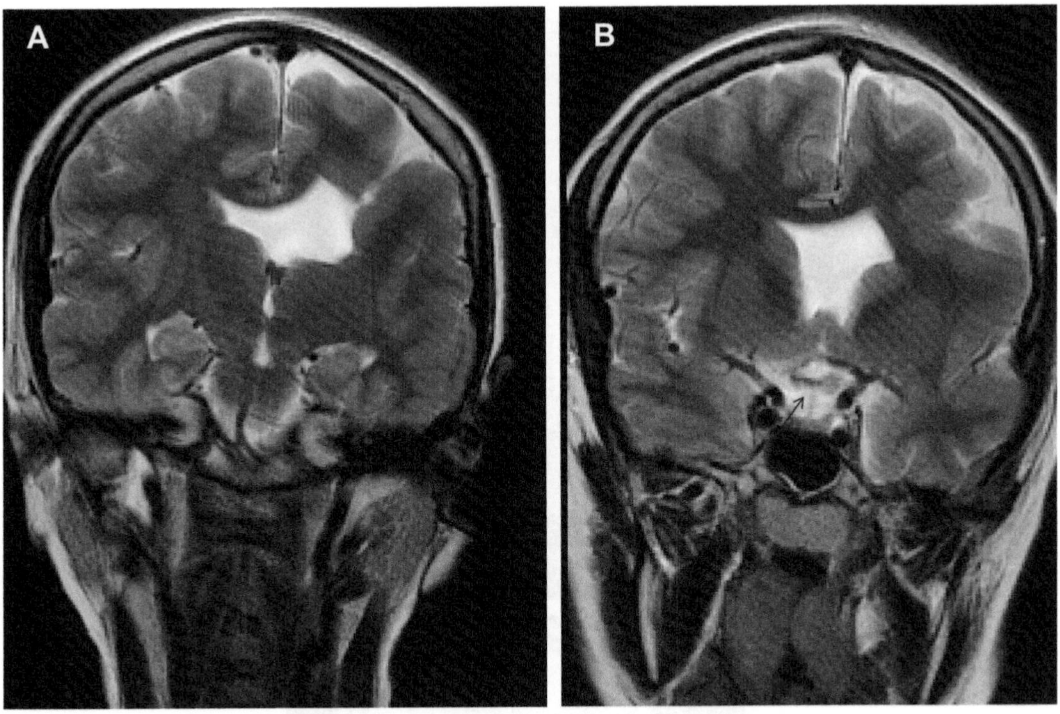

Fig. 21. (*A, B*) Septo-optic dysplasia with schizencephaly: coronal T2-weighted MR images. Square and inferior pointed frontal horns, septum pellucidum absence, right optic nerve hypoplasia (*arrow*).

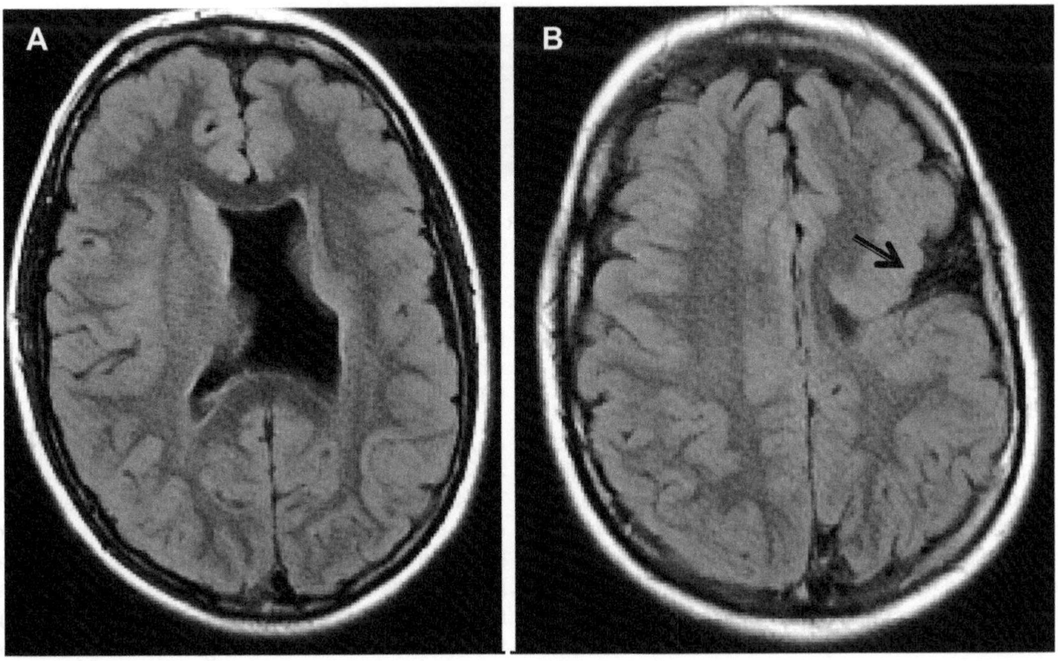

Fig. 22. (*A, B*) Septo-optic dysplasia with schizencephaly: axial T2-weighted MR images (FLAIR). Square and hypoplastic frontal horns, septum pellucidum absence, left frontal schizencephaly (*arrow*).

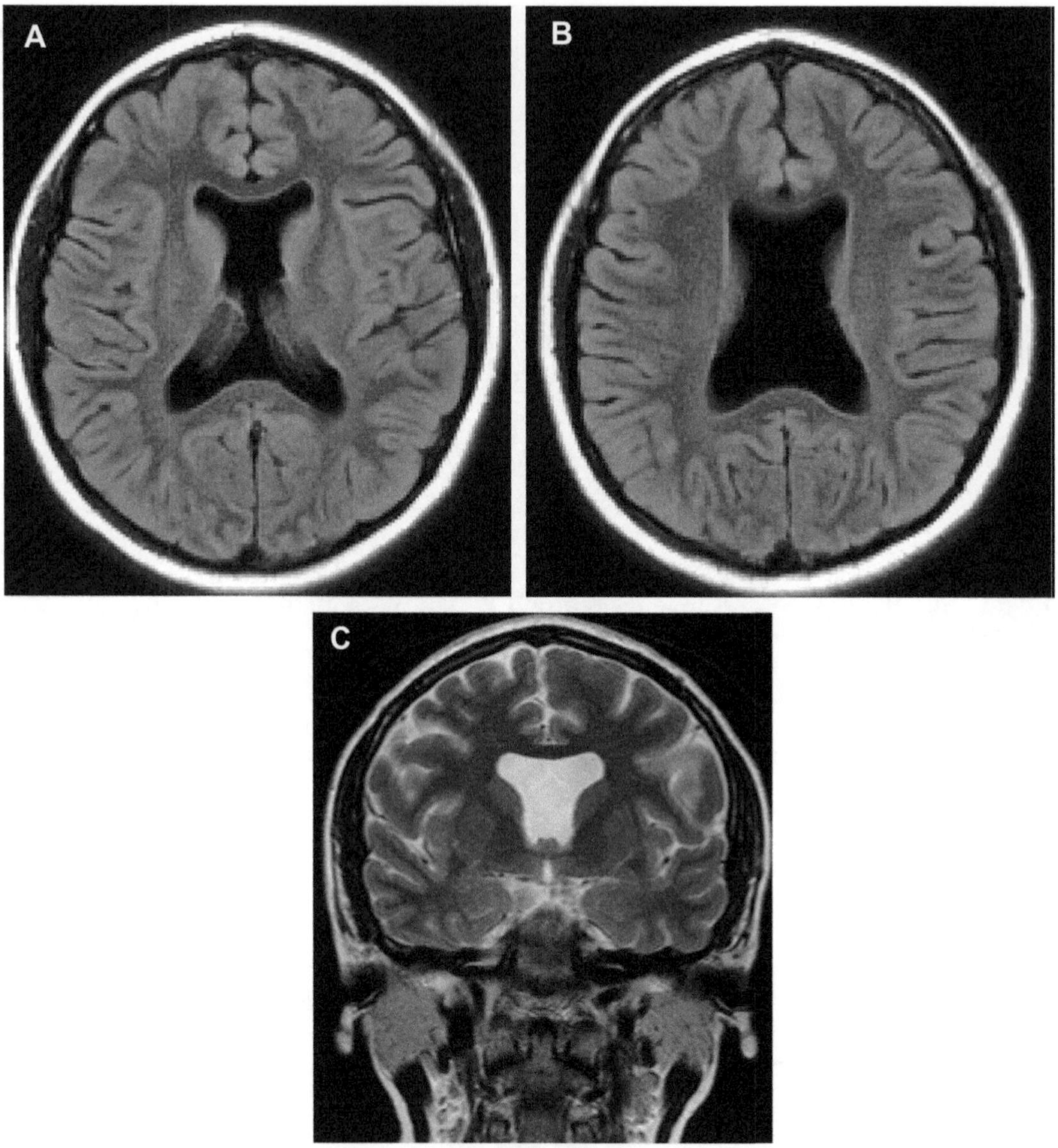

Fig. 23. Isolated septum pellucidum absence. (*A, B*) FLAIR-weighted axial MR images. (*C*) Coronal T2-weighted image.

Pituitary Absence or Aplasia

Pituitary absence is a rare anomaly, with absence of the anterior posterior pituitary and sometimes of the pituitary stalk. The importance of making this diagnosis in the newborn is in avoiding neurologic and developmental consequences of panhypopituitarism by hormone replacement therapy. Symptoms such as severe hypoglycemia, seizures, apnea, and cardiovascular complications could appear in the first hours after delivery.

Hormonal laboratory examinations and MR imaging provide the diagnostic clues. Absence of the pituitary gland, and no visualization of the bright spot on the neurohypophysis associated with a flattened and small sella are findings on MR images.[65]

Tuber Cinereum-Hypothalamic Hamartoma

These masses could be located in the tuber cinereum or adjacent to it (parahypothalamic), and histopathologically they contain glial and neural normal cells similar to hypothalamic ones.[66] Their limits are well defined in relation to the floor of the third ventricle. The signal intensity is the same as that of the brain, and there is no cyst calcification or contrast enhancement (**Fig. 27**).

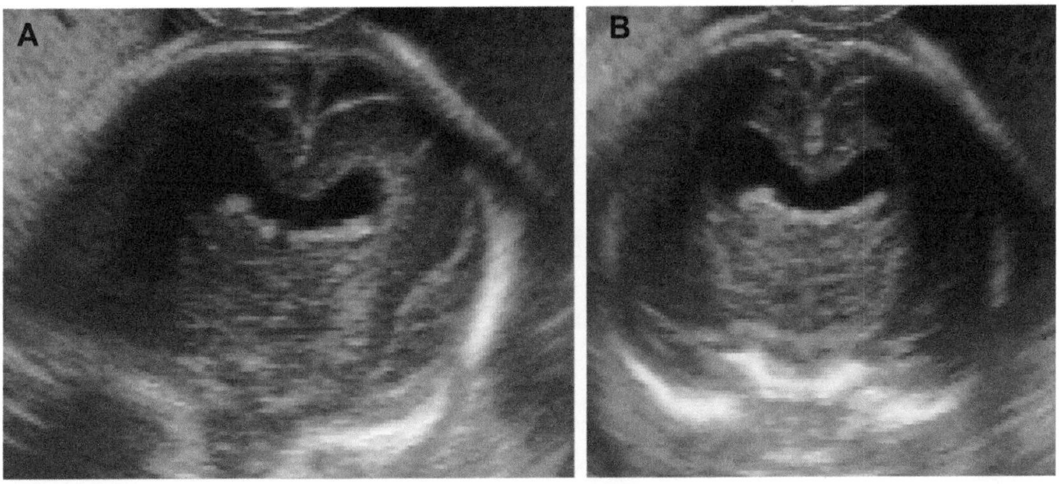

Fig. 24. (*A, B*) Congenital absence of the septum pellucidum: obstetric ultrasound coronal view. Mild ventriculomegaly without septum pellucidum.

During the first or second decade of their lives, patients may clinically present with gelastic seizures, precocious puberty, obesity, and/or diabetes insipidus, or be asymptomatic.[67]

Germinoma

The most common place of this developmental benign tumor in the CNS is the pineal gland. In the hypothalamic region it usually occurs in relation to the pituitary stalk. The tumor involving the pituitary stalk is homogeneous without cysts or calcifications. Its MR imaging signal is similar to the gray matter in T1-weighted sequences and relatively higher in T2-weighted sequences, and enhances with contrast injection (**Fig. 28**). Because of the blockage of the pituitary stalk function, the high signal of the posterior pituitary may be absent.

Rathke Cleft Anomalies: Craniopharyngioma and Cyst

Both the craniopharyngioma and the cyst originate from the remains of the Rathke pouch, and can be located in its embryologic pathway along the suprasellar portion of stalk in the suprasellar cistern and/or in the sella. The cystic form, Rathke

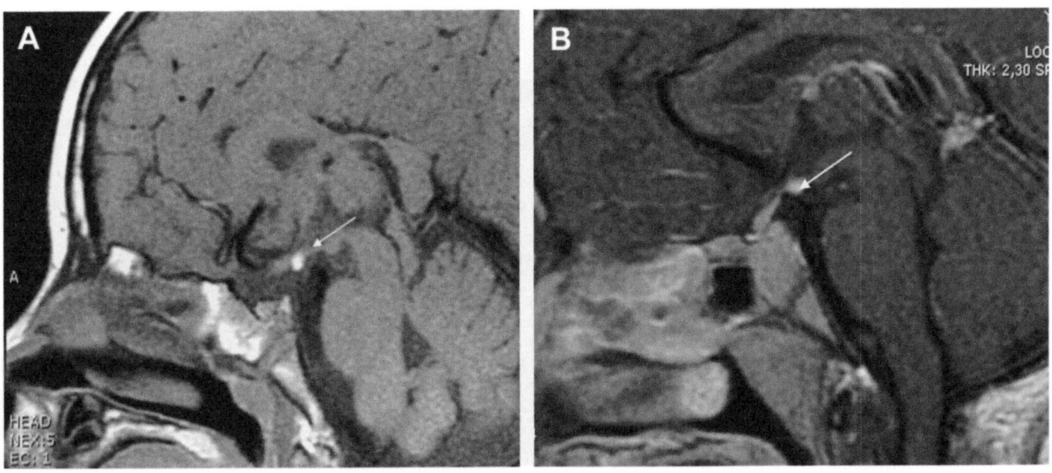

Fig. 25. Posterior pituitary ectopy (PPE) in a 5-year-old boy: T1-weighted sagittal images before (*A*) and after (*B*) contrast medium: PPE is represented by a hypothalamic bright spot in the tuber cinereum (*arrows*) and hypoplastic, anterior pituitary gland.

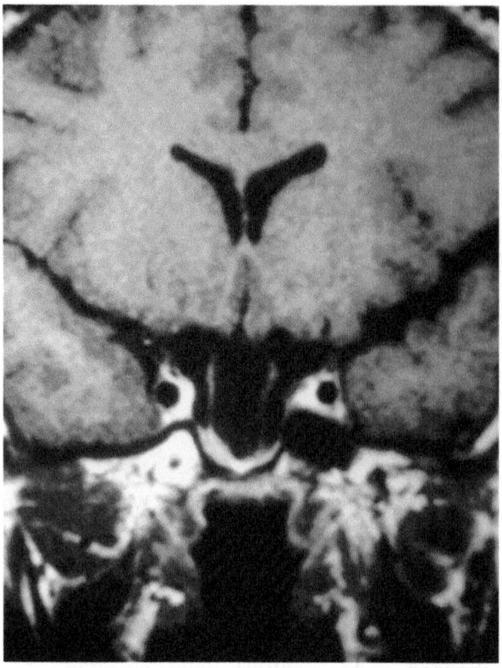

Fig. 26. Duplication of pituitary stalk: coronal T1-weighted MR image.

cleft cyst, is usually well defined, round, or oval. It is located in the midline of the anterior pituitary or typically between the anterior and posterior lobe, anterior to the pituitary stalk. Its MR imaging signal is very similar to that of the CSF or is higher in relation to its protein concentration; it does not enhance with contrast and a small node may be present, but usually without calcifications (**Fig. 29**).

Craniopharyngioma tumor, a generally lobulated, suprasellar tumor, has a mixed signal due to its cystic, solid, and calcified components. The cystic components usually have a high signal in T1-weighted and T2-weighted sequences, due to cholesterol and proteins. The solid components and the tumor wall usually enhance with contrast injection. Its calcifications are displayed on CT or in susceptibility sequences as small low signal areas. On histopathology, two different types could be distinguished: the adantinomatous form, the most common in the first or second decades of life, with predominant cystic components; and the papillary form, the most common form found in patients in their forties or fifties, with predominant solid components. Symptoms are usually related to the compression of the adjacent structures such as the optic way, the third ventricle, or the pituitary gland.

Kallmann Syndrome

This X-linked autosomal dominant anomaly consists of the absence of olfactory nerve bulb, and sulci that produce anosmia in association with hypogonadotropic hypogonadism. There are osseous anomalies, such as midline craniofacial defects and brachiphalangism due to short fourth metacarpals, renal agenesis, cryptorchidism, and some cardiovascular anomalies.

The clue to diagnosis is an MR image that shows the absence of the olfactory nerves in a coronal plane, with a flattened gyrus rectus due to the absence of the olfactory sulci.[68]

POSTERIOR FOSSA CONGENITAL ABNORMALITIES

On a complex congenital malformation of the posterior fossa, the detailed information on the cerebellum is generally undervalued. Nevertheless, because anomalies of the cerebellum are

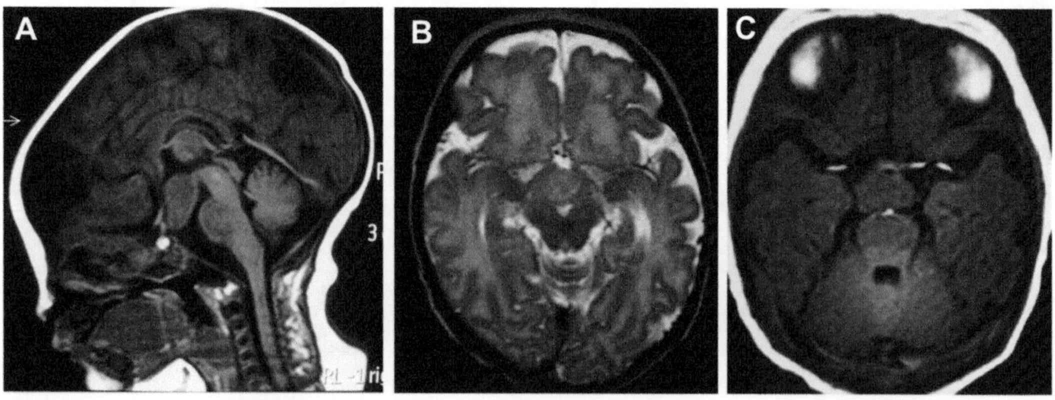

Fig. 27. Tuber cinereum hamartoma. (*A*) Sagittal T1-weighted MR image. (*B, C*) Axial T2-weighted (FLAIR and spin echo) images. Oval well-defined suprasellar mass anterior to mammillary bodies that widen the interpeduncular cistern.

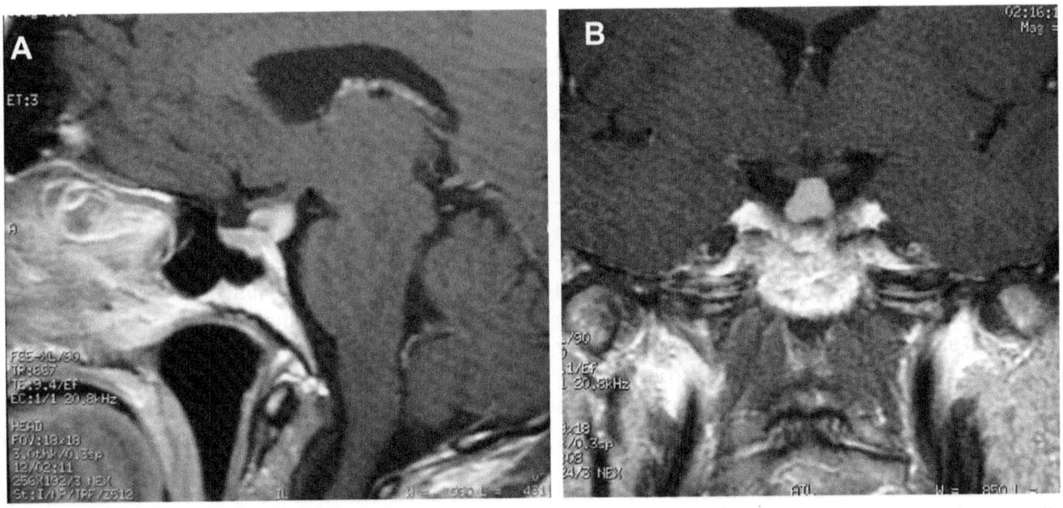

Fig. 28. Germinoma: (*A*) coronal and (*B*) sagittal T1-weighted images with gadolinium. Lobulated suprasellar mass with homogeneous contrast enhancement.

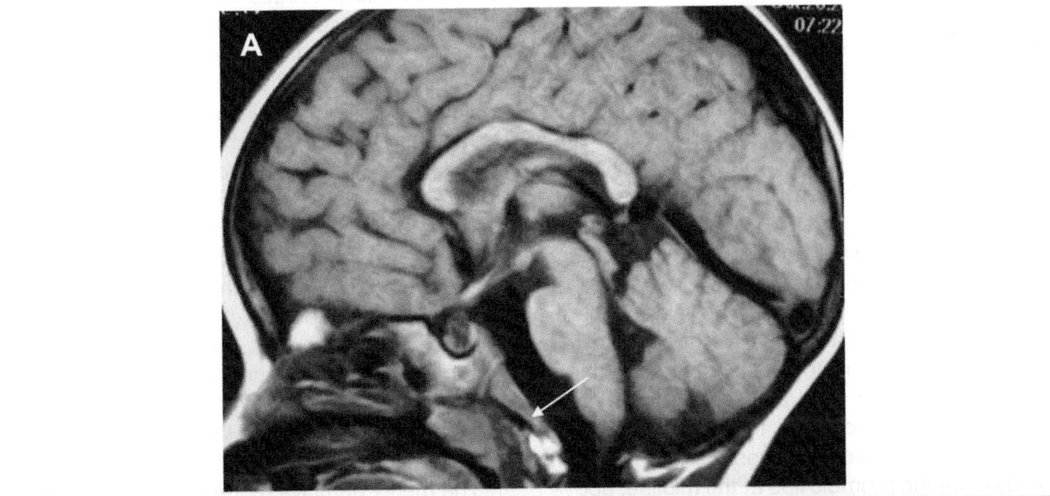

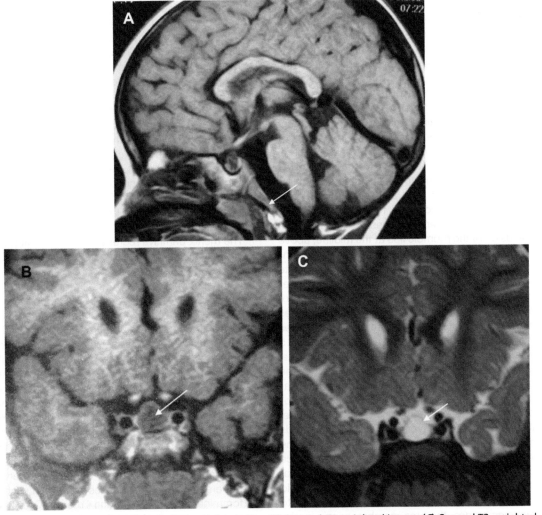

Fig. 29. Rathke cleft cyst. (*A*) Sagittal T1-weighted view. (*B*) Coronal T1-weighted image. (*C*) Coronal T2-weighted image. Cystic round lesion between neurohypophysis and adenohypophysis (*arrows*).

related to alterations in coordination, motor learning, higher cognitive function, and language development, as well as with autism, it is mandatory to review the embryologic development to better understand malformations, as well as the impact these might have on the patient.

An embryonic organizer within the neuroepithelium, which is localized at the isthmic constriction or isthmic organizer, adjacent to hindbrain rhombomere 1, controls the patterning of the midbrain and the anterior hindbrain. Some genes and signaling molecules such as murine genes, netrins and their receptors, and the WnT family play a role in cerebellar development.[69,70] By 24 to 27 days GA, the neural tube divides into 3 primary brain vesicles: the prosencephalon, mesencephalon, and rombencephalon. This early differentiation of the neural tube is called patterning, a mechanism that is partially understood. The metencephalon and myelencephalon stem from the rombencephalon. The metencephalon is located under the mesencephalon and evolves into the protuberance and the cerebellum. The myelencephalon evolves into the medulla oblongata. At 4 weeks GA, there is a proliferation of cells in the alar plate in the rostral and lateral aspects of the metencephalon. The alar plate hypertrophies at its medial aspect and creates the rhombic lips at 5 weeks GA. The cerebellum originates entirely from the first rhombomere (upper rhombic lip), and the hindbrain from rhombomeres 2 to 8 (lower rhombic lip). The neuroepithelial zones, in the roof of the fourth ventricle and the rhombic lips, are the locations of the germinal matrices where the cells of the cerebellum and many brainstem nuclei will form. The cerebellar primordium or tuberculum cerebelli derive from the fusion of the rhombic lips at the midline, above the roof of the fourth ventricle and anterior to the choroid plexus. The flocculus and the nodule originate from this fusion at 9 weeks GA. The small cerebellum covers the most rostral portion of the roof of a prominent fourth ventricle. The fusion continues in a caudal and mediolateral direction, and creates the rest of the cerebellum and the vermis by 15 weeks GA. The fourth ventricle acquires its normal and definitive relations by 24 weeks GA. When the pontic flexure (dorsal pontomesencephalic angulation) emerges at 5 weeks GA, the roof of the rhombencephalon widens and attains a diamond shape, thus forming a transverse crease that extends across the rhombic vesicle perpendicular to the long axis of the neural tube, giving rise to the plica choroidea. The plica invaginates into the lumen of the fourth ventricle and forms a rudimentary choroid plexus that divides the rhombencephalic roof into two membranes: the area membranacea superior and the area membranacea inferior. Active multiplication continues at the cerebral cortex and generates the fastigium in the roof of the fourth ventricle, anterior to the cerebellum, which is an open anterior "V" shape on the sagittal plane. The superior subdivision, limited on its inferior aspect by the plica choroidea, thickens in the craniocaudal direction and forms the vermis. Intense neuroblastic activity during the third month produces extraventricular prominence of the cerebellum that starts to subdivide. The first subdivision is the flocculonodular fissure that separates the flocculus from the cerebellar hemispheres and the nodule from the vermis. The flocculonodular lobe is the most primitive part of the cerebellum (archicerebellum). The primary fissure, which is located between the culmen and the declive in the adult brain, then forms at 10 weeks GA. The anterior (superior) lobe is anterior to the primary fissure and the flocculonodular posterior to this fissure. The development of the vermis precedes the development of the cerebellar hemispheres by approximately 30 to 60 days GA. Hence the flocculus and the vermis (pyramid, uvula, central lobule, and culmen) are called the paleocerebellum. The other cerebellar hemispheres and posterior lobule (without pyramid and uvula) constitute the neocerebellum. The fissures and main subdivisions of the cerebellum can be identified by 4 months GA. Anatomically there are 9 vermian lobes. Three constitute the anterior lobe: the lingula, the central lobe, and the culmen. Five comprise the posterior lobe: declive, folium, tuber, pyramid, and uvula; and one comprises the flocculonodular lobe (**Figs. 30** and **31**). Access videos online for animations of axial view and sagittal view of the development of the 4th ventricle at www.neuroimaging.theclinics.com.

The menix primitiva regresses during the fifth to seventh week of gestation, so the cisterna magna is formed by the end of week 7. Simultaneously, when these changes take place in the roof of the rhombencephalon (7–10 weeks GA), the meninx primitiva that surrounds the neural tube differentiates into the pia mater and dura mater, and both the production of cerebrospinal fluid and of the subarachnoid space, which at first are independent from the fourth ventricle, begin. The inferior area membranacea, an ependymal membrane, expands posteriorly to form a recess (Blake's pouch) that then disappears, leaving a median aperture (Blake pouch metapore), precursor of the foramen of Magendie, around 8 weeks GA. Disorders in this process result in cysts of the posterior fossa. At the same time of gestation, the tentorium and the different infratentorial sinuses form. The Luschka foramina appear later, around 4 months GA. This period of formation of the infratentorial structures corresponds to the end of the prosencephalic

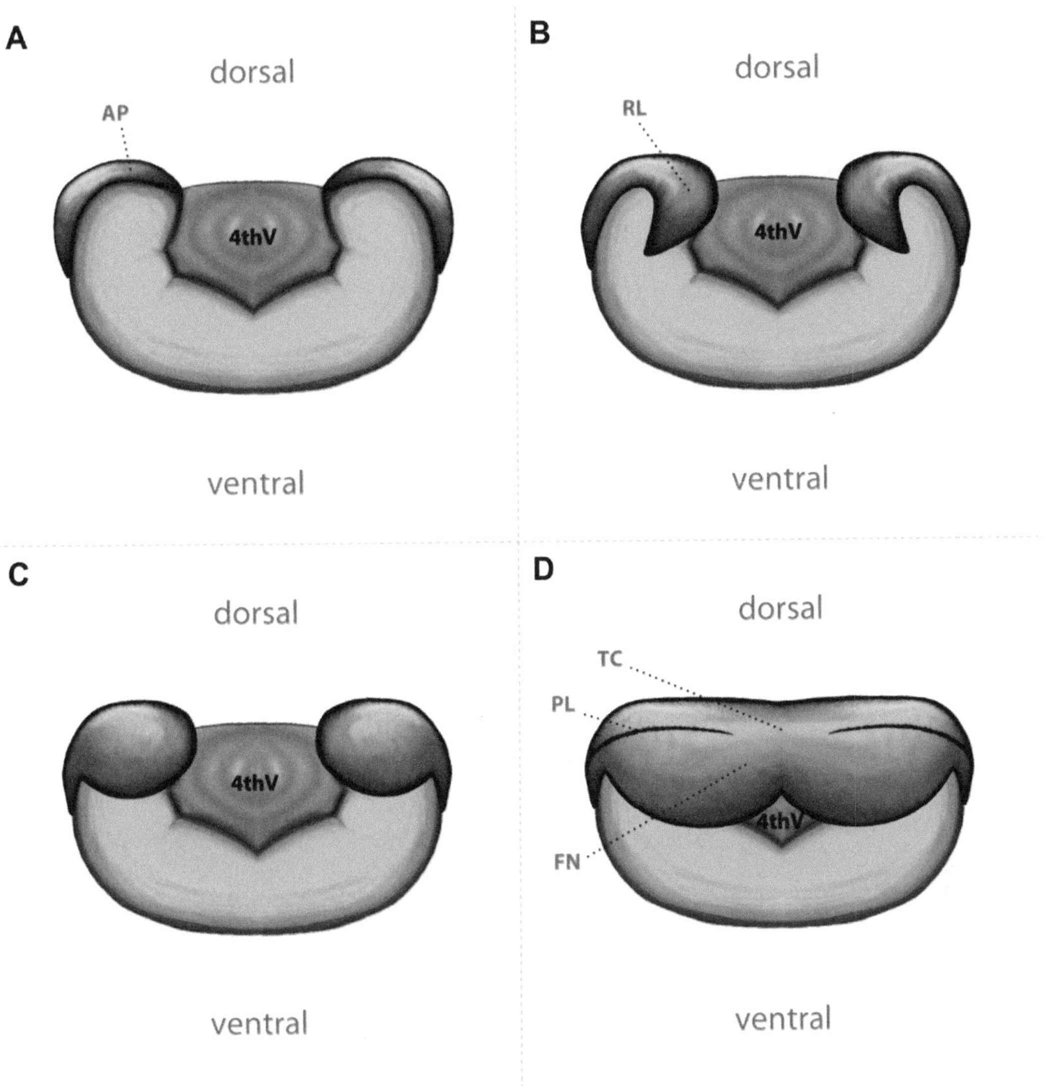

Fig. 30. Axial view of metencephalon. (*A*) Four weeks GA. Allar plate (AP) cell proliferation in the most rostral aspect of the metencephalon. (*B*) Five weeks GA. The AP hypertrophy at its medial aspect creates the rhombic lips (RL). (*C*) Cerebellum originates entirely from rhombomere 1. (*D*) Fusion of the RL at the midline creates the cerebellar primordium or tuberculum cerebelli (TC). PL, posterolateral fissure; FN, flocullonodular lobule.

diverticulation and to the beginning of the supratentorial commissural formation.

The histogenesis of the cerebellar cortex starts around 7 weeks GA, when neuroblasts migrate tangentially from the germinal zone, in the lateral aspect of the rhombic lips to the cerebellar surface, forming a temporal external granular layer that later differentiates to form the external molecular layer. The cells that form the deep paired cerebellar nuclei and the Purkinje layer migrate radially in a lateral direction from the germinal matrix to their definitive location in the cerebellar hemispheres. Some cells present an inward migration to form the internal granular layer. Finally, the cerebellar cortex achieves a 3-layered histologic composition: outer molecular layer, middle Purkinje layer, and inner granular layer. The intense cell proliferation in the inner and external granular layers develops the folia. At birth the cerebellum is morphologically identical to that of the adult, but differentiation, late migration, and organization continues after birth, until the middle of the second year; thereafter, the only change is enlargement.[69,71]

It is also important to be fully familiar with the terminology, and to understand the anomalies of the posterior fossa (**Box 15**). The distinction

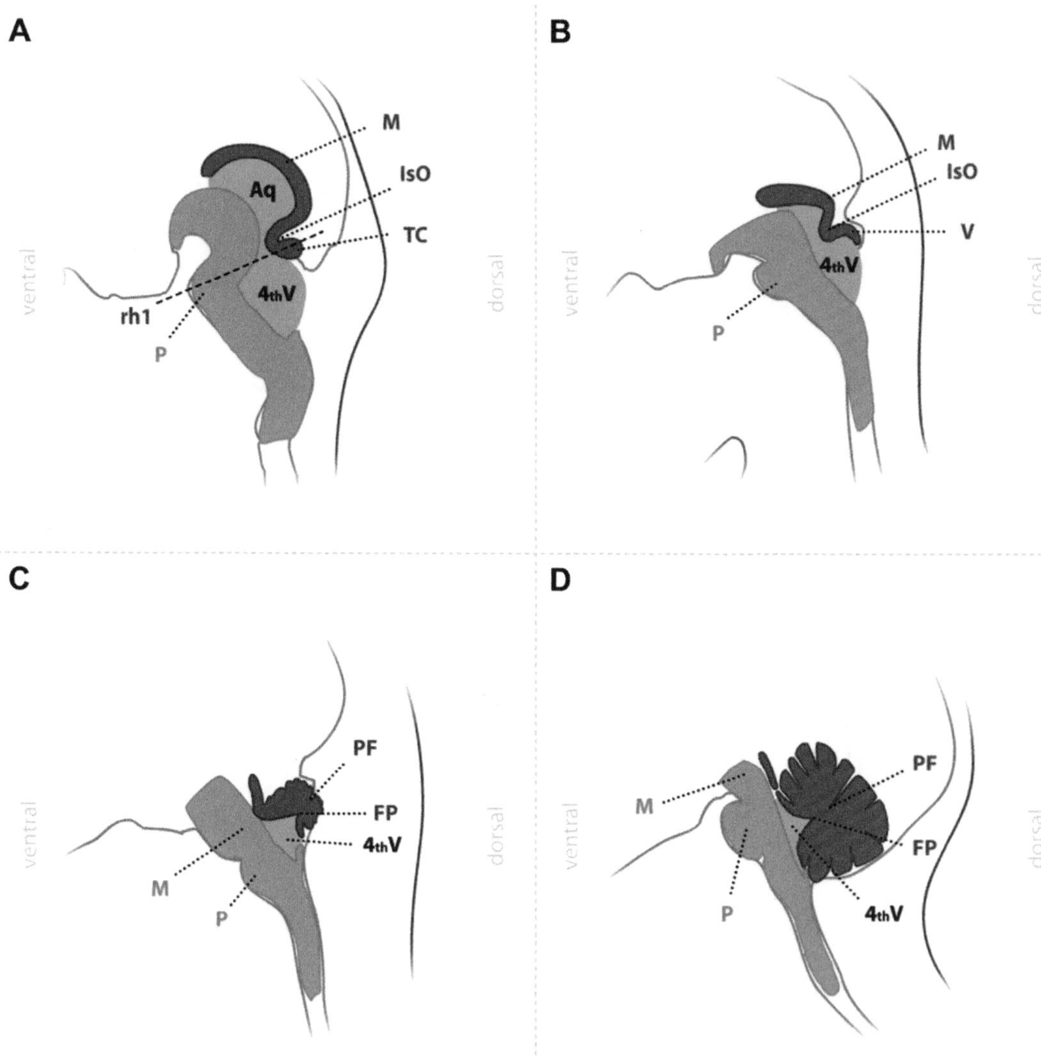

Fig. 31. Sagittal view. (*A*) Tuberculum cerebellum at most rostral roof of fourth ventricle. (*B*) Fusion continues in a caudal and mediolateral direction. (*C*) At 13 to 14 weeks GA. Active proliferation continues at the cerebellar cortex and generates the fastigium. (*D*) The fourth ventricle acquires its normal and definitive relations by 24 weeks GA. M, mesencephalon; IsO, isthmic organizer; rh1, rhombomere 1; Aq, aqueduct; TC, tuberculum cerebelli; V, vermis; P, pons; PF, primary fissure; FP, fastigial point.

between hypoplasia and atrophy is not always clear, because they could be superimposed (eg, in congenital disorders of glycosylation).

Cerebellar Malformations

Because cerebellar embryology is complex and poorly understood, and a limited number of histologic and genetic studies are available, it is often difficult to know whether an abnormal cerebellum represents atrophy, hypoplasia, or malformation. Various classifications and descriptions of posterior fossa malformations can be found in the published medical literature.[29,71–74] Imaging classification is usually based on morphology; sometimes, many terms are used to describe the same abnormality, or a single term is used to indicate a variety of interpretations. Although a classification based on images is practical, it has limitations. Truly developmental malformations are sometimes placed in the same category as disruptions. The delineation of many cerebellar malformations and syndromes will still be somewhat arbitrary, until the pathogenetic mechanism is understood and there is enough molecular genetic knowledge of posterior fossa malformations. An integrated classification of such

Box 15
Terminology of anomalies of the posterior fossa

1. Hypoplasia. Disorder of formation with reduction or early termination of cellular production and migration (incomplete formation). Cerebellar hypoplasia implies a small cerebellum with normal-size fissures as compared with the folia.
2. Dysplasia. Abnormal cellular migration and abnormal cortical organization that produce morphologic alteration in the folia and fissures (abnormal formation).
3. Atrophy. Small, shrunken cerebellum, with enlarged fissures, usually secondary to a neurodegenerative process. Atrophy indicates a progressive metabolic injury and not a congenital anomaly.

malformations based on morphologic appearance, embryology, and molecular neurogenetics will be helpful.[69,71–73]

When one has to analyze an image with a possible posterior fossa malformation, it is useful to consult some criteria and follow some steps (**Box 16**; **Figs. 32** and **33**).[75,76]

The classifications of posterior fossa malformations, which include both morphologic and genetic criteria, such as those proposed by Barkovich, and by Sarnat based on the genetic patterning (gradients) of the neural tube, have evolved to the latest classification by Barkovich and colleagues that integrates both previous and new information.[71,77,78]

Cerebellar Hypoplasia

Cerebellar hypoplasia could be the consequence of a variety of causes, both malformations and disruptions, particularly neocerebellar compromise.[79] It is usually asymmetric, and can be seen in heterogeneous conditions such as prenatal vascular injury prenatal infections (cytomegalovirus), prenatal exposure to teratogens, chromosomal aberrations, metabolic disorders, isolated (genetic) cerebellar hypoplasias, complex (genetic) malformations, (genetic) migration disorders, some types of congenital muscular dystrophies, and pontocerebellar hypoplasias (**Fig. 34**).

Cystic Malformations of the Posterior Fossa

These malformations overlap clinically, radiologically, and pathologically. There is no consensus on the criteria for their diagnosis in the published literature. Following the initial description many modifications have been proposed by different investigators. The ability to distinguish them based on neuroimaging criteria alone is limited. Differential diagnosis may be difficult or even impossible. Rather than fitting the lesion into a specific classification,[17,28,78,80] identifying it as well as the

Box 16
MR imaging criteria for evaluation of the posterior fossa

1. Vermis and cerebellar hemisphere anomaly, compromise: focal or generalized
2. Vermis and cerebellar folial pattern: normal or abnormal
3. Fastigial point: normal or abnormal
4. Craniocaudal vermian axis: normal or rotated
5. Ratio anterior/posterior vermian lobes 47%/53%[74]
6. Vermis and cerebellar hemispheres characteristics: dysplastic, hypoplastic, or absent
7. Brainstem development: normal, hypoplastic, or dysplastic
8. Posterior fossa CSF collection: present or absent
9. Size of the posterior fossa: reduced, normal, or increased
10. Mass effect: present or absent

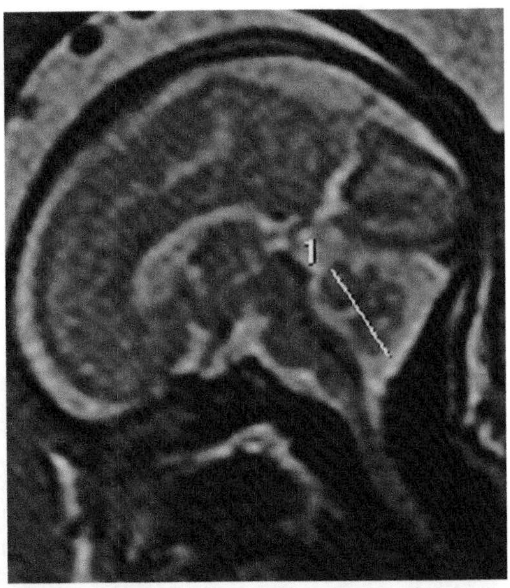

Fig. 32. Normally oriented craniocaudal vermian axis. Sagittal single-shot fast spin echo (SSFSE) T2-weighted fetal image.

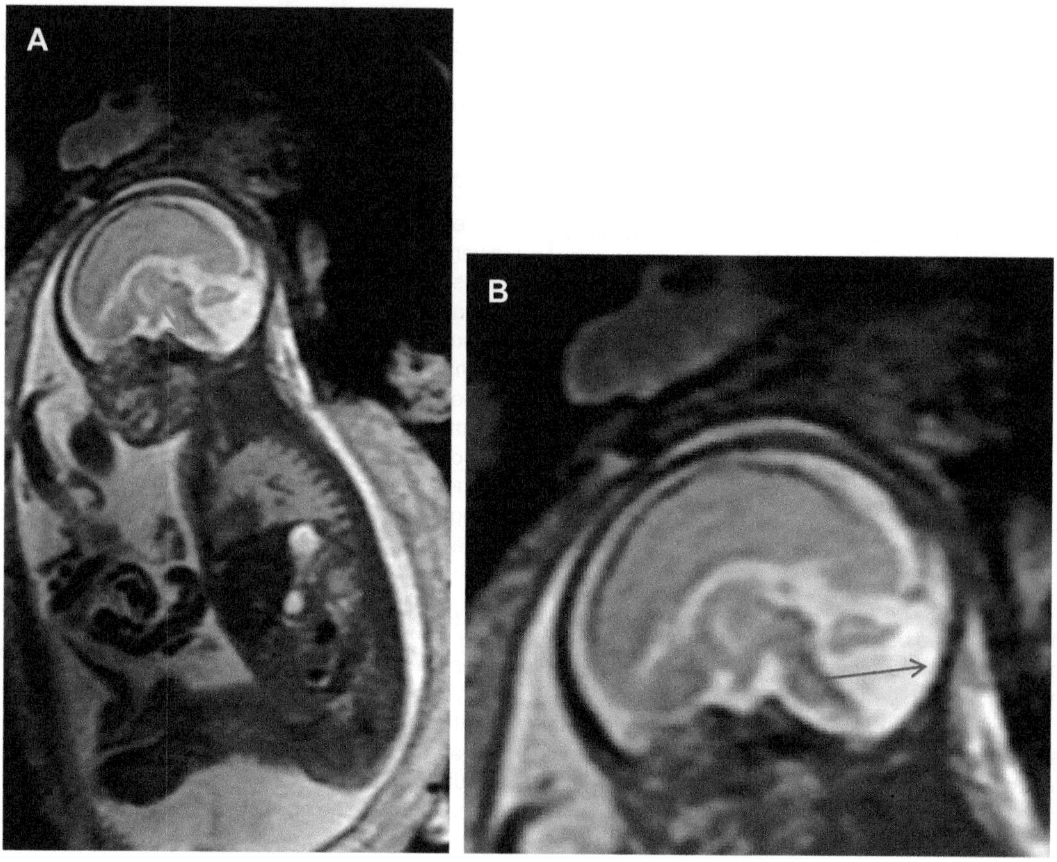

Fig. 33. (*A*, *B*) Abnormally upward rotated craniocaudal vermian axis. Sagittal SSFSE T2-weighted fetal images. The normal axis should be parallel to the brainstem (*blue arrow*). The abnormal upward cerebellar axis is shown by the red arrow.

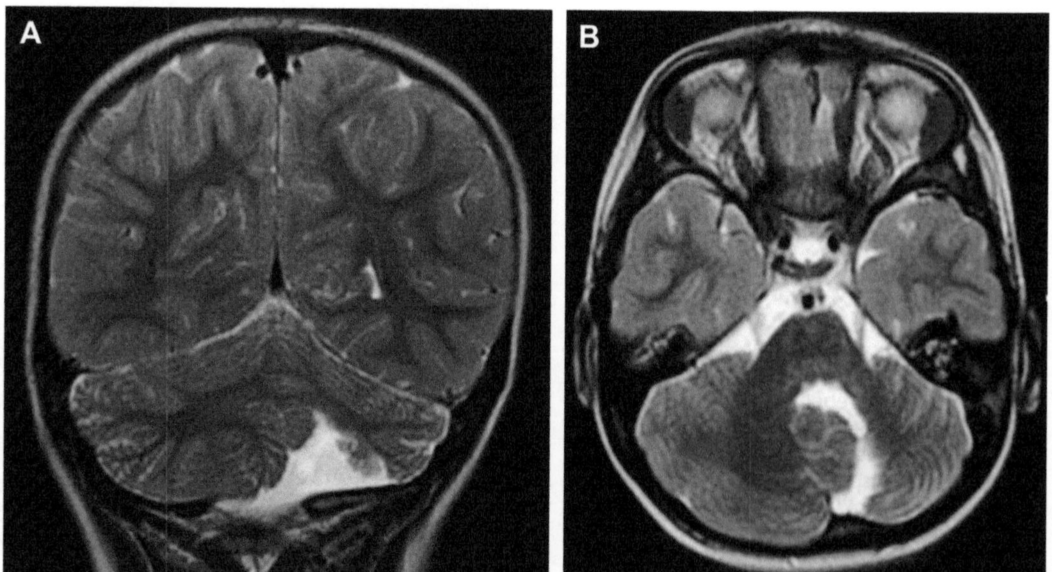

Fig. 34. Hypoplastic and dysplastic left hemispheric cerebella and middle cerebellar peduncle. (*A*) Coronal and (*B*) axial T2-weighted images.

Box 17
Cystic posterior fossa malformations

1. Malformations of the cerebellum
   a. Dandy-Walker continuum or Dandy-Walker complex
      i. Classic Dandy-Walker malformation
      ii. Cerebellar vermian hypoplasia-dysplasia (CVH) or Dandy-Walker variant
   b. Blake pouch cyst
   c. Mega cisterna magna
2. Malformation of the meninges
   a. Arachnoid cyst

associated developmental lesions and giving a detailed description must be the goals (**Box 17**).

DANDY-WALKER CONTINUUM OR DANDY-WALKER COMPLEX

Classic Dandy-Walker malformation

There is great confusion about the definition and limits of this syndrome, which was first described in 1914 by Dandy and Blackfan, and further defined in 1942 by Taggart and Walker. Afterwards in 1954, Benda suggested the accepted name of Dandy-Walker malformation. D'Agostino and colleagues and Hart and colleagues defined the characteristic triad (**Box 18**; **Fig. 35**).

The cause of this anomaly is unknown and heterogeneous. Most cases are sporadic, and the risk of sibling recurrence is less than 5% for the isolated form of the disease. The insult occurs around the seventh to tenth week of GA, resulting from a defect in the development of the superior mesenteric artery. There are some predisposing factors such as gestational exposure to rubella, cytomegalovirus, toxoplasmosis, coumadin, and alcohol.

Hydrocephalus should be considered a complication and not a part of the malformation itself. Associated CNS anomalies are present in approximately 68% of the cases. The most common is dysgenesis of the corpus callosum. Brainstem dysplasias, especially pontomedullary hypoplasia and aqueductal stenosis, may also be associated. Neuronal heterotopias, polymicrogyria, agyria, schizencephaly, lipomas, cephaloceles, and lumbosacral meningoceles are also associated, and usually seen when there is great cerebellar compromise. On contrasting with lesser degrees of posterior fossa enlargement, the finding is usually an isolated callosal anomaly. Associated peripheral malformations, such as cleft lip and palate, cardiac anomalies, and urinary tract abnormalities have been reported in 20% to 33% of cases.[29,71] The patient usually presents with characteristic dolicocephaly with a bulging occipital region and macrocrania secondary to hydrocephalus, or the presence of the posterior fossa cyst itself.

Box 18
Classic Dandy-Walker triad

1. Dysgenesis, complete or partial agenesis of the vermis
2. Cystic dilatation of the fourth ventricle
3. Enlarged posterior fossa with upward displacement of the venous sinuses, tentorium, and torcula

The neurologic signs usually present in the neonate are poor head control, retarded motor development, spasticity, and respiratory failure. In older children cranial nerve palsies, nystagmus, and truncal ataxia may be present. Those who present with milder variants in this continuum can have mild or no symptoms, with a normal neurologic examination. Medical literature reports normal intellectual development in approximately 50% to 75% of patients.[29,71] If there are associated supratentorial anomalies, the prognosis is less favorable.

In approximately 25% of patients there is an absent vermis and in the majority there is only hypoplasia. A dysplastic vermis is rotated posterosuperiorly, compressed, and sometimes attached to the tentorium, best assessed by midsagittal MR images. The cerebellar hemispheres are hypoplastic, asymmetric, or symmetric, and pushed superolaterally, and the medulla oblongata pushed anteriorly by the cystic fourth ventricle. The cyst membrane has 3 layers: an inner ependymal layer adjacent to the ependyma of the fourth ventricle, an outer pial layer, and an intermediate layer of neuroglial tissue, which may be calcified in approximately 7% of the cases. Anomalies of the posterior inferior cerebellar arteries may be present as well, such as absence of the inferior vermian branches and absence of the inferior vermian vein. The falx cerebelli is absent.

Cerebellar Vermian Hypoplasia-Dysplasia or Dandy-Walker Variant

CVH describes a group of posterior fossa congenital malformations that are clinically and radiologically difficult to differentiate. Confusion still exists in the literature, because it may be similar to the

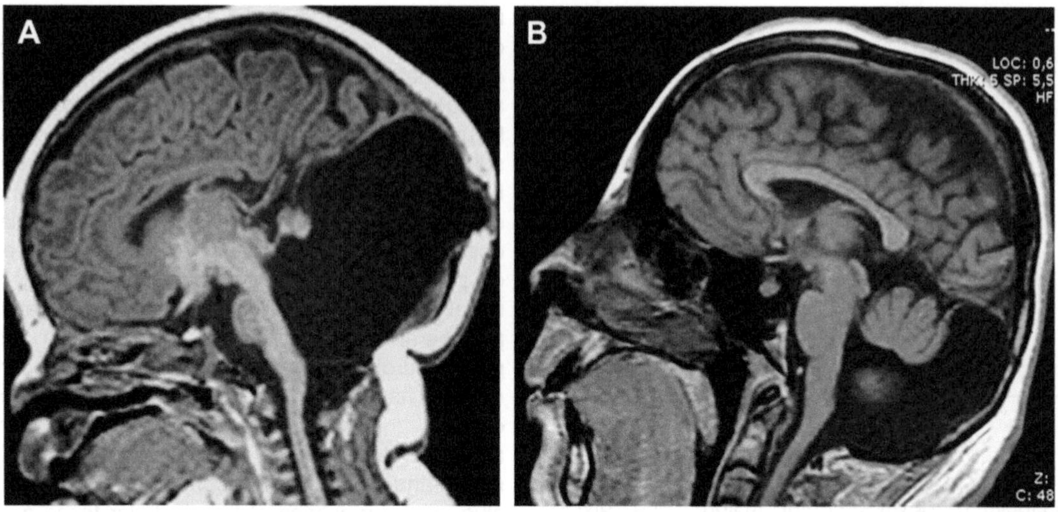

Fig. 35. Classic Dandy-Walker malformation (DWM). (*A, B*) Sagittal T1-weighted images. Dysgenesis and superior rotation of the vermis associated with a cystic dilatation of the fourth ventricle, enlarged posterior fossa with upward displacement of tentorium. (*A*) Associated small occipital meningocele. (*B*) Classic DWM; patient with less severe expression in the continuum malformation.

classic Dandy-Walker malformation but may differ by the degree of enlargement of the posterior fossa itself. Harwood-Nash first used the term Dandy-Walker variant; Sarnat and Alcala, and afterwards Raynaud, used the same term with some differences in the description of the pathology. Barkovich and colleagues used the term Dandy-Walker complex that includes the classic Dandy-Walker malformation, Dandy-Walker variant, and mega cisterna magna, based on the belief that these conditions represent steps on a continuum of developmental anomalies. Parisi and Dobyns proposed a new classification scheme, and do not advocate the term Dandy-Walker variant. Other investigators recommend abandoning the term because in the majority of cases they do not believe that it corresponds to the same spectrum of Dandy-Walker malformation and it presents variable definitions, lack of specificity, and induces confusion with the classic Dandy-Walker malformation. Heterogeneity in these conditions is quite broad, reflecting the lack of knowledge of a specific etiology. CVH is more common than the classic Dandy-Walker malformation and represents approximately one-third of all posterior fossa malformations (**Box 19**; **Fig. 36**).

All the changes are less severe than in the classic malformation; the tentorium is located in a normal position without trocular-lambdoid inversion. The cerebellar vermis is poorly or abnormally formed; sometimes its appearance is more dysplastic than hypoplastic.

Associated supratentorial anomalies such as corpus callosum agenesis, diencephalic cysts, heterotopias, gyral malformations, holoprosencephaly, septo-optic dysplasia, and occipital meningoencephaloceles can also be found, as in the classic anomaly, indicating that the intrauterine noxa occurs in the same embryologic period. Ventriculomegaly is present in approximately 32% of patients with secondary macrocrania. Developmental delay is associated with the presence of supratentorial anomalies. Another clinical manifestation often present is mild ataxia (**Figs. 37–39**).

Box 19
Radiologic and pathologic findings for CVH

1. Posterior fossa normal in size
2. Varying degrees of CVH (never agenesis)
3. Normal position of the vermis relative to the brainstem or minimal upward rotation
4. Prominent cerebrospinal fluid, retrocerebellar space that communicates freely through a prominent vallecula with a normal or minimal dilated fourth ventricle, not a cyst
5. Normal position of the tentorium cerebelli

Data from Brown MS, Sheridan-Pereira M. Outlook for the child with a cephalocele. Pediatrics 1992;90(6):914–9; and Naidich TP, Altman NR, Braffman BH, et al. Cephaloceles and related malformations. AJNR Am J Neuroradiol 1992;13(2):655–90.

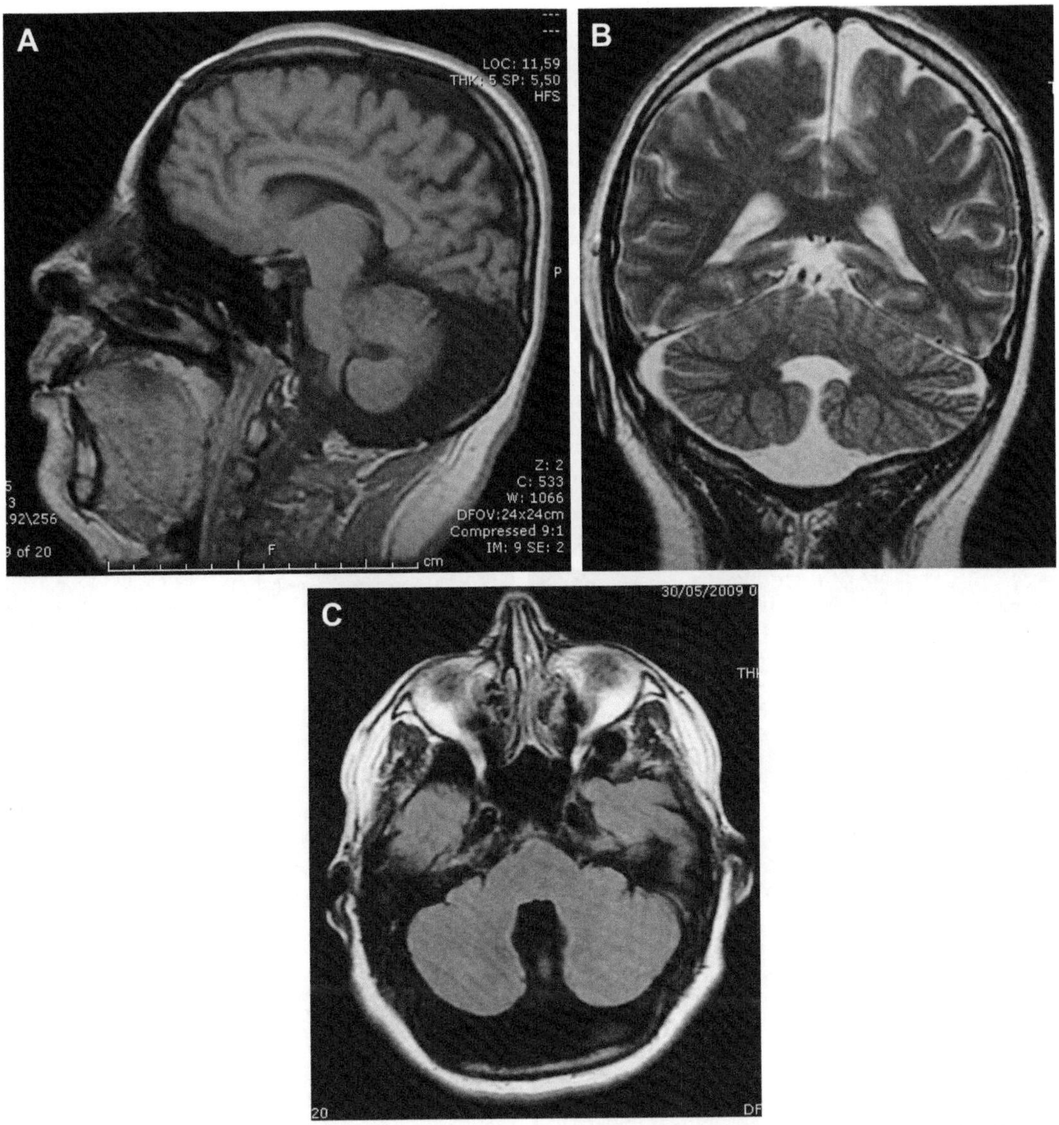

Fig. 36. DWM, milder variant in this continuum. (*A*) Sagittal T1-weighted image. (*B*) Coronal T2-weighted image. (*C*) Axial FLAIR image. Less severe vermian/cerebellar hypoplasia, slight elevation of the tentorium, and prominent CSF retrocerebellar space that communicates freely through a prominent vallecula, with a normal or minimal dilated fourth ventricle.

MEGA CISTERNA MAGNA

The term mega cisterna magna proposed by Gonsette and colleagues, is considered inaccurate by other investigators. The mega cisterna magna is a common developmental variation of the posterior fossa and does not necessarily indicate a malformation. It is characterized by a posterior fossa cystic space with expansion of the cisterna magna. The cisterna magna is completely formed within the leptomeninges. Anatomically, it occupies the vallecula cerebelli and extends inferiorly; the posterior limit is the arachnoid membrane, which extends from the upper cervical cord to the posteroinferior surface of the cerebellum at the level of the vermian pyramid. The posterior part of the cistern is divided by the falx cerebelli in 60% of cases. The arachnoid separates the cisterna magna from the supravermian cistern. There are no definitive measurements for the size (**Box 20**; **Fig. 40**).

The cystic collection can be very large and may extend beyond the normal anatomic limits of the cisterna magna or extend supratentorially, with

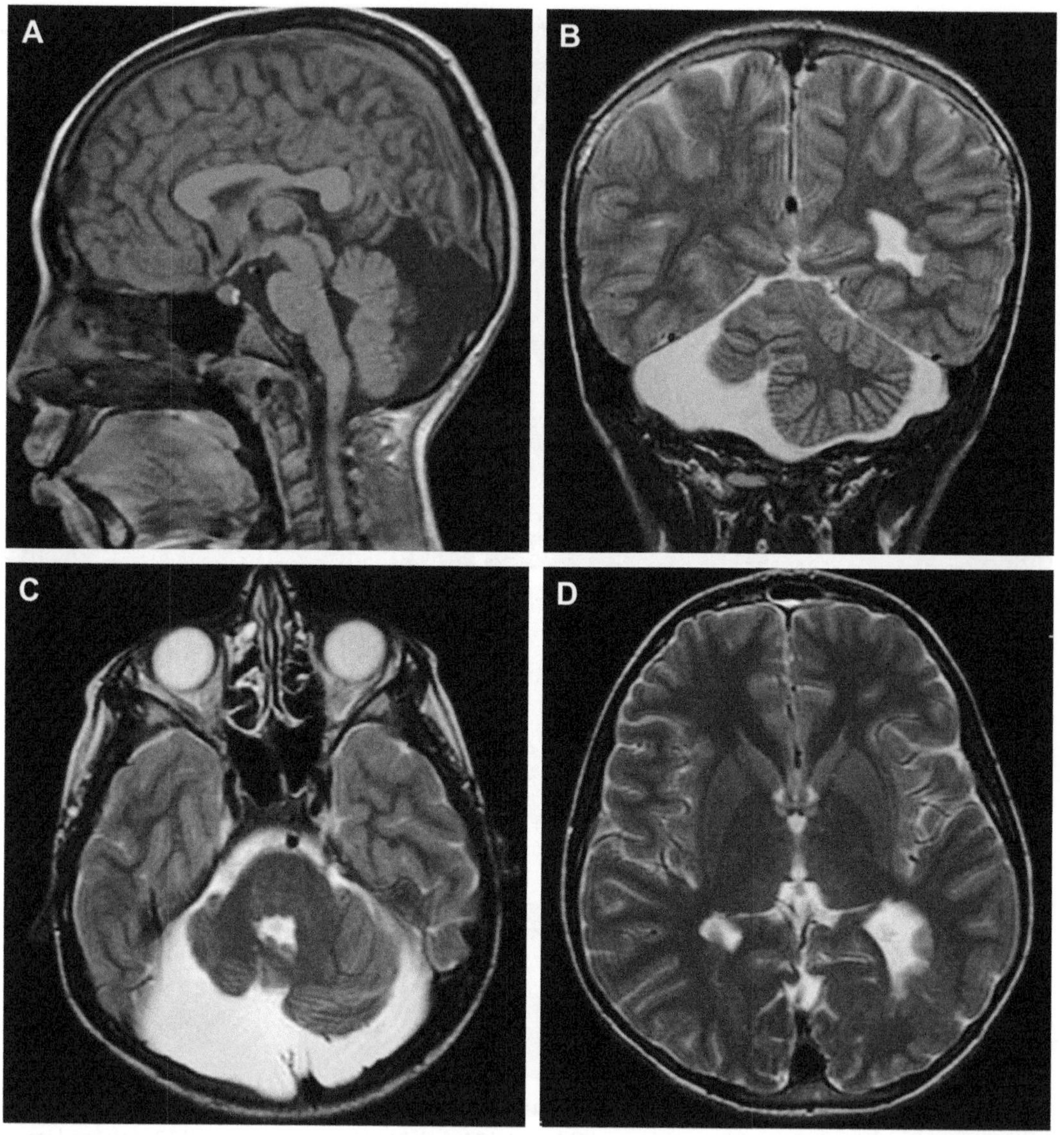

Fig. 37. Cerebellar vermian hypoplasia-dysplasia (CVH) or Dandy-Walker variant. (*A*) Sagittal T1-weighted image shows a posterior fossa of normal size, prominent CSF retrocerebellar space, normal position of the vermis relative to the brainstem, and normal position of the tentorium cerebelli. (*B*) Coronal T2-weighted image and (*C, D*) axial T2-weighted images show a vermian cerebellar hypoplasia-dysplasia, with right predominance. (*C*) and (*D*) show associated occipital nodular heterotopias.

a high position of the tentorium, cases in which the radiological differentiation with Dandy-Walker malformation and CVH is difficult. Most cases are detected incidentally. However, some investigators have reported that patients may present with hydrocephalus.

BLAKE POUCH CYST

This posterior fossa malformation is believed to derive from the persistence of the transient Blake pouch that arises from the area membranacea inferior that normally regresses at 5 to 8 weeks GA. The cyst protrudes through either the Magendie or Luschka foramina (**Box 21**).

ARACHNOID CYST

The arachnoid cyst is a benign developmental cavity of the subarachnoid space containing a fluid with similar composition to CSF. Derived from the meninx primitiva, it is believed that the developing

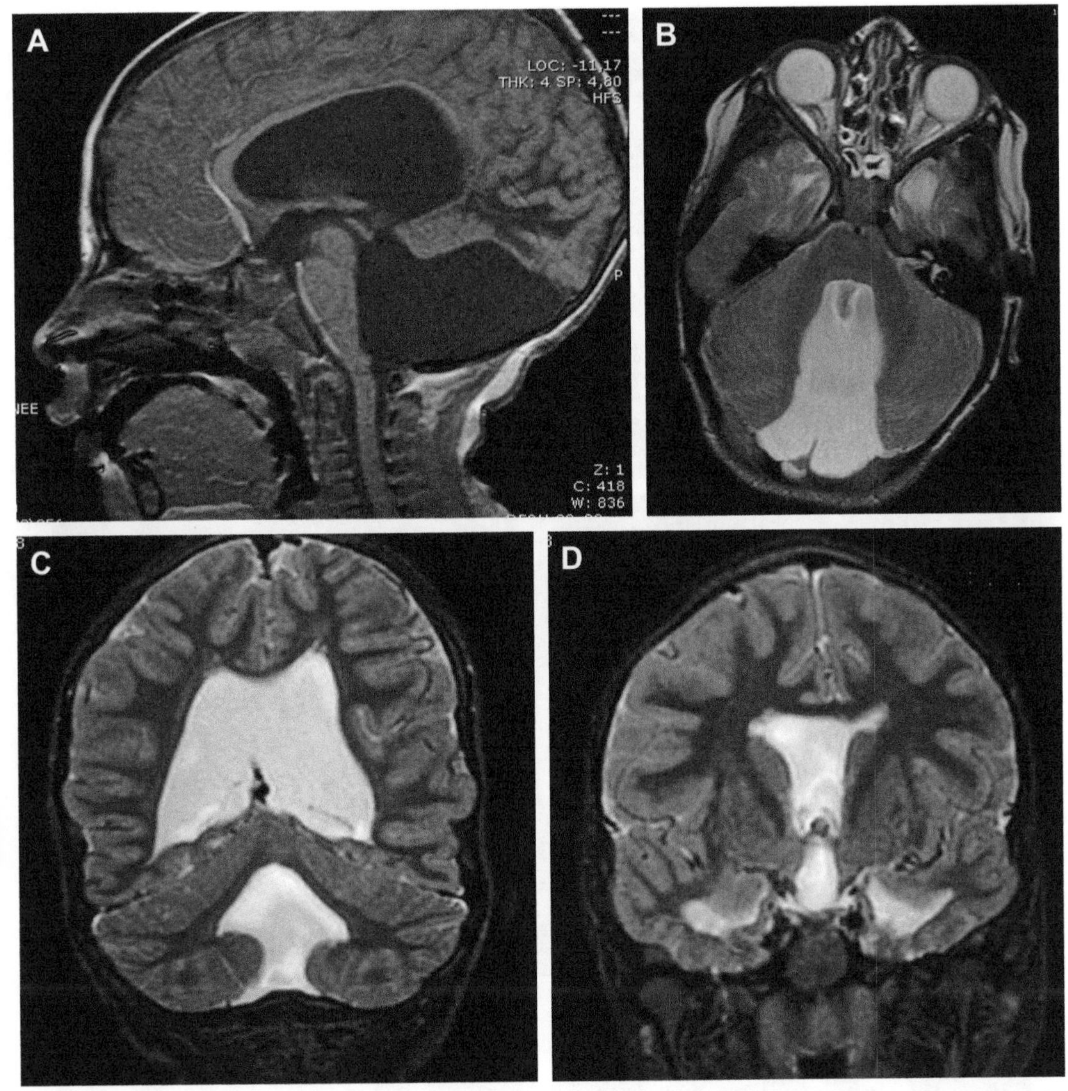

Fig. 38. Dandy-Walker continuum or Dandy-Walker complex with associated septo-optic dysplasia. (*A*) Sagittal T1-weighted image shows a dysgenetic corpus callosum, dysgenetic, hypoplastic, and posterosuperiorly rotated vermis with dolicocephaly, cystic dilatation of the fourth ventricle, and hydrocephalus that communicates freely through a prominent vallecula. (*B*) Axial T2-weighted image shows partially formed tentorium cerebelli and wide vallecula that communicates with the cyst. (*C*) Coronal T2-weighted image also shows hypoplastic vermis with hydrocephalus, and absent septum pellucidum. (*D*) Coronal T2-weighted image. (*A, D*) Hypoplastic hypophysis and optic nerves.

arachnoid membrane may split and secrete fluid into the cleft. The cyst does not communicate with the subarachnoid space or the fourth ventricle; nevertheless, this is a matter of controversy. Some investigators postulate that the arachnoid cyst could be the sequel of a failed attempt at formation of an arachnoid villus. It presents with an infratentorial location in 16% to 23% of the cases and a retrocerebellar location in 9% to 16% (**Box 22**, see **Fig. 12**).

In some cases, imaging diagnosis of the posterior fossa cystic malformations is not possible. There is no characteristic image that allows the differential diagnosis among the minimally expressed Dandy-Walker malformation, mega cisterna magna, and Blake pouch cyst; hence the existing concept of a continuum in cystic congenital anomalies of the posterior fossa.[7] Infratentorial cysts may present a similar appearance, if the position of the torcula, anomalies of the vermis,

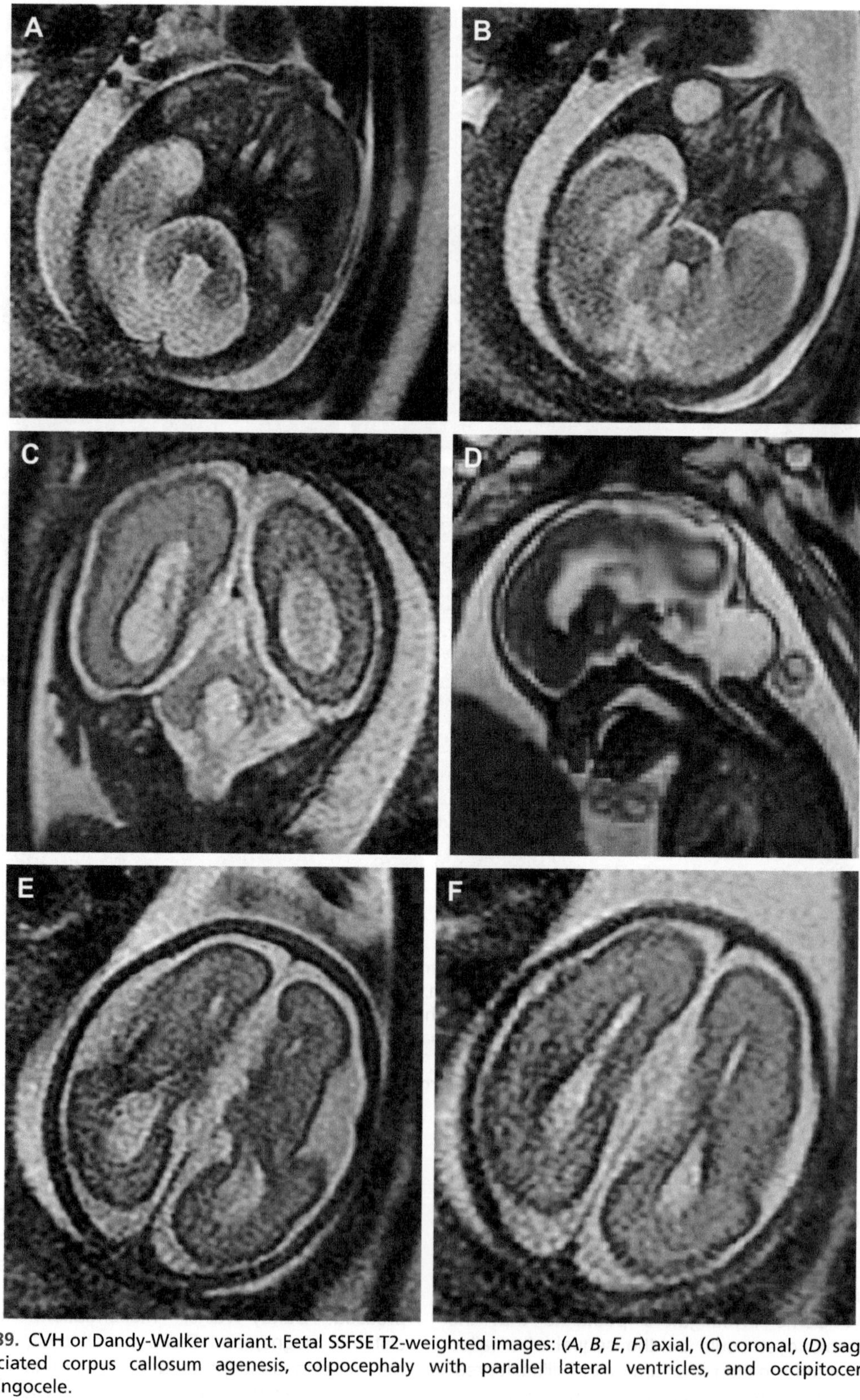

Fig. 39. CVH or Dandy-Walker variant. Fetal SSFSE T2-weighted images: (*A*, *B*, *E*, *F*) axial, (*C*) coronal, (*D*) sagittal. Associated corpus callosum agenesis, colpocephaly with parallel lateral ventricles, and occipitocervical meningocele.

Box 20
Radiologic and pathologic findings for mega cisterna magna

1. Large posterior fluid collection that freely communicates with the subarachnoid perimedullary spaces, and ventricular system
2. Normal vermis and cerebellar hemispheres
3. Lined by arachnoid
4. No compressive effects on the cerebellum

Box 21
Radiologic and pathologic findings for Blake pouch cyst

1. Develops behind and around the cerebellum and pushes the tentorium into a high insertion
2. Freely communication with the fourth ventricle, separated from the subarachnoid spaces
3. Includes widening of the valleculum and separation of the cerebellar hemispheres
4. Normal vermis and cerebellar hemispheres
5. Consistently associated with hydrocephalus
6. Cystic collection lined by ependyma and glia
7. Choroid plexus pushed anteriorly and superiorly within the cyst wall

or the mass effect on the cerebellum and the occipital bone are taken separately. Some investigators propose that determining either the location of the choroid plexus in the fourth ventricle or the histology of its wall is the suggested pointer to establish the true nature of the cyst. A normal choroid plexus is present in arachnoid cysts, absent in the classic Dandy-Walker malformation, or displaced inside the superior wall of the cyst in Blake pouch cyst. These investigators also consider and propose using the term "retrocerebellar cyst or collection" on the radiologic report if the histology of the cyst wall is unknown, and suggest "speculative terms" such as Dandy-Walker variation, mega cisterna magna, or arachnoid cyst be avoided.[3] The radiologist should describe the cyst according to its position: retrocerebellar, supracerebellar, infracerebellar, and so forth; and the secondary effects: present or absent local mass effect, obstruction of the ventricular system. Blake pouch cyst, arachnoid duplication cyst, and the acquired variety are generally indistinguishable by imaging methods. The radiologist should also give an opinion based on the patient's medical picture. Patients with isolated hypoplasia of the vermis or cerebellar unilateral hypoplasia may present with normal intelligence, just as in mega cisterna magna, Blake pouch cyst, and congenital arachnoid cyst.

PONTOCEREBELLAR HYPOPLASIAS

Pontocerebellar hypoplasias are a group of autosomal recessive neurodegenerative disorders

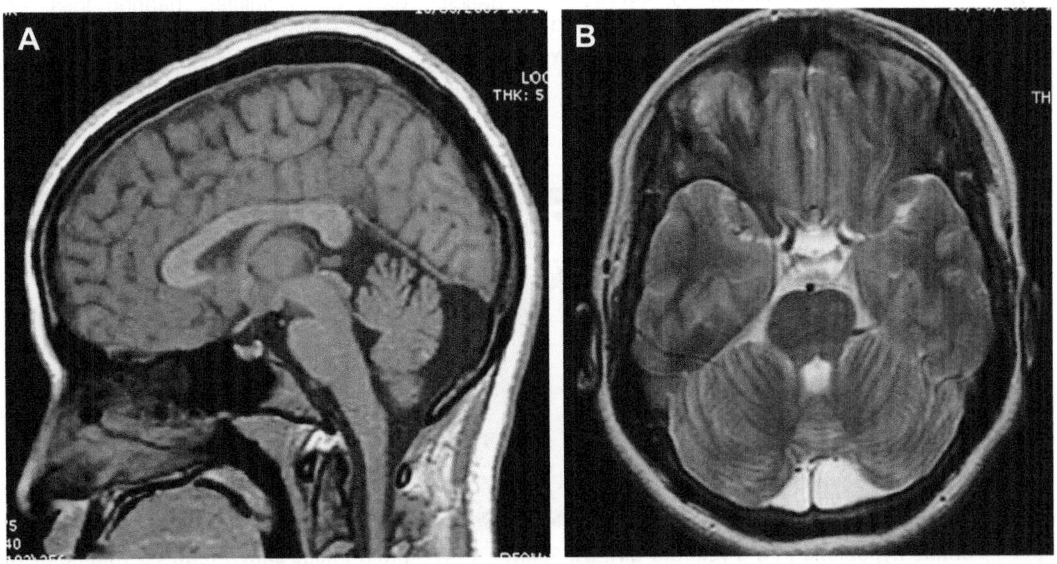

Fig. 40. Mega cisterna magna. (*A*) Sagittal T1-weighted image. Retrocerebellar fluid collection that freely communicates with the subarachnoid space, normal vermis, and no rotated craniocaudal vermian axis. (*B*) Normal cerebellar hemispheres and vermis, with tentorium cerebelli present.

Box 22
Radiologic and pathologic findings for arachnoid cyst

1. Choroid plexus in its usual location within the fourth ventricle
2. Cyst lined by a membrane of true arachnoid cells (intra-arachnoid cyst)
3. May exert mass effect on adjacent brain or bone
4. Posterior fossa may present bone remodeling and increase volume
5. Normal vermis and cerebellar hemispheres

described by Barth in 1993. He suggested two main types.

Type 1 (PCH-1) is associated with spinal anterior horn cell degeneration. Clinical findings are congenital contractures, microcephaly, gross delay milestones, peripheral motor system involvement, and early death. There is concomitant spinal muscular atrophy. Type 2 (PCH-2) is dominated by microcephaly, There is no spinal anterior horn cell compromise, and dystonia is a major feature. It also presents with swallowing impairment, seizures, extrapyramidal dyskinesia, and mental retardation.

Both entities are associated with moderate pons hypoplasia, with compromise of cerebellar hemispheres and vermis, often with preserved lobulation. Types 1 and 2 cannot be distinguished by neuroimaging findings alone.

Type 3 PCH is characterized by cerebellar atrophy with progressive microcephaly, mapped to chromosomes 7q11–q21. Types 1 to 3 show progressive thinning of the corpus callosum.[81]

Type 4 PCH (fatal infantile encephalopathy with olivopontocerebellar hypoplasia), Type 5 PCH (fetal-onset olivopontocerebellar hypoplasia), and Type 6 PCH (fatal infantile encephalopathy with mitochondrial chain defects), have also been described (**Fig. 41**).

BRAINSTEM ANOMALIES

Developmental Clefts

Developmental clefts were classified by Barkovich and colleagues as a regional developmental defect that affects the brainstem and cerebellum. The cleft can be present in the midline surface of the pons (dorsal or ventral). Clefts are most commonly ventral longitudinal in the pons, and can be associated with brainstem hypoplasia, cerebellar hypoplasia, or dysplasia,[14] or with a normal cerebellum. It is believed that clefts are due to the absence of the decussation of the middle cerebellar peduncles and the transverse pontine axons that connect the cerebellar cortex with pontine nuclei. Dorsal midline clefts are probably secondary to an abnormal development of the median longitudinal fasciculus. Congenital horizontal gaze palsy with associated progressive scoliosis is a known condition in this group of midline malformations (**Fig. 42**).[28,82]

Pontine Tegmental Cap Dysplasia

Pontine tegmental cap dysplasia is a severe, rare, regional developmental defect, recently described, probably secondary to abnormal axonal path finding. It may present with motor and cognitive deficits, gaze abnormalities, hearing loss, and seizures. This malformation is characterized by a hypoplastic flat ventral pons, as a consequence of the absence of normal ventral decussation of

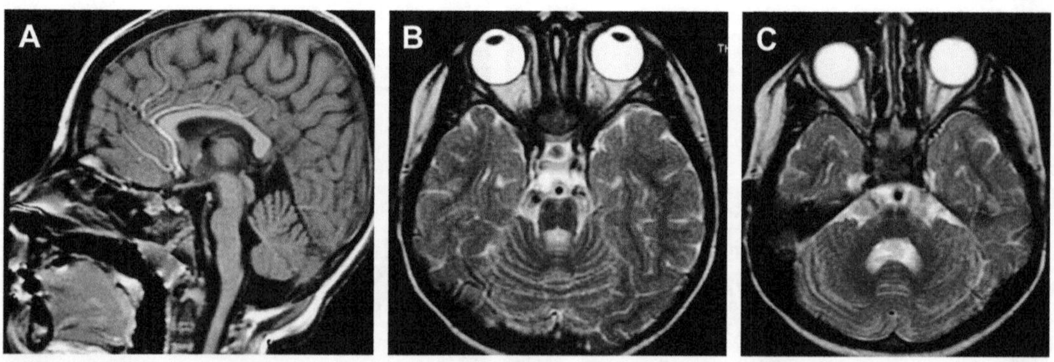

Fig. 41. Pontine hypoplasia in a 3-year-old girl. (*A*) Sagittal T1-weighted image shows reduced volume of the brainstem, especially the pons. (*B, C*) Axial T2-weighted image. Reduced pons size with middle cerebellar peduncle hypoplasia. There is also a midline cleft in the ventral surface of the pons, and a flattened floor of fourth ventricle.

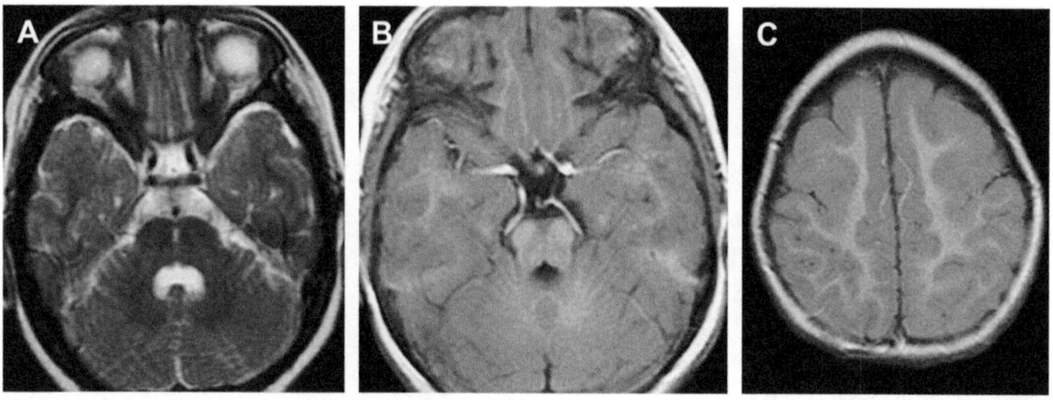

Fig. 42. Pontine cleft. (*A*) Axial T2-weighted image of midline central pontine cleft at the level of the middle cerebellar peduncles. (*B*) Axial T1-weighted image at the level of the superior cerebellar peduncles shows a midline cleft. (*C*) Axial T1-weighted image. In the frontal lobes the cortex is thick and the white matter is reduced secondary to a pachygyria.

the middle cerebellar peduncles, with a band of horizontally oriented axons and a vaulted dorsal pons projecting into the fourth ventricle, hypoplasia of the middle cerebellar peduncles, hypoplasia and malformation of the vermis, short mesencephalic isthmus with molar tooth sign, and hypoplasia of the seventh and eighth cranial nerves and the internal auditory meati (**Fig. 43**).[28,69]

CEREBELLAR FOCAL DYSPLASIAS

Rhombencephalosynapsis

Rhombencephalosynapsis is a rare cerebellar malformation, first described by Obersteiner, that results from a disturbed development at 28 to 41 gestational days and that mainly affects the midline cerebellar structures, with a frequency of about 0.13%.[83] All the published cases have been sporadic. Clinical findings are variable; there is no correlation between them and neuroimaging findings. Associated anomalies seem to be responsible for the neurologic and cognitive impairments. Children with isolated rhombencephalosynapsis may present with normal cognitive and language function; severely affected patients present with mental retardation, epilepsy, spasticity, and strabismus. Most patients die in their infancy or early childhood (**Box 23**).

Neuroimaging diagnosis is best confirmed in a posterior coronal MR slice. There is absence or hypogenesis of the vermis, and some investigators describe a poorly differentiated vermis. The rostral vermis is more severely hypoplastic. There is also dorsal fusion of the cerebellar hemispheres. The dentate nuclei may be fused or partially fused. Small fused superior cerebellar peduncles, middle peduncles, tectum, or a small brainstem might be seen, as well as slight to moderate cerebellar hemisphere hypoplasia. There are also supratentorial anomalies such as the absence of the septum pellucidum in almost 50%, ventriculomegaly or hydrocephalus, fused thalami and fornices, reduced white matter, hypoplastic anterior commissure and temporal lobes, and polymicrogyria.[9] The fourth ventricle is characteristically diamond or keyhole-shaped on axial images (**Fig. 44**).

Molar Tooth Malformations

Molar tooth malformations were first described by Jourbert and colleagues in 1969. Joubert syndrome is an autosomal recessive disorder. An increased prevalence of consanguineous parents has been found; in some series there is a clear male preponderance and genetic heterogeneity has been accepted, though the cause is not known. There are some MR imaging and CT criteria for diagnosis, observed at the level of the midbrain, especially on the axial view (**Box 24**).

Enlarged superior cerebellar peduncles are caused by the lack of decussation of peduncular fiber tracts. The peduncles follow a more horizontal course as they extend perpendicularly between the pons and the cerebellum. There is a deep interpeduncular fossa, and absence of decussation of the central pontine tracts.

The fourth ventricle communicates with the magna cisterna through a thin cleft, or sometimes through large defects with wide separations of the cerebellar hemispheres, that look like a Dandy-Walker cyst, especially in those cases with an

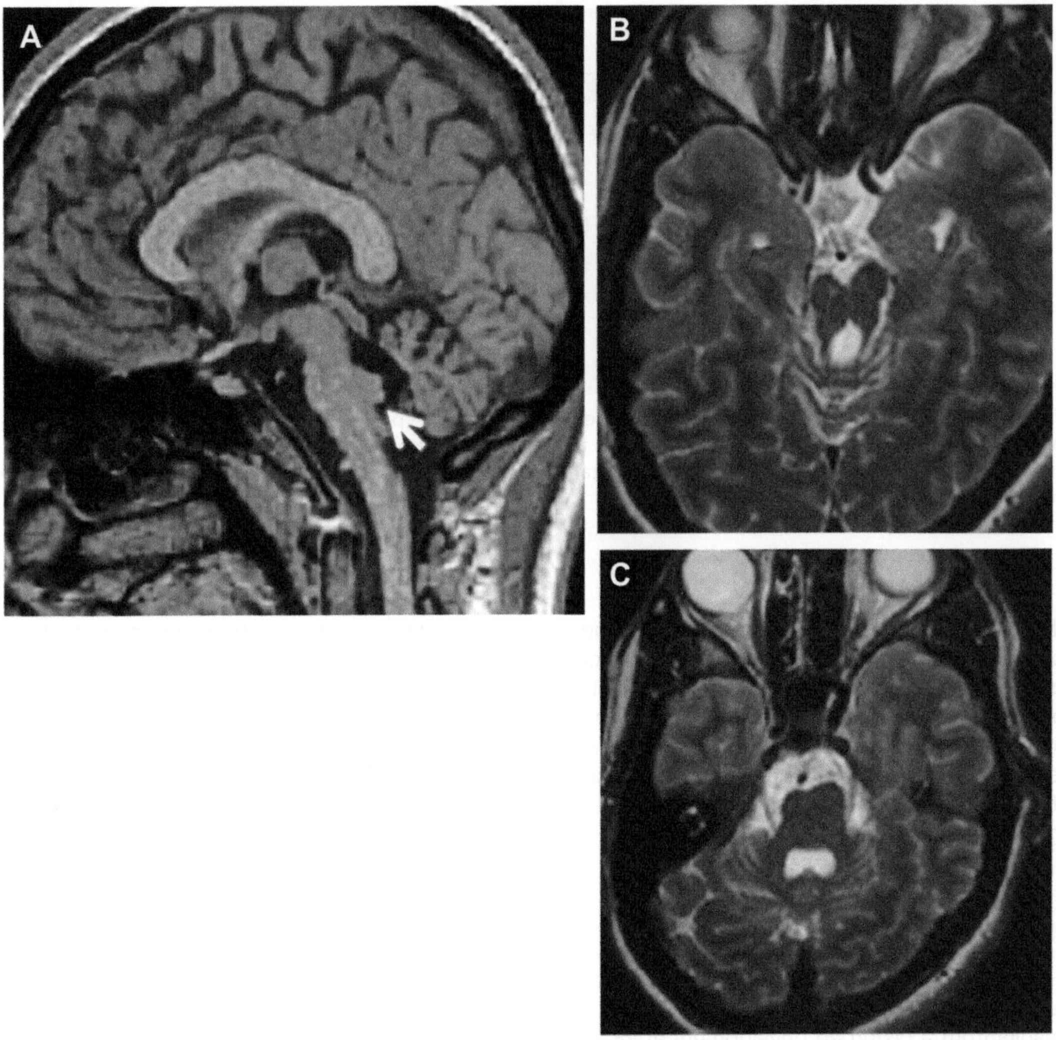

Fig. 43. Pontine tegmental cap dysplasia. (*A*) Sagittal T1-weighted image. Hypoplastic brainstem, with flattened ventral pons and a dorsal tegmental cap (*white arrow*). Hypoplastic and dysplastic vermis with abnormal vermian foliation and fastigial point. (*B, C*) Axial T2-weighted images. Hypoplastic pons, and superior and middle cerebellar peduncles with dysplastic vermis.

elevated tentorium. When the fourth ventricle is normal in appearance, the diagnosis may be difficult: the flocculus looks prominent and so do the cerebellar hemispheres to some degree; the folial pattern can be more vertical. The brainstem can also be abnormal, with a deep interpeduncular fossa (lack of decussation), reduced volume of the pons with a pontomesencephalic cleft, and a thin junction. All these changes are consistent with the resemblance of a molar tooth in an axial view. Other common pathologic findings include dentate nuclei distortion, dysplastic inferior olivary and paraolivary nuclei, anomalies of the dorsal column nuclei, near total absence of pyramidal decussations, and a reduced volume of the cervicomedullary union. Associated abnormalities include unsegmented midbrain tectum and agenesis of the corpus callosum. This malformation is of poor prognosis. Muscle hypotonia, ataxia,

Box 23
Radiologic and pathologic findings for rhombencephalosynapsis

1. Axial plane: fused cerebellar hemispheres, absent/hypoplastic vermis, narrow diamond or keyhole-shaped fourth ventricle, fused dentate nuclei
2. Sagittal plane: lack of primary vermian fissure, abnormal fastigial point

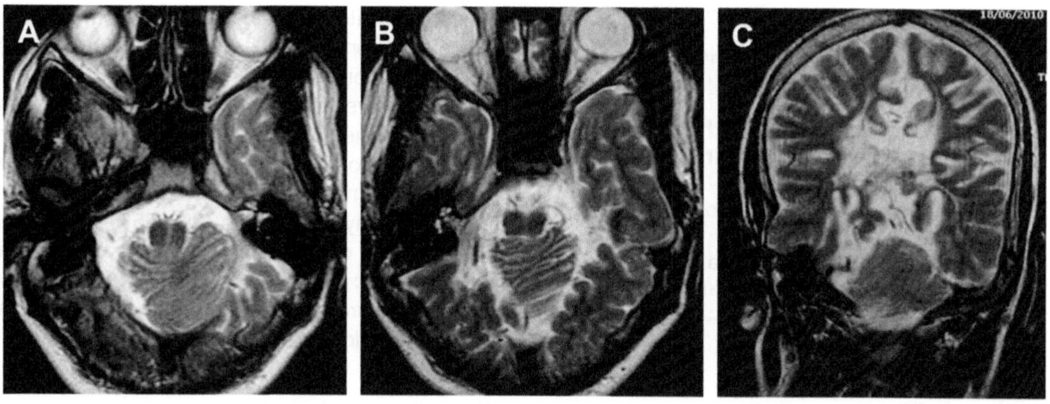

Fig. 44. Rhombencephalosynapsis in a 13-year-old boy presenting with mental retardation. (*A, B*) Axial T2-weighted images. Fused and hypoplastic cerebellar hemispheres, absent vermis, hypoplastic pons with a midline cleft. (*C*) Sagittal plane: lack primary vermian fissure, abnormal fastigial point. Small fussed superior cerebellar peduncles, middle peduncles, tectum or a small brainstem might be seen, as well as slight to moderate cerebellar hemisphere hypoplasia.

developmental delay, and cognitive impairment are common and are consistent abnormalities present in all patients. An abnormal breathing pattern, retinal dystrophy, oculomotor apraxia, upgaze palsy, and ptosis are frequently associated but not consistent. Occipital meningocele, polydactyly, short stature, scoliosis, congenital cataract, hydrocephalus, hepatic fibrosis, and nephronophthisis are rarely present. In infancy respiratory disturbances such as episodes of hyperopnea or apnea, and abnormal eye movements are present. In older children, ataxia and psychomotor retardation are often seen. Patients tend to have large heads, a prominent forehead, dysmorphic facies, hemifacial spasm, retinopathy, coloboma, tongue hamartomas and tongue protrusion, multicystic kidney disease, congenital heart disease, campodactyly, and syndactyly.

Box 24
Radiologic and pathologic findings for molar tooth malformations

1. Enlarged horizontal superior cerebellar peduncles
2. Severe hypoplasia and clefting or vermian agenesis
3. Enlarged fourth ventricle (bat wing or triangular configuration)
4. Molar tooth appearance at the level of midbrain in an axial view
5. Thin isthmic region (in sagittal view)

ARNOLD-CHIARI MALFORMATIONS

Arnold-Chiari malformations were first described in 1891 by Hans Chiari, who published the findings of 3 malformations of the hindbrain associated with hydrocephalus. Five years later, he published a second type of malformation and described a new fourth type.[28]

Chiari Type I Malformation

Several theories that explain the pathogenesis of the Chiari type I malformation have been proposed. Downward displacement is usually an acquired phenomenon, and labeling it a "malformation" is problematic. The term tonsillar ectopia would be more suitable.[5] Various processes that decrease the capacity of the posterior fossa result in caudal tonsillar displacement. There is a correlation between the size of the posterior fossa and the degree of tonsillar ectopia. A bony malformation that causes a small posterior fossa is considered the primary abnormality, and the neural malformation the secondary. This malformation is characterized by signs listed in **Box 25**.

Either a symmetric extension or pointing of at least 3 to 5 mm of the cerebellar tonsils below the foramen magnum, or an asymmetric caudal extension of the tonsils is considered for the diagnosis. Some investigators use the McRoe line on sagittal images to confirm the diagnosis; others, however, use coronal T1-weighted or T2-weighted MR imaging through the foramen magnum; they consider that this plane readily demonstrates the inferior pole of the tonsils and

Box 25
Radiologic and pathologic findings for Chiari type I malformation

1. Inferior displacement of the cerebellar tonsils, and sometimes the inferior vermis below the foramen magnum
2. Flat and small posterior fossa (occipital dysplasia)
3. No caudally displaced medulla
4. No associated supratentorial anomalies

clearly demarcates the inferior plane of the foramen magnum.

The degree of cerebellar herniation in Chiari type I correlates positively with the amount of bone thickening. High incidence of complex craniosynostosis, skull base and cervical spine anomalies, such as Klippel-Feil syndrome, cervical and craniovertebral fusion, platybasia, and skeletal dysplasias are associated. With the increasing access to neuroimaging, incidental cases are also on the increase. Chiari type I may be associated with syringohydromyelia and hydrocephalus. Related signs and symptoms include chronic headache, neck pain, torticollis, lower cranial nerve palsies, nystagmus, ataxia, motor and sensory deficits, scoliosis, sleep apnea, seizures, psychiatric complaints, and unexplained episodes of unconsciousness. Phase-contrast cine-MR imaging shows reduced or absent posterior fossa CSF flow in the subarachnoid space either posteriorly or anteriorly to the cervicomedullary junction.

Spinal MR imaging for the assessment of concurrent syringohydromyelia (25%–65%) is useful. Suboccipital craniectomy is not indicated in asymptomatic patients, but decompressive surgery may prevent permanent neurologic deficits in symptomatic patients (**Figs. 45** and **46**).[82,84–86]

Chiari Type II Malformation

The Chiari II malformation is complex, and involves the spinal cord and the hindbrain. A causative gene has not been found. This malformation is often associated with supratentorial anomalies; nearly all cases present with myelomeningocele at birth.[87] Primary causes of NTD are variable and still debated. Prenatal closure of the tube defect has shown to reduce or reverse the hindbrain herniation, thus this malformation could be the result or a partial consequence of a CSF leak and abnormal CSF dynamics. Intrauterine hydrocephalus and hydromyelia leading to herniation has also been proposed, as have abnormal traction by tethering of the distal spinal cord, primary

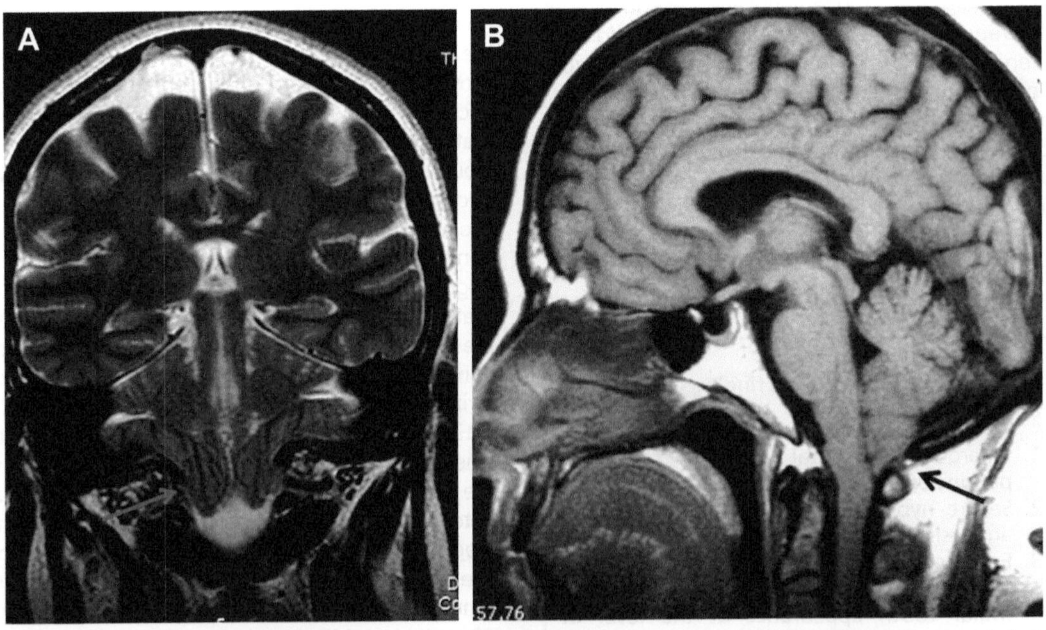

Fig. 45. Chiari type I malformation. (*A*) Coronal T2-weighted image, (*B*) Sagittal T1-weighted image. Inferior displacement of the cerebellar tonsils below the foramen magnum (*red arrow* in *A* and *black arrow* in *B*). Flat and small posterior fossa (occipital dysplasia). No associated supratentorial anomalies.

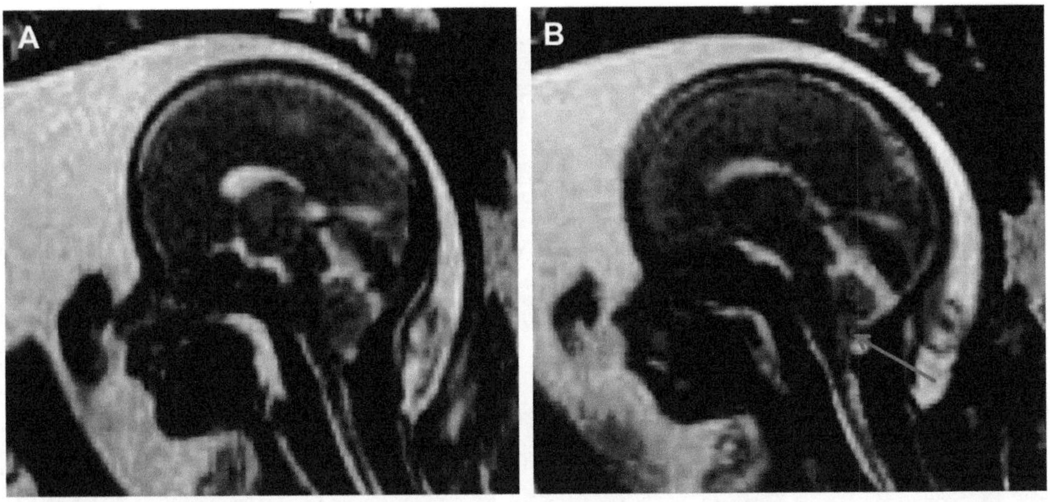

Fig. 46. Chiari type I malformation. (*A, B*) Fetal coronal SSFSE T2-weighted images. Inferior displacement of the cerebellar tonsils below the foramen magnum (*red arrow* in *B*). Flat and small posterior fossa (occipital dysplasia). No associated supratentorial anomalies.

hindbrain dysgenesis, and a primary mesodermal defect (**Box 26**).

The vermis degenerates in areas where it is compressed by bony or fibrous structures. No cerebellum may be present. The fourth ventricle could be trapped and isolated from the rest of the ventricular system as a result of aqueductal narrowing or scarring, and look like a "normal fourth ventricle," but the fourth ventricle in Chiari II malformations is always slit-like. On the contrary, this appearance could be secondary to the malfunction of the shunt or to an isolated fourth ventricle. Anomalies of the supratentorial brain can also be present. The corpus callosum is abnormal in 75% to 90% of cases. Hypogenesis and distortion occurs secondarily to hydrocephalus, the splenium is nearly always hypoplastic or absent, and in severe cases there could be agenesis of the corpus callosum with subsequent colpocephaly. Absence of the septum pellucidum could be present. The gyral pattern is abnormal in the posterior parietal and occipital regions, giving the configuration termed "stenogyria," with multiple small gyri within a cortex of normal thickness. Caudate heads and massa intermedia are frequently enlarged. Gyri interdigitation through fenestrations of the falx cerebri are also frequent. All these findings are not always present; they depend on the severity of the case. The degree of deformity varies widely (**Figs. 47** and **48**).

Box 26
Radiologic and pathologic findings for Chiari type II malformation

1. Herniation of the inferior vermis, medulla, pons, and fourth ventricle into the cervical or thoracic spinal canal
2. Osseous abnormalities: small posterior fossa, lacunar skull 85%, petrous and clivus scalloping, enlargement of the foramen magnum
3. Dural anomalies: hypoplasia and fenestration of the falx, low insertion of the tentorium, tentorial hypoplasia with wide incisura
4. The quadrigeminal plate is stretched inferiorly and posteriorly, resulting in the typical beaked shape
5. The cerebellum can wrap itself around the brainstem
6. The medulla buckles posterior to the cervical spinal cord in severe cases

Chiari III malformation

The Chiari III malformation is very rare (**Fig. 49**), characterized by occipital cephalocele that includes cerebellum, brainstem, and sometimes upper cervical cord (**Box 27**).

The herniation must encompass both the low occipital and upper cervical regions for the diagnosis. The cephalocele sac variably includes the brainstem, occipital lobes, subarachnoid or ventricular CSF spaces, and the dural venous sinuses. Hypoplasia or agenesis of the corpus callosum, occipital and cervical osseous defects,

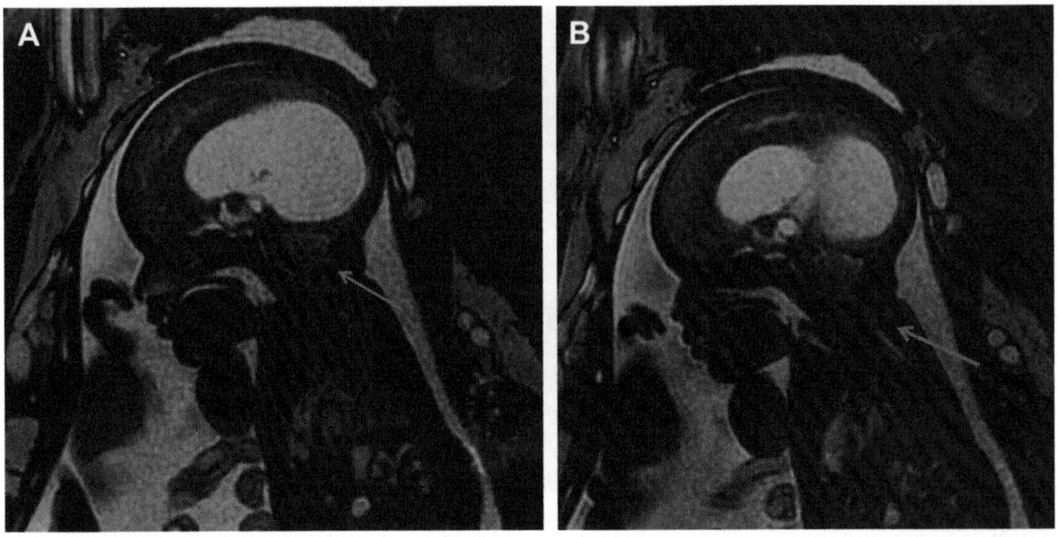

Fig. 47. Chiari type II malformation. (*A*, *B*) Sagittal SSFSE T2-weighted images of 22-week-old infant. Inferior displacement of the cerebellar tonsils (*red arrow* in *A*), and the inferior vermis below the foramen magnum, up to the middle cervical spinal canal level (*blue arrow* in *B*). Flat and small posterior fossa (occipital dysplasia). Hydrocephalus.

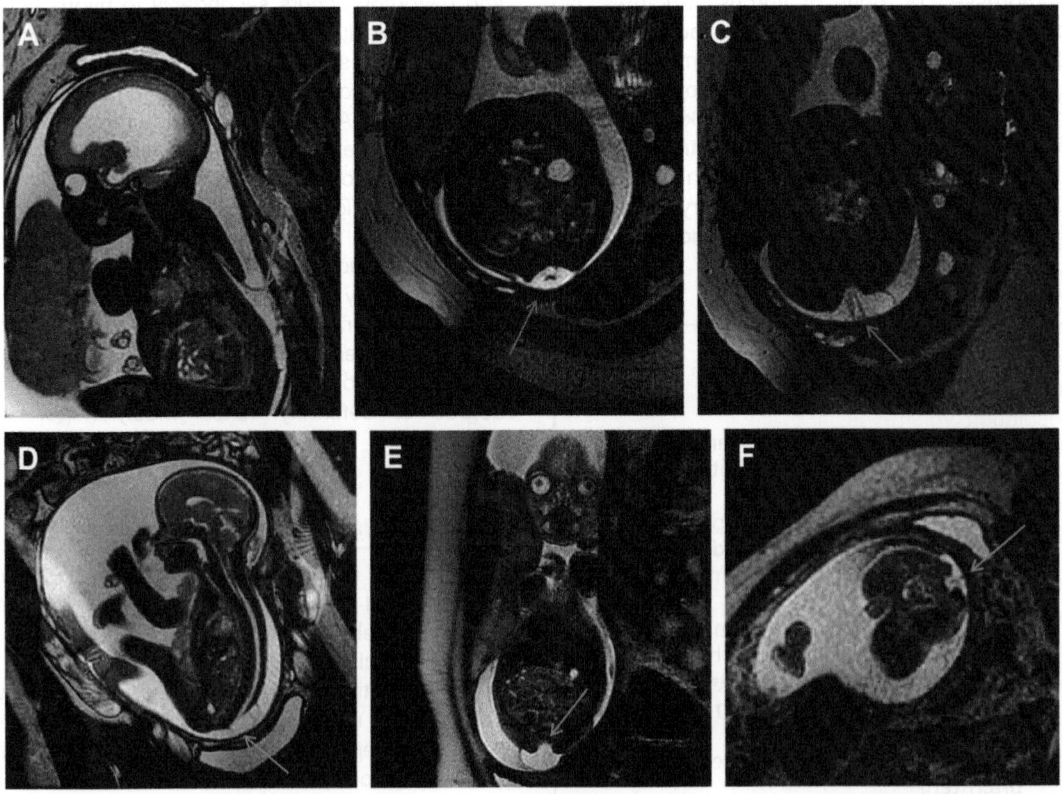

Fig. 48. Chiari type II malformation with myelomeningocele. Fetal MR imaging. (*A*) Sagittal T2-weighted image; (*B*) axial T2-weighted image; (*C*) axial SSFSE T2-weighted image. Thoracolumbar level (*red arrow*). (*D–F*) Lumbosacral level (*blue arrow*).

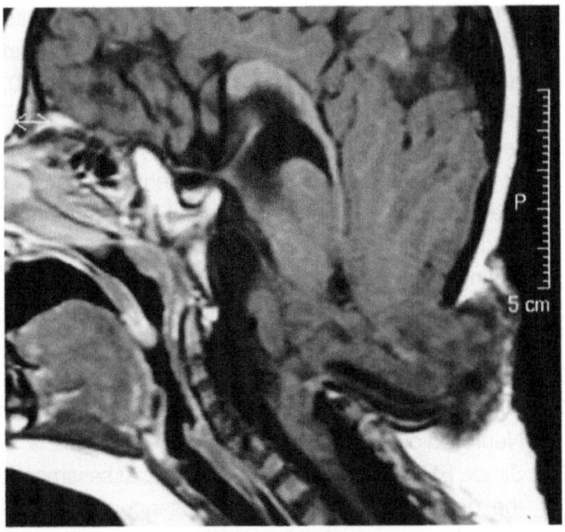

Fig. 49. Chiari type III malformation. Sagittal T1-weighted image. Severe alteration of craniocervical anatomic relations, caudal medullary displacement, and caudal cerebellar herniation through the foramen magnum with dorsal herniation of occipital lobes and cerebellar hemispheres through a cervical spina bifida, resulting in an encephalocele.

dorsal clivus and petrous bones scalloping, as well as craniolacunia could be associated.

Considering Chiari type IV to be a distinct malformation and not a form of severe hypoplasia or agenesis is controversial and, as some believe, of doubtful utility.[78]

In summary, classifying the different midline malformations is difficult. Progress in understanding embryology, developmental biology, and the creation of multidisciplinary expert groups with a clinical, neuroimaging, and molecular genetics approach may be successful in the future.[73]

One should not forget the importance of obtaining high-quality images, with thin sections, high-resolution volumetric acquisitions, and views of sagittal as well as axial and coronal planes, when performing the different modalities of diagnostic imaging (ultrasonography or MR imaging),so as to avoid erroneous diagnosis such as vermian or cerebellar hypoplasia. The advent of new technology such as diffusion tensor imaging with color fractional anisotropy maps offers important information for easy identification of malformations.

Box 27
Radiologic and pathologic findings for Chiari type III malformation

1. Caudal medullary displacement
2. Caudal cerebellar herniation through the foramen magnum
3. Dorsal cerebellar herniation through a cervical spina bifida resulting in an encephalocele

REFERENCES

1. Mahapatra AK, Suri A. Anterior encephaloceles: a study of 92 cases. Pediatr Neurosurg 2002;36(3):113–8.
2. Brown MS, Sheridan-Pereira M. Outlook for the child with a cephalocele. Pediatrics 1992;90(6):914–9.
3. Naidich TP, Altman NR, Braffman BH, et al. Cephaloceles and related malformations. AJNR Am J Neuroradiol 1992;13(2):655–90.
4. Patterson RJ, Egelhoff JC, Crone KR, et al. Atretic parietal cephaloceles revisited: an enlarging clinical and imaging spectrum? AJNR Am J Neuroradiol 1998;19(4):791–5.
5. Czech T, Reinprecht A, Matula C, et al. Cephaloceles—experience with 42 patients. Acta Neurochir (Wien) 1995;134(3–4):125–9.
6. Lowe LH, Booth TN, Joglar JM, et al. Midface anomalies in children. Radiographics 2000;20(4):907–22 [quiz: 1106–7, 1112].
7. Suwanwela C, Suwanwela N. A morphological classification of sincipital encephalomeningoceles. J Neurosurg 1972;36(2):201–11.
8. Martinez-Lage JF, Poza M, Sola J, et al. The child with a cephalocele: etiology, neuroimaging, and outcome. Childs Nerv Syst 1996;12(9):540–50.
9. David DJ, Proudman TW. Cephaloceles: classification, pathology, and management. World J Surg 1989;13(4):349–57.
10. Hoving EW. Nasal encephaloceles. Childs Nerv Syst 2000;16(10–11):702–6.
11. Trovato M, D'Armiento M, Lavra L, et al. Expression of p53/HGF/c-met/STAT3 signal in fetuses with neural tube defects. Virchows Arch 2007;450(2):203–10.
12. Langman J. Second week of development: trilaminar germ disc 65. In: Sadler TW, Langman J, editors. Langman's medical embryology. 9th edition. Philadelphia: Lippincott Williams & Wilkins; 2004. p. 534.
13. Barkovich AJ. Congenital malformations of the brain and skull. In: Barkovich AJ, editor. Pediatric neuroimaging. 4th edition. United Kingdom: Lippincott William and Wilkins; 2005. p. 291–405.
14. Padmanabhan R. Etiology, pathogenesis and prevention of neural tube defects. Congenit Anom (Kyoto) 2006;46(2):55–67.
15. Blustajn J, Netchine I, Fredy D, et al. Dysgenesis of the internal carotid artery associated with transsphenoidal encephalocele: a neural crest syndrome? AJNR Am J Neuroradiol 1999;20(6):1154–7.

16. Diebler C, Dulac O. Cephaloceles: clinical and neuroradiological appearance. Associated cerebral malformations. Neuroradiology 1983;25(4):199–216.
17. Krajewski A, Borch S, Khan A, et al. Surgical management and reconstruction of sincipital encephalocele presenting in adulthood. Eur J Plast Surg 2009;32(1):39–45.
18. Hofmann E, Behr R, Schwager K. Imaging of cerebrospinal fluid leaks. Klin Neuroradiol 2009;19(2): 111–21.
19. Kotil K, Kilinc B, Bilge T. Diagnosis and management of large occipitocervical cephaloceles: a 10-year experience. Pediatr Neurosurg 2008;44(3):193–8.
20. Morioka T, Hashiguchi K, Samura K, et al. Detailed anatomy of intracranial venous anomalies associated with atretic parietal cephaloceles revealed by high-resolution 3D-CISS and high-field T2-weighted reversed MR images. Childs Nerv Syst 2009;25(3): 309–15.
21. Brunelle F, Baraton J, Renier D, et al. Intracranial venous anomalies associated with atretic cephalocoeles. Pediatr Radiol 2000;30(11):743–7.
22. Hedlund G. Congenital frontonasal masses: developmental anatomy, malformations, and MR imaging. Pediatr Radiol 2006;36(7):647–62 [quiz: 726–7].
23. Narasimhan K, Coticchia J. Transsphenoidal encephalocele in a neonate. Ear Nose Throat J 2006; 85(7):420, 422.
24. Allbery SM, Chaljub G, Cho NL, et al. MR imaging of nasal masses. Radiographics 1995;15(6):1311–27.
25. Castillo M. Neuroradiology. Philadelphia: Lippincott Williams & Wilkins; 2002.
26. Moron FE, Morriss MC, Jones JJ, et al. Lumps and bumps on the head in children: use of CT and MR imaging in solving the clinical diagnostic dilemma. Radiographics 2004;24(6):1655–74.
27. Utsunomiya H, Ogasawara T, Hayashi T, et al. Dysgenesis of the corpus callosum and associated telencephalic anomalies: MRI. Neuroradiology 1997;39(4):302–10.
28. Caruso P, Robertson R, Setty B, et al. Disorders of brain development. In: Atlas S, editor. 4th edition, Magnetic resonance imaging of the brain and spine, vol. 1. China: Lippincott Willians & Wilkins; 2009.
29. Kollias SS, Ball WS Jr, Prenger EC. Cystic malformations of the posterior fossa: differential diagnosis clarified through embryologic analysis. Radiographics 1993;13(6):1211–31.
30. Chen CF, Lee YC, Lui CC, et al. Posterior pericallosal lipoma extending through the interhemispheric fissure into the scalp via the anterior fontanelle. Neuroradiology 2004;46(8):692–5.
31. Yildiz H, Hakyemez B, Koroglu M, et al. Intracranial lipomas: importance of localization. Neuroradiology 2006;48(1):1–7.
32. Alfonso I, Papazian O, Sinisterra S. Cerebral malformation in the newborn: holoprosencephaly and agenesis of the corpus callosum. Rev Neurol 2003; 36(2):179–84 [in Spanish].
33. ten Donkelaar HJ, Lammens M, Cruysberg JRM, et al. Development and developmental disorders of the forebrain. In: ten Donkelaar HJ, Lammens M, Hori A, editors. Clinical neuroembryology. Berlin: Springer-Verlag; 2006. p. 345–511.
34. Thakur S, Singh R, Pradhan M, et al. Spectrum of holoprosencephaly. Indian J Pediatr 2004;71(7): 593–7.
35. Fitz CR. Holoprosencephaly and related entities. Neuroradiology 1983;25(4):225–38.
36. Simon EM, Hevner R, Pinter JD, et al. Assessment of the deep gray nuclei in holoprosencephaly. AJNR Am J Neuroradiol 2000;21(10):1955–61.
37. Hahn JS, Plawner LL. Evaluation and management of children with holoprosencephaly. Pediatr Neurol 2004;31(2):79–88.
38. Oba H, Barkovich AJ. Holoprosencephaly: an analysis of callosal formation and its relation to development of the interhemispheric fissure. AJNR Am J Neuroradiol 1995;16(3):453–60.
39. Barkovich AJ. Apparent atypical callosal dysgenesis: analysis of MR findings in six cases and their relationship to holoprosencephaly. AJNR Am J Neuroradiol 1990;11(2):333–9.
40. Barkovich AJ, Simon EM, Clegg NJ, et al. Analysis of the cerebral cortex in holoprosencephaly with attention to the sylvian fissures. AJNR Am J Neuroradiol 2002;23(1):143–50.
41. Hahn JS, Barnes PD. Neuroimaging advances in holoprosencephaly: refining the spectrum of the midline malformation. Am J Med Genet C Semin Med Genet 2010;154C(1):120–32.
42. Barkovich AJ, Quint DJ. Middle interhemispheric fusion: an unusual variant of holoprosencephaly. AJNR Am J Neuroradiol 1993;14(2):431–40.
43. Khandelwal G, Bathla G, Jain R, et al. Syntelencephaly, a lesser known variant of holoprosencephal. The Internet Journal of Radiology 2008;9(1).
44. Barkovich AJ, Fram EK, Norman D. Septo-optic dysplasia: MR imaging. Radiology 1989;171(1):189–92.
45. Miller SP, Shevell MI, Patenaude Y, et al. Septo-optic dysplasia plus: a spectrum of malformations of cortical development. Neurology 2000;54(8):1701–3.
46. Necula G, Antochi F. Septo-optic dysplasia. Romanian Journal of Neurology 2008;3:114–6.
47. Cameron FJ, Khadilkar VV, Stanhope R. Pituitary dysfunction, morbidity and mortality with congenital midline malformation of the cerebrum. Eur J Pediatr 1999;158(2):97–102.
48. Riedl S, Vosahlo J, Battelino T, et al. Refining clinical phenotypes in septo-optic dysplasia based on MRI findings. Eur J Pediatr 2008;167(11):1269–76.

49. Supprian T, Sian J, Heils A, et al. Isolated absence of the septum pellucidum. Neuroradiology 1999;41(8): 563–6.
50. Belhocine O, Andre C, Kalifa G, et al. Does asymptomatic septal agenesis exist? A review of 34 cases. Pediatr Radiol 2005;35(4):410–8.
51. Jellinger K, Gross H, Kaltenback E, et al. Holoprosencephaly and agenesis of the corpus callosum: frequency of associated malformations. Acta Neuropathol 1981;55(1):1–10.
52. Pinto N, Latorre A, Latorre A, et al. Diagnóstico prenatal de holoprosencefaliaalobar. Rev Colomb Radiol 2003;14(3):1421–2.
53. Blaas HG, Eriksson AG, Salvesen KA, et al. Brains and faces in holoprosencephaly: pre- and postnatal description of 30 cases. Ultrasound Obstet Gynecol 2002;19(1):24–38.
54. Nowell M. Ultrasound evaluation of septo-optic dysplasia in the new born. Report of a case. Neuroradiology 1986;28(5–6):491–2.
55. Blaas HG, Eik-Nes SH, Vainio T, et al. Alobar holoprosencephaly at 9 weeks gestational age visualized by two- and three-dimensional ultrasound. Ultrasound Obstet Gynecol 2000;15(1):62–5.
56. Golja AM, Estroff JA, Robertson RL. Fetal imaging of central nervous system abnormalities. Neuroimaging Clin N Am 2004;14(2):293–306, viii.
57. Levine D, Barnes PD, Robertson RR, et al. Fast MR imaging of fetal central nervous system abnormalities. Radiology 2003;229(1):51–61.
58. Rollins N. Semilobar holoprosencephaly seen with diffusion tensor imaging and fiber tracking. AJNR Am J Neuroradiol 2005;26(8):2148–52.
59. Salmela MB, Cauley KA, Nickerson JP, et al. Magnetic resonance diffusion tensor imaging (MRDTI) and tractography in children with septo-optic dysplasia. Pediatr Radiol 2010;40(5):708–13.
60. Simon EM, Hevner RF, Pinter JD, et al. The middle interhemispheric variant of holoprosencephaly. AJNR Am J Neuroradiol 2002;23(1):151–6.
61. Wahl M, Barkovich AJ, Mukherjee P. Diffusion imaging and tractography of congenital brain malformations. Pediatr Radiol 2010;40(1):59–67.
62. Maintz D, Benz-Bohm G, Gindele A, et al. Posterior pituitary ectopia: another hint toward a genetic etiology. AJNR Am J Neuroradiol 2000;21(6):1116–8.
63. Kelly WM, Kucharczyk W, Kucharczyk J, et al. Posterior pituitary ectopia: an MR feature of pituitary dwarfism. AJNR Am J Neuroradiol 1988;9(3):453–60.
64. Vittore CP, Murray RA, Martin LS. Case 79: pituitary duplication. Radiology 2005;234(2):411–4.
65. Cervantes LF, Altman NR, Medina LS. Case 102: pituitary aplasia. Radiology 2006;241(3):936–8.
66. Saleem SN, Said AH, Lee DH. Lesions of the hypothalamus: MR imaging diagnostic features. Radiographics 2007;27(4):1087–108.
67. Georgakoulias N, Vize C, Jenkins A, et al. Hypothalamic hamartomas causing gelastic epilepsy: two cases and a review of the literature. Seizure 1998; 7(2):167–71.
68. Knorr JR, Ragland RL, Brown RS, et al. Kallmann syndrome: MR findings. AJNR Am J Neuroradiol 1993;14(4):845–51.
69. Barkovich AJ, Millen KJ, Dobyns WB. A developmental and genetic classification for midbrain-hindbrain malformations. Brain 2009;132(Pt 12):3199–230.
70. Patel S, Barkovich AJ. Analysis and classification of cerebellar malformations. AJNR Am J Neuroradiol 2002;23(7):1074–87.
71. Parisi MA, Dobyns WB. Human malformations of the midbrain and hindbrain: review and proposed classification scheme. Mol Genet Metab 2003;80(1–2):36–53.
72. Nelson MD Jr, Maher K, Gilles FH. A different approach to cysts of the posterior fossa. Pediatr Radiol 2004;34(9):720–32.
73. Alkan O, Kizilkilic O, Yildirim T. Malformations of the midbrain and hindbrain: a retrospective study and review of the literature. Cerebellum 2009;8(3):355–65.
74. Robinson AJ, Blaser S, Toi A, et al. The fetal cerebellar vermis: assessment for abnormal development by ultrasonography and magnetic resonance imaging. Ultrasound Q 2007;23(3):211–23.
75. Paladini D, Volpe P. Posterior fossa and vermian morphometry in the characterization of fetal cerebellar abnormalities: a prospective three-dimensional ultrasound study. Ultrasound Obstet Gynecol 2006; 27(5):482–9.
76. Adamsbaum C, Moutard ML, Andre C, et al. MRI of the fetal posterior fossa. Pediatr Radiol 2005;35(2):124–40.
77. McGraw P. The molar tooth sign. Radiology 2003; 229(3):671–2.
78. Sarnat HB. Molecular genetic classification of central nervous system malformations. J Child Neurol 2000;15(10):675–87.
79. Poretti A, Prayer D, Boltshauser E. Morphological spectrum of prenatal cerebellar disruptions. Eur J Paediatr Neurol 2009;13(5):397–407.
80. Caldemeyer KS, Boaz JC, Wappner RS, et al. Chiari I malformation: association with hypophosphatemic rickets and MR imaging appearance. Radiology 1995;195(3):733–8.
81. Takanashi J, Arai H, Nabatame S, et al. Neuroradiologic features of CASK mutations. AJNR Am J Neuroradiol 2010;31(9):1619–22.
82. dos Santos AV, Matias S, Saraiva P, et al. MR imaging features of brain stem hypoplasia in familial horizontal gaze palsy and scoliosis. AJNR Am J Neuroradiol 2006;27(6):1382–3.
83. Pasquier L, Marcorelles P, Loget P, et al. Rhombencephalosynapsis and related anomalies: a neuropathological study of 40 fetal cases. Acta Neuropathol 2009;117(2):185–200.

84. Naidich TP, Pudlowski RM, Naidich JB, et al. Computed tomographic signs of the Chiari II malformation. Part I: skull and dural partitions. Radiology 1980;134(1):65–71.
85. McLeary RD, Kuhns LR, Barr M Jr. Ultrasonography of the fetal cerebellum. Radiology 1984; 151(2):439–42.
86. Poretti A, Leventer RJ, Cowan FM, et al. Cerebellar cleft: a form of prenatal cerebellar disruption. Neuropediatrics 2008;39(2):106–12.
87. Boltshauser E. Cerebellum—small brain but large confusion: a review of selected cerebellar malformations and disruptions. Am J Med Genet A 2004; 126(4):376–85.

Development and Dysgenesis of the Cerebral Cortex: Malformations of Cortical Development

Charles Raybaud, MD*, Elysa Widjaja, MD

KEYWORDS

- Cortex, development • Focal cortical dysplasia
- Microcephaly • Macrocephaly • Lissencephaly
- Cobblestone brain • Nodular heterotopia • Schizencephaly
- Polymicrogyria

The development of the cerebral cortex results from complex and overlapping processes of cellular proliferation, differentiation, and apoptosis, of migration, and of organization (development of neuronal connections). The term malformation of cortical development (MCD) describes the structural abnormality resulting from any defect affecting any stage of this development. From a terminological point of view, it is now preferred to the name "migration defect," which is too specific (the cortex may be malformed even when the cells have migrated normally). The term cortical dysgenesis would be appropriate as well. The term "cortical dysplasia" would be acceptable, but it has been in use since as early as 1971 to describe a specific variety of cortical malformation.[1]

MCD have been known for a long time (see Refs.[2,3] for review), but it is only after the introduction of modern imaging modalities (computed tomography [CT], but above all magnetic resonance [MR] imaging) that their clinical importance has been recognized as a major cause of developmental delay, refractory epilepsy, and cerebral palsy. When the development of the brain was not yet clearly understood, they were described by pathologists according to the morphologic feature that was the most striking when looking at the brain, such as the size or the appearance of the brain surface (eg, small or big: microencephaly or megalencephaly; smooth: lissencephaly-agyria-pachygyria, cobblestone brain; too many small gyri: polymicrogyria; cavities: porencephaly-schizencephaly). This terminology has remained despite a much better understanding of the pathogenetic processes. As soon as the present model of development was established, with its phases of proliferation-apoptosis, migration, and organization,[4,5] the malformations were classified accordingly, while the names were retained[6]: microencephaly and megalencephaly as proliferation disorders; heterotopia and later lissencephaly as migration disorders; polymicrogyria and schizencephaly (which includes polymicrogyric cortex) as organization disorders. It must be mentioned that such a classification introduces a bias in the understanding of the MCD, as it suggests that the malformations would develop sequentially: proliferation disorders early, migration disorders later, and organization disorders last, which would be an oversimplification.

In the last two decades the progressive unraveling of the role of specific genetic cascades that

Division of Neuroradiology, Hospital for Sick Children, 555 University Avenue, Toronto, ON M5G1X8, Canada
* Corresponding author.
E-mail address: charles.raybaud@sickkids.ca

Neuroimag Clin N Am 21 (2011) 483–543
doi:10.1016/j.nic.2011.05.014
1052-5149/11/$ – see front matter

control the development of the cortex, and the identification in several entities of corresponding genetic defects, have opened new avenues to understanding the MCD.[7] Putting all those facts together, Barkovich and colleagues[8] have proposed a morphologic and tentatively pathogenetic classification of MCD, which includes the developmental glioneuronal tumors in MCD (like the classification of Raymond and colleagues[9] before) and subdivides focal cortical dysplasia (FCD) into two clearly separate groups depending on whether they present with dysmorphic/balloon cells (considered as malformed cells related to an abnormal neuronal and glial genesis), or with architectural changes only (considered the result of an abnormal cortical organization). This classification, updated in 2001 and 2005, is the most widely accepted today (**Box 1**).[10,11]

Although this article fully adheres to this classification, the authors mildly diverge from it in dealing with FCD: it is described first and separately as a single group because (whatever their pathogenesis) all present in a similar and specific clinical, radiological, and surgical context. The authors then resume the classical approach and proceed with the groups of disorders of proliferation/apoptosis, of migration disorders (including the lissencephalies), and of schizencephaly and polymicrogyria. Before that, an introductory review of the imaging approach and of the development is provided.

THE IMAGING APPROACH

What to Look for

MCD are primarily disorders of the cerebral cortex, and imaging therefore should carefully investigate the cortex: sulcal/gyral pattern (all primary and secondary sulci bear names and can be identified; they are essentially symmetric) and depth (symmetric); cortical thickness (normally 1 mm in the depth of the sulcus, 2–3 mm at the crown of the gyrus) and demarcation from the white matter; T1 and T2/fluid-attenuated inversion recovery (FLAIR) signals. In addition, the white matter originates from and is functionally associated with the cortex, and it is traversed by the migration path of the cortical cells: it may have become dysplastic together with the cortex (abnormal cellularity, heterotopic neurons or monstrous cells, abnormal connectivity) as a part of the cortical malformation, or its development may have been secondarily altered by the cortical abnormality (distorted plasticity); it may also have become abnormal as a late result of the seizure activity of the overlying cortex (demyelination, gliosis). As the connectivity often is decreased, so is the volume of the white

Box 1
Malformations of cortical development

1. Malformations due to abnormal neuronal and glial proliferation or apoptosis
   a. Abnormality of brain size: decreased proliferation/increased apoptosis or increased proliferation/decreased apoptosis:
      i. Microcephaly with normal to thin cortex
      ii. Microlissencephaly (extreme microencephaly with thick cortex)
      iii. Microcephaly with extensive polymicrogyria
      iv. Macrocephalies
   b. Abnormal proliferation
      i. Nonneoplastic
         1. Cortical tubers of tuberous sclerosis
         2. Focal cortical dysplasia with balloon cells
         3. Hemimegalencephaly
      ii. Neoplastic (associated with disordered cortex)
         1. Dysembryoplastic neuroectodermal tumor (DNET)
         2. Ganglioglioma
         3. Gangliocytoma
2. Malformations due to abnormal neuronal migration
   a. Lissencephaly/band heterotopia spectrum
   b. Cobblestone cortex complex
   c. Heterotopia
      i. Periventricular nodular heterotopia
      ii. Subcortical nodular heterotopia
      iii. Marginal glioneuronal heterotopia
3. Malformation due to abnormal cortical organization/late neuronal migration
   a. Polymicrogyria and schizencephaly
      i. Bilateral polymicrogyria syndromes
      ii. Schizencephaly (polymicrogyria with clefts)
      iii. Polymicrogyria or schizencephaly as part of multiple congenital anomaly/mental retardation syndromes
   b. Focal cortical dysplasia without balloon cells
   c. Microdysgenesis
4. Malformations of cortical development not otherwise classified
   a. Malformations secondary to inborn errors of metabolism
      i. Mitochondrial and pyruvate metabolic disorders
      ii. Peroxisomal disorders
   b. Other unclassified malformations
      i. Sublobar dysplasia
      ii. Others

Data from Barkovich AJ, Kuzniecky RI, Jackson GD, et al. A developmental and genetic classification for malformations of cortical development. Neurology 2005;65:1873–87.

matter: this may be expressed by the volume of the brain, of one hemisphere or lobe, by the size and morphology of the ventricle(s), or by the asymmetry of the brainstem. Finally, many of the genes that control the cellular migration to and fate in the cerebral cortex may also control the development of the basal ganglia,[12] thalami, and brainstem nuclei, of the cerebellar cortex, and of the cord. Some even may be involved in the development of extraneural tissues (eg, cobblestone cortex and deficient white matter associated with congenital muscular dystrophy).

The Tools

Conventional imaging

The clinical importance of the MCD appeared as soon as CT became the primary diagnostic modality in Neuroradiology (mid-1970s), but in this field like elsewhere, the imaging modality of choice is MR. The "best protocols" are many, depending on the type of equipment available, on the technological advances, and on the familiarity of the neuroradiologist with the pathology.[13–19] Whatever is preferred, the study should always be multisequential and multiplanar, using high spatial definition and high contrast resolution (high signal-to-noise [S/N]). Because the abnormalities often are subtle, the most recent and most efficient machine should be used, and older cases of "nonlesional" epilepsies should be reinvestigated when the equipment is changed or updated. Obviously 3-T magnets have a better resolution power than 1.5-T magnets; multiple-phased array coils with parallel imaging are better than conventional coils, providing high S/N images while keeping the acquisition time within reasonable limits. Most modern neuroimaging centers are now equipped with PACS (picture archiving and communications system); if not, digital storage of the image is mandatory, rather than conventional films, because small, subtle lesions may escape the first review of the images and may be identified after repeated and careful review only. As much as possible, the examination should be directed by the clinical and electrographic/magnetoencephalographic (MEG) data, and if available, the results of the functional studies (single-photon emission CT [SPECT], positron emission tomography [PET]): an oriented study is more likely to be productive than a blind study.[16]

The basic conventional sequences are T1, T2, and FLAIR. T1 images ideally should be from volumic acquisition (MP-RAGE/TFE/SPGR), with 1- to 1.5-mm partitions to minimize the partial volume effects. The thickness and demarcation of the cortical ribbon are better appreciated, and focal cortical signal changes can be securely identified. The typical acquisition plane is the sagittal plane, with reformatting in whatever other plane is felt necessary, even curvilinear planes. The images provide an excellent spatial resolution and an excellent gray-white contrast, allowing for a superb anatomic study. To analyze the suprasylvian sulcal pattern, the sagittal and axial planes are the best; for the temporal structures, especially the mesial ones, coronal slices perpendicular to the long axis of the hippocampus are optimal. The cortical-subcortical definition, however, is poor in infants between the ages of a few weeks and at least 1 year.

T2 imaging is still important for anatomy, and to evaluate the microstructural changes in the parenchyma. The plane(s) should be adapted to the location of the expected abnormality; in a routine protocol, coronal and axial planes are usually chosen. Some groups prefer using true T2 spin echo (T2SE), whereas most use conventional T2 fast-spin echo (T2FSE). Some also advocate the use of 3-dimensional (3D)-FSE with 1-mm partition, and slices certainly should not be thicker than 2 to 3 mm, depending on the equipment available. In the neonatal and in the mature brain, T2-weighted imaging (T2WI) is excellent at showing the cortical involvement, the cortical thickness, and the cortical-subcortical blurring, if any.

FLAIR imaging certainly is the sequence most sensitive to structural changes, but its spatial resolution is not as good as that of T2 turbo-spin echo (T2TSE), with artifacts from flowing blood or cerebrospinal fluid (CSF) being more common. Yet it is practically the first sequence to be looked at, as it will readily demonstrate any significant abnormality of signal. Like conventional T2WI, 2- to 3-mm slices should obtained, typically axial and coronal, or even 1-mm slices using 3D FLAIR.[20] It demonstrates changes in both the cortex and the white matter, and a cortical blurring as well. It is of limited use, however, in young children. Some groups like to use proton density images instead, or in complement of FLAIR.[20]

Besides the main conventional sequences, other sequences may be useful in specific instances. Susceptibility sequences (SWI) are useful to demonstrate that an epileptogenic dysplasia is associated with vascular abnormalities such as a cavernoma or a meningoangiomatosis. Diffusion imaging (DWI/ADC) is not very contributive in the assessment of MCD: it is typically not sensitive enough to show the microstructural changes of the tissue, which will be much more confidently evaluated by quantitative diffusion tensor imaging (DTI); however, it may demonstrate restriction due to cytotoxic edema in case of refractory seizure activity. MR venography may be used to illustrate venous abnormalities commonly associated with some MCD such as a polymicrogyria (PMG), whereas MR arteriography may show abnormal arterial patterns.

Imaging in infants

In infants and young children (as well as in developmentally delayed children) good MR imaging implies the use of sedation/general anesthesia. During the first months of life the structure of the immature brain tissue is different and the T1 relaxation time is much longer than in the mature brain, so that adapted sequences should be used. T1-weighted (T1W) sequences need a longer repetition time (TR), and T2W sequences need longer TR and echo time. Also, as mentioned earlier, if the cortex is exquisitely delineated at birth on T1 and T2, the contrast becomes lost with advancing myelination, until after 1 year on T1, and 2 years on T2. On FLAIR images the evolution is still more complex: at birth, the very high water content of the white matter is cancelled by the saturation pulse and the appearance is somewhat similar to T1; in the following weeks the myelin precursors accumulate and the signal increases to look more like a conventional T2. However, it remains fairly heterogeneous for a much longer time than on ordinary T2 sequences, as the mature pattern is not reached until about the age of 3 to 4 years. In summary, the optimal time to identify a cortical dysplasia in an infant is either early in the first weeks or much later when the mature pattern is established after 2 years, and FLAIR imaging is of limited use in young children.

Another specificity of epileptic infants is the possible occurrence of a focally accelerated myelination. Many investigators have observed that when FCD is diagnosed in the first months of life the white matter under the dysplastic cortex displays a low T2 signal,[21–25] which eventually disappears while maturation proceeds.[25] Most assumed that this appearance was a feature inherent to FCD, a reflection of an associated white matter dysplasia, and/or possibly microscopic calcification, but it was also suggested that it could result from the seizure activity itself.[26] This idea is supported by the experimental evidence that electrical activity in the axons induces the myelination, and that increasing this activity increases the myelination,[27] a process mediated by astrocytes.[28] Accelerated myelination is observed in other epileptogenic conditions such as the Stürge-Weber syndrome.[29] Finally, it explains why the change is no longer apparent when myelination is completed: this would not be expected to happen in the case of white matter dysplasia. It is important to keep in mind that as a consequence, the early myelination points to an epileptogenic focus and not necessarily to an FCD.

Special MR imaging techniques

Because of the high percentage of lesions that are not well demonstrated on MR imaging, different approaches have been proposed to increase the diagnostic yield. Various MR techniques are available to provide more insight into the structure, function, and metabolism of the epileptic brain affected with an MCD. Quantitative MR demonstrates that T2 correlates with the neuronal density in the cortex.[30] Volumetric studies suggest a relative defect of the white matter, hence of the connectivity.[31] DTI is being used extensively. Quantitative DTI is more sensitive than DWI/ADC to demonstrate a decreased diffusivity postictally, matching the epileptic focus, apparently related to a cellular swelling due to the metabolic exhaustion.[32] It also identifies an increased diffusivity interictally, which may be due to neuronal loss and gliosis in both gray and white matter,[16,33,34] as well as to a dysgenetic structural alteration.[16] DTI tractography demonstrates more extensive changes in the brain organization and connectivity beyond the cortical lesion.[35–39] Proton spectroscopy (^{1}H-MRS) is not very useful for the diagnosis of an MCD composed of normal if ill-located or ill-organized neurons and glia, but it provides insights on their metabolism. *N*-Acetylaspartic acid (NAA) appears largely unchanged or only mildly decreased in heterotopia and PMG,[40–42] choline appears either increased or normal,[41,42] and glutamate and γ-aminobutyric acid (GABA) appear increased in patients with epileptogenic heterotopias and PMG.[42] In lesions made of poorly differentiated cells such as in FCD or in the tubers of tuberous sclerosis complex (TSC), NAA appears significantly decreased[41,43] and choline increased, but less so than in cerebral tumors.[43] Perfusion also is low in cortical tubers but normal in PMG.[44] Despite it having been proved useful in the evaluation of the cortical and white matter dysplasia in tuberous sclerosis,[45–47] there is no report on the potential use of magnetization transfer imaging (MTI) in MCD in general, and in FCD in particular. One report, however, indicates that in acquired and developmental epileptogenic lesions, significantly reduced magnetization transfer ratio (MTR) was found within the MR-visible lesions (presumably gliosis with low myelin content) as well as in normal-looking white matter. These areas concurred with the electrographic epileptic activity and the clinical seizure semiology.[48]

Cortical Function and White Matter Organization In and Around MCD: Presurgical Assessment

Imaging has become essential in preparing for epilepsy surgery, if warranted. It is expected to show the lesion, identify its nature and, as much as possible, its extent. Quantitative DTI shows microstructural changes beyond the abnormalities seen on conventional MR images, in good correlation with the MEG abnormalities.[35–39,49]

Imaging is also expected to tell whether the lesion is functional or not. MCD have an intrinsic epileptogenicity, which implies that they are interconnected with the rest of the brain; some patients with MCD present with reflex epilepsy, which means that the lesion can be activated by outside stimuli (for review see Ref.[50]). Using functional imaging (fMRI), one study demonstrated that 64% of MCD are activated by simple sensory motor or visual stimuli (71% if they are located in the corresponding eloquent areas), but only 40% become involved in complex cognitive tasks.[50] However, the response of the dysgenetic cortex depends on the severity of the malformation: all cases of organization disorders (PMG, schizencephaly, and FCD type I) become activated by simple tasks against only 47% of cases of FCD type II (Taylor) and heterotopias; this is in good agreement with the current classification of MCD (see **Box 1**).[11]

MR imaging techniques are also used to locate the main cognitive functions and white matter tracts. fMRI has, in practice, completely supplanted the sodium amobarbital Wada test.[16,51,52] It is used to locate the motor function when surgery in the sensory-motor area is considered, and to locate the language representation when the lesion to be operated on is in the so-called dominant hemisphere, as language representation is commonly atypical not only in MCD but more generally in refractory epilepsy.[37,53,54] Assessment and lateralization of memory functions can be done, but need validation and are not performed routinely as yet.[16,51,52] Finally, DTI tractography is an efficient way of locating the major axonal tracts such as the corticospinal tract[16,52,55] or the optic radiations.[16,52,56] Some groups are attempting to demonstrate the language networks[37,52] and the memory networks[16,52] as well.

As mentioned earlier, a focused MR study is more efficient than a blind one, and a multimodality approach enhances the diagnostic efficacy in demonstrating the lesional as well as the epileptogenic area: clinical semiology, scalp electroencephalography (EEG), coregistered MEG and magnetic source imaging (MSI),[57] or functional neuroimaging such as postictal/interictal SPECT[58] and PET[59] are extremely productive. A new approach using EEG-correlated fMRI is being developed and seems promising.[51,60]

DEVELOPMENT OF THE CEREBRAL CORTEX

Cortical Anatomy

The cerebral cortex comprises the trilayered olfactory paleocortex and hippocampal archicortex, and an extensive 6-layered neocortex (90% of the cortical surface in human). In advanced mammals and especially in humans, it is conspicuously folded, two-thirds of the cortical surface being located inside the sulci; cortical folding is related to the development of the connectivity. The sulci have been classified into primary sulci (pericallosal, cingulate, parieto-occipital, hippocampal sulci) and secondary sulci (such as the central, precentral and postcentral, intraparietal, frontal, temporal, calcarine and occipital sulci). The primary and secondary sulci may vary in shape slightly but are constant and symmetric in location. The sulci delineate the gyri, which more or less reflect the functional areas of Brodmann. The primary sulci become apparent shortly after mid-gestation, and the secondary sulci appear between 25 and 30 weeks. Tertiary sulci are branches of the primary and secondary sulci and appear mostly after birth; they are extremely variable.

The thickness of the neocortex varies from 1 to 3 mm, thinner in the depth of the sulci and thicker at the crown of the gyri. Pyramidal neurons (glutamatergic, excitatory) are the most numerous (80%) and establish long-range connections; interneurons (GABAergic, inhibitory) establish local, intracortical connections between the pyramidal neurons. The neurons are primarily organized in columnar units, but because of the intracortical course of the connecting fibers they become organized in layers. From the surface to the depth, the neocortical layers are as follows, albeit with some overlapping between them:

- Layer 1 or molecular layer contains mostly local connecting fibers
- Layer 2 receives corticocortical afferents (association and commissural fibers)
- Layer 3 sends corticocortical efferents (association and commissural fibers)
- Layer 4 or granular layer receives the corticothalamic afferents

- Layer 5 or pyramidal layer sends the cortico-subcortical efferents (to the striatum, brainstem, and cord)
- Layer 6 or polymorphic layer sends the corticothalamic efferents.

The 6-tier layering of the cortex is due to the predominantly horizontal organization of the intracortical fiber tracts. The most prominent fiber layers are in layer 1, in layer 4 (external band of Baillarger), and between layers 5 and 6 (internal band of Baillarger). If the general cortical pattern is constant, the proportion between the layers varies according to the cortical location, resulting in the various histologic patterns that characterize the cortical functional areas of Brodmann.

Formation of the Cortex

In the last 4 decades a considerable amount of information has accumulated regarding the development of the cortex, notably in the last decade (for reviews see Refs.[4,5,61–68]) (**Fig. 1**). The early central nervous system emerges from the surface ectoderm as a band of dorsal midline neuroepithelium or neural plate during the third week (for review see Ref.[69]). This neural plate forms a groove with neural folds and closes to form the neural tube (NT) during the fourth week (neurulation); 3 cerebral vesicles (forebrain, midbrain, and hindbrain) become apparent during the fifth week, and the lateral evaginations of the cerebral hemispheres develop from the forebrain during the sixth week.[70] Under the influence of ventralization and dorsalization factors, the hemispheric vesicles become divided into a basal part or subpallium (future basal ganglia) and a dorsal part or pallium (future cortex and white matter), each with its own germinal zone, the dorsal one producing pyramidal neurons and the basal one (ganglionic eminence) producing the cortical interneurons as well as the neurons of the basal ganglia (in humans interneurons may come from the pallial germinal zone as well). The division is clearly apparent during the seventh week.[70]

Proliferation of neuroepithelial, truly neural stem cells already begins in the fourth week in the neural plate.[69] As the NT closes, its whole thickness forms a proliferating zone where the cells divide in a symmetric way (one stem cell produces two stem cells) (see **Fig. 1**A).[67] At the end of the fifth week the proliferation process switches to asymmetric divisions (one stem cell produces one stem cell and one neuron) and the differentiated neurons accumulate at the periphery: as a consequence the wall of the NT contains a deep germinative zone, which is called the ventricular zone (VZ), and a peripheral zone with the first neurons, which is called the primordial plexiform layer or preplate (PP) (see **Fig. 1**B).[62,71] The distance between the ventricular and the meningeal surfaces of the NT is short in the early stages and the differentiated cells are able to migrate by somal translocation (nucleokinesis): from the germinal zone where they are born they extend a process toward the meningeal surface, the nucleus migrates into this process toward the surface while the ventricular process shortens and loses its ventricular contact. One of the genes that controls this nucleokinesis is the *LIS1* gene, whose defect is associated with one major form of lissencephaly.[63] The process of translocation is used by the neurons of the PP and possibly by the early neurons (future layer 6) of the cortical plate (CP).[64] The PP contains Cajal-Retzius cells and other neurons that are the first to establish extracortical connections.[68] When the cortical plate appears on about day 50 (end of week 7), it divides the PP into two layers: the superficial layer or marginal zone (MZ) contains the reelin-positive Cajal-Retzius cells (in addition to various other neurons), and the subcortical layer forms the subplate (SP) and contains reelin-negative neurons (see **Fig. 1**C).[67] Cajal-Retzius cells play a major role of controlling the migration of the neurons in the CP; the subplate is essential also, as it directs outgoing axons and maintains transient connections with the incoming axons until the cortex becomes ready.

Radial migration of glutamatergic pyramidal neuron to the CP begins at the end of week 7 in the lateral part of the telencephalon, and a week later in its posteromedial aspect; the peak migratory activity lasts until mid-gestation (weeks 20–22) and migration is essentially complete before the third trimester.[67] Radial migration uses specialized cells, the radial glia, to guide the pyramidal neuron from the germinal zone to the CP. Each radial glial cell has a process anchored on the ventricular surface, and a radial process that extends to the pial basement membrane (where it often makes contact with vessels[65]), so that the radial glia forms a scaffolding across the mantle. The newly generated neurons travel perpendicular to the surface, from the pallial VZ along the glial fibers to the CP, where they are induced to detach from the radial glia by the signal (Reelin) provided by the Cajal-Retzius cells. As a consequence early-migrating cells are in the deep cortical layers and late-arriving cells are close to the surface: this is called the inside-out pattern (see **Fig. 1**C–E). A first wave of migration toward the deep layer 6 develops at about 7 to 11 weeks; a second wave toward layer 5 occurs at about 12 to 16 weeks; a third and last wave to the more superficial layers

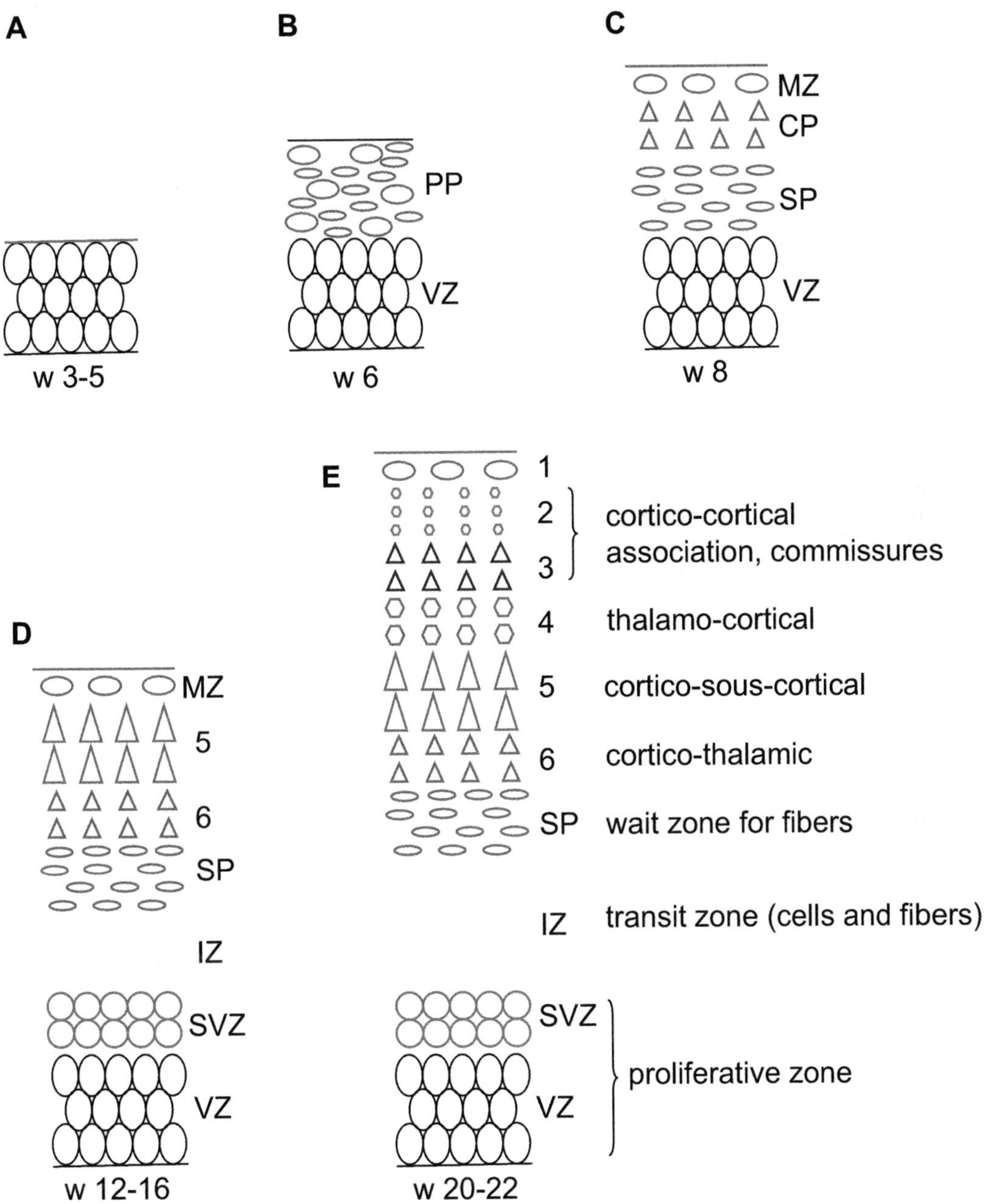

Fig. 1. Pyramidal neuronal migration to the cortex. (*A*) Weeks 3 to 5. Pseudostratified epithelium of proliferating cells. (*B*) Week 6. The pallium is subdivided into a deep proliferative layer (ventricular zone, VZ) and a superficial layer of early postmitotic neurons, the primordial plexiform layer or preplate (PP). (*C*) Week 8. Radial migration of neurons to the surface forms the cortical plate (CP), which divides the PP into a superficial marginal zone (MZ) containing the Cajal-Retzius cells (C-R) and a subcortical subplate (SP). C-R stop the migrating neurons before they reach the surface, which results in the inside-out arrangement whereby young neurons are more superficial and older ones are in the depth of the cortex. The subplate neurons guide the outgoing axons, and make transient connection with the incoming axons until their final targets are ready to become connected. (*D*) Weeks 12 to 16. More neurons migrate to the periphery after making a stop in the subventricular zone (SVZ) where they make contact with other pyramidal neurons and interneurons. An intermediate zone (IZ) develops between the SVZ and the SP: it contains radial glial fibers, migrating neurons, and early axons. (*E*). Weeks 20 to 22. Neuronal migration is essentially complete. The deep layers 5 and 6 contains neurons that project axons to the subcortical structures; layer 4 starts receiving axons from the thalamus (until then connected in the transient subplate); layers 2 and 3 later receive the long association and commissural fibers first, then around and after birth, the subcortical short association fibers.

occurs after 16 weeks.[5] This last wave is prominent in primates, including man, and corresponds to the neurons that will develop corticocortical connections.[67] Late migration of individual neurons may continue even after the end of the cellular proliferation until after birth.[5] As a consequence of the radial migration, all neurons using a single radial cell form a single column in the CP.[5] The glia-guided migration depends on the cellular microfilament network, and involves the *FLN1* gene (whose defect has been demonstrated in specific varieties of gray matter heterotopia), as well as on two proteins associated with the regulation of the actin network, Cdk5 and p35.[63] Doublecortin (DCX) also is involved with radial radiation, and defects of the *DCX* gene are associated with some human lissencephalies (for review see Ref.[63]).

Besides their role of guidance, the radial glia recently have been shown to be stem cells and to produce neuronal progenitors.[65] In a rather complex process, they divide asymmetrically in the VZ, producing another radial glial cell and a neuronal progenitor. The neuronal progenitor moves to the subventricular zone (SVZ) (phase 1) where it stays for up to 24 hours, becomes multipolar, and establishes multiple cellular contacts, moves tangentially free from radial glial attachment, and becomes dispersed within the SVZ before dividing symmetrically (phase 2). The new neurons may migrate directly to the cortex along the radial glia, but most translocate back to the VZ (phase 3), from where they make their final journey toward the CP along the radial glial fibers (phase 4).[64,65]

Tangential migration of the GABAergic inhibitory interneurons occurs in close association with the radial migration of the pyramidal neurons (the first interneurons are seen at about weeks 6–7, even before the appearance of the CP[67]). These neurons typically originate in the ventral VZ of the medial ganglionic eminence (MGE; the primordium of the globus pallidus[63]) and travel parallel to the surface of the hemisphere toward the pallium. Like the radial migration, the tangential migration is complex (for review see Ref.[64]). Studies in rodents show that there are primarily two migration streams, one along the MZ and the other along the deep IZ/SVZ (the intermediate zone [IZ] is the portion of the pallium that is located between the SP and the germinal SVZ). From their MGE origin, some interneurons disperse into the IZ/SVZ before reaching the CP either radially or obliquely; some travel along the MZ and enter the CP from above; some travel in the IZ/SVZ, then reach the MZ radially across the CP, disperse into the MZ, and enter the CP from above. However, the majority of interneurons (70%) travel through the IZ/SVZ and dive toward the ventricle to enter the VZ, where they pause before resuming their course and migrating radially to the CP.[63,65] In this process, the interneurons are likely to acquire laminar address information,[64,65] possibly mediated by GABA information.[65] The partial convergence during their migration of at least some pyramidal neurons and interneurons might allow transmission of positional information. Pyramidal neurons pause in the SVZ, become multipolar, and may contact interneurons there. The different migration speed—10 μm/h for the radial migration, 50 μm/h for the tangential ones—may favor birth-date related encounters, and cellular birth date relates to laminar position precisely. What guides the interneurons—guiding glia, axons projecting from the CP—is not clear, but the process has been shown to involve class 3 semaphorins, neuropilins, cell-adhesion molecules, neuroregulins, and the slit/robo complex.[63,64]

The organization of the pallium changes and becomes more complex as it develops (**Table 1**), and so does the terminology (see **Fig. 1**).[67] In weeks 4 to 5 the pallium is a simple homogeneous pseudostratified neuroepithelium. Between week 5 and week 7 (before the appearance of CP) it comprises a deep germinal zone VZ and a superficial postmitotic zone PP. After the CP divides the PP during week 8, the postmitotic zone is made up of 3 layers (MZ, CP, and SP), the germinal zone is made up of 2 layers (VZ and SVZ), and an IZ in between contains migrating cells, radial glia processes, and early incoming and outgoing axons. After peaking before mid-gestation, migration stops at about 25 to 27 weeks. The radial glia loses contact with the ventricle, migrates toward the cortex, and forms astrocytes (changing its nestin and PAX6 expression for glial fibrillary acidic protein). The pallial VZ disappears leaving the unicellular layer of ependyma only, but the SVZ persists and contains stem cells even in the adult brain, presumably a potential source of brain tumor cells. The germinal zone of the lateral ganglionic eminence remains prominent for some time (the so-called germinal matrix of the premature brain), before vanishing progressively during the last prenatal weeks. After a peak of complexity between 18 and 28 weeks, the cellularity of the MZ, notably the Cajal-Retzius cells, regresses and disappears before term. On the contrary, the SP expands significantly until the third trimester, being largest at week 28,[62] particularly under the frontal associative cortex, and then attenuates until about term, leaving interstitial neurons only in the white matter. As connectivity develops, white matter fibers progressively invade both the IZ and the SP area, which together form the final hemispheric white matter.

Table 1
Development of the pallium

Age in Weeks	Forebrain	Cellular Processes	Organization of Pallium	White Matter	Metabolic Supply/ Vasculature
3	Neural plate	Stem cell proliferation	Pseudostratified	—	Amniotic fluid
4	Anterior neural plate neural tube closure	Stem cell proliferation	Pseudostratified	—	Primitive meninges
5–6	Prosencephalon then hemispheres (pallium/ subpallium)	First peripheral primordial neurons	VZ and PP	—	Choroid plexus
7–9	Pallium	Translocation First wave to layer 6	Postmitotic: MZ, CP, SP Germinal: VZ	Corticothalamic Corticospinal	Choroid plexuses First perforators to VZ/MGE
10–12	Pallium	Radial glia Progenitors Second wave to layers 5–4	Postmitotic: MZ, CP, SP Intermediate: IZ Germinal: VZ–SVZ	First thalamocortical in SP	Choroid plexuses Rich germinal plexus SVZ/VZ/MGE
16–20	Pallium	Third wave to layers 3–2	—	Thalamocortical in SP Commissural and association in SP	Rich germinal plexus SVZ/VZ/MGE
22–26	Pallium Primary and early secondary sulci	End of migration and of radial glia	Disappearance of VZ Ependyma	Thalamocortical in layer 4 Early commissural and association to layers 2–3	Rich germinal plexus SVZ/MGE Early branches in deep cortex
27–32	Pallium Secondary sulci	—	Reaches mature appearance Prominent SP	Layer 1 and Baillarger Commissural and association to layers 2–3	Germinal plexus recedes in SVZ Growing vasculature in deep cortex
33–40	Pallium Developing tertiary sulci	—	SP recedes White matter in IZ/SP	Short association to layers 2–3	Radial vasculature in superficial cortex End of germinal plexus SVZ/MGE
42–47	Pallium Developing tertiary sulci	—	End of frontal SP	Short association to layers 2–3	Steep increase of CBF

Abbreviations: CBF, cerebral blood flow; CP, cortical plate; IZ, intermediate zone; MGE, medial ganglionic eminence; MZ, marginal zone; PP, preplate; SP, subplate; SVZ, subventricular zone; VZ, ventricular zone.

Cellular apoptosis cannot be dissociated from proliferation and organization. The number of neurons in the brain peaks at week 28, but as many as 50% die through apoptosis before the end of the adolescence.[72] Two main periods of apoptosis occur prenatally. The first lasts from week 7 to week 13, and involves proliferating progenitors and young neurons in the VZ.[72] The second, regulated by synaptic activity, cellular contacts, and glial and neuronal trophic factors, eliminates neurons within the CP itself between week 19 and week 23.[72]

Cortical Organization and Developing Connectivity

The period after 22 weeks is the period of organization and differentiation of the cortex (**Fig. 2**).[67] Neuronal proliferation and migration are essentially complete, while many neurons become eliminated.[69,72] Yet from 80 g at mid-gestation, the mass of the brain increases to 350 g at birth, 950 g at 1 year, and 1300 to 1400 g in adulthood. This enormous increase is related to the development of an intense synaptogenesis, which results in a mild thickening but a huge tangential growth of the hemispheric cortex, thus leading to the development of the sulcation/gyration and in a spectacular brain expansion. Each neuron develops one axon only, but axons leaving their temporary connections in the subplate elongate and develop many collateral axons to reach their cortical targets, while the dendritic tree expands dramatically as well (it is estimated that at maturity, each neuron becomes connected with approximately 10,000 neurons, which means as many axonal collaterals). In the late fetal and early postnatal months, a massive increase of the number of oligodendrocytes ("myelination gliosis") takes place, followed by an equally massive development of the myelin and of the supporting cells (astrocytes, microglia). In addition, the increasing brain diameter leads to more elongation of the axons with more myelin and more supporting tissue. The increase in volume is mostly peripheral (elongation of long-projection, commissural and association tracts; late development of the short, subcortical association tracts) while the absolute measurements of the lateral ventricular diameters remain quite stable until after birth.

Within the cortex, the developing connectivity transforms the columnar organization into a laminar pattern. In the motor cortex the cortical neurons at 5 months (22 weeks) are still organized in columns; most early synapses are within the columns and the first horizontal connections use layer 1 to travel to other columns[5,61,72]; horizontal, likely afferent fibers originating from the internal capsule and from the corpus callosum are found in the deep portion of the IZ.[61] At 7 months (about 30 weeks) the laminar pattern is better defined, especially in the deeper cortical layers, with well-defined horizontal fiber tracts in layer 1, in the developing layer 4 (future external band of Baillarger) and between layers 5 and 6 (future internal band of Baillarger).[61] Two weeks later (32 weeks, 7.5 months), the neurons have become more mature in all layers and the horizontal stratification is well apparent[61,67,72] (demonstrated by DTI at week 36[73]). At term, the cellular maturation is complete and the horizontal pattern fully established, with afferent corticocortical fibers present in layer 3. Only the complexity of the organization changes in the following months.[61] In the ferret and the cat, it has been shown that the lateral expansion of the cortex originates at the crown of the gyrus, corresponding to the late cellular maturation, organization, and connections there while the bottom of the sulci would represent relatively fixed points, and apoptosis would be more important in the sulci than at the crown of the gyri.[74–76]

The development of the white matter is related to the development of the cortex, and accordingly connectivity proceeds from the deeper layers (corticothalamic, corticospinal, thalamocortical) to the superficial ones (long-association and commissural tracts, then short-association tracts). The single most important structure in the development of the white matter is the SP. The SP plays the essential role of a wait zone by guiding efferent axons and establishing transient connections with efferent axons until their cortical target cells are mature enough to become connected. The SP expands markedly during the gestation, assumedly both by dispersion due to accumulating incoming axons and by the addition of new cells.[67] It is most prominent about week 28, and especially so in the highly associative areas such as the anterior frontal cortex.[62,67,69,72,77] SP neurons send axons to both the cortex and the subcortical structures, which serve to guide the cortical and subcortical fibers,[77,78] and connect transiently with incoming fibers. The first efferent axons to leave the cortex are likely to be the corticothalamic axons from future layer 6 and the corticospinal (pyramidal) axons from future layer 5, although not much is found in the literature regarding their development in man. It should occur early because the corticothalamic fibers, originating from the deepest layer, are likely to be the first, while the corticospinal fibers are seen at the pyramidal decussation as early as 8 weeks[79] (before the neuronal body reaches layer 5); both are likely to be guided to the internal capsule by SP neurons (see **Fig. 2**A).[80] On the other hand, the first afferent axons to approach the cortex are the thalamocortical axons: pioneer fibers are seen in the SP as early as week 12,[67] more are seen accumulating in the superficial SP at week 22,[69,77,81] and cortical layer 4 becomes connected by week 26 (see **Fig. 2**B, C).[69] Commissural and long-association fibers reach the SP between weeks 24 and 29[77] and extend to the cortex itself about 33 to 35

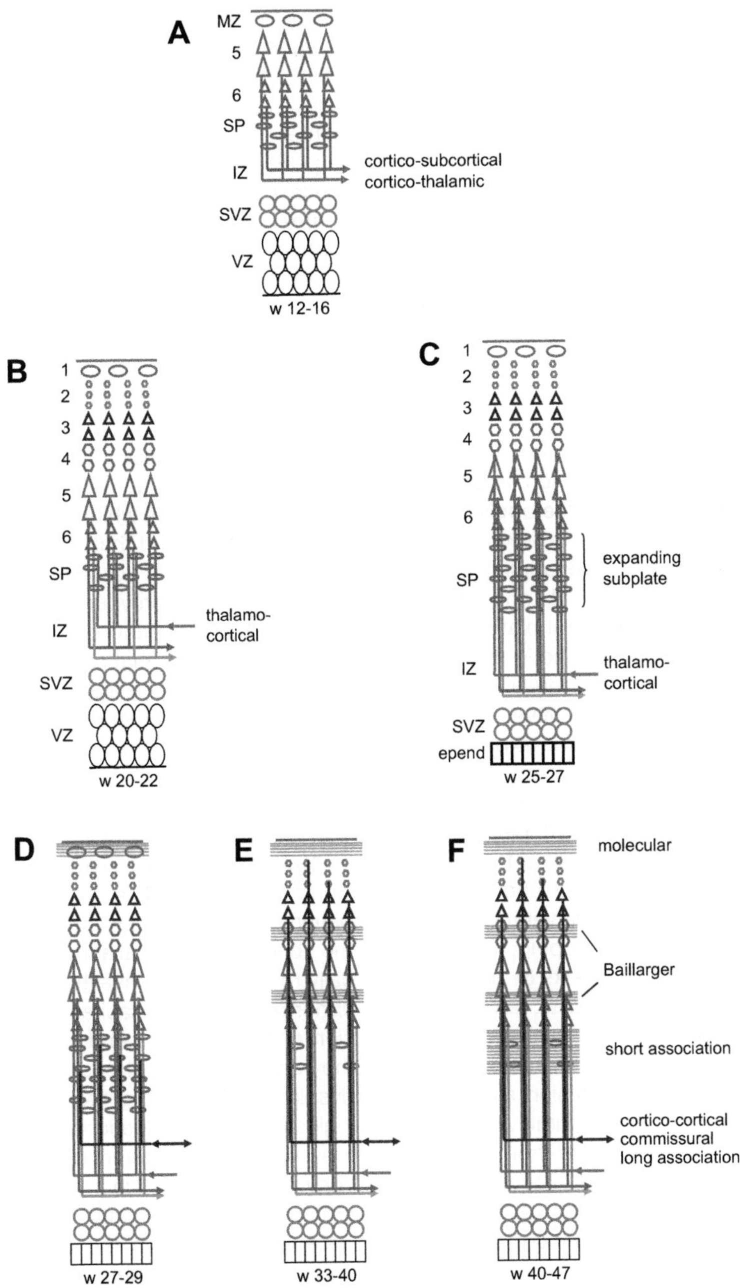

Fig. 2. Development of the connectivity. (*A*) Weeks 12 to 16. The cortico-subcortical fibers (to the thalamus, striatum, brainstem, and cord) are already present even before the neurons reach their layers 6 and 5. (*B*) Weeks 20 to 22. The neuronal migration is complete but the thalamocortical fibers are still in the SP. (*C*) Weeks 25 to 27. The thalamocortical fibers reach layer 4 from week 22 until it is complete by week 26. This is a crucial event in the maturation of the cortex, as local circuits become organized along the radial columns; the SP wait-zone reaches its maximum expansion at 28 weeks, and the thickness of the IZ increases with the number of fibers. The radial glia disappears, as well as the VZ, which leaves the ependymal lining only. (*D, E*) Weeks 27 to 40. The corticocortical fibers, including the interhemispheric commissural fibers, become connected to the SP first, then after 32 weeks to the superficial layers 2 to 3 while the SP attenuates. Intracortical connections develop as well, in the molecular layer and in the bands of Baillarger. (*F*) Weeks 40 to 47. Around and after term, and while the SP progressively vanishes, the short subcortical association fibers connect within layers 2 to 3.

weeks while the SP starts receding (see **Fig. 2**D, E). At the same time, the thalamocortical afferents are promoting local intracortical circuits, and short-association fibers start connecting with layers 2 and 3.[77] The development of these short corticocortical association fibers continues until postnatal week 7 and is related to the late persistence of the SP in the high-level associative areas (see **Fig. 2**F). During the first postnatal years the number of synapses increases considerably; later on, however, about age 4 to 6 years, a cortical areal specialization occurs with a corresponding pruning of the axonal branches in excess.

Development of Cortical Vascularization

During development, vascularization is continuously precisely adapted to the metabolic needs of the moment (see Ref.[82] for review) (**Fig. 3**). Vascularization evolves in 4 overlapping phases of amniotic, meningeal, choroidal, and intrinsic capillary supply.[83] The open neural plate in week 4 is fed by diffusion from the amniotic fluid. After its closure at the end of week 4, the NT is fed by diffusion from the surrounding primitive meningeal capillaries (see **Fig. 3**A, B). With the expansion of the brain vesicles and the enlargement of the ventricles, the primitive meninge invaginates into the ventricles to form the choroid plexuses: in addition to the peripheral supply from the meningeal network, oxygen, glucose, and other nutrients now diffuse from the plexus to the ventricular wall where the germinal tissue is developing; this corresponds to the preplate stage (weeks 6–7) (a major role for the choroid plexuses persists, however, as they reach their maximal size at 11 weeks[84]). After week 7, as the CP appears the NT becomes too thick to be fed by extrinsic diffusion alone, and the first intrinsic vessels, actually primitive sinusoid capillaries, enter the brain tissue from the periphery toward the deep germinal areas (VZ first and then SVZ) (see **Fig. 3**C). These vessels cross the CP without giving it any branch, and form arteriovenous loops in the germinal zone, which expand and develop into a rich vascular plexus by 12 to 15 weeks (see **Fig. 3**D). The first horizontal branches to enter the deep cortical layers appear at 20 weeks (see **Fig. 3**E), and progressively become more numerous until 27 weeks (see **Fig. 3**F). New short radial branches emerge from the superficial network during the last trimester to feed the superficial layers (see **Fig. 3**G).[82] The development of the cortical vascular system therefore reflects and is adapted to the progressive development of the connectivity during the second half of gestation, especially the last trimester, advancing from the deep to the superficial layers. However, this does not mean that the blood flow is significantly increased. The cerebral blood flow (CBF) measurements performed in prematures (allowing for the limitations inherent to the clinical context in such patients) seem to indicate that the CBF remains low at 10 to 20 mL/100 g/min in the last trimester until term (see Ref.[85] for review). A steep increase of the CBF values occurs after birth, peaking at 70 mL/100 g/min at 5 years before declining to adult levels of 50 mL/100 g/min at the end of the adolescence.[86,87] Surprisingly, the increase seems to occur at the same time after birth in premature and in term infants, and therefore seems to relate to the conditions of extrauterine life rather than to gestational age.[88] These figures represent an average of the blood flows of the gray and white matter: assuming that the blood flow of the white matter does not change much over time and that white matter represents 50% of the brain in volume, the perfusion values of the gray matter in young children are still more remarkable. (Quantitative blood flow data, however, are scarce in that age range and sometimes discordant, given the fragility of the patients and the use of different technical approaches.)

FOCAL CORTICAL DYSPLASIA

Definition and Classification of FCD

In 1971, Taylor and Falconer with Bruton and Corsellis published a series on 10 epileptic patients, in which the parts of the brain where the abnormal electrical activity existed were surgically removed.[1] The investigators noted histologic abnormalities, which lacked the tumor-like expansion of hamartomata and which, for that reason, they called "a particular form of localized cortical dysplasia." The lesions were characterized histologically by "congregations of large, bizarre neurons which were littered through all but the first cortical layer" with "in most but not all cases, grotesque cells, probably of glial origin, [which] were also present in the depth of the affected cortex and in the subjacent white matter." The study noted that in all cases the brain surface was normal with no tuber-like appearance; when cut, the cortex looked macroscopically normal in 7 of 10 cases but was wide with blurred junction with the white matter in 3 of 10 cases. Microscopically there was disorganization of the laminar architecture with large aberrant neurons scattered randomly, which stood out by their number, large size, and bizarre structure, and the common presence (7 of 10 cases) of large, multinucleated cells in the deep cortical layers and the white matter. There were reactive astrocytes but no fibrous gliosis, and sometimes a reduction of the myelinated fibers

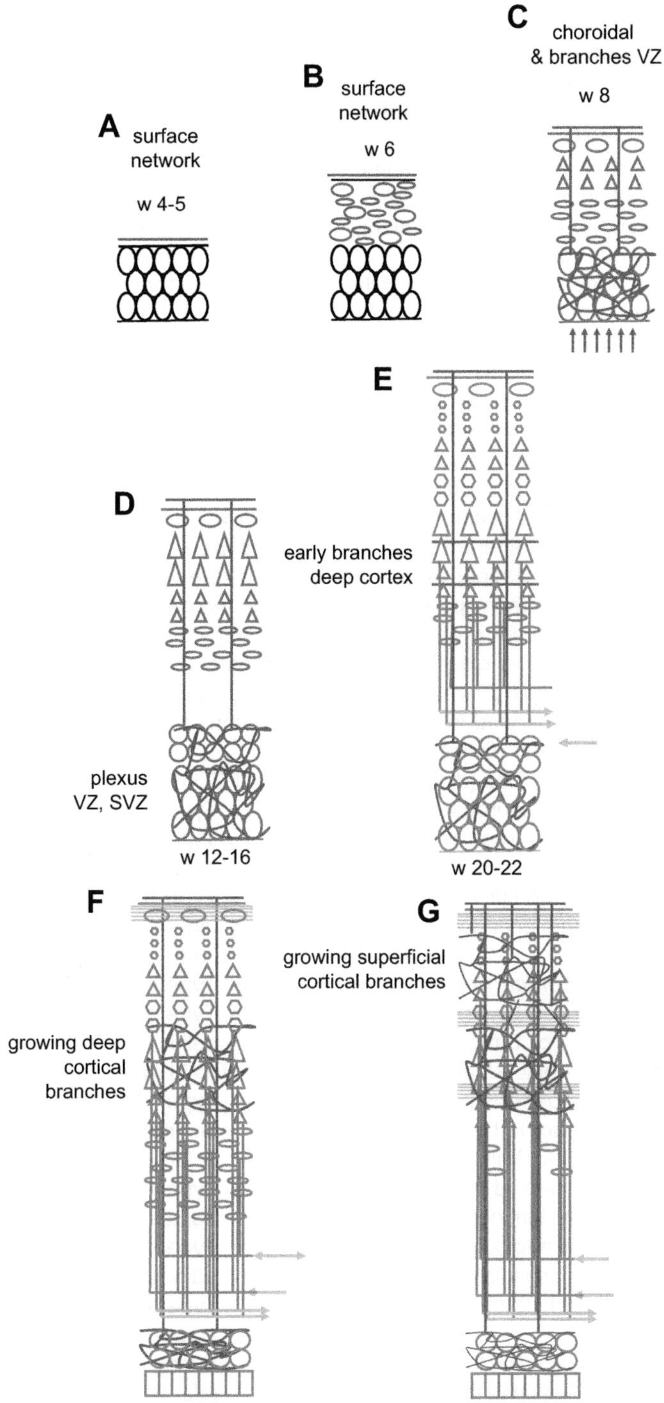

Fig. 3. Development of the vascularity. (*A*, *B*) Weeks 4 to 6. After the neural tube closes, a leptomeningeal network surrounds the brain, from which the nutrients diffuse in the neural tissue. (*C*, *D*) Weeks 8 to 16. About week 7, the choroid plexuses develop so that nutrients may diffuse from the CSF into the VZ. In addition at week 8, perforators from the surface network penetrate into the neural parenchyma toward the proliferative VZ and SVZ, and develop a rich vascular plexus there while the cortex remains essentially avascular. (*E*) Weeks 20 to 22. After midgestation a few horizontal branches develop in the deep cortical layers. (*F*) Weeks 27 to 29. Once the thalamocortical connections are established, a rich vascular network develops in the deep cortical layers. (*G*) Weeks 33 to 40. Superficial cortical vessels develop together with the corticocortical connections in the superficial layers, both from the long perforant vessels and from the pial vessels. The plexus in the proliferative zone regresses.

in the underlying white matter. The investigators mentioned previous reports of findings somewhat similar to theirs, that had been related to formes frustes of tuberous sclerosis, only to mention that their patients did not present the features, either clinical (family history, intellectual delay, other stigmata), radiologic (subependymal nodules, calcification), or histologic (tuber appearance, cellular depopulation), which characterize tuberous sclerosis.[1]

From the perspective of epilepsy surgery in children this article, which defined the entity "focal cortical dysplasia (FCD)," was probably the most seminal in the past half-century. FCD is the single most important cause of focal refractory epilepsy in children, histologically proved in almost 50% of children undergoing epilepsy surgery (20% of adults).[89] With time, it became obvious that it was a heterogeneous entity, with distinct clinical and imaging characteristics, and different surgical responses,[89–93] the surgical indications and the prognosis being closely related with the pathologic subtype, so that classifications were proposed to provide more consistency.[94–96] The classification most widely used until recently ("Cleveland" or Palmini classification[95]) was proposed in 2004 by a panel of experts. It made a clear distinction between the architectural abnormalities (dyslamination, heteropic and misoriented neurons) and the cytologic abnormalities (giant neurons, immature neurons, dysmorphic neurons, balloon cells), with the following 3-tiered classification (from the milder to the more severe histologic changes).

- *Mild malformations of cortical development (mMCD)* are characterized by ectopic neurons located in (type I) or outside (type II) layer 1 (this subgroup replaced the previous subgroup of microdysgenesis). Cases of mMCD were assumed not to be detectable by the then current MR techniques.
- *FCD type I* are characterized by architectural abnormalities (dyslamination of the cortex without or with additional features of mMCD), which may be isolated (type IA) or associated with giant or immature neurons (type IB).
- *FCD type II* are characterized by the presence of monstrous cells in addition to the architectural abnormalities, either dysmorphic neurons only (type IIA) or dysmorphic neurons and balloon cells (type IIB). FCD type II are often referred to as Taylor-type FCD.

This classification has 3 main limitations, the first being that such a grading system suggests different degrees of severity in the same disease entity. The second limitation was revealed by a blinded evaluation of interobserver and intraobserver reproducibility of histologic diagnosis in mMCD-FCD (26 specimens rotated among 8 neuropathologists), which showed that whereas the reproducibility rate was high for FCD type II (especially IIB), it was quite low for mMCD and FCD type I, meaning that except for the monstrous cells of type II, the other subgroups lack an unequivocal morphologic definition.[97] The third limitation is that the classification did not take into account the FCD associated with other disorders including obviously acquired diseases such as sequelae of perinatal hypoxic ischemic encephalopathy, trauma, infection, or strokes.[98–104] For these reasons, a more refined classification is proposed by the Diagnostic Method Commission of the International League Against Epilepsy (ILAE) (which includes the Cleveland classification experts as well).[105] Considering the FCD only (the mMCD is evaluated later), this new classification retains the group of FCD type IIA and type IIB, as it is clearly defined by the monstrous dysmorphic neurons and balloon cells. It better defines type I and introduces a new type III FCD, associated with another, principal lesion.

- FCD type I (isolated)
    - Type IA: abnormal radial cortical lamination
    - Type IB: abnormal tangential cortical lamination
    - Type IC: abnormal radial and tangential lamination
- FCD II
    - Type IIA: dysmorphic neurons
    - Type IIB: dysmorphic neurons and balloon cells
- FCD III (associated with principal lesion)
    - Type IIIA: abnormal temporal cortical lamination associated with hippocampal sclerosis (HS)
    - Type IIIB: abnormal cortical lamination adjacent to a glial or glioneuronal tumor
    - Type IIIC: abnormal cortical lamination adjacent to a vascular malformation
    - Type IIID: abnormal cortical lamination adjacent to any other lesion acquired during early life (eg, trauma, ischemia, infection).

Note that should an FCD type II be associated with another lesion, it would not be considered a subgroup of FCD III but the association of two principal lesions. Also, it is proposed that by convention the use of the term "dual pathology" be restricted to cases of HS presenting with a second principal lesion of the brain (tumor, vascular malformation, glial scar, encephalitis, MCD including FCD type II), even outside the ipsilateral temporal lobe.

As is implicit in the classification, FCD are pathogenetically heterogeneous. FCD type II is characterized by monstrous cells and is assumed to be truly developmental (this is supported by the similarities between FCD type II and TSC brain lesions). The dysmorphic neurons may present with either a pyramidal or an interneuronal phenotype,[105] so that apparently the cellular dysplasia may affect different cellular lineages. The balloon cells are consistent with dysplastic glia,[105,106] which is the same lineage as the pyramidal dysmorphic neurons. White matter changes may be mild or severe, and have been related to a heterotopic distribution of dysplastic cells and neurons along the path of migration, a lack or loss of myelin, inflammation, oligodendrocytic satellitosis, and astrocytosis.[107] In the classification of MCD,[11] FCD type II accordingly is understood as a defect of proliferation/apoptosis. Moreover, there is some evidence that it could result from an excessive neurogenesis and retention of preplate cells in the late phases of late corticoneurogenetic (first half of second trimester).[108] FCD type I and mMCD are classified as organization disorders[11]: abnormal retention of the radial cortical pattern, lack of tangential lamination, and giant and immature neurons may relate to a true dysplasia or to a disruption of the normal cortical development occurring as late as during the neonatal period.[98–104]

Imaging of FCD

In clinical situations, FCD is the most difficult MCD to diagnose with MR imaging. Various strategies have been suggested over the years to improve the detection rate of the lesion using MR, electroclinical data, and complementary functional/metabolic imaging modalities.[49,58,59,109–115] As a rule, the less severe the dysplastic changes, the more likely the MR is to appear normal.[116] The diagnostic efficacy obviously depends on better equipment (high magnetic fields, multiple phased array coils) and greater expertise of the neuroradiologist.

FCD type II presents the most characteristic appearances (**Figs. 4–8**)[22]: an increased cortical thickness with a blurring of the cortical-subcortical junction (see **Fig. 4**); a high T2/FLAIR signal of the cortex; a low T1, high T2/FLAIR signal in the subcortical white matter (see **Fig. 5**), sometimes tapering from the cortex to the ventricular wall, so reproducing the migration path (this "transmantle dysplasia" is practically pathognomonic of a FCD type IIB[117]) (see **Fig. 6**). The lesion may be small, sulcal, centered at the very bottom of a sulcus that is deeper than its contralateral

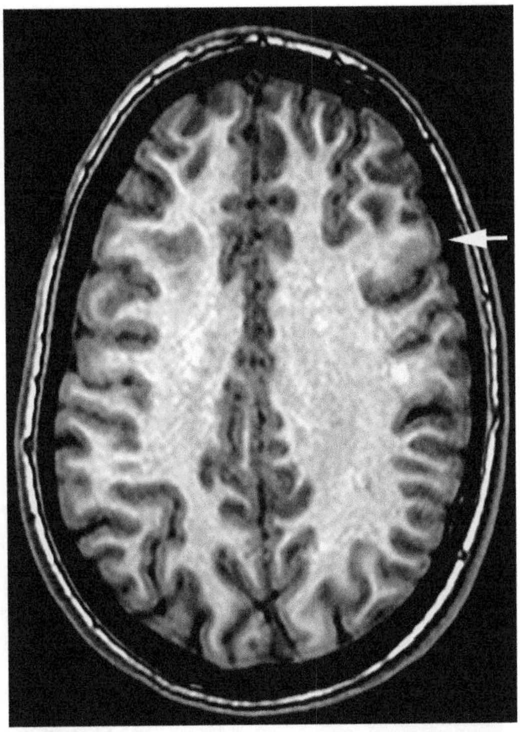

Fig. 4. Left frontal FCD II. T1 high-definition image demonstrates a cortical thickening with cortical-subcortical blurring on the sulcal side of the gyrus (*arrow*).

counterpart[118]; there it may appear as a focal, strictly cortical clear-cut bright T1 signal (see **Fig. 7**). The lesion may extend along the walls of the sulcus, or may affect the crown of the gyrus, or the whole gyrus between 2 sulci; the gyrus then may be somewhat bulky. It may uncommonly mimic a tuber (see **Fig. 8**). Large FCD type II may also be multigyral or lobar, usually with an abnormal gyration pattern. It may rarely also be multiple, unilateral or bilateral.[119] When large FCD type II lesions are so large as to occupy a large part of the hemisphere, they are referred to as partial, or lobar, hemimegalencephalies (HME). FCD type IIB presents only rarely without any MR abnormalities (4%); this occurs more often with FCD type IIA (22%).[116] However, as mentioned earlier, a normal-appearing white matter may reflect mild pathologic changes[107] with increased diffusivity and decreased fat attenuation only.[39,112,120]

FCD type I, when typical, is different (**Figs. 9–11**). The main features are a diffusely bright T2/FLAIR signal of the white matter as compared with the other side, with a consequent loss of the gray/white contrast (often designated as a blurring of the gray-white junction, different from the progressive gradient of cellularity that is seen in

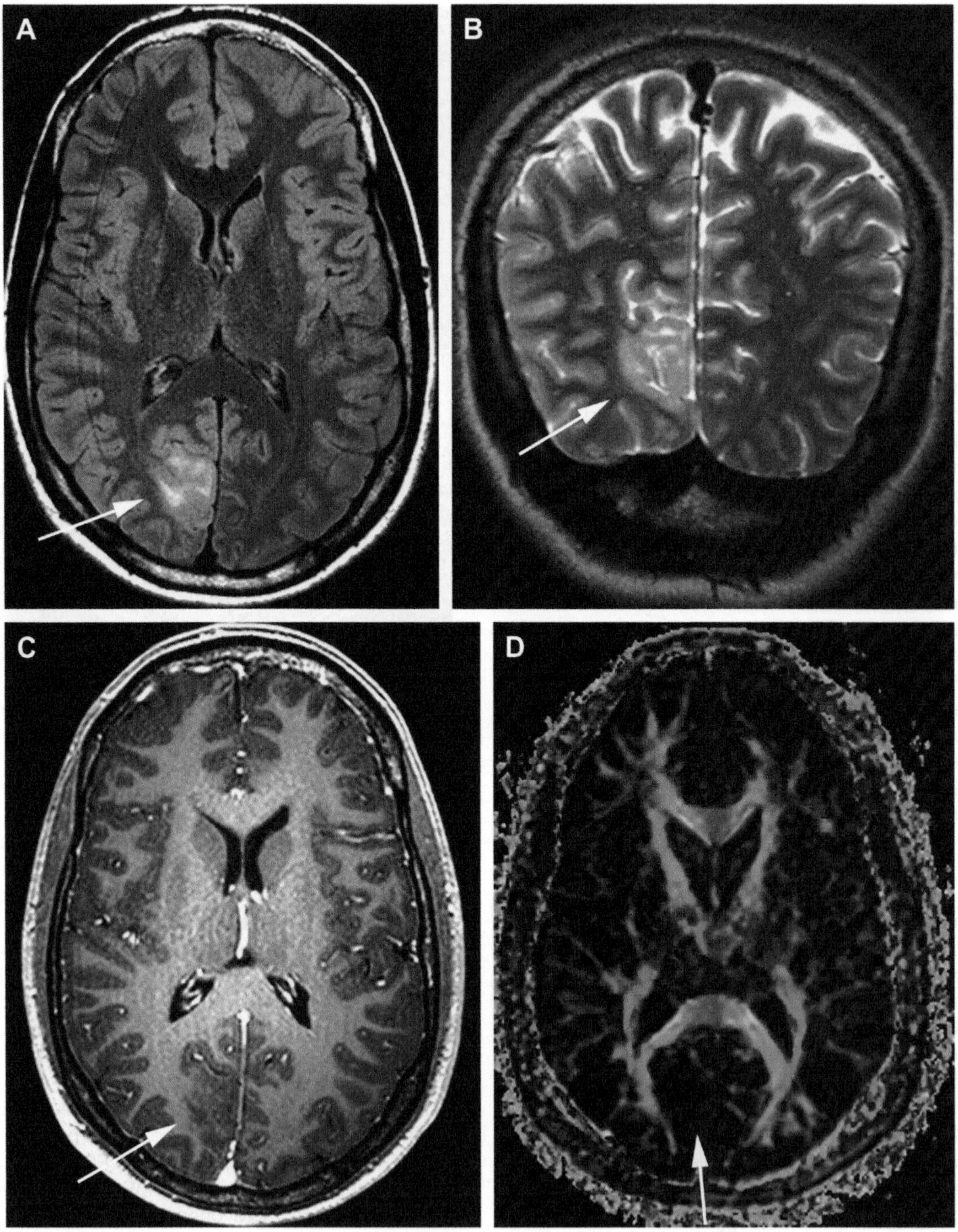

Fig. 5. Right occipital FCD II. (*A*) Bright FLAIR signal in the white matter and cortex of the cuneus (*arrow*). (*B*) Similarly bright signal on T2TSE (*arrow*). (*C*) Low T1 signal of the white matter blurring the cortico-subcortical junction (*arrow*); no contrast enhancement. (*D*) Fractional anisotropy (FA) color map demonstrates a lack of transverse fascicular organization in the white matter of the cuneus (*arrow*).

FCD type II) (see **Fig. 9**) and a smaller volume of the involved portion of the brain (this is more evident when it affects the temporal lobe). The lesion is usually extensive, and its limits are not clear: multilobar or hemispheric involvement are more common in FCD type I than in FCD type II,[116] with a more common cognitive impairment. The cortex may present a high T2/FLAIR signal, though less commonly than in FCD type II,[116] and a well-defined transmantle dysplasia is never

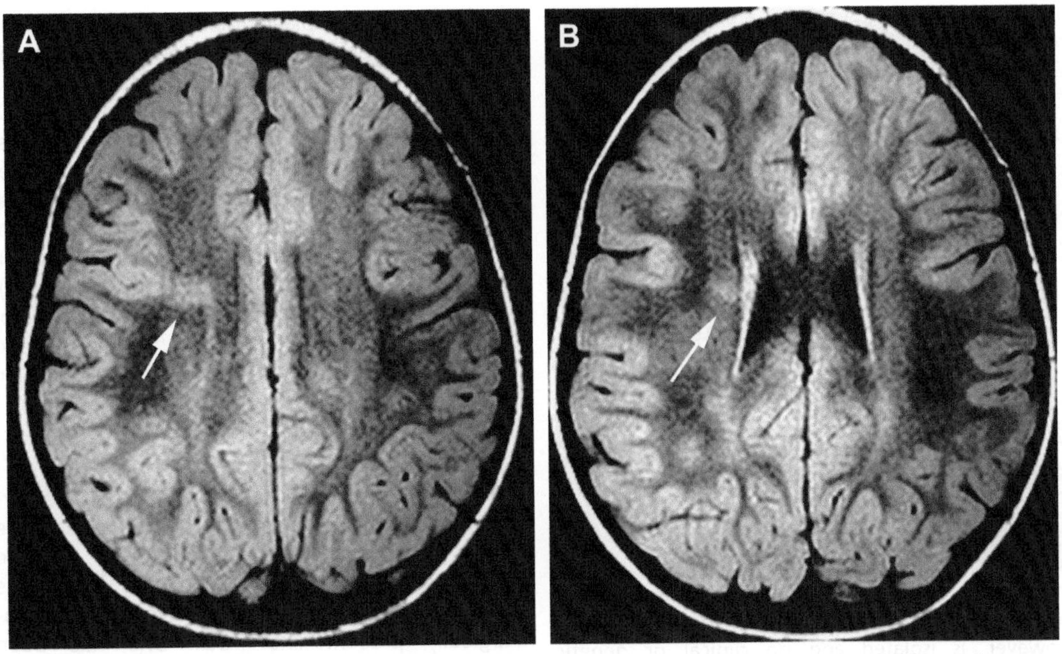

Fig. 6. Transmantle dysplasia (FCD IIB). (*A, B*) Axial FLAIR. There is cortico-subcortical blurring of the right precentral cortex with a streak of high FLAIR signal extending from the depth of the sulcus to the ventricular wall (*arrow*). This pattern is practically pathognomonic for FCD IIB (with balloon cells).

found in FCD type I. The brain may appear normal in 20% to 29% of the cases (see **Fig. 10**), which is not different from type IIA (22%). There is no way to differentiate the 3 subtypes of FCD type I.

FCD type III is characterized by the association of a FCD type I with a principal lesion adjacent to it[105] (**Figs. 12–16**), which may be a HS (FCD type IIIA) (see **Fig. 12**), a developmental tumor such

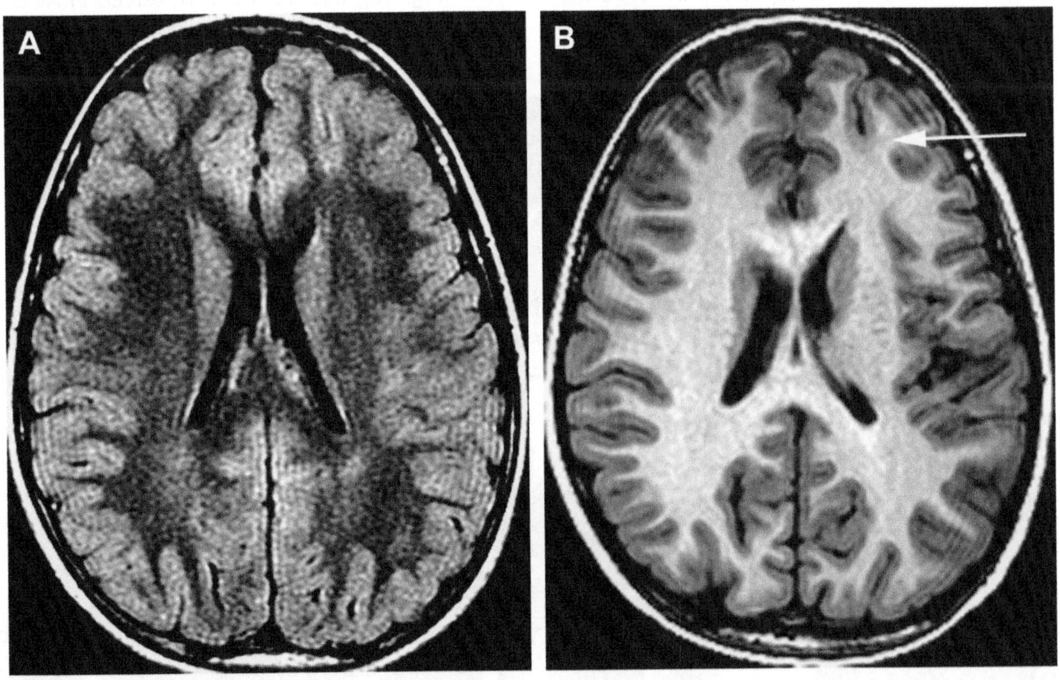

Fig. 7. Bottom-of-the-sulcus FCD II. (*A*) Axial FLAIR. The image is essentially unremarkable except that the superior frontal sulcus on the left side appears to be deeper than on the right side. (*B*) Thin T1 imaging demonstrates a bright T1 signal of the cortex in the bottom of this abnormal sulcus (*arrow*); this is highly suggestive of FCD II.

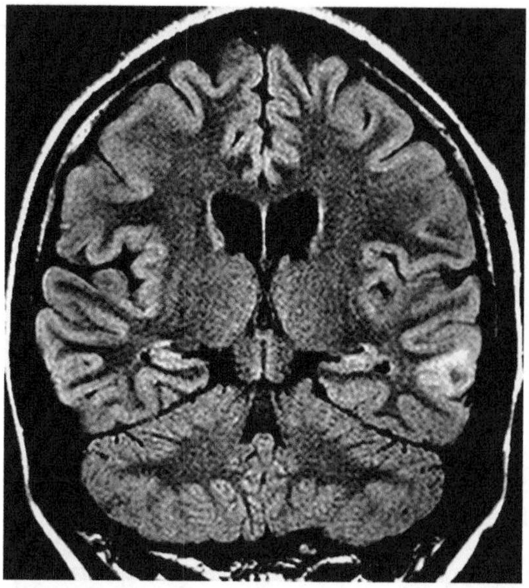

Fig. 8. Tuber-like FCD II. The appearance of the lesion would suggest a cortical tuber of TSC. The lesion, however, is isolated and no clinical or genetic evidence of TSC is found. Therefore, the name "forme fruste of TSC" is not appropriate.

as a DNET or a ganglioglioma (FCD type IIIB) (see **Fig. 13**), a vascular malformation such as a meningioangiomatosis or a cavernoma (FCD type IIIC) (see **Fig. 15**), or a destructive lesion such as an encephalomalacia or porencephaly (FCD type IIID) (see **Fig. 16**). Diffuse lesions that are not adjacent to the cortical dysplasia (periventricular leukomalacia, hydrocephalus, nonspecific atrophy, ventriculomegaly, and gliosis) are not uncommon and are associated mostly with FCD type I and mMCD.

mMCD (formerly cortical microdysgenesis) presents with normal MR more often than the other forms of cortical dysplasia (50%).[116] The most usual findings otherwise are a diffuse bright signal in the white matter effacing the contrast between gray and white, and a lobar hypoplasia (25%), which is usually not as extensive (multilobar or hemispheric) as in FCD type I[116] (**Figs. 17** and **18**). The cortex is never thick and never bright on T2/FLAIR.[116]

Other microdysgeneses

Besides the neuronal heterotopia that characterizes mMCD, other histologic abnormalities have been demonstrated in the cortex of epileptic patients, which are usually included as variants of microdysgenesis and may clinically and radiologically present like FCD. One has been described as a cortical perivascular satellitosis or perivascular clustering, in which the cortical vessels are surrounded by rounded neural cells, presumably oligodendrocytes.[121,122] Another one is characterized by unique cortical astrocytic inclusions in young patients who presented with developmental delay and seizures in the first year of life, with intracellular accumulation of Filamin A[123] (**Fig. 19**); this has been observed in Aicardi syndrome as well.[124] A last epileptogenic disorder

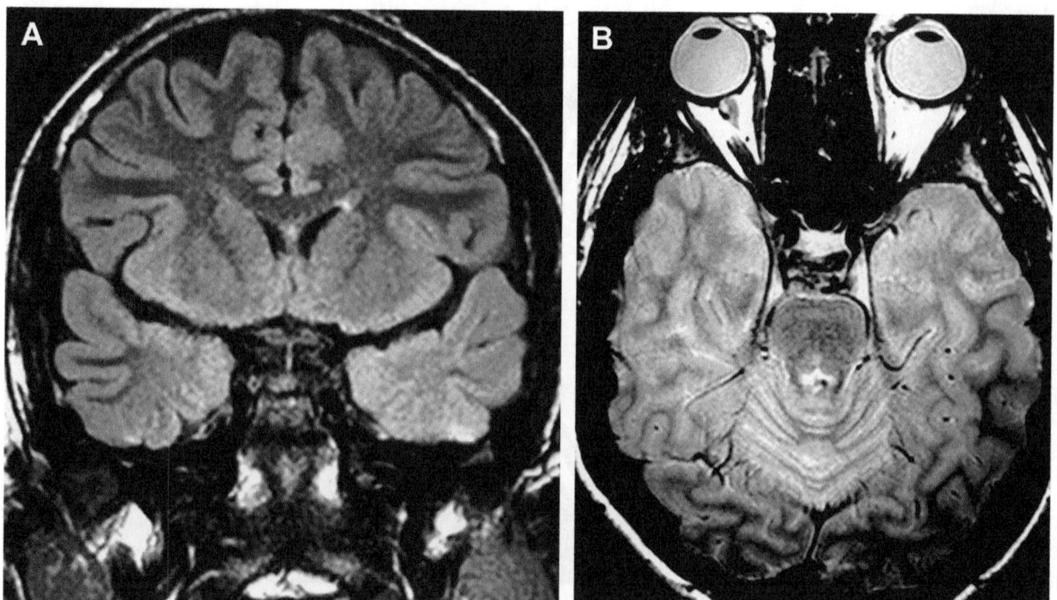

Fig. 9. Left temporal FCD I. (*A*) Coronal FLAIR. As compared with the right side, the gyral digitations of low signal appear effaced on the left. (*B*) This is also apparent on this axial PD image.

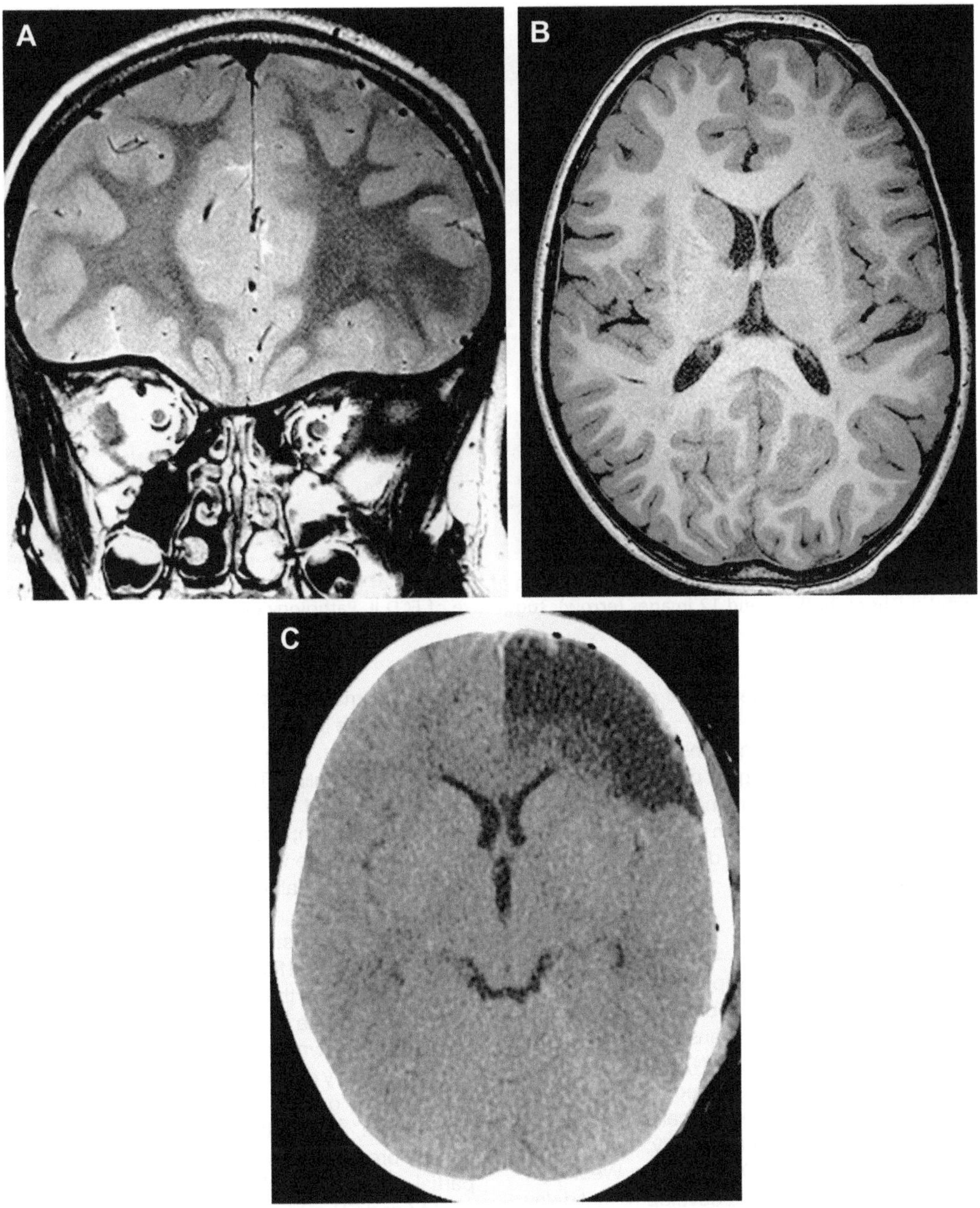

Fig. 10. FCD I, normal appearance. (*A*) Coronal PD. No abnormality was found in this patient who presents with a left frontal seizure focus. (*B*) Axial high-definition T1. No abnormality is found here either. (*C*) Postsurgical CT. The patient was operated on according to the MEG abnormalities, with large anterior frontal lobectomy. Pathology demonstrated diffuse abnormalities consistent with FCD I.

presenting like an FCD on MR imaging is oligodendroglial hyperplasia, which is an infiltration of the juxtacortical white matter by nonneoplastic oligodendrocytes (**Fig. 20**).[125]

The features to look for in the diagnosis of mMCD/FCD are summarized as follows:

- The cortical thickness, the gradual cortical blurring, the excessive depth of a sulcus as compared with its contralateral homolog, the bright T1, T2, and FLAIR cortical signal changes, the focal, often wedge-shaped low T1, bright T2, and FLAIR T2

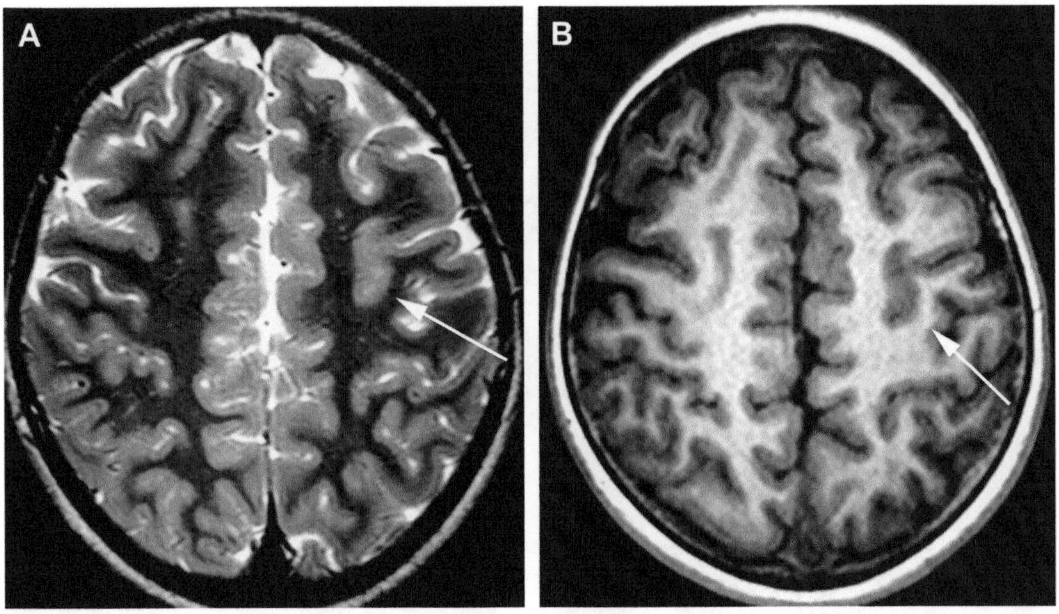

Fig. 11. FCD I. (*A, B*) Abnormal thickness and blurring of the cortex of the posterior segment of the left superior frontal sulcus on both T1 and T2 images (*arrow*), suggestive of FCD II. Pathology disclosed an FCD I, however.

signal of the white matter all suggest an FCD type II

- A normal cortical thickness, a diffusely (eg, lobar) increased signal of the white matter on T2/FLAIR, and a smaller lobe or smaller hemisphere suggest an mMCD or FCD type I
- A normal MR image does not exclude an FCD.

Hemimegalencephaly

HME is considered a hemispheric variety of FCD type II. The malformation is unilateral, characterized by the asymmetric expansion of all or most of the hemisphere (**Figs. 21–24**). Although a right predominance has been reported,[126] either hemisphere may be affected. The clinical picture associates an asymmetric macrocephaly; early onset, severe epilepsy (often Ohtahara or West syndrome); a unilateral deficit; a developmental delay; and a poor functional and vital prognosis.[126–128] The only possible treatment is an anatomic or functional hemispherectomy.[128] There are 3 groups of HME, all sporadic (except for NF1): the isolated HME (restricted to the hypertrophic/dysplastic hemisphere), the syndromic HME in which the malformation is part of a neuroectodermal syndrome (epidermal nevus/linear nevus sebaceous; hypomelanosis of Ito; Proteus; Klippel-Trénaunay; NF1; TSC) (see **Fig. 24**), and the total HME in which the ipsilateral half of the brainstem and cerebellar hemisphere are augmented as well.[126–130] The pathology, imaging, and clinical features are essentially the same in all 3 groups.

Histologically, the abnormalities are both neuronal and glial. The cortex is dislaminated with a blurring of the gray-white junction and an abnormal gyration; giant neurons are scattered in the cortex and the white matter; the glia is hypertrophic and glial balloon cells also are distributed in cortex and white matter; the hypertrophic white matter may demonstrate demyelination with association of Rosenthal fibers.[127,131] The abnormalities are so widespread that the lesion has been considered a hamartoma or a tumor.[127,131] The origin of HME is not known, and has been proposed to be an early primary disorder of neuroepithelial lineage and cellular growth with secondary migratory disturbance,[132] or on the contrary an overproliferation of progenitor cells in later cell cycles, with partial failure of postneurogenesis apoptosis in the MZ and SP.[133]

Imaging of HME rests on MR and, to a lesser extent, CT. The appearance of the brain may be very different in different patients: sometimes large but morphologically close to normal, sometimes grossly dysmorphic (see **Figs. 21–24**). The hemispheric involvement also may be only partial, either anterior or, more commonly, posterior (see **Figs. 21** and **22**).[134] The main radiological features are as follows.

- Asymmetry between the hemispheres, the large one sometimes being grossly dysmorphic. The occipital lobe may be so

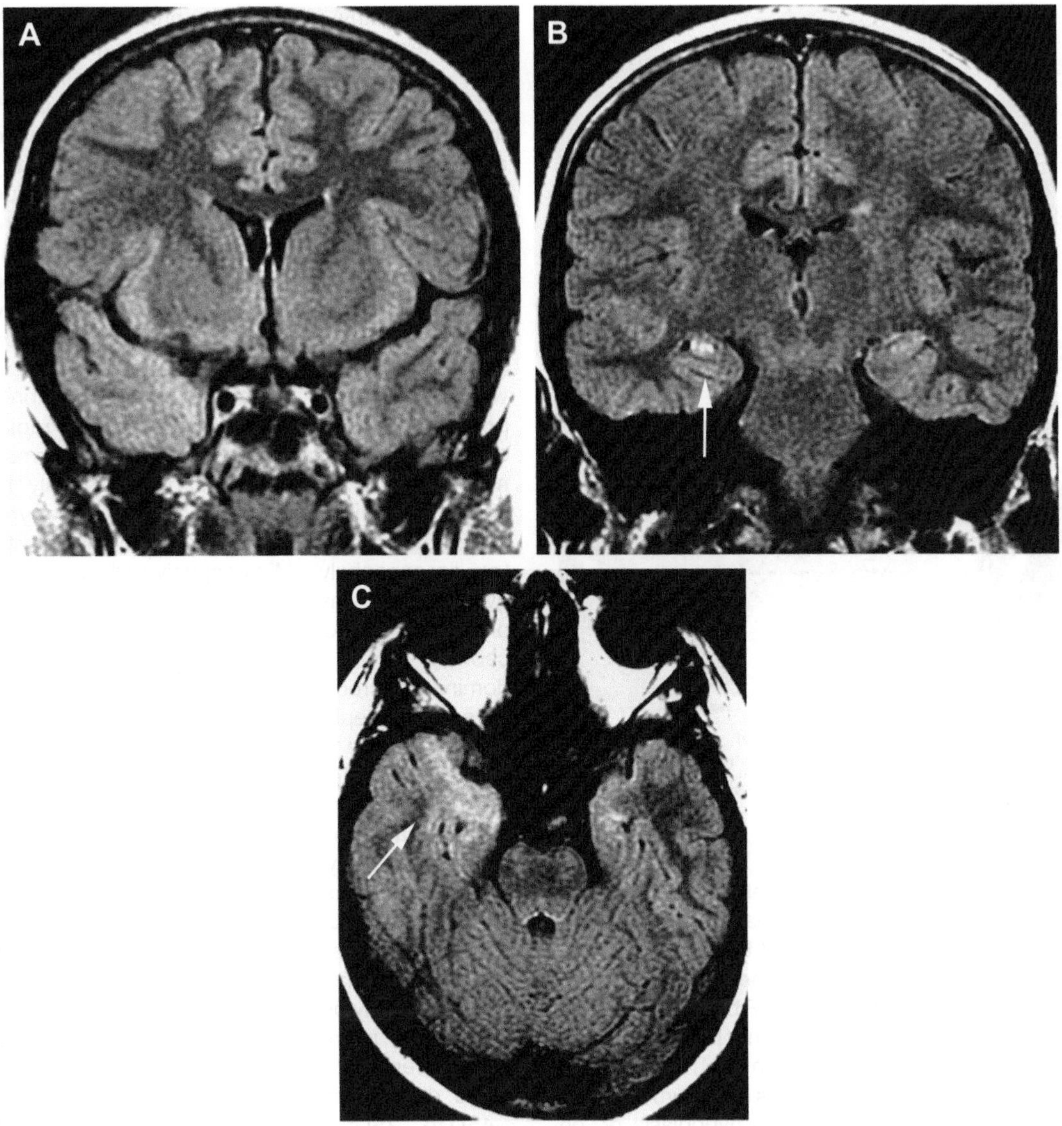

Fig. 12. FCD IIIA. (*A*) Coronal FLAIR. The normal low signal of the anterior temporal white matter is lost on the right side. (*B*) Coronal FLAIR. This posterior coronal image demonstrates a bright signal and atrophy of the right hippocampus (*arrow*). This association of hippocampal sclerosis and adjacent likely FCD of the temporal lobe characterizes FCD IIIA. (*C*) Axial FLAIR. Ill-demarcated bright signal of the anteromedial temporal pole (*arrow*).

disproportionately prominent as to be displaced with the falx across the midline toward the other side. It must be noted that in rare cases, the large hemisphere may develop atrophy, presumably because of the severe epilepsy with repeated episodes of status epilepticus.[135]

- The ipsilateral ventricle is typically enlarged (see **Figs. 21** and **23**), although it may rarely be small. It is sometimes markedly deformed, due to poor organization of the hemisphere. The frontal horn may be straightened and even effaced, presumably because of abnormal adjacent white matter tracts. The atrium may be colpocephalic.
- The gyral pattern is abnormal, often with shallow sulci, and may associate areas that resemble lissencephaly, pachygyria, and/or PMG (see **Figs. 21**, **22**, and **24**). Gray matter heterotopias also are common. The cortical ribbon usually is thick with a blurred cortico-subcortical junction (see **Fig. 23**).

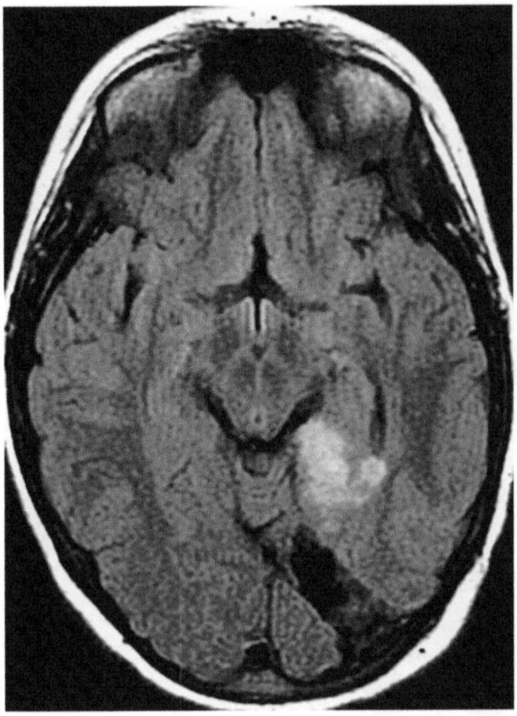

Fig. 13. FCD IIIB. Left posterior temporal DNET. Removal of the adjacent cortex disclosed an FCD. The association of a developmental tumor with adjacent FCD defines the FCD IIIB.

- The white matter is typically hypertrophied. In infants it may show early myelination,[136] presumably an effect of the seizure activity. On the contrary, in older children it may remain bright on T2/FLAIR because of absent or incomplete myelination. If looked for, calcification is not uncommon on CT, presumably dystrophic. The corpus callosum may be dysmorphic, with partial hypoplasia or, on the contrary, prominent. The septum pellucidum may be dislocated toward the abnormal frontal lobe and abnormally thick, which has been related to an abnormal fascicle of white matter (see **Fig. 22**).[137,138] The ipsilateral olfactory and optic nerves (which are truly white matter) may also be enlarged in a significant number of cases.[139]
- The contralateral hemisphere is insufficiently developed in patients with HME.[133]

DISORDERS OF PROLIFERATION/APOPTOSIS: MICROCEPHALY, MACROCEPHALY

Microcephaly

Terminology

Microcephaly describes a small head, which may be due to a destructive process (hypoxic-ischemic encephalopathy), a disruptive process (TORCH), a degenerative process, or a primary malformation. Over the last decades, the evolving terminology introduced to clarify the concept of primary malformation has resulted in some confusion. Among the attempts at finding a proper name was the early introduction of the term "microcephalia vera" (true microcephaly) to stress the developmental nature of the abnormality against any instance of prenatally or postnatally acquired microcephaly. The term "microencephaly" instead of microcephaly was meant to make it clear that it was the brain (encephalon) that was too small, not the head; it was not retained. "Radial microbrain" was proposed to express the fact that it was the radial expansion of the brain that was primarily abnormal, not so much its shape, and "microlissencephaly" to stress the importance of the simplified gyral pattern, leading, however, to some confusion with true lissencephaly. "Microcephaly with simplified gyral pattern" was then suggested, but is now replaced with "autosomal recessive primary microcephaly" (MCPH) (OMIM #251200), "autosomal dominant microcephaly" (OMIM #156580), and "X-linked microcephaly" (OMIM #309500).[140] These terms describe conditions in which the microcephaly is isolated, as opposed to the syndromic microcephalies in which the small brain is part of a constellation of features.[140,141] Finally, the use of term "primary microcephaly" should be restricted to the cases in which the small size of the brain is the principal abnormality: this restriction eliminates the instances of small brains that result from another malformation such as, for example, a lissencephaly or a holoprosencephaly.

Clinically, microcephaly is defined by a head circumference at −3SD below the mean (there is some disagreement, and the mark varies from −4SD to −2SD). The body height and weight must be close to normal and if less, not in proportion to the microcephaly. Children present with a stable mental retardation, mostly affecting speech but allowing for the majority of self-care. There should be no spasticity, but seizures may occur.[142] From a neuropathological point of view, descriptions are scarce and do not help in the definition of the disease: the cerebral hemispheres are small and the convolutional pattern is simplified; this seems related to a poorly expanded cortex and white matter while the central gray matter is better preserved; the cerebellum may or may not be involved; there may be minor abnormalities of the cortical architecture, such as a retained columnar arrangement and occasional heterotopia.[2] The genetics are better known. Eight loci of MCPH have been identified.[143] Mutations in the gene *ASPM* (on MCPH5, 1q31.3) account for 50% of cases and

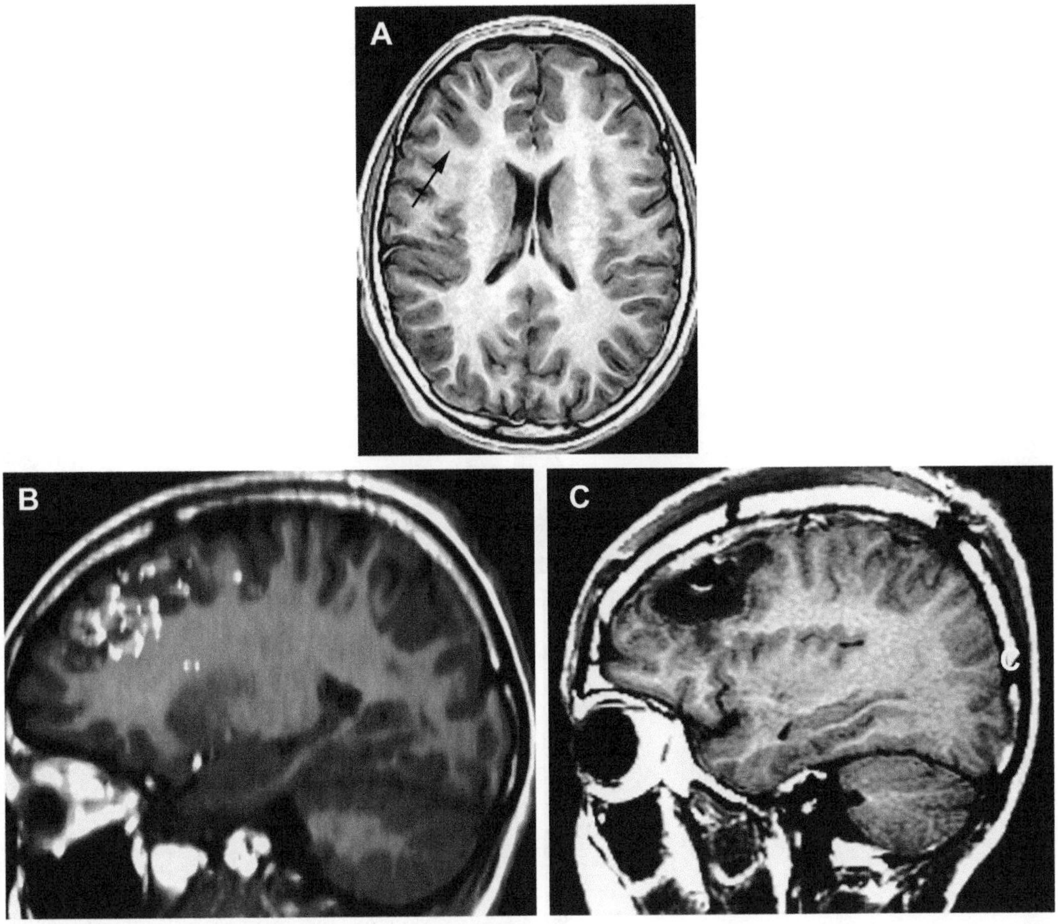

Fig. 14. FCD IIIB. (*A*) Axial high-definition T1. Thick cortex with cortico-subcortical blurring suggests FCD II (*arrow*). (*B*) MEG demonstrates an extensive epileptogenic zone. (*C*) Large frontal corticectomy. In addition to a FCD II corresponding to the abnormal cortex shown by imaging, pathology demonstrated extensive adjacent cortical changes consistent with FCD I.

mutations of MCPH2 (gene not identified) for 10%.[143] Other genes identified are *microcephalin* on MCPH1 (8p23), involved in DNA damage repair; *CDK5RAP2* on MCPH3 (9q33.2), *CENPJ/CPAP* on MCPH6 (13q12.12), and *STIL/SIL* on MCPH7 (1p33). These genes are all involved, like *ASPM* on MCPH5, in the processes of cellular mitosis.[143]

Pathogenesis

The malformation results from a disorder of brain growth. It has been observed by ultrasonography of microcephalic fetuses that the head measurements were normal until 20 weeks, while microcephaly was patent by 32 weeks and persisted afterwards.[142] Given this fact, and that the genes mutated are involved in the processes of cellular division of the radial glia and neuronal progenitors, it is assumed that the primary cause is an insufficient neurogenesis. As most of the brain growth is due to the connectivity, and therefore to the multiplication of the axonal branching within the cortex, a defective pool of neurons would result in a defective tangential growth of the cortex (less gyrus formation) and in a reduced volume of the white matter, while the cortical thickness would be grossly unchanged.

Imaging

If the child presents the features of a syndrome of which microcephaly is a defining feature, brain imaging aims to assess the brain rather than make the diagnosis.

On the contrary, the main purpose of imaging the isolated microcephaly is to rule out what is not a primary microencephaly: acquired disorders include sequelae of prenatal brain infections, perinatal injury, or a degenerative disease. Malformations in which the microcephaly is prominent without being the defining feature, such as holoprosencephaly, classical or atypical lissencephaly,

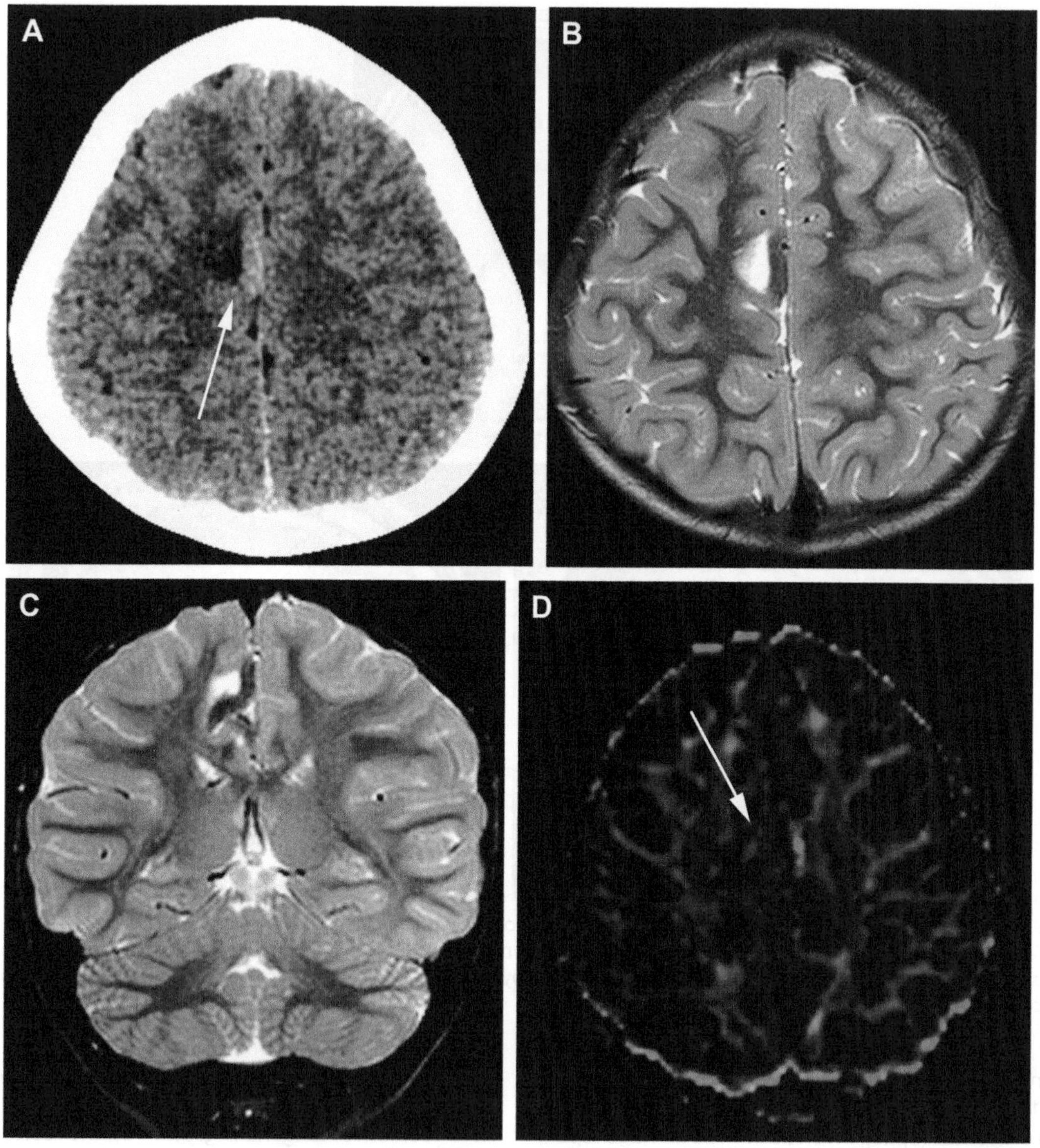

Fig. 15. FCD IIIC. Meningoangiomatosis. (*A*) Unenhanced CT. Small focal area of low attenuation with adjacent dense, likely calcified medial frontal cortex (*arrow*). (*B*) Axial T2. Demonstration of the corresponding MR image, with low signal of the calcified cortex and bright signal of the white matter. (*C*) Coronal T2. The lesion affects both the superior frontal and the cingulate gyri. (*D*) FA color mapping. The lack of parasagittal fibers of the cingulum in the lesion is demonstrated (*arrow*).

cobblestone cortex, polymicrogyria, or schizencephaly, should be excluded as well.

Once these diagnoses are ruled out the microcephaly is likely to be primary, therefore genetic. There are very few radiologic descriptions of MCPH, but in a recent study Adachi and colleagues[144] retrospectively analyzed a large series of 119 clinically diagnosed cases of presumably primary microcephaly. These investigators found that the gyral pattern could be considered as normal in 16 of 119 cases and severely abnormal in 27 of 119, and that the degree of severity globally reflected the severity of the microcephaly. The lack of volume of white matter also grossly correlated with the severity of the microcephaly. The corpus callosum was normal in 28 of 119 patients, thin in 59 of 119, and incomplete or absent in 26 of 119. These findings match the assumption that the disorder results from a deficient pool of neurons with a consequent lack of

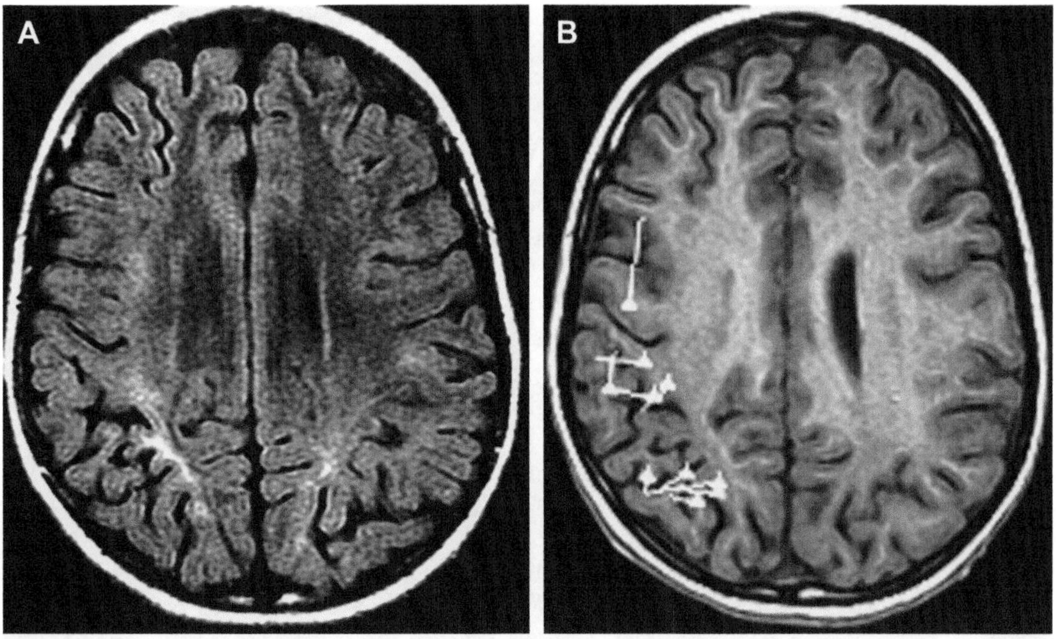

Fig. 16. FCD IIID (perinatal hypoglycemic injury). (*A*) Axial FLAIR. Bilateral parieto-occipital parasagittal bands of gliosis and ulegyria in a child who suffered from a severe hypoglycemia shortly after birth. (*B*) MEG demonstrated a unilateral, right-sided epileptogenic focus. The child was operated on and an FCD associated with the gliotic scar was demonstrated.

connectivity. Periventricular heterotopia was found in few cases (7/119); myelination was delayed in 32. The finding that the majority of patients have normal basal ganglia and thalami would suggest that in general, the pathogenesis of microcephaly relates to a disorder of the dorsal pallial germinal matrix. However, the finding that 30 of 119 patients present small basal ganglia and/or thalami may define a subgroup with a defect of the germinal matrix of the ganglionic eminence as well. Similarly, the fact that the cerebellum may be in proportion to the brain (45 cases), small relative to the brain (19 cases) or, on the contrary, large (54 cases), may also suggest different disease processes. No correlation with genetic studies could be done in this retrospective study, but the radiological phenotype of primary microcephaly appears somewhat heterogeneous (Figs. 25 and 26).[144]

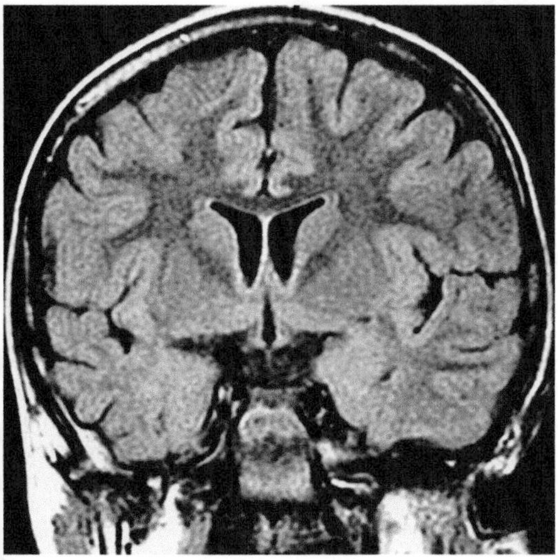

Fig. 17. mMCD (formerly microdysgenesis). This coronal FLAIR image demonstrates a loss of white matter signal in the temporal lobe and a small right hemisphere. After surgery, pathology disclosed mMCD (although the diffuse atrophy would rather suggest FCD I).

Besides the presentation of the classical "proportionate" microcephaly, a mention should be made of patients who come to MR with a diagnosis of developmental delay without a formal microcephaly, present a lack of white matter with ventriculomegaly and abnormal corpus callosum, and demonstrate a poor development of the anterior portion of the temporal lobes (this can be identified by drawing two lines along the superior and inferior borders of the temporal lobes: these line should be parallel—there is underdevelopment of the temporal lobes if they converge anteriorly).[145]

Macrocephaly/Megalencephaly Syndromes

There is no isolated primary megalencephaly, but megalencephaly may be a salient feature of many syndromes.[141,146] As a consequence, the

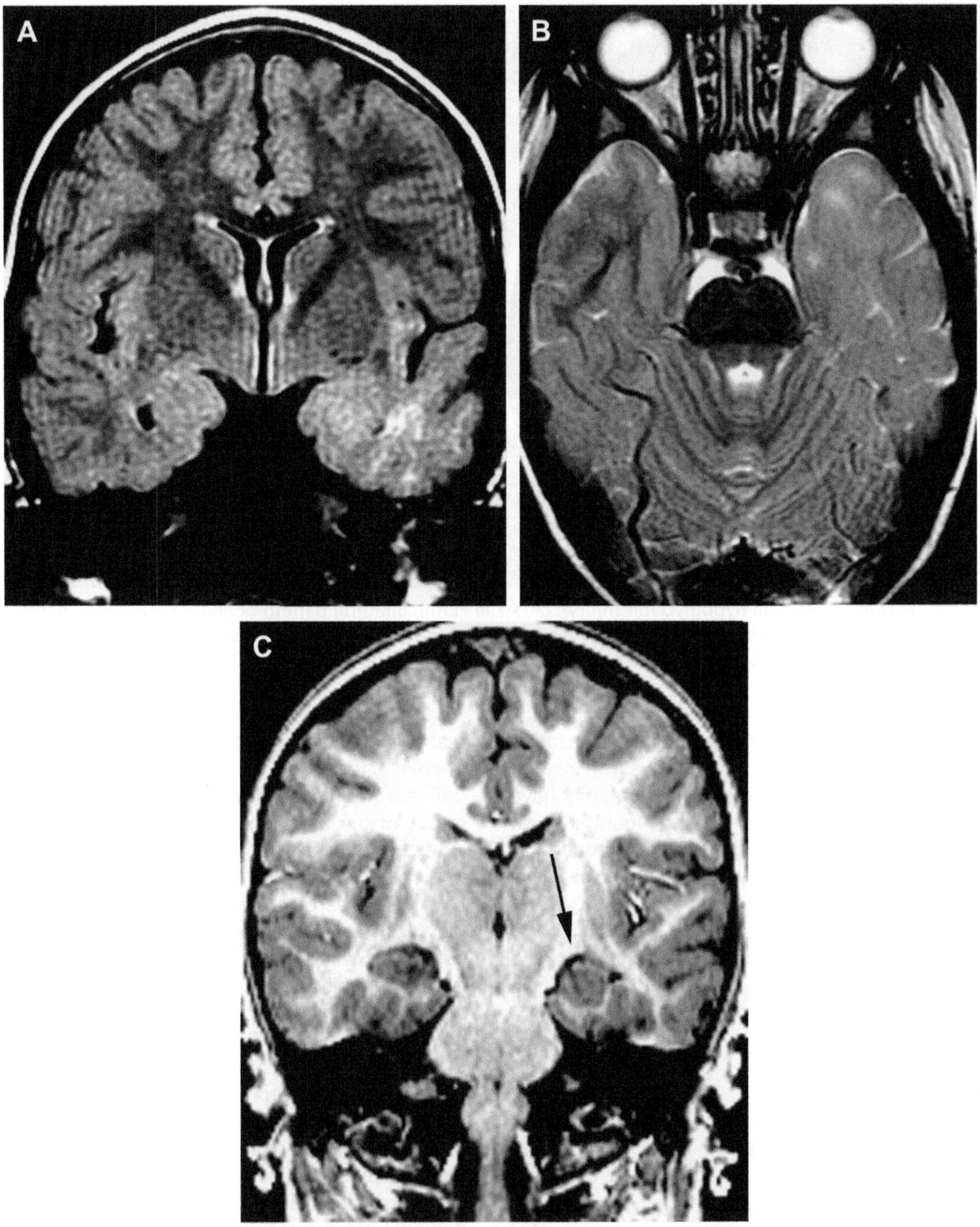

Fig. 18. mMCD (formerly microdysgenesis) associated with hippocampal dysplasia. (*A*) Coronal FLAIR demonstrates diffuse bright signal of the anterior left temporal lobe with some loss of volume. (*B*) Axial T2 demonstrates the diffuse loss of contrast between the cortex and the white matter in the left temporal lobe. (*C*) Coronal high-definition T1 demonstrates a rounded, bulky, dysplastic hippocampus (*arrow*). After surgery, pathology disclosed mMCD of the temporal lobe and dysplasia of the hippocampus.

role of imaging is either to rule out a nonmalformative cause for a macrocephaly without or with megalencephaly (thick calvarium and other skull bone dysplasia, hydrocephalus, metabolic diseases such as Alexander or Canavan, storage diseases), or to assess the brain in case of syndromic megalencephaly. The diagnosis of benign familial megalencephaly is made clinically because there is no neurologic or neurocognitive impairment. Clinically and pathologically, unilateral

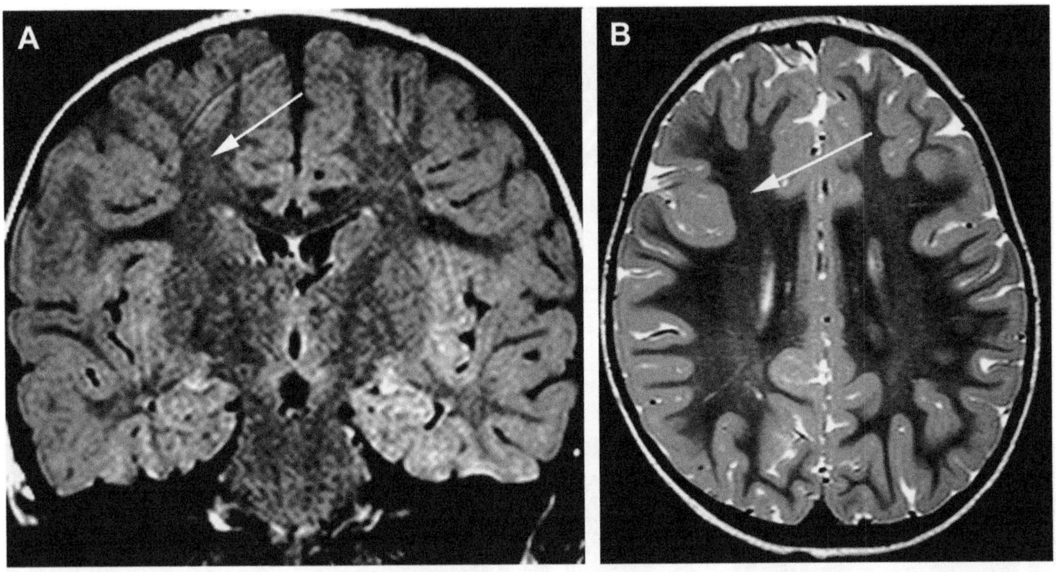

Fig. 19. Cortical dysplasia with astrocytic inclusion of filamin A. (*A, B*) Coronal FLAIR and axial T2 demonstrate an abnormal deep sulcation in the right lateral frontal lobe (*arrow*). Pathology demonstrated a dysplastic cortex and white matter, with astrocytic inclusions corresponding to intracellular accumulation of filamin A.

megalencephalies (hemimegalencephaly), either isolated or syndromic, belong to the group of the cortical dysplasia type II.

From a morphologic point of view, megalencephaly is defined by the head circumference being above 98% (+2SD), explained by the presence of a proportionately large brain parenchyma. Pathologically the volume of the brain is increased, with bulky gyri. The cerebellum typically is large (and may obliterate the foramen magnum, leading to the development of hydrosyringomyelia). The thickness of the cortex and the volume of the white matter are increased; the corpus callosum may be thick, or on the contrary thin or dysgenetic.[2] There is no clear evidence of histologic abnormality, although there has been some unconfirmed suggestion of hypercellularity.[2] It seems that the malformation would result from a true overproduction of brain cells, possibly related to a defect in the normal developmental process of apoptosis.[2]

Patients with syndromic megalencephaly present clinically with a large head already present before birth and persisting over the years. Patients may also demonstrate macrosomia, developmental delay, hypotonia, and an increased risk of developing a neoplastic disease.[146]

The radiologic abnormalities of the brain have been well described in Sotos syndrome only, the most common type of megalencephaly (**Fig. 27**). These findings associate a ventriculomegaly, a thin or defective corpus callosum, persistent midline cava (cava septi pellucidi, vergae and veli interpositi), macrocerebellum (possible cause of a Chiari I deformity), and occasional gray matter heterotopias.[147] Grossly, similar changes are mentioned in other syndromes, albeit with some specific features: a vermian hypoplasia in Simpson-Golabi-Behmel syndrome; prominent gray matter in relation to white matter (notably caudate) in the Fragile-X syndrome; hypervascularity in the Weaver syndrome; and interhemispheric and other arachnoid cysts in acrocallosal syndrome. By contrast, the brain is radiologically normal in the Bannayan-Ruvalcava-Riley syndrome.[146]

MIGRATION DISORDERS: LISSENCEPHALIES, BAND HETEROTOPIA, AND COBBLESTONE BRAIN

Although it is anything but simple, the migration process is easy to apprehend, and the concept of migration disorder is intuitively evident. The migration disorders or heterotopias are remarkable also in that many of them can be related to specific genetic defects, with a good correlation between phenotypes and genotypes. Depending on what they look like, heterotopias are described as laminar (also called band-heterotopia) or nodular; depending on where they sit, they are described as periventricular, transcerebral, subcortical, cortical, marginal (in molecular layer 1), and even extracortical meningeal (cobblestone brain). Histologically they may present a rudimentary laminar organization, with a cell-free zone

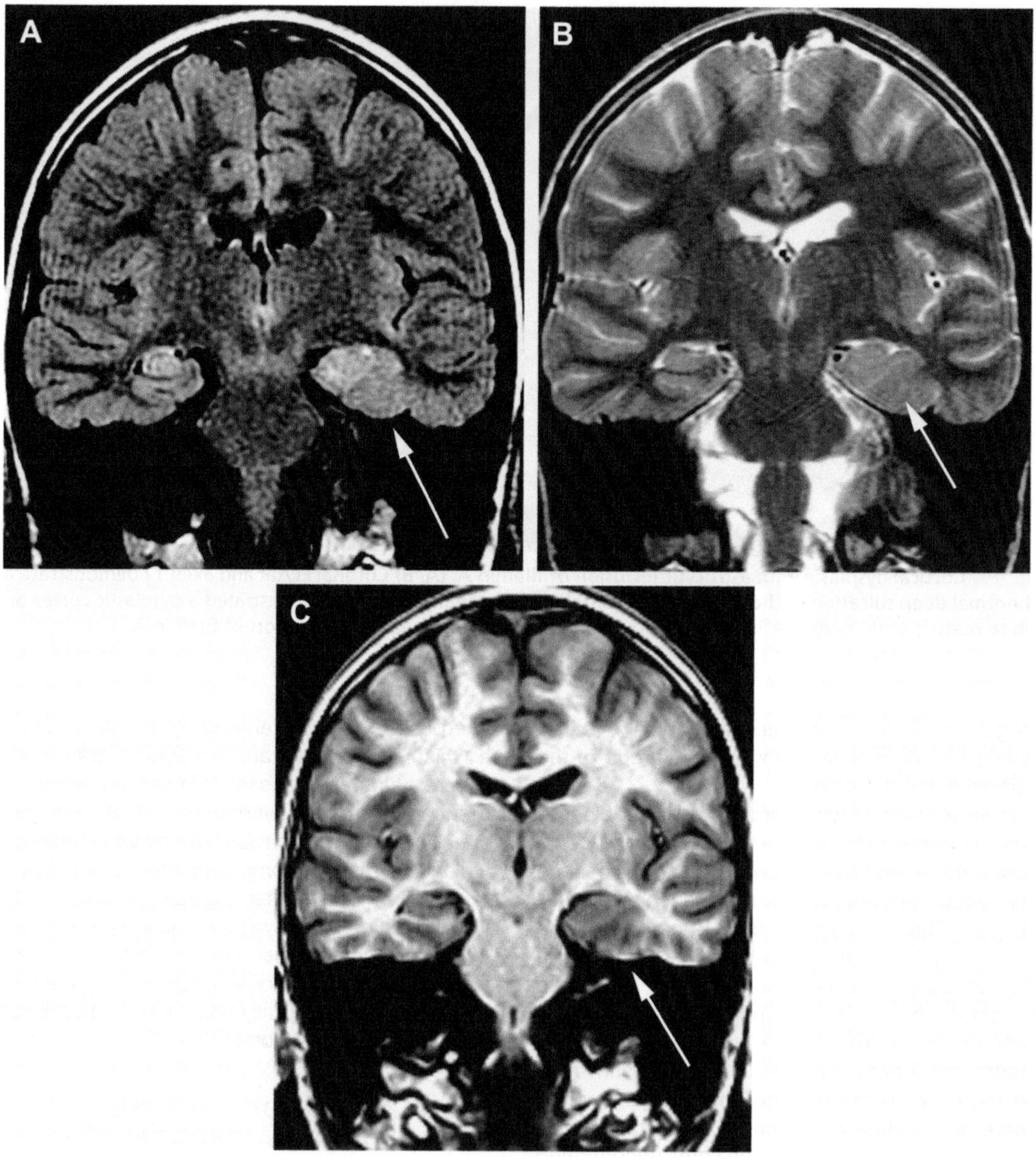

Fig. 20. Cortical dysplasia with oligodendroglial hyperplasia. (*A–C*) FLAIR, T2, and T1 coronal imaging demonstrate swelling of the left mesial temporal lobe with increased T2/FLAIR and decreased T1 signals of both cortex and white matter (*arrow*). Pathology demonstrated infiltration by nonneoplastic oligodendrocytes.

mimicking the molecular layer 1, and contain normal looking if typically disorganized pyramidal neurons and interneurons[148–150]; the architecture of the heterotopia, however, is usually different in different genetic disorders.

Heterotopias are functional and integrated in the neuronal functional loops[50,151–154]; they are typically easy to diagnose on MR imaging as nodules or band of otherwise normal-looking gray matter (identical to cortex in every sequence), located where they should not be. However, not all heterotopias can be seen radiologically: heterotopic neurons obviously, but also cortical or subpial heterotopias, and even the subcortical lentiform heterotopia found in the temporal lobes in association with FCD[105,155] cannot be identified with current clinical MR machines. Heterotopia due to undermigration (periventricular or subcortical) are caused by disorders, typically genetic, implicating genes that are involved in the homeostasis of the cellular microtubules[156] and therefore the nuclear translocation. Heterotopias due to

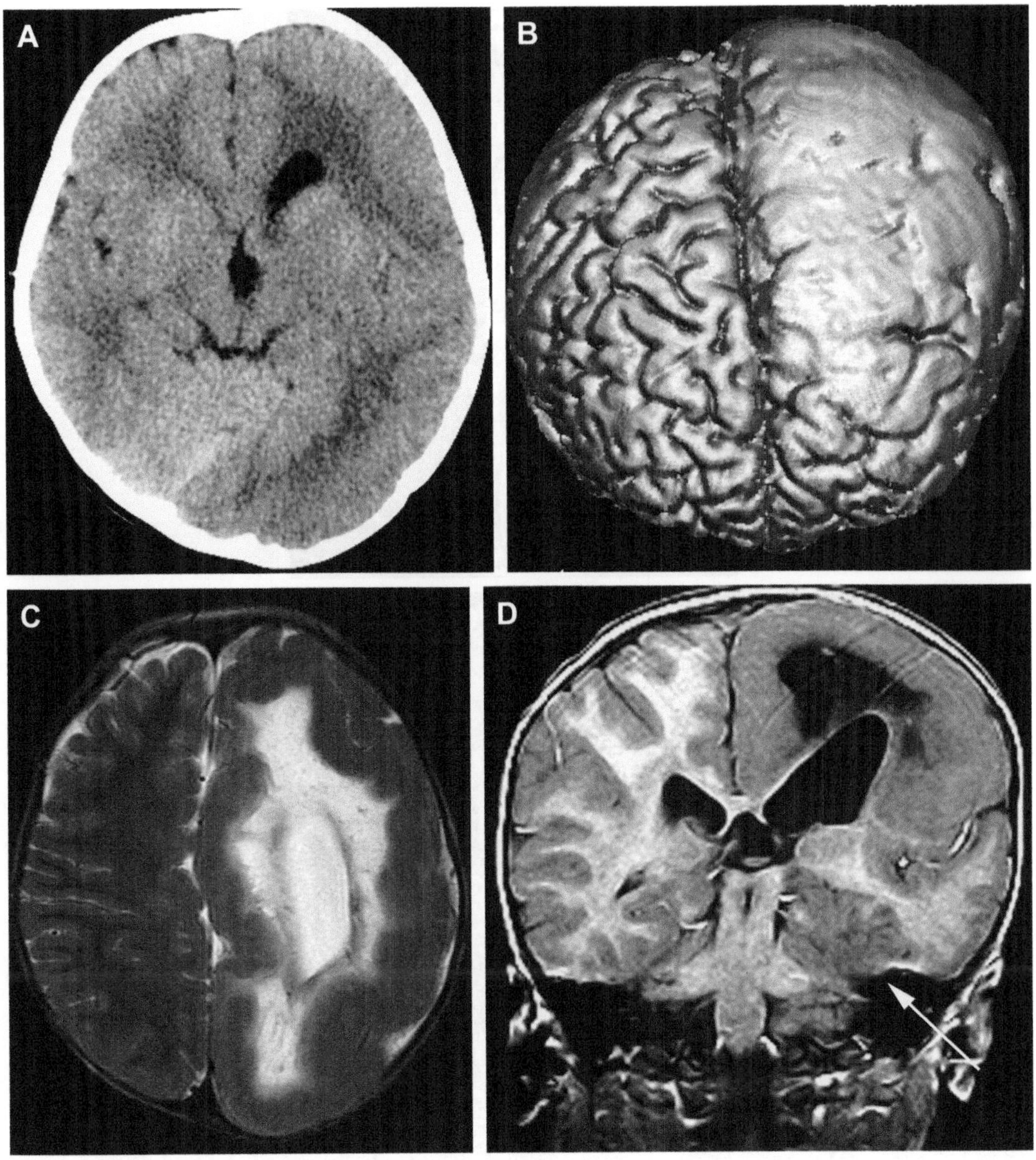

Fig. 21. Left HME. (*A*) CT image demonstrates a huge dysplastic left hemisphere with large ventricle and prominent occipital lobe. The posterior falx is dislocated to the right. (*B*) Tridimensional volume rendering shows the essentially agyric portion of the abnormal hemisphere. (*C*) Axial T2. Diffuse agyria with thick cortex and dysplastic, unmyelinated white matter; note the abnormal appearance of the right hemisphere as well, with straightening of the sulci in the rolandic area. (*D*) Coronal T1. Massive enlargement of the ventricle; the temporal lobe is relatively spared, but its medial aspect shows massive dysplasia (*arrow*).

overmigration, or an abnormal cortical layering, may be due to a defect of the reelin signaling or to defects in the pial basement membrane.

Lissencephalies

Lissencephalies have been known for a long time, and it was recognized that band heterotopia (or laminar heterotopia, or double cortex) are part of lissencephalies.[3] In the last two decades it has been demonstrated that most are related to specific gene defects,[157–159] discoveries that paved the way for further understanding of their pathogenesis.[160,161] All lissencephalies are characterized by an absence or a paucity of sulcation, and by a disorganized cortex with heterotopic gray matter that may appear as a thick cortex or as a subcortical-band heterotopia. In all, the white

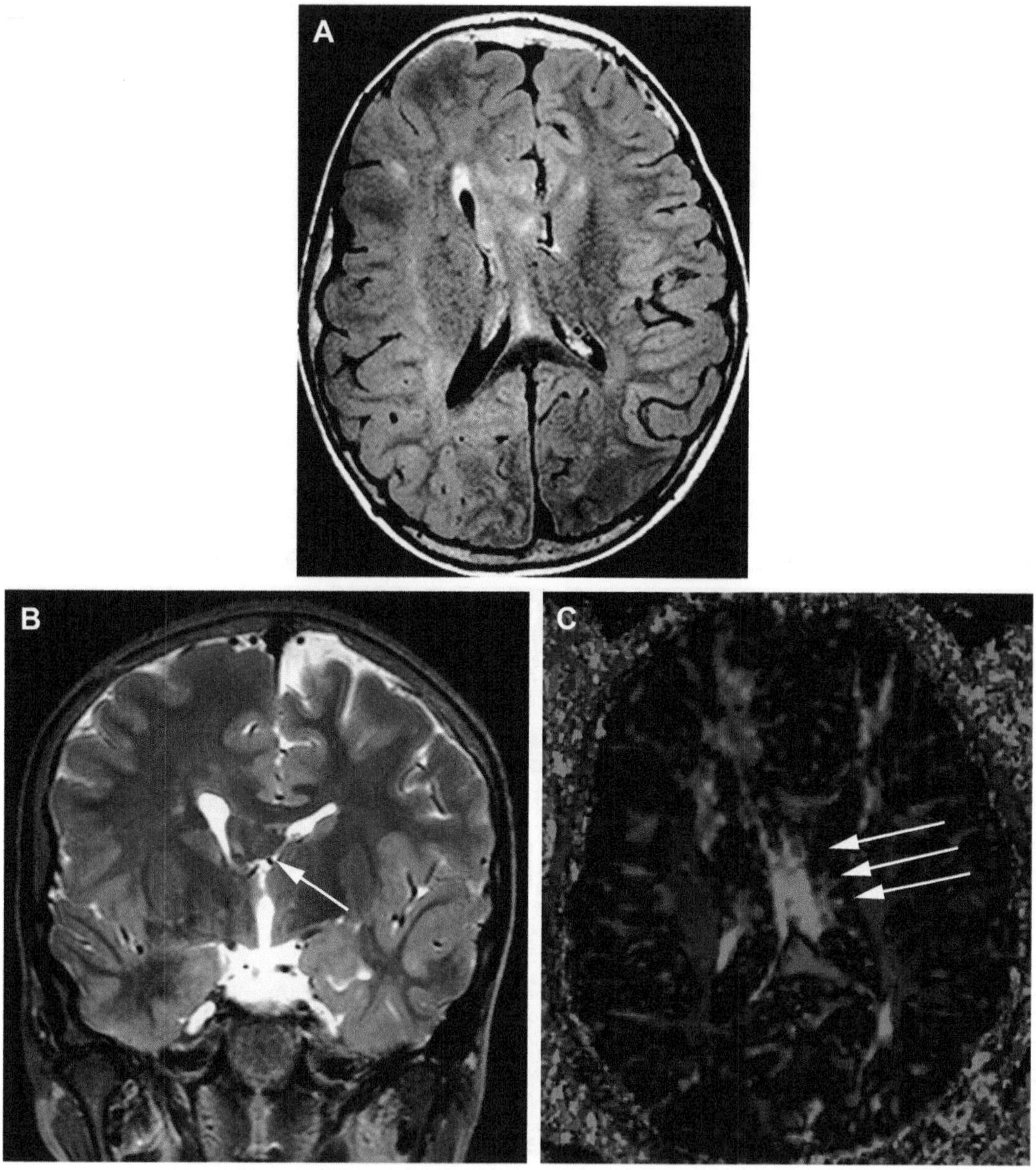

Fig. 22. Right anterior HME. (*A*) Axial FLAIR. Hypertrophy and dysplasia of the right hemisphere, predominantly its anterior portion; the signal of the white matter is heterogeneous; cortex appears thick over the whole lateral convexity, with poor gyration anteriorly; massive dysplasia of the septum pellucidum, which also appears "pulled" toward the abnormal right frontal lobe. (*B*) Coronal T2 better depicts the heterogeneous appearance of the hypertrophic septum pellucidum (*arrow*). (*C*) FA color mapping demonstrates that the septum pellucidum conveys a huge abnormal tract of white matter (*arrows*) that extends from the posterior left hemisphere to the anterior right HME.

matter is deficient as well, with a ventriculomegaly, usually a thinning of the commissures, and often a hypoplastic brainstem and cerebellum. Pathologically the cortical dysgenesis has been classified as being 4-layered (from the surface to the depth: molecular layer, cellular layer with neurons, cell-sparse layer, heterotopic layer with disorganized neurons), 3-layered (hypercellular molecular layer, no sparse cell layer), or 2-layered (molecular layer and single heterotopic layer), which correlates well with the different genetic defects identified.[162]

Classical lissencephaly (agyria, pachygyria, band heterotopia): LIS1, DCX

Clinically, patients with classical lissencephaly present during the first year of life with poor

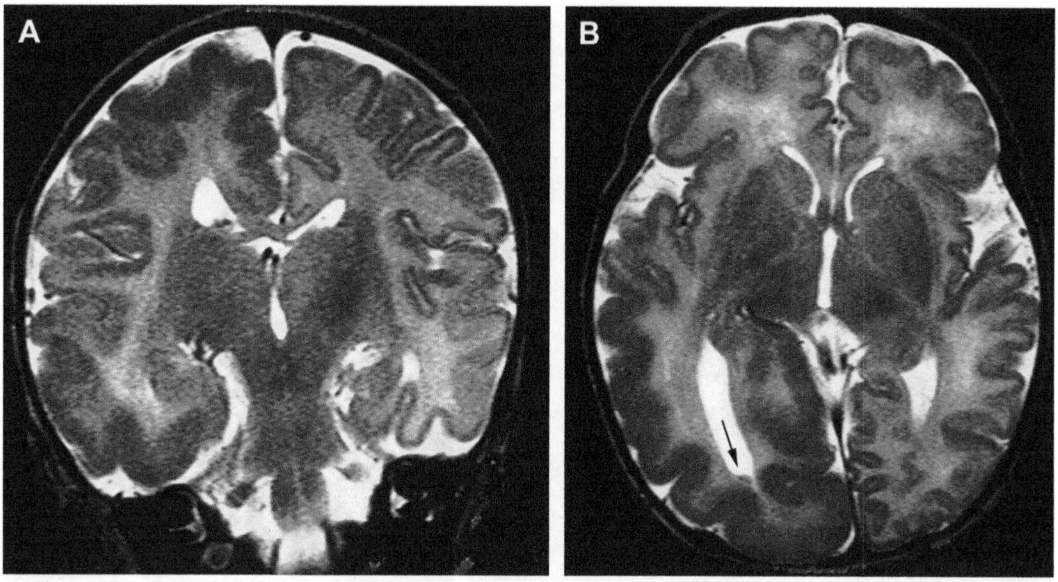

Fig. 23. Right HME in an infant. (*A, B*) In this 1-month-old infant, coronal and axial T2 demonstrate a large right hemisphere with large ventricle. Cortical abnormalities, predominantly posterior with dislocation of the falx, are characterized by a significant thickening of the cortical ribbon and diffuse blurring of the cortico-subcortical junction. Note the presence of a single periventricular nodular heterotopia (*arrow*).

feeding, hypotonia, opisthotonos, delayed acquisition of the developmental milestones, and epilepsy (often and characteristically infantile spasms). Depending on the severity of the malformation, however, the clinical manifestations may be milder.

Morphologically and radiologically, classical lissencephaly is characterized by the complete or partial lack or gyration, and by an excessively thick cortex (**Figs. 28–30**). The sulci are totally absent in agyria and the sylvian fissure widely open with no operculation. When present (pachygyria) the sulci are few, shallow, but are normal sulci symmetrically placed in normal locations, and can be designated by their specific names (mostly primary and main secondary sulci) (see **Fig. 29**). The cortex is very thick, up to 12 to 20 mm in complete agyria and 8 to 10 mm in pachygyria (see **Figs. 28–30**). Macroscopically the classical lissencephalic cortex presents a 4-layer organization. Its deep border is smooth and regular, well demarcated from the white matter. This cortical band does not follow the cortical pattern but rather is deeply indented by the sulci. This excessive thickness of the cortex is the cardinal feature of classical lissencephaly, which allows the MR-recognition of the disorder even in young fetuses, and makes the difference from the simplified gyral pattern of the primary microcephaly, in which the cortex is of normal or of decreased thickness. In the lesser form of classical lissencephaly, the subcortical-band heterotopia (also called laminar heterotopia, or double cortex—hence the name of doublecortin for the *DCX* gene product), the bilateral and symmetric band of heterotopic gray matter is clearly separate from an apparently normal cortical ribbon, with a more or less normal gyral pattern (**Figs. 31** and **32**).

In addition, other abnormalities are found. The white matter is not well developed and the defect correlates with the severity of the cortical malformation (ie, more severe in agyria, less severe in band heterotopia); this is apparent from the ventriculomegaly and from the appearance of the commissures, which typically are thin, although the corpus callosum may appear, paradoxically, too thick in some cases.[163–165] There is no comprehensive explanation given for this lack of white matter.[163,165] Both the molecular layer 1 and the abnormal intermediate layer 3 contain tangential fibers with presumably short-range connections. One may assume that because the neurons are dislocated and disorganized, the proper connections to and from the subpallium and with the long association and commissural fibers may fail; the location of the heterotopic layer 4 may interfere with the development, organization, and function of the subplate itself. Typically the brainstem is small also, which reflects a poor development of both the intrinsic gray matter and the long fascicles. The cerebellum may be hypoplastic, but this finding by itself is not specific or necessarily

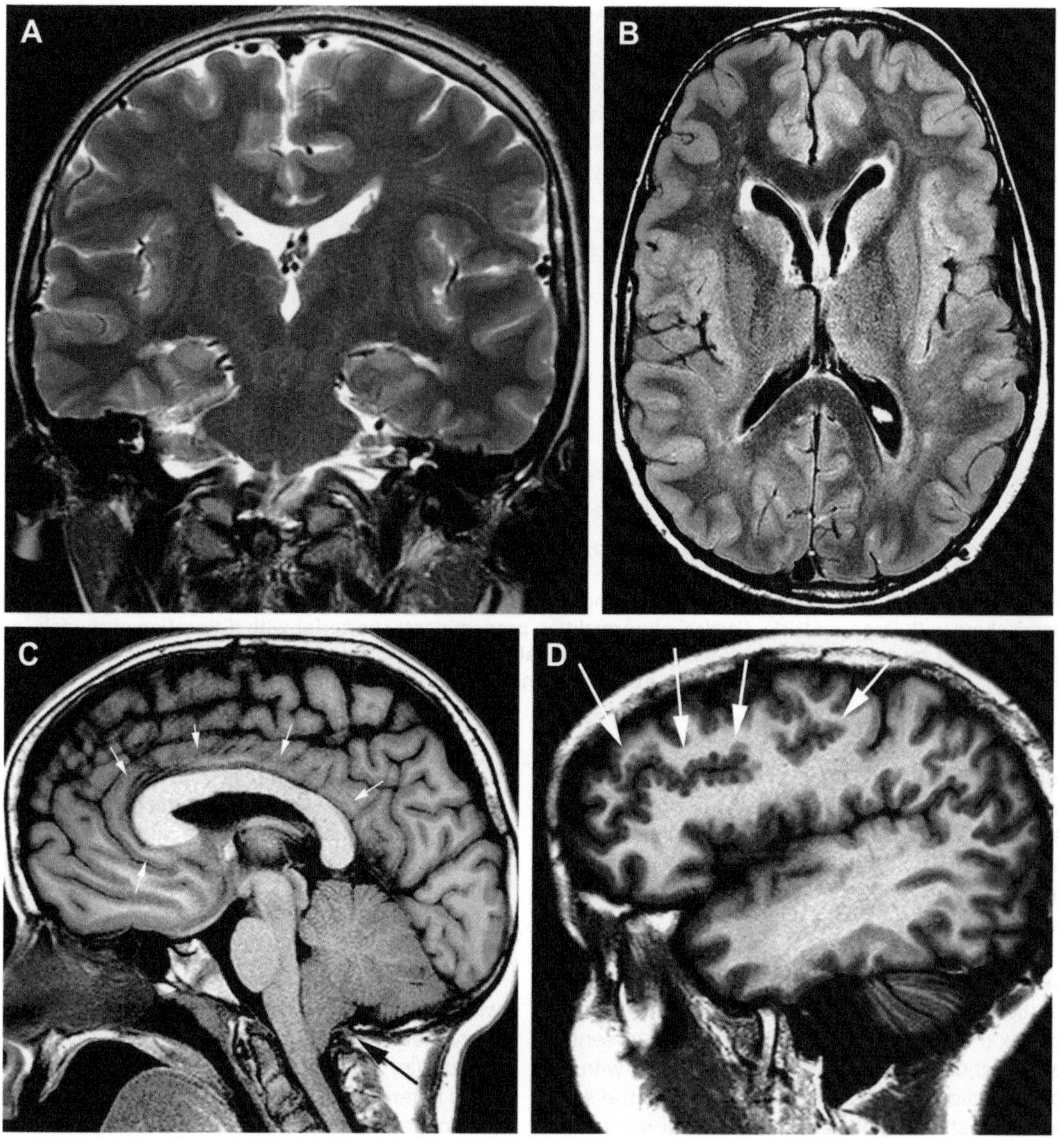

Fig. 24. Left HME, Proteus syndrome. (*A*) Coronal T2. Mild hypertrophy of left hemisphere with dysplasia of the mesial temporal lobe; prominent and ill-shaped ventricles bilaterally. (*B*) Axial FLAIR. Heterogeneous signal in the white matter and periventricular bright signals, bilaterally; note a prominent vessel in the scalp over the left parietal area. (*C*) Midline sagittal T1 demonstrates prominent corpus callosum (*white arrows*) and a Chiari I deformity (*black arrow*). (*D*) Left lateral sagittal cut demonstrates a "curly," polymicrogyric appearance of the cortex (*white arrows*) along the otherwise normally located inferior frontal gyrus.

significant in a context of lissencephaly.[166] Good correlation, however, was found between the severity of the supratentorial abnormalities and the defects of the midbrain and hindbrain, and between the callosal agenesis and the vermian hypoplasia; posterior fossa defects were more common in DCX lissencephaly (for details see Ref.[167]).

Beyond the similarities, and importantly, the appearances of the brain are different morphologically, radiologically, and neuropathologically, depending on whether the malformation results from a mutation of *LIS1* or of *DCX*.[168] In the LIS1 lissencephaly (17p13.3) and except in the rare form of complete agyria, the abnormalities are more prominent in the posterior portion of the hemisphere, more agyric posteriorly and more pachygyric anteriorly. In cases of band heterotopias the band is located posteriorly below the parieto-occipital and posterior temporal cortex; this pattern is observed mostly in males (see **Figs. 29** and **31**).[169] On the contrary, the

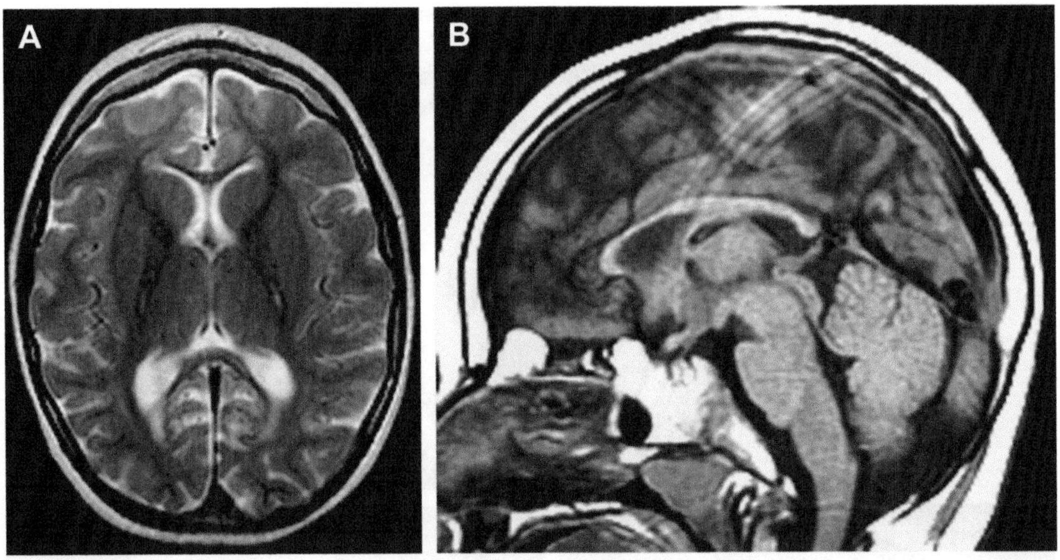

Fig. 25. Primary microcephaly. (*A*) Axial T2. Relatively normal-looking brain, apart from the size. Abnormal signal in the posterior limbs of the internal capsules. Note some excessive thickness of the anterior calvarium, pointing to a failure of cerebral growth. (*B*) Sagittal T1. The hindbrain looks normal but too large in proportion to the forebrain. The corpus callosum is thin, expressing the lack of white matter.

dysgenesis is more prominent anteriorly in the frontal lobes in cases of DCX lissencephaly (Xq22.3–q23); a complete agyria is exceptional and is seen in boys only; band heterotopia is more common and affects almost exclusively girls (with a second X chromosome) (see **Figs. 30** and **32**).[168]

Pathologically a similar 4-layer cortex was found in both genetic defects, with similar layer 1 (with Cajal-Retzius cells), and a pyramidal layer 2 grossly similar but thinner and less cellular in DCX lissencephaly, in contrast with layers 3 and 4 that contain more pyramidal cells in DCX. Below the abnormal cortex in the deep white matter, subcortical heterotopias appear more commonly and prominently in DCX, while both types share the same abnormalities in the pons (neuronal depopulation) and the medulla (simplified and heterotopic olives).[162] Grossly similar findings were reported in a second study of a DCX band heterotopia.[170] A third report found a more organized heterotopic layer in DCX.[171] At least in LIS1 lissencephaly, the severity of the malformation typically depends on the extent of the genetic defect: large deletions result in the most severe phenotypes and milder phenotypes result from intragenic mutations.[172]

Other lissencephalies

Lissencephaly associated with TUBA1A mutations (12q13.12) Patients with this variety of lissencephaly present clinically with microcephaly, severe mental delay, significant motor deficit and, commonly, epilepsy. Morphologically and radiologically, agyria, pachygyria or, less commonly, band heterotopia may be observed, more prominent in the posterior part of the hemisphere. This finding is commonly associated with white matter disorders associating ventriculomegaly and thin, dysgenetic, or agenetic corpus callosum with no or small Probst bundles, abnormal hippocampi, and significant degrees of midbrain and hindbrain hypoplasia (**Fig. 33**).[173] In a neuropathologic study of 4 fetuses, abnormal lamination with a thin, 2-layered cortex, disorganized hippocampi, abnormal white matter (including missing internal capsule and hypoplastic brainstem), immature cerebellar cortex, heterotopias in the cerebral and cerebellar white matter, fragmented dentate, and heterotopic olivary nuclei were observed.[174] As in other lissencephalies, the mutated gene *TUBA1A* (*Tubulin Alpha 1A*) is involved in the control of the cellular tubulin network.[173–175]

X-linked lissencephaly with absent corpus callosum and ambiguous genitalia Clinically, affected patients are genotypic males and present with profound mental retardation, early neonatal (prenatal, even) severe epilepsy with any type of partial or generalized seizures, temperature instability, feeding problems, epilepsy, ambiguous genitalia, and early death. On gross morphology and imaging there is microcephaly, lissencephaly more prominent posteriorly, a mildly thick cortex (5–7 mm), a defective white matter with a ventriculomegaly, a complete commissural agenesis with

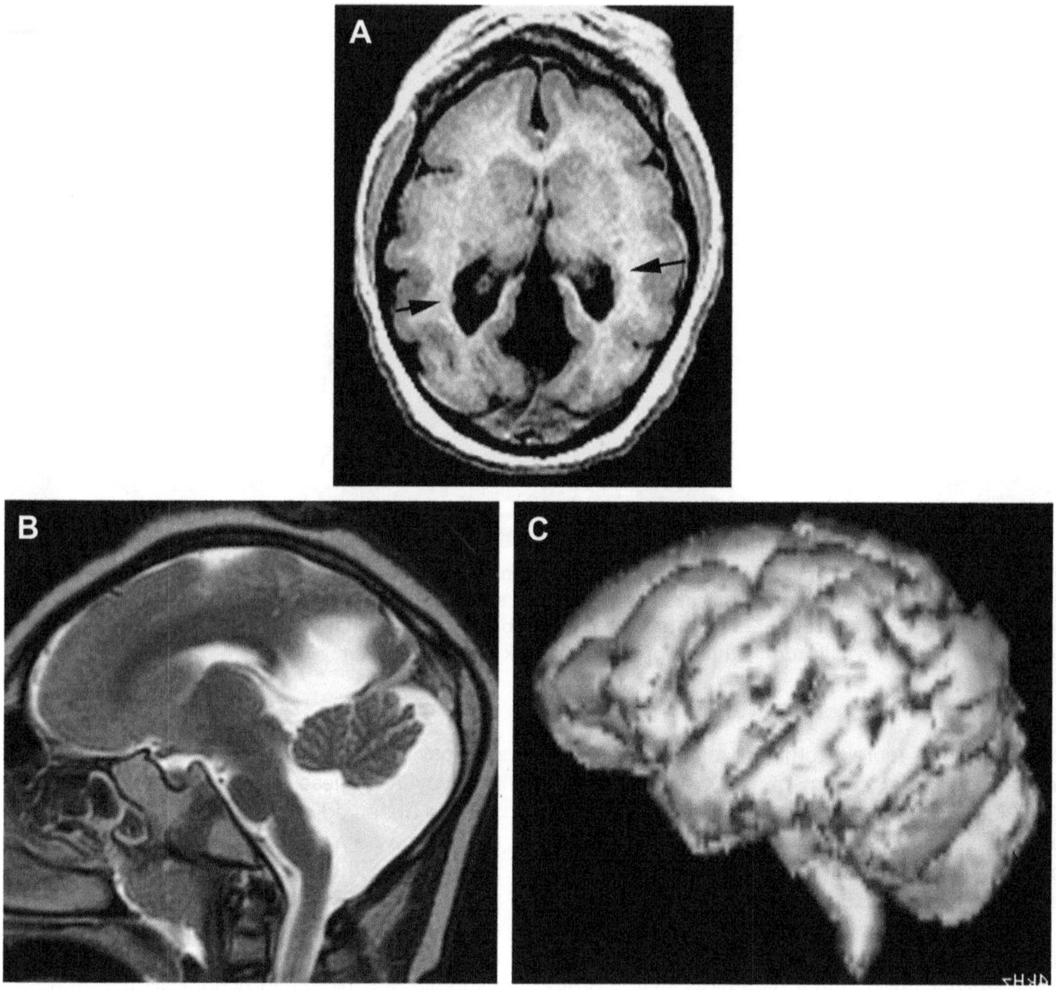

Fig. 26. Primary microcephaly. (*A*) Axial T1. Poorly developed forebrain, with markedly simplified gyral pattern. Bilateral periventricular nodular heterotopia (*black arrows*). Note the excessive thickness of the frontal calvarium, again reflecting the failure of the forebrain to grow. (*B*) Midline sagittal T2. Exceedingly small forebrain. Abnormal posterior fossa with high tentorium (due to lack of growth of the forebrain?) with rotation and inferior hypoplasia of the vermis. (*C*) Surface rendering of the brain.

no Probst bundles, no olfactory bulbs, small and disorganized basal ganglia and hypothalamus, but normal posterior fossa[176,177] (or not, see Ref.[167]). The disorder is related to a mutation of *ARX* (Xq22.13), a gene that is involved in the proliferation, differentiation, and migration of the interneurons within the germinal zone of the medial and lateral ganglionic eminence, leading to aberration in the basal ganglia, hypothalamus, and CP.[178,179] Pathologically the malformed cortex is 3-layered with a unique hypercellularity of the molecular layer and no cell-sparse layer.[162] In another study severe dysplasia of the hypothalamus, globus pallidus, putamen, thalamus, and hypothalamic nucleus was observed, with a hypoplastic pyramidal tract.[180]

The last group of lissencephalies with an identified genetic defect is the Reelin (and/or its receptors VLDLR and APOER2) lissencephaly.[181] Reelin is the substance that characterizes the Cajal-Retzius cell, and the absence of the *RELN* gene (7q22) is responsible for the neurologic disorder that characterizes the strain of Reeler mice. It controls the neuronal migration to the cortex and notably the inside-out pattern. Affected children present with microcephaly, developmental delay, and early epilepsy. On imaging the brain is small, there is a pachygyria that is more severe anteriorly than posteriorly, a moderately thick cortex of 5 to 10 mm, malformed hippocampi, mild brainstem hypoplasia with a cerebellar hypoplasia, and significant foliation defect.[166,167]

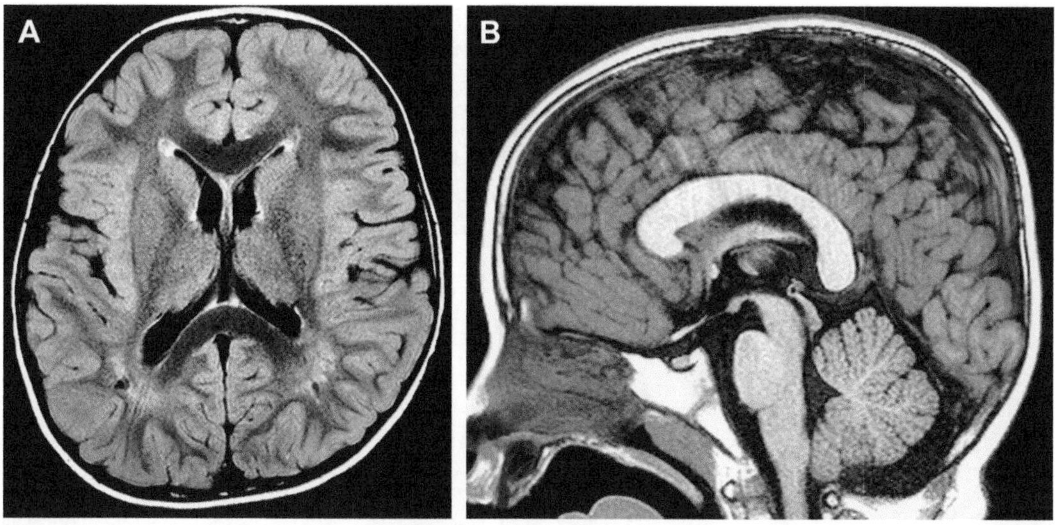

Fig. 27. Primary macrocephaly (Sotos syndrome). (*A*) Axial FLAIR. Large head, large slightly asymmetric hemispheres, prominent ventricles. Some gliotic/cystic changes in the deep posterior white matter are nonspecific. (*B*) Midline sagittal T1 demonstrates a thick corpus callosum (bulky white matter).

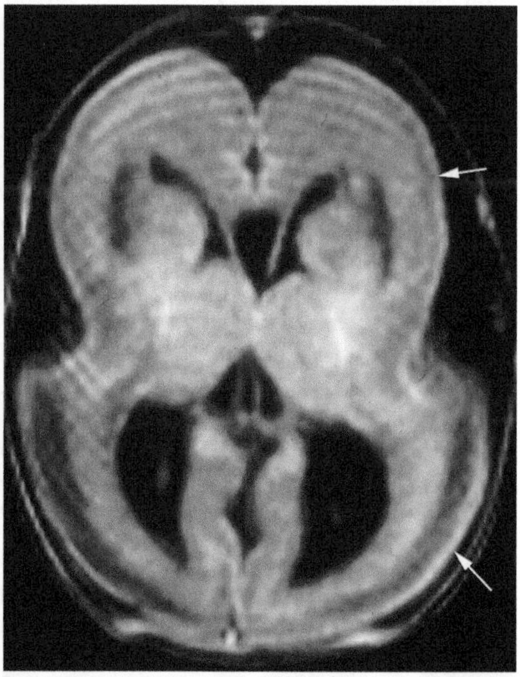

Fig. 28. Complete agyria (Miller-Dieker syndrome, *LIS1*). Axial T1. Four-layered cortex: the molecular layer cannot be seen but the thin cortex, the cell-sparse layer, and the thick heterotopic layer are well apparent (*arrows*). Note the colpocephaly (lack of white matter).

Many other isolated cases of lissencephaly with or without cerebellar hypoplasia and with or without commissural agenesis have been reported in the literature, as well as cases apparently related to fetal cytomegalovirus (CMV) infections.

Abnormalities of the Pial Basement Membrane: Cobblestone Brain and Related Disorders

Dystroglycanopathies with cerebral involvement

Dystroglycanopathies are, above all, a group of severe muscular diseases, the congenital muscular dystrophies (CMD). Considerable advances in the understanding of the pathogenesis of these diseases have occurred in the last two decades (see Refs.[182,183] for review). The defects result from mutations of the genes that encode for glycosyltransferase enzymes with a reduction of the glycosylated α-dystroglycan. Involvement of the brain and eyes results from the defective glycosylation preventing the linking of the α-dystroglycan with laminin $\alpha 2$, a major constituent of the glial basement membrane (also known as glial limiting membrane). In the developing brain α-dystroglycan is expressed in the VZ and in the pial basement membrane, and seems to participate in the neuronal proliferation, in the constitution of the meningeal layers, and in the migration and lamination processes as the radial glia is attached to the pial limiting membrane. In mouse models of dystroglycan defects, the disease leads to the rupture of this membrane and results in a cobblestone appearance.[183] Six genes have been identified

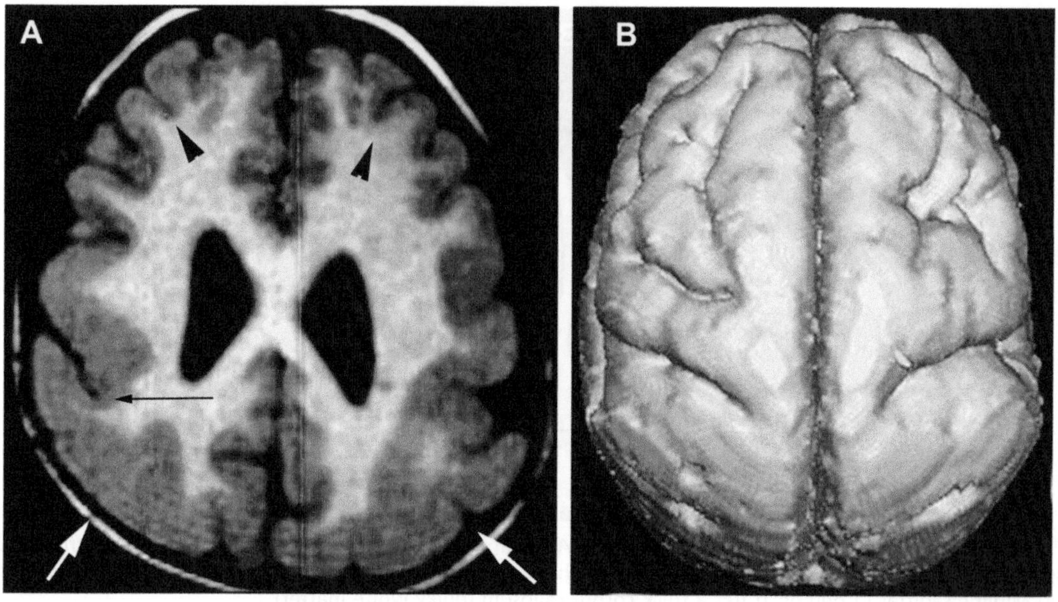

Fig. 29. Posterior pachygyria (presumably *LIS1*). (*A*) Axial T1. Very thick cortex (*white arrows*) contrasting with the more normal anterior cortex (*black arrowheads*). Note that the sulci indent the thick heterotopic cortical layer deeply (*thin black arrow*). (*B*) Surface rendering. The sulci are few but normally located and symmetric (can be named).

whose mutation may result in cerebral involvement: *Fukutin* (*FKTN*, 9q31), *Fukutin*-related protein (*FKRP*, 19q13.3), Protein-*o*-mannosyl transferase 1 (*POMT1*, 9q34.1), Protein-*o*-mannosyl transferase 2 (*POMT2*, 14q24), Protein-*o*-mannose 1,2-*N*-acetylglucosaminyltransferase (*POMGnT1*, 1p33–34), and *LARGE* (22q12.3–q13.1).[183,184] Although it was initially assumed that there was a correlation between the genotype and the phenotype (eg, *Fukutin* with Fukuyama; *POMT1* with muscle-eye-brain [MEB] disease; *POMT1* or *POMT2* with Walker-Warburg syndrome) it appears today that there is a wide range of variation of severity whatever the genotype, the most severe phenotype being the Walker-Warburg syndrome,[182–184] so that the clinical features may vary from a complete clinical and radiological normality, a clinical normality with minimal MR changes, to various combinations of supratentorial and infratentorial malformations and possibly to major syndromes.[182–184]

Clinically the range of variations is broad: all patients present with variable muscular weakness.

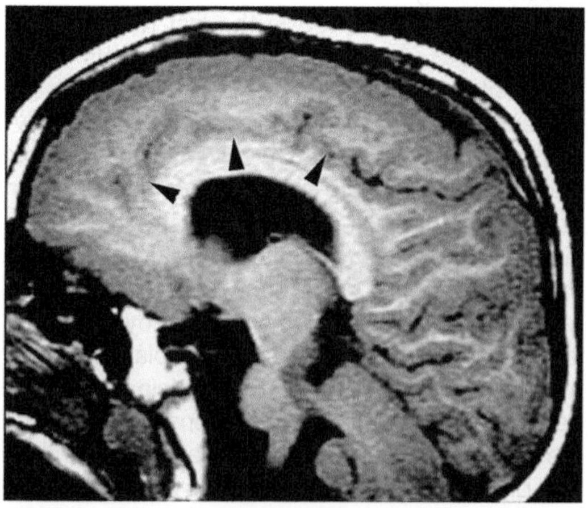

Fig. 30. Anterior pachygyria (*DCX*). Parasagittal T1. Note the paucity of sulcation in the superior frontal gyrus (*arrowheads*) contrasting with the normal parieto-occipital cortex.

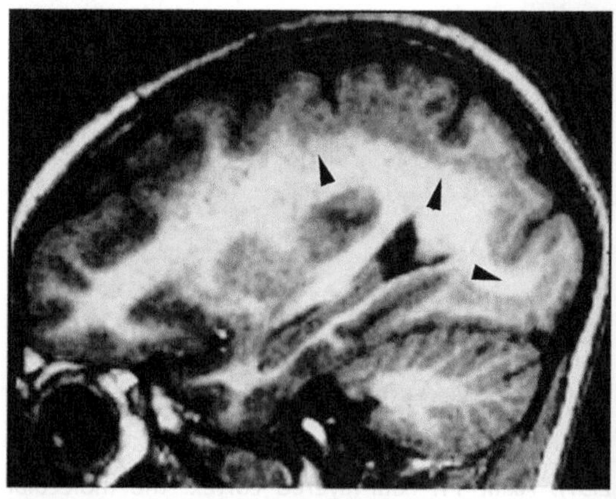

Fig. 31. Posterior band heterotopia (double-cortex) in a boy (*LIS1*). Sagittal T1. Parieto-occipital band heterotopia under an almost normal-looking cortex (*black arrowheads*).

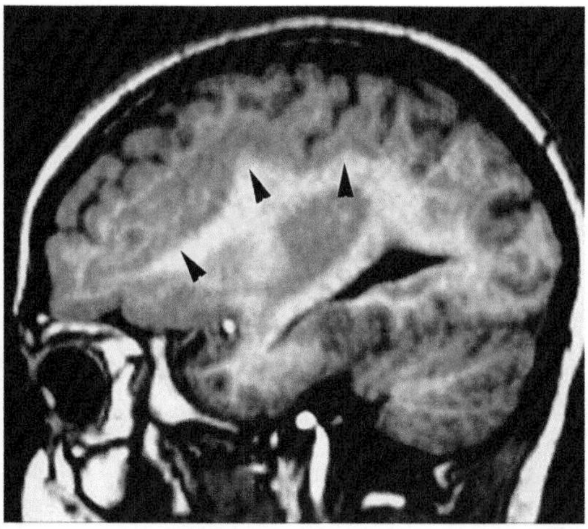

Fig. 32. Anterior band heterotopia (double cortex) in a girl (*DCX*). A thick band of subcortical heterotopic gray matter underlines the frontal and the perirolandic cortices (*arrowheads*).

Neurologically they may be normal, or present variable degrees of cognitive delay, more or less severe seizures, feeding difficulties, and premature death.

Morphologically the spectrum of abnormality was well described by Clement and colleagues.[184] The brain may be normal, or show mild deep white matter changes and/or ventriculomegaly. There may be isolated cerebellar hypoplasia, or cerebellar cysts or hypoplasia with pontine hypoplasia, There may be bilateral frontoparietotemporal polymicrogyria without any posterior fossa abnormality. There may be cortical dysgenesis with cerebellar dysplasia and posteriorly concave brainstem, with normal pons. The classic phenotypes are not the most frequent[184] but they are the most severe expressions of the genetic disorders.[182]

The classical Fukuyama phenotype corresponds to the gene mutation as it is found in Japan (where it is the most complete) (**Fig. 34**). It seems to correlate well with the *Fukutin FKTN* mutation. It includes cerebral and cerebellar PMG, fibroglial proliferation of the leptomeninges and interhemispheric fusion, and hypoplasia of the corticospinal tracts, but hydrocephalus is rare. The white matter abnormalities are present but may be transient, and the posterior part of the hemisphere may appear as a cobblestone cortex. Hypoplasia of the pons and vermis, and cerebellar cysts may be present.

In the classical MEB disease the cortex may variably appear agyric, pachygyric, or polymicrogyric with white matter changes, in association with cerebellar hypoplasia and flat brainstem (**Fig. 35**). The MEB phenotype does not correlate well with any gene mutation: besides *POMGnT1*, it can be observed in association with a mutation of *FKRP*, *Fukutin FKTN*, *POMT1*, and *POMT2.*

Finally, the classical Walker-Warburg syndrome is the most severe, clinically (no survival beyond 3 years) and morphologically (**Fig. 36**). It can be observed with the mutation of any of the dystroglycanopathy genes: *FKTN*, *FKRP*, *POMT1*, *POMT2*, *POMGnT1*, and *LARGE*. The neuronal overmigration results in a diffuse cobblestone brain appearance with heterotopic neurons, leptomeningeal

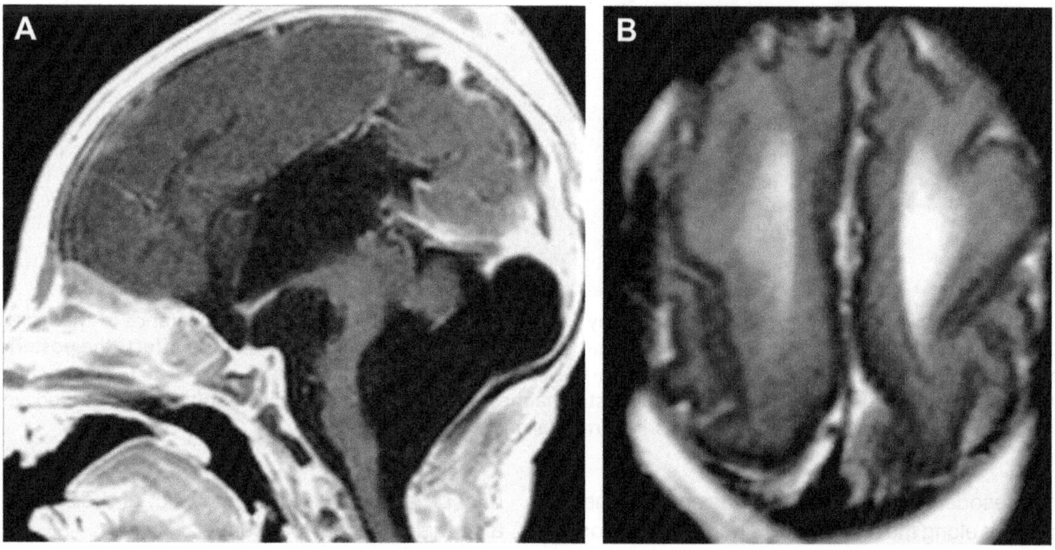

Fig. 33. Lissencephaly with microcephaly, absent commissures, and hindbrain hypoplasia (presumably *TUBA1A*). (*A*) Sagittal T1 demonstrates the lack of any commissure (anterior, hippocampal, callosal), the gross pachygyria, and the posteriorly concave brainstem with pontocerebellar hypoplasia. The tentorium is deficient posteriorly. (*B*) Axial T2. Pachygyria with thin cortex and ventriculomegaly.

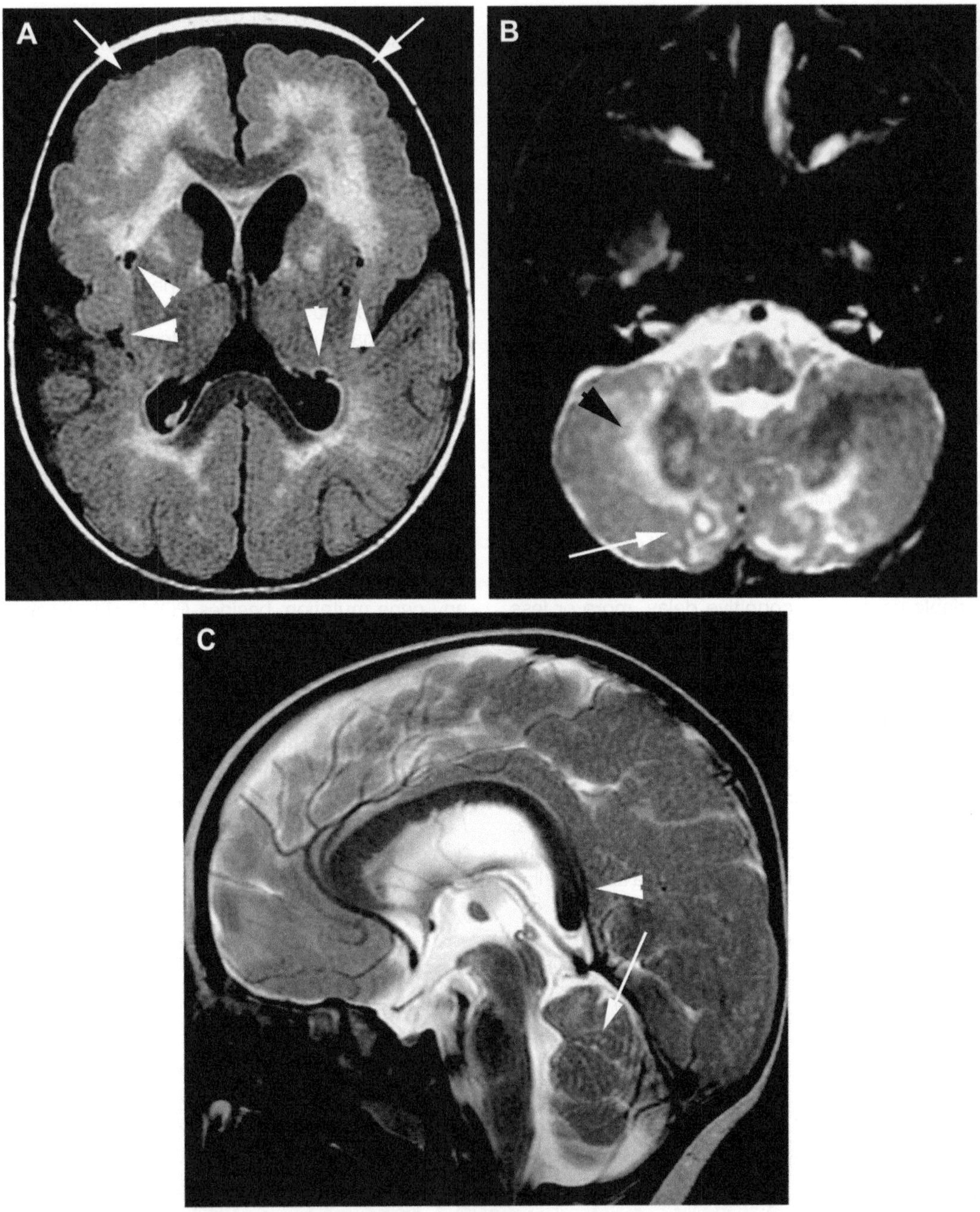

Fig. 34. Fukuyama congenital muscular dystrophy. (*A*) Axial FLAIR. Polymicrogyria-like appearance of the frontal cortex bilaterally (*arrows*), with abnormal myelination that predominates anteriorly but also affects the posterior part of the hemisphere. Microcysts are seen in the external capsules (*arrowheads*). (*B*) Axial T2, cerebellum. Abnormal myelination (*black arrowhead*) and cystic changes (*white arrow*). (*C*) Midline sagittal T2. Extended, verticalized splenium (*arrowhead*); microcysts in vermis (*arrow*).

gliomesodermal proliferation, a fusion of the hemispheres along the midline and a huge ventriculomegaly with or without hydrocephalus, a commissural agenesis, a pontocerebellar hypoplasia with a hypoplastic concave brainstem (Z appearance), and midline clefting of the pons. The fourth ventricle may be enlarged and even cystic, and classically a cephalocele may be found.

Bilateral frontoparietal polymicrogyria

Bilateral frontoparietal polymicrogyria (BFPP) is not a real polymicrogyria, nor a dystroglycanopathy,

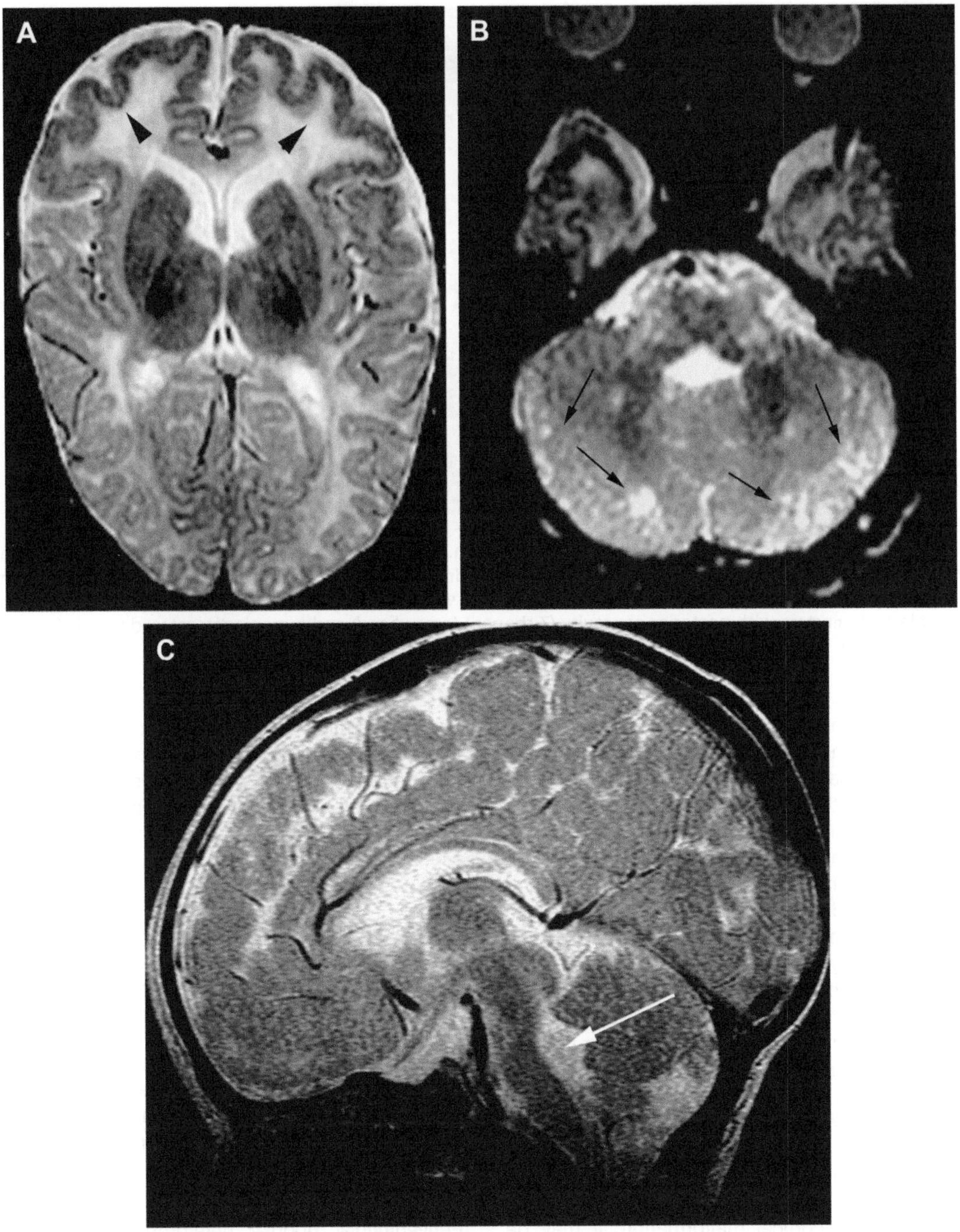

Fig. 35. MEB syndrome. (*A*) Axial T2, forebrain. Polymicrogyria-like changes of the frontal cortex bilaterally (*arrowheads*). Abnormal appearance of the frontal white matter in this 5-month-old infant (compare with the posterior part of the hemispheres). (*B*) Axial T2, cerebellum. Diffuse microcystic changes (*arrows*). (*C*) Midline sagittal T2. Thin corpus callosum, posterior concavity of the brainstem (*arrow*).

but it does result from gaps in the pial basement membrane and has close similarities with cobblestone brain pathogenetically, morphologically, and clinically.[185]

Pathogenetically, BFPP is related to a mutation of the *GPR56* gene (16q13), which encodes a G-protein–coupled receptor that is expressed in radial glial endfeet and presumably participates

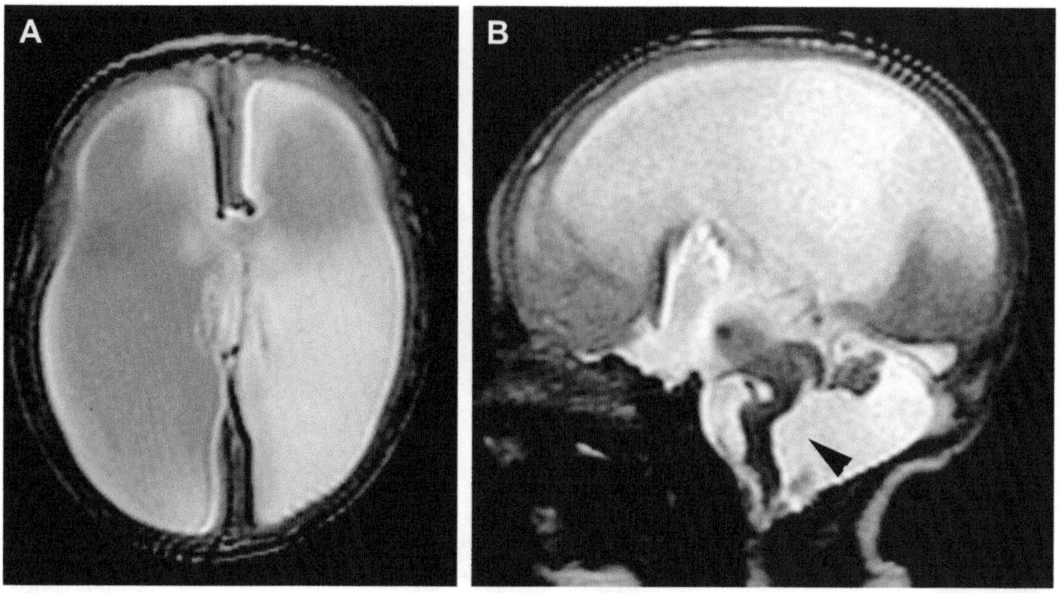

Fig. 36. Walker-Warburg syndrome. (*A*) Axial T2, forebrain. Extremely thin cortex and white matter. Huge ventriculomegaly, due to both a lack of white matter and hydrocephalus. Corpus callosum and septum pellucidum are absent. (*B*) Midline sagittal T2. Huge ventriculomegaly with markedly dilated third ventricle. Very abnormal hypoplastic brainstem with posterior concavity (Z-shaped) (*arrowhead*) and hypoplastic, rotated vermis (pseudo Dandy-Walker).

in the maintenance of the pial basement membrane. In a knocked-out mouse model, there is a major regional lamination defect in the frontoparietal areas with leptomeningeal cortical ectopia containing neurons from both the deep and the superficial layers; this overmigration can be explained by the breaches in the pial basement membrane, by the disorganization of the radial glia with abnormal anchorage of the glial endfeet into the ectopia, and by the fact that the Cajal-Retzius cells are dislocalized into the ectopia as well.[186]

Clinically the patients present with an early hypotonia with pseudo-myopathic features, then a severe motor and mental retardation, and later pyramidal and cerebellar symptoms with abnormal eye movements and severe generalized epilepsy.[185]

Radiologically the hemispheres are severely abnormal with a bilateral symmetric polymicrogyria-like cortical malformation; it may be typically frontoparietal but more often extends to most of the hemisphere, with an anterior to posterior gradient (A>P). There is a lack of white matter with ventriculomegaly and thin, dysgenetic corpus callosum; in addition the myelination is abnormal, with marked hypomyelination in infants evolving toward a pattern of patchy areas of bright T2/FLAIR signal; these abnormalities are prominent in the parieto-occipital subcortical white matter.[185] In the posterior fossa there is disorganization of the superior vermian foliation, subpial and cortical vermian and hemispheric cysts, and poor demarcation and flattening of the ventral pons with in some cases a posterior concavity of the brainstem.[185]

MIGRATION DISORDERS: NODULAR HETEROTOPIA

Nodular heterotopia are different from band heterotopias in that they form gray matter nodules that may be unilateral or bilateral but never perfectly symmetric; they are often consistent with a normal intelligence, and epilepsy typically develops late (second decade). Depending on their location, they are classified as periventricular nodular heterotopia (PVNH) and subcortical nodular heterotopia (SCNH), which are usually transcerebral.

Periventricular Nodular Heterotopia

Periventricular nodular heterotopia typically encroach on the ventricular lumen, and for this reason the authors believe that the term subependymal heterotopia that is sometimes used is not appropriate (however, this term may apply to the extremely uncommon occurrence of a deep laminar heterotopia that lines the ventricular wall).

Morphologically, PVNH are aggregates of neurons organized in nodules of gray matter: on CT, but now preferably on MR, their appearance is similar to that of the cortex, whatever the modality or the sequences used. They are never calcified, and they never enhance (different from the subependymal nodules of the TSC, which typically have signals always different from those of the gray matter on MR imaging, are calcified, and enhance). There is no mass effect and no surrounding edema. Their location is important: they develop from the germinal zone of the pallium, and therefore are never found on the ventricular surface of the basal ganglia, but always on the ventricular surface of the white matter except, importantly, on the septum pellucidum and the callosal roof of the lateral ventricles. The fact that they protrude into the ventricles suggests that they developed within the VZ and were left there after the ventricular zone disappeared at week 26.

PVNH may be single, multiple, or diffuse; they may be uni- or bilateral but, as mentioned earlier, they are asymmetrical even when distributed along symmetric portions of the ventricles (**Figs. 37–41**). When unilateral they seem to be preferentially located on the right side.[187] PVNH affect the posterior part of the ventricles (atrium/occipital horns, temporal horns) more commonly than the body, and especially than the frontal horns[187,188] (where they appear squeezed between the head of the caudate and the corpus callosum). Often they are sporadic, but they also occur in families (then typically affecting girls[187,188]), or in syndromes. PVNH may be associated also with a remarkably high frequency in some brain malformations: Chiari II, cephaloceles, commissural agenesis, and septo-optic dysplasia (de Morsier type). When familial, they are often associated with a mega cisterna magna.[189] Among the MCD they are more commonly associated with microcephaly, subcortical nodular heterotopia, schizencephaly, and polymicrogyria.[188] FCD type I in the overlying cortex has been identified on specimens of surgical cases of PVNH with refractory epilepsy.[155] Volumetric studies have shown a negative correlation between the volume of the PVNH and that of the gray matter, suggesting that the arrested neurons should have belonged to the overlying cortex.[190]

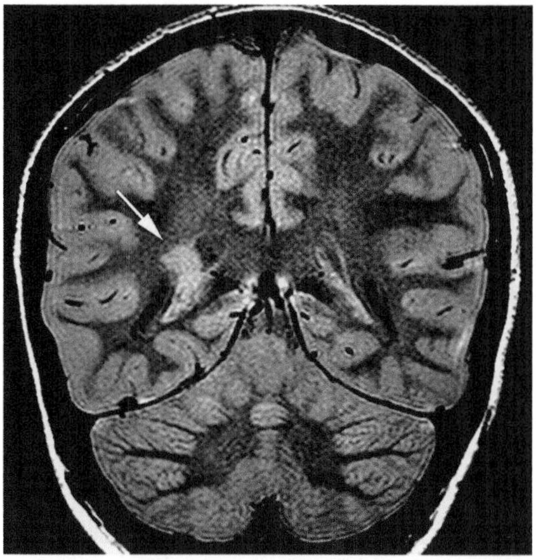

Fig. 38. Isolated large periventricular nodular heterotopia (*arrow*) (proton density).

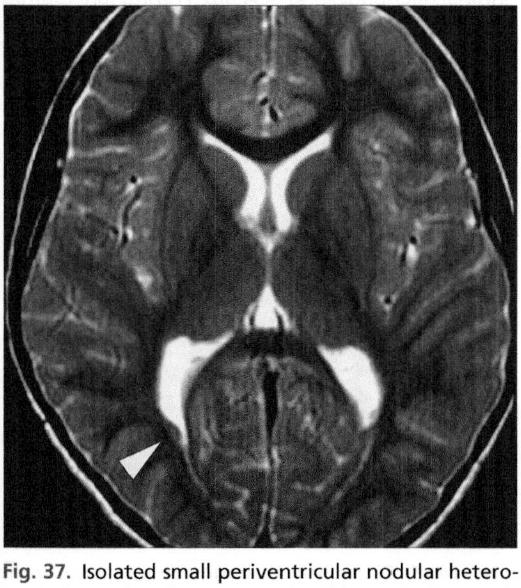

Fig. 37. Isolated small periventricular nodular heterotopia (*arrowhead*). Associated mild ventriculomegaly (T2 axial).

Pathogenesis

For years it has been considered that PVNH would result from an insult to the VZ and occur late in the

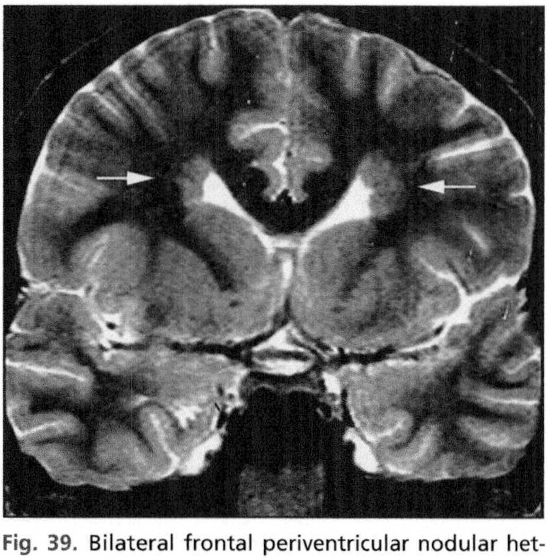

Fig. 39. Bilateral frontal periventricular nodular heterotopia between the corpus callosum and the caudate nuclei (*arrows*) (T2 coronal).

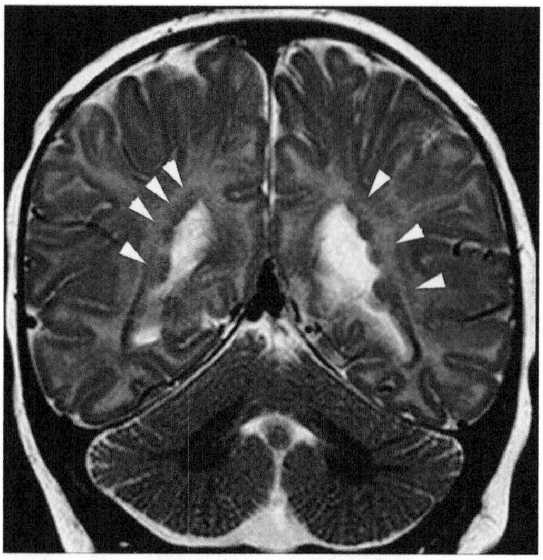

Fig. 40. Multiple bilateral periventricular nodular heterotopia in an infant girl (*arrowheads*), possibly due to *FLNA* mutation (T2 coronal).

process of migration. However, the occurrence of the malformations in families and the preponderance of affected females in most of the series made a genetic defect likely. A locus on Xq28 was identified in 1996,[191] and the responsible gene *filamin 1* (*FLN1*), now *filamin A* (*FLNA*), in 1998.[192] *FLNA* encodes for a protein that is essential in the cross-binding of intracellular actin. It plays a crucial role in angiogenesis, coagulation, cellular migration (notably melanocytes), and neuronal migration.[192] Boys affected with the mutation tend to die in utero from hemorrhages, whereas girls survive but present with PVNH: among the patients with the mutation, 93% are female and only 7% male.[193] The mutation is found in 49% of patients with bilateral PVNH as a group (see **Fig. 40**), but in 100% of the familial cases against only 26% of the sporadic cases. The mutation is found also in patients in whom PVNH is part of an Ehlers-Danlos syndrome. It is extremely uncommon (4%) in the other phenotypes, including those in which the PVNH are isolated, unilateral, or associated with other MCD.[193] The mutation has never been reported in cases where the PVNH are associated with commissural agenesis, septo-optic dysplasia, cephaloceles, or Chiari II malformation.

Subcortical Nodular Heterotopia

Subcortical nodular heterotopia (SCNH) may appear as small nodules of gray matter distributed between the ventricular wall and the cortex (typically multiple, rarely single) or, more commonly, as transcerebral aggregates of gray matter extending from the ventricle to, and continuous with the cortex, which typically is dysgenetic over the malformation (**Figs. 42–47**). Such transcerebral SCNH may be bulky, or may form relatively thin streaks of gray matter crossing the white matter, often bilateral and symmetric. SCNH may be found isolated, or in association with other MCD, notably schizencephaly and polymicrogyria (which confirms that these two entities involve migration disorders in addition to the poor organization of the cortex[11]), but also PVNH (see **Fig. 45**). Together with a polymicrogyria-like cortical dysgenesis, SCNH are a prominent feature

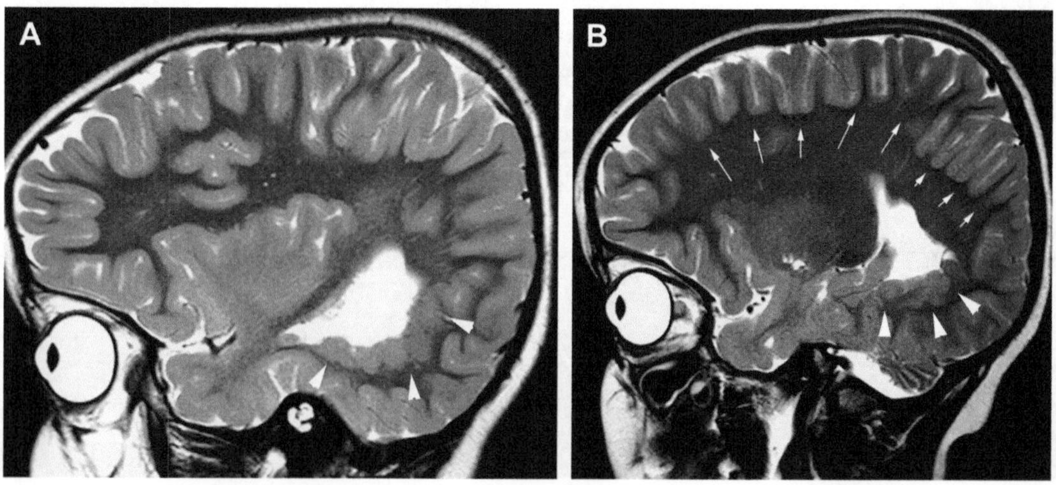

Fig. 41. Diffuse bilateral periventricular nodular heterotopias. (*A, B*) T2 sagittal through the temporal horns demonstrates the continuous coating of the ventricular wall (*arrowheads*). Note the dislocated hippocampus and associated cortical polygyria (*arrows*).

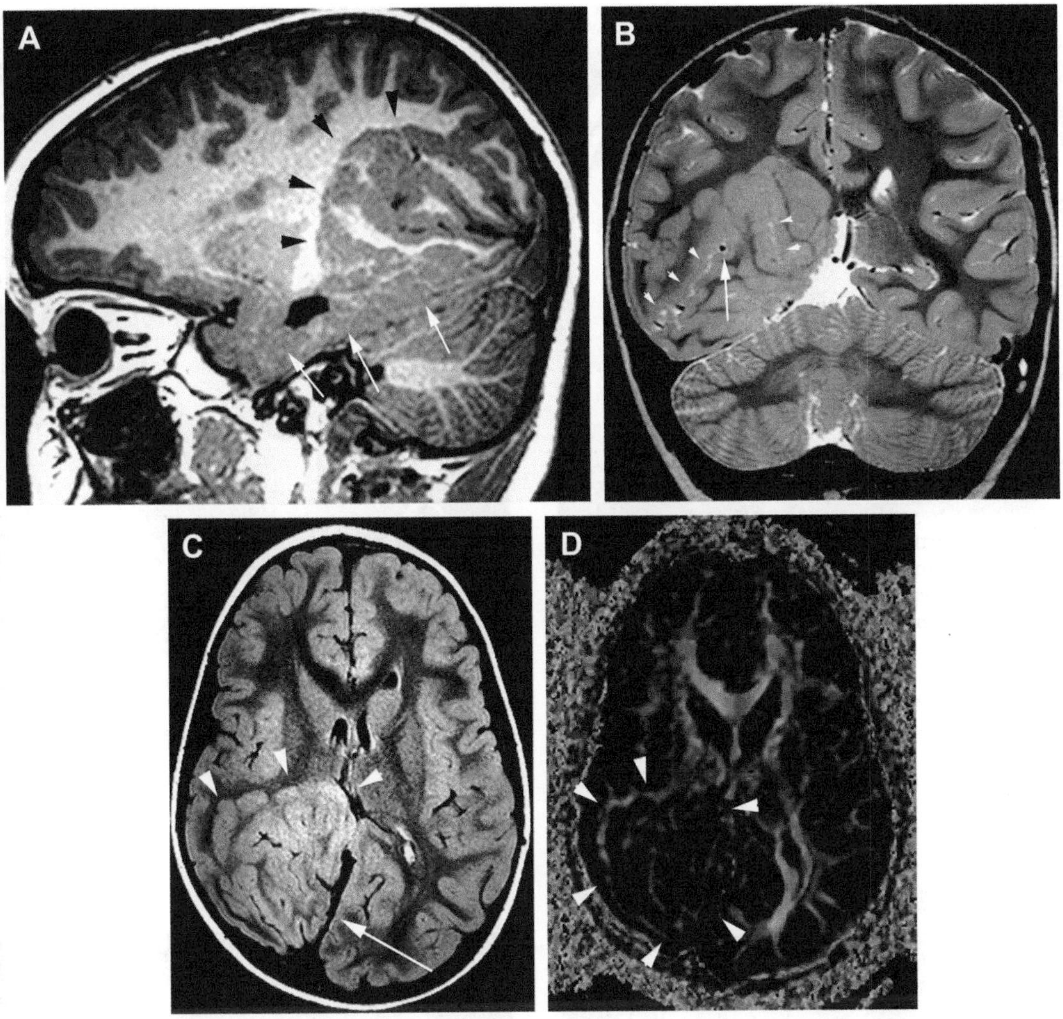

Fig. 42. Subcortical nodular heterotopia. (*A*) Lateral sagittal T1. Large nodular conglomerate of intermingled gray and white matter (*black arrowheads*); the malformation extends along the inferior aspect of the temporal lobe (*arrows*). (*B*) Coronal T2. Besides cortical-like gray matter and the associated white matter, the malformation presents with a deep CSF-containing and vessel-containing fissure (*arrowheads*). (*C*) Axial FLAIR. Despite its volume, the SCNH (*arrowheads*) is associated with focal hypoplasia of the hemisphere with dislocated falx (*arrow*). (*D*) FA color mapping. The hemispheric white matter fascicles are disorganized at the level of the SCNH (*arrowheads*), but within the heterotopia, the white matter appears organized in a coherent fashion (appearing mostly *green*—dorsoventral, or *blue*—craniocaudal, in this image).

of the commissural agenesis with interhemispheric dysplastic cysts (including the Aicardi syndrome).

Small SCNH, except for location, are no different from PVNH: well-circumscribed nodules of gray matter, without any mass effect or edema, never calcified, never enhancing with contrast media. Small SCNH may be bilateral but not symmetric. Typically the hemisphere, including the cortex and the ventricle, looks otherwise normal.

Large SCNH look different (see **Fig. 42**),[194] and are almost always unilateral. Large SCNH always extend from the ventricular wall to the cortex and have no anatomically consistent topography: they may be sublobar, lobar or interlobar, or multilobar. When they sit on the medial aspect of the frontoparietal lobes they are typically associated with a partial or complete commissural agenesis (see **Fig. 43**).[195] Their appearance is unusual, as they are made of intermingled gray and white matter, may contain signal void indicating the presence of prominent vessels (larger than the usual transcerebral perforators), and even bright CSF-like signals, which is assumed to be from perivascular spaces accompanying the vessel

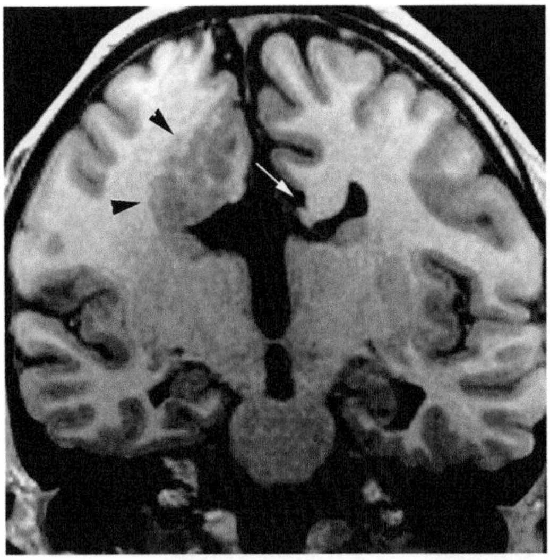

Fig. 43. Subcortical nodular heterotopia with callosal dysgenesis. Coronal T1. The SCNH lies at the level of the cingulate gyrus and ventricular roof (*arrowheads*). Assumedly it prevented the development of the corpus callosum as well as of the septum pellucidum (septocingulate fibers), as well as of a bundle of Probst (compare with left side, *white arrow*). Hippocampi appear dysplastic.

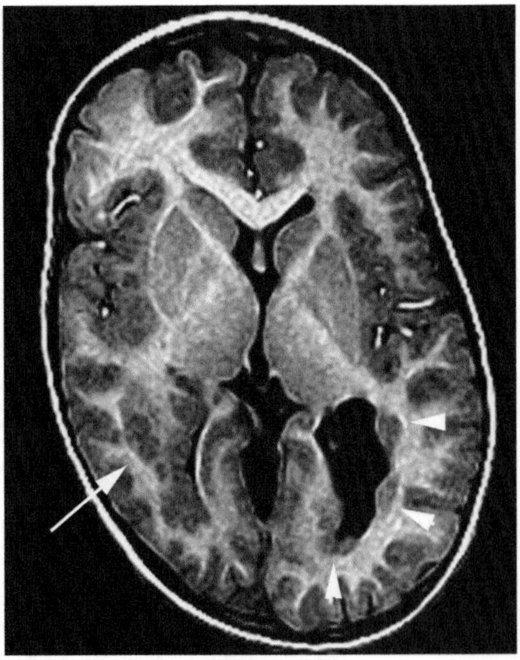

Fig. 45. Associated subcortical and periventricular nodular heterotopia. Axial T1. The SCNH extends medially to coat the ventricular wall (*arrow*), and is associated with contralateral PVNH (*arrowheads*).

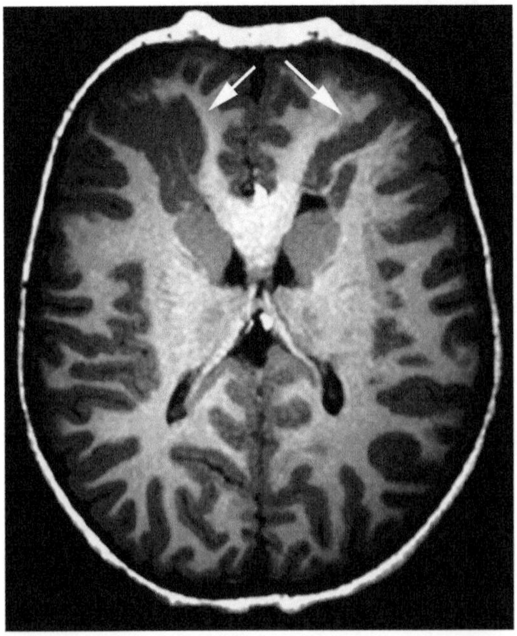

Fig. 44. Bilateral streak-like subcortical nodular heterotopia. Axial T1. Patient with frontonasal dysplasia, interhemispheric lipoma, and callosal dysgenesis. Bilateral streaks of gray matter extending from the frontal horns to the frontal cortex (*arrows*).

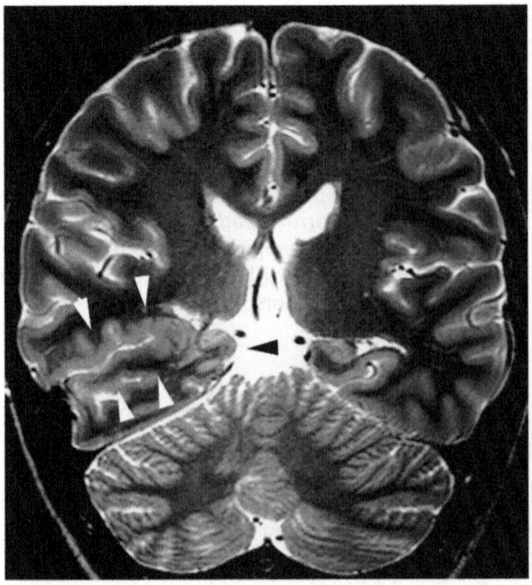

Fig. 46. Subcortical nodular heterotopia. Coronal T2. The SCNH extends to the ventricle (*arrowheads*) and is centered by a deep sulcus which, however, does not open in the ventricle; therefore it is not a true schizencephaly (although the pathogenesis may be similar). Note the right hippocampal dysplasia.

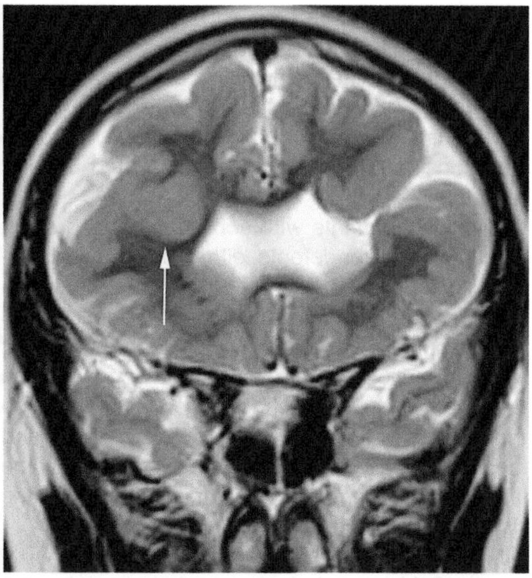

Fig. 47. Subcortical nodular heterotopia and schizencephaly. Coronal T2. This pattern of left frontal schizencephaly with contralateral SCNH (*arrow*) suggests a common pathogenesis.

within the heterotopia[194] (different, however, from the usual Virchow-Robin spaces as are ordinarily seen in the normal white matter) (see **Fig. 42**). Large SCNH often encroach on the ventricle, and the ventricle is deformed accordingly, sometimes narrowed but most often enlarged, likely because of lack of white matter. The cortex continuous with and overlying the SCNH is dysgenetic with abnormal sulcation, sometimes described as "polymicrogyria." The basal ganglia often are dysplastic as well. Independent small SCNH and/or PVNH may be seen in the white matter adjacent to the main SCNH or along the ventricle, and even contralaterally.[196] The hemisphere is typically smaller on the affected side: this is likely due to a lack of volume of the white matter, which cannot connect properly in such a dysmorphic hemisphere[194] (whether there is a specific abnormality of the subplate is not known, but it would seem likely). Sometimes, however, the SCNH may be giant, resulting in an enlargement of a portion the affected hemisphere.[197] The gray-white matter mixture of the heterotopia sometimes has the pseudo-brain appearance of a glioneuronal heterotopia.

Whereas PVNH are common in patients with the classical form of commissural agenesis, SCNH are more common in patients with commissural agenesis with multiple dysplastic interhemispheric cysts.[195] In a subgroup of such patients the heterotopia and the associated cortical dysgenesis are on the medial aspect of the hemisphere, adjacent to the interhemispheric cysts. Besides callosal agenesis, the white matter abnormalities include unilateral absence of the septum pellucidum and of the Probst bundle: it seems logical to assume that the dysplastic gray matter in that location may prevent the axonal pathfinding. In fact a similar SCNH and callosal agenesis may be seen uncommonly without interhemispheric cysts (see **Fig. 43**).[195] In other cases the SCNH may be small and dispersed, apparently unilaterally.

Uncommonly a streak-like SCNH can be seen, which appears as a relatively thin streak of gray matter that crosses the hemisphere from the ventricular wall to the surface; it may be bilateral and quite symmetric (see **Fig. 44**). Like every heterotopia, it presents with the same signals as the cortex on all sequences, which differentiates it from the "transmantle dysplasia" of some FCD type IIB; also it has parallel borders rather than being wedge shaped. It may be confused with a closed-lip schizencephaly, but there is no dimple on the ventricular end and no converging sulci around the pial end (see **Fig. 46**). Yet there are rare instances in which such a streak-like SCNH can be seen contralateral to a true schizencephaly, so that both types of lesions may actually overlap pathogenetically (see **Fig. 47**).

SCHIZENCEPHALY AND POLYMICROGYRIAS

Schizencephaly and classical PMG share many features, and one may wonder whether they are different degrees of the same pathology. Above all, the cortex lining a schizencephalic cleft, and extending more or less over the hemispheric surface, is typically polymicrogyric. Both types of lesion are usually located in the perisylvian regions. Both may be unilateral or bilateral, but when bilateral are usually not perfectly symmetric. Their clinical manifestations are similar: epilepsy, neurologic deficits, spasticity and, when extensive, developmental delay. In most instances, both schizencephaly and PMG are idiopathic, but both may develop in similar contexts such as a fetal CMV infections, or (in relatively frequent if anecdotal gestational records) following second-trimester incidents such as maternal trauma, bleeding, anoxia, or other potential causes of fetal injury. There are significant differences, however. Specific phenotypes of familial/genetic PMG have been identified, while it is still uncertain whether specific genes or loci are involved in schizencephaly. Another difference is that while the definition of schizencephaly is clear (a transcerebral cleft lined with cortex with a pial-ependymal seam), the definition of PMG is much less specific ("too many small gyri") and used to describe very different disorders.

Schizencephaly

Porencephaly (transcerebral cavities from the ventricle to the surface) was initially described by Heschl (quoted in Ref.[198]). In the following decades it became evident that some of the porencephalies were lined with gliotic white matter and therefore occurred late, whereas others were lined with microgyric cortex, therefore occurring relatively early before the end of the fourth month or earlier (for review see Ref.[198]). To make a clear distinction between destructive and what they considered to be agenetic porencephalies, Yakovlev and Wadsworth, in two articles published in 1946, promoted the use of the term schizencephaly for the latter, and described two subtypes, one with closed lips (no real porus)[199] and one with open lips (CSF-containing cavity),[200] and they maintained that both variants were agenetic in origin, for identical reasons: mostly because they share the "same embryonic relationship between the cortical gray matter and the ventricular ependyma," the same "pial-ependymal seam," the same identity of location, and the same associated heterotopia (they also describe a same early myelination that the authors now assume to be secondary to the seizure activity).[200]

In opposition to these arguments, and reflecting the "adult" cerebrovascular diseases, the proponents of the encephaloclastic pathogenesis argued for the location of the clefts in the territories of the main cerebral arteries.[198,201] A proximal occlusion of one of the main cortical arteries however is unlikely, as on angiography of patients with schizencephaly the arterial branches can be seen coursing over the roof of an open schizencephalic cleft to supply the cortex beyond it.[202] As a CP lines the whole cleft, it may be assumed that the defect developed before the end of the neuronal migration, which is a time when the SVZ-VZ only is vascularized. As an initial lesion, a portion of the proliferative zone must have been absent or destroyed: obviously, a vascular lesion is a possibility (arterial or venous) but so also is a focal hemorrhage or an infection (eg, CMV). Such a lesion has been experimentally induced in hamsters by injection of mumps virus.[203] In humans, it may occur in the period between 10 weeks (when vessels proliferate in the germinal tissue) and 16 weeks (before the start of the third wave of migration). The cleft would be due to the agenetic/destructive event and the PMG to an incomplete migration/distorted connection. In the distinction between malformative disorder (inborn), disruptive disorder (distorted anatomy due to injury during development), and acquired disorder (scarring process), classical schizencephaly may be considered an early disruptive lesion, although it is generally idiopathic. In addition, familial cases have been reported.[204,205] From a genetic point of view a role for a germline mutation in the *EMX2* gene was considered,[206] but is not supported by later reports.

Clinically, patients with schizencephaly present mostly with motor defects, either unilateral or bilateral. A second common feature is epilepsy, which may develop late during the second decade, and may become refractory in a significant number of cases. Developmental delays vary depending on the extent of the lesions (not only the cleft but also the commonly associated surrounding PMG), and their unilaterality or bilaterality. Speech may be significantly altered both in the motor and the comprehension aspects.

Morphologically the diagnosis is relatively simple.[207] Schizencephaly is characterized by the presence of a transcerebral cleft extending from the ventricle to the surface and completely lined with cortex, so that the cortical pial surface is continuous with the ventricular ependymal lining, the pial-ependymal seam of Yakovlev and Wadsworth (see **Fig. 47**; **Figs. 48–52**).[199,200] The cleft may be closed (fused lips), with no visible CSF in it (see **Figs. 48**, **50**, and **52**); or it may be open (see **Figs. 47**, **49**, and **51**). Even when it is closed, a dimple on the ventricular surface and often an umbilication with converging sulci on the hemispheric surface may be seen. The cortex lining

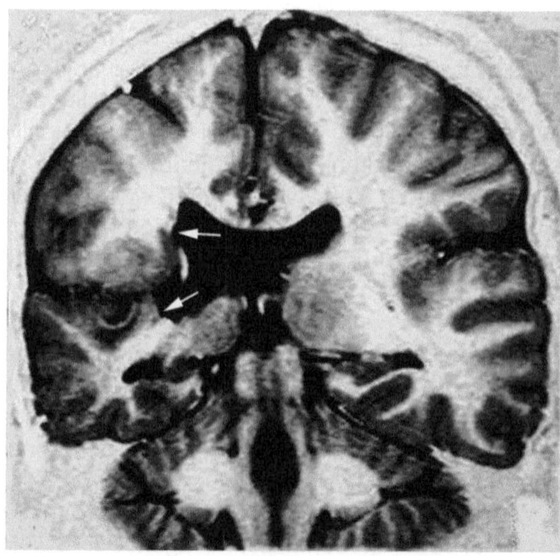

Fig. 48. Unilateral closed-lips schizencephaly. Coronal T1. Deep transcerebral cleft on the right side, lined with cortex so that the cortical ribbon joins the ependyma (*arrows*). Right hemispheric hypoplasia and absent pellucidum.

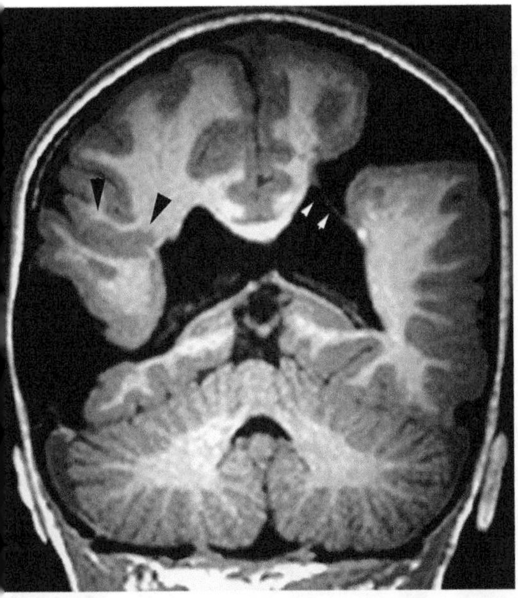

Fig. 49. Multiple bilateral schizencephaly. Coronal T1. Left parietal and right temporal open clefts, the latter with a thin closing membrane (*white arrowheads*), right parietal closed cleft (*black arrowheads*).

the cyst is polymicrogyric, as well as, often, the cortex surrounding the cleft on the hemispheric surface. The most common location of the clefts is suprasylvian, but they can be found anywhere on the lateral, medial, or inferior surface of the hemispheres. The clefts may be unilateral or bilateral, and sometimes more than 2 clefts may be seen when the images are carefully analyzed (eg, anterior temporal lobes, inferior occipital lobes). When bilateral, the clefts are usually not strictly symmetric, and may present as a closed cleft on one side and an open cleft on the other. Strictly symmetric schizencephalies may be seen, however (see **Figs. 50** and **52**) and may well be genetic (not all familial schizencephalies, however, are symmetric or even bilateral). Also, unilateral schizencephaly may present with a contralateral PMG, or even with a contralateral transmantle streak-like SCNH (see **Fig. 47**).

As in most MCD, the white matter is affected and its volume is reduced so that the brainstem may be hypoplastic. More specifically, the pellucidum is characteristically absent when the clefts are suprasylvian, either unilaterally or bilaterally.[208] There is no ready explanation for this, as the fibers that constitute the septum pellucidum are limbic, not neocortical.[195] Together with the pellucidum, the anterior optic pathway may be hypoplastic, suggesting that at least some variants of schizencephaly could be complex forms of septo-optic dysplasia[209]; it may also be that optic and pituitary hypoplasia may be nonspecifically associated with diverse disorders. More consistently with what is known of brain development, the corpus callosum may be at least partially defective when the schizencephalic clefts involve the medial aspect of the hemisphere (see **Fig. 50**). Of interest, PVNH may be observed lining the ventricle around the ventricular opening of the cleft as well as at some distance from it.

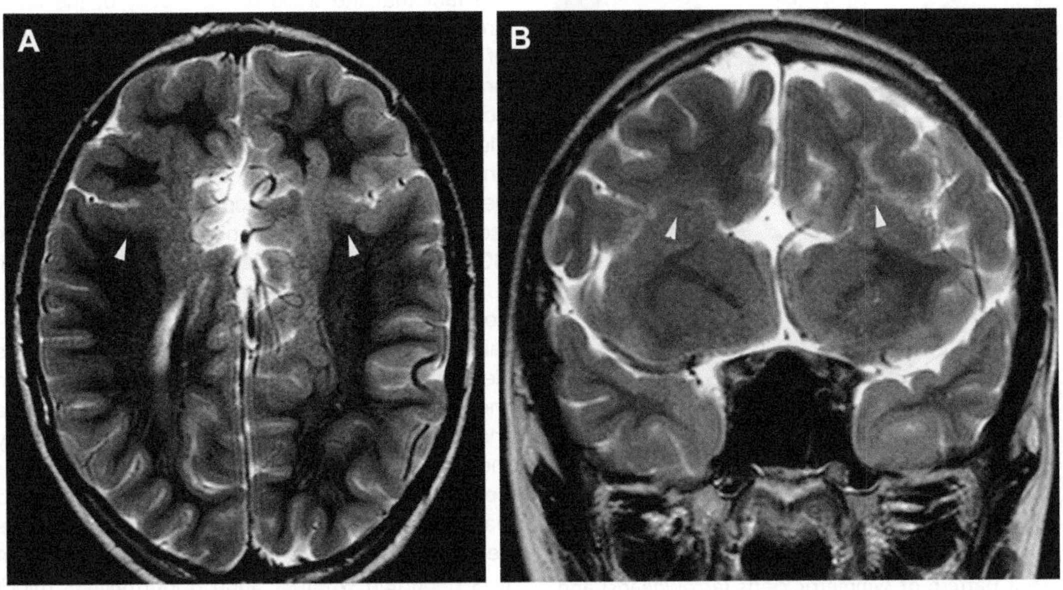

Fig. 50. Schizencephaly with commissural agenesis. (*A*, axial and *B*, coronal T2). The bilateral clefts extend to the medial cortex and cingulate gyrus (*arrowheads*), thereby preventing the development of the commissural plate.

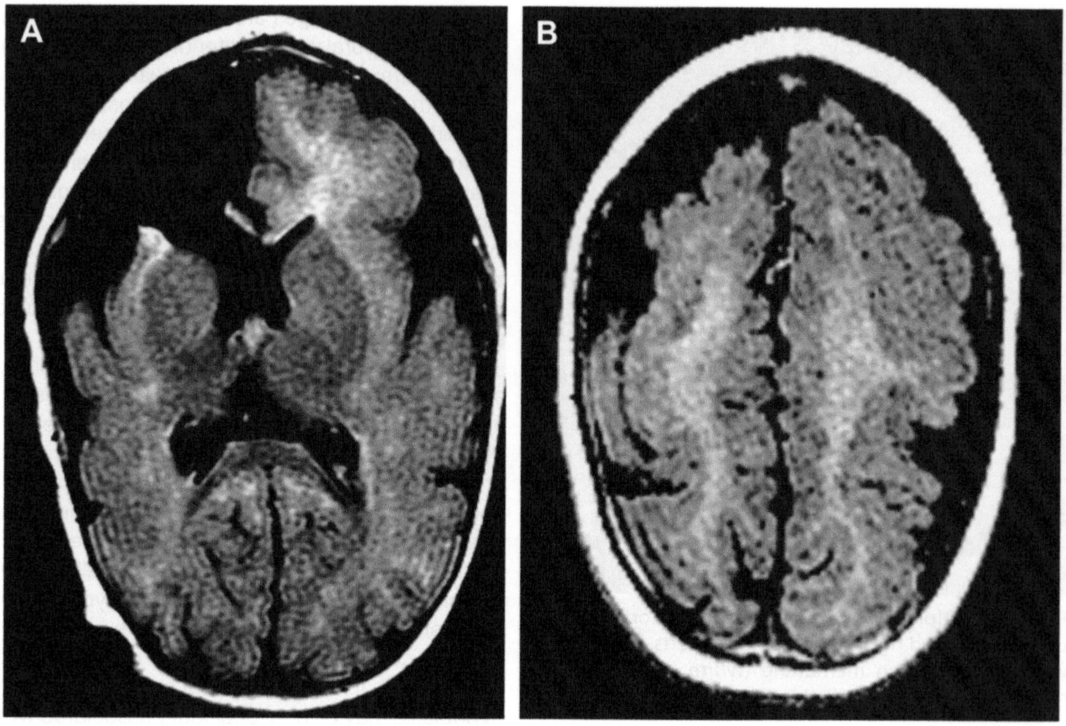

Fig. 51. Fetal brain infection with cytomegalovirus. (*A, B*) Axial T1. Right frontal open cleft with diffuse polymicrogyria.

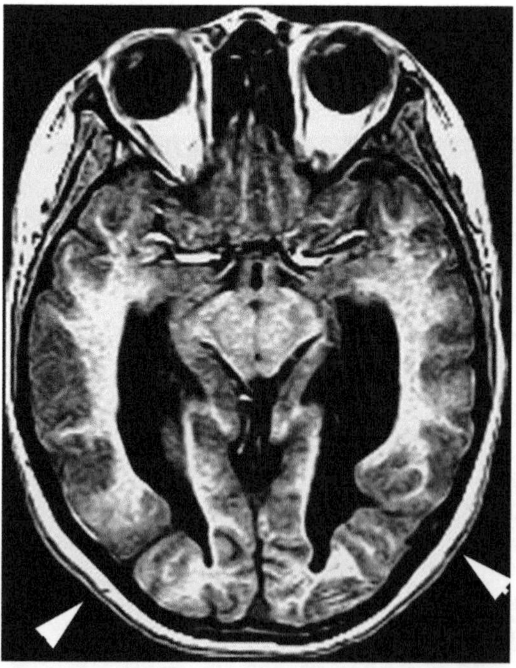

Fig. 52. Bilateral symmetric schizencephaly. Axial T1. Such a pattern of symmetric clefts (*arrowheads*) and the temporo-occipital location are unusual, and may suggest a genetic origin.

The differential diagnosis of schizencephaly is both easy—the anatomic definition of the lesion is clear—and difficult, as the pathogenesis is uncertain. Obviously it can be differentiated from congenital encephaloclastic porencephalies by the fact that the walls of the cavity of the latter are made of white matter, not cortex. In the case of fetal infection with CMV, the importance of the brain alteration (especially the microcephaly) sometimes makes it difficult to tell whether the cleft is lined with cortex or not: the diffuse PMG and the common white matter abnormality suggest that it is a real, if acquired, schizencephaly (see **Fig. 51**). As mentioned before, streak-like SCNH can be differentiated by the absence of a ventricular dimple, but the 2 entities may be somewhat related. A common source of uncertainty is when a sulcus lined with PMG extends deep into the hemisphere, being separated from the ventricle by a thin layer of subcortical white matter only: this is technically not a schizencephaly (no pial-ependymal seam), but a complete or incomplete layer of white matter has been described partially forming the floor of the cleft in true schizencephaly (compare **Figs. 46** and **49**),[207] so that it is uncertain whether such abnormalities might be intermediate degrees of severity in a wide spectrum of schizencephaly-PMG.

The Polymicrogyrias

Histopathologically, polymicrogyria is a specific disorder: under a smooth (but irregular, compared with a cauliflower or with morocco leather) and pachygyric-like surface, PMG is made of a piling upon each other of numerous small, somewhat irregular folds under a fused surface.[3] The development of these irregular undulations does not correspond to the normal mechanism of gyration-sulcation, as the abnormality may be observed as early as 18 gestational weeks,[210] well before the first normal primary sulci form after mid-gestation: it is rather an early primary dysplastic development of the CP, resulting in an undulated, serrated appearance under the preexisting MZ/molecular layer. Because it is a primary cortical disorder that antecedes their development, the connectivity and the related gyration/sulcation become severely abnormal in classical PMG. In addition, the meninges overlying the PMG are commonly

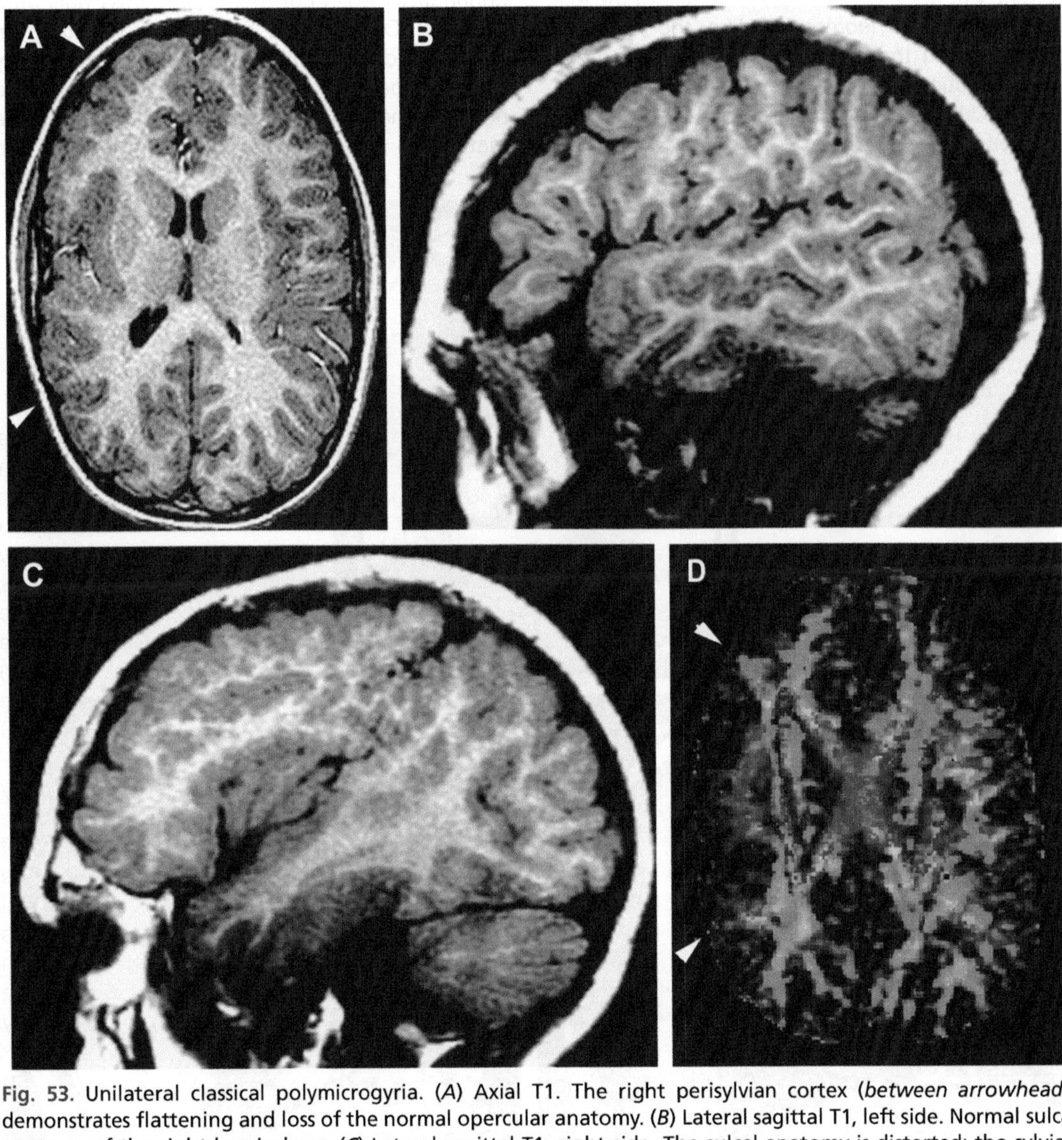

Fig. 53. Unilateral classical polymicrogyria. (*A*) Axial T1. The right perisylvian cortex (*between arrowheads*) demonstrates flattening and loss of the normal opercular anatomy. (*B*) Lateral sagittal T1, left side. Normal sulcal anatomy of the right hemisphere. (*C*) Lateral sagittal T1, right side. The sulcal anatomy is distorted: the sylvian fissure extends into the rolandic-parietal region; the sulci present are aberrant. (*D*) FA color mapping. Disorganization of the fascicular pattern; possibly because of the flattening of the lateral hemispheric cortex, the subcortical fibers all appear transverse (*between arrowheads*).

abnormal and thickened, with (unexplained) vascular proliferation[3,210] and leptomeningeal heterotopia.[210] The PMG cortex is described as either 4-layered or unlayered. It is characterized by an abnormal arrangement of the cell layers and intracortical fiber plexus, and by an excessive folding of the upper or all cellular layers under the continuous smooth molecular layer. The 4-layered cortex is made of the molecular layer, an upper dense cell layer, a layer of low cellular density with horizontal myelinated fibers, and a deep cell layer.[3] The neurons may be small, even immature. The molecular layer may contain too many fibers. The CP is thinner than normal, but does appear thick because of the excessive folding[3] (something like the Spanish collar worn in the sixteenth century). The gray-white junction may be either sharp or histologically blurred by heterotopic neurons or nodules.[210]

More severe (unlayered) patterns associate a molecular layer with a single cellular layer. Abnormal persistence of Cajal-Retzius cells has been described in the molecular layer and in the leptomeningeal heterotopia, as well as in the apparently normal adjacent surrounding cortex[211] to the best of the authors' knowledge, there is nothing in the literature regarding the subplate in PMG. The undulation involves the CP but not the smooth molecular layer (normal gyration involves the cortical plate and the molecular layer together)[3,210]; this may be due to different rates of expansion of the cellular layers[3] but cannot be due to an abnormal connectivity, as the afferent connectivity does not reach the cortex until after week 22. On the other hand, PMG results in an abnormal connectivity that is demonstrated by a poor, aberrant sulcation (the sulci cannot be named) and by a decreased volume of white matter in the corresponding portion of the

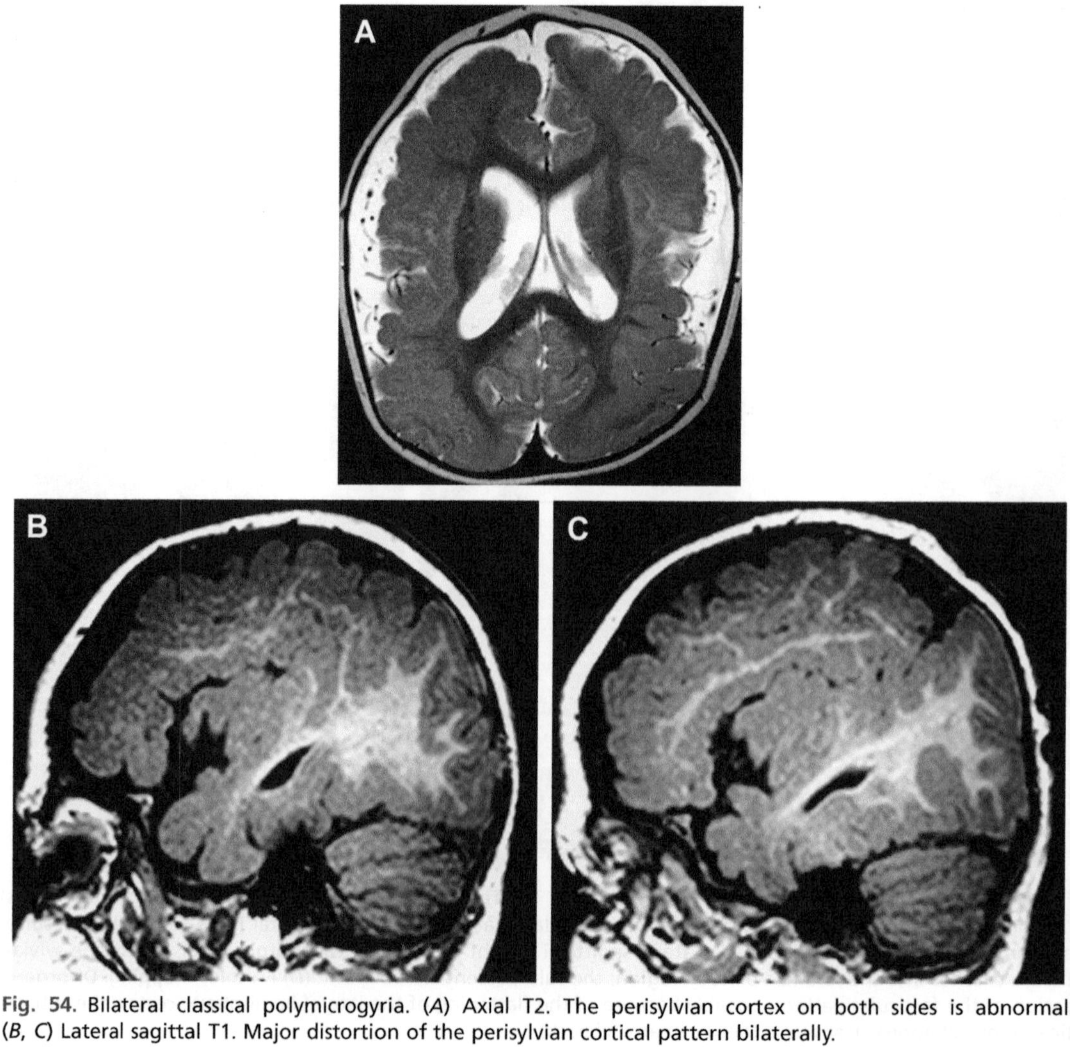

Fig. 54. Bilateral classical polymicrogyria. (*A*) Axial T2. The perisylvian cortex on both sides is abnormal. (*B, C*) Lateral sagittal T1. Major distortion of the perisylvian cortical pattern bilaterally.

hemisphere and the brainstem. This pattern corresponds to that of classical PMG, which assumedly is a specific malformation. However, the diagnosis of PMG is not made by pathology but mostly by MR imaging, and the name PMG (many small gyri) is commonly used as a descriptive term to designate a multiplicity of likely different entities, such as the cortical abnormalities seen in Zellweger syndrome, hemimegalencephaly, the cortex overlying a giant SCNH, the cobblestone cortex resulting from pial basement membrane defects (eg, Fukuyama, MEB, "bilateral frontal polymicrogyria" due to *GPR56* mutation), and even in Chiari II malformation (for which a special name, stenogyria, has been coined to describe a specific cortical pattern): all are different diseases from, and not variants of, PMG.

What causes a PMG? There are many well-defined genetic PMG syndromes,[212,213] but the vast majority of PMG cases observed in clinical practice are idiopathic. Because of the common location of the abnormalities in the perisylvian regions, and because of anecdotal reports of possible anoxic-ischemic injury in the second trimester, a hemodynamic mechanism is commonly proposed, as for schizencephaly. Yet it should be remembered that there is no cortical vascularization before week 22, so that any vascular event before that time would affect the germinal zone, not the cortex, and would be consistent with PMG being considered a milder form of a group of injuries of which schizencephaly could be the most severe form. An event occurring during the third wave of neuronal migration (after week 16) and before 18 weeks would sound logical, as definite PMG can be seen at this gestational age: yet it seems odd that the most common cortical malformation would result from an event occurring within such a very limited period of 2 weeks in the early third trimester. Therefore, PMG may be the end result of many events occurring at any time during the neuronal migration before 18 weeks (or less).

Beyond the "many small gyri," Barkovich proposed a distinction between "coarse" PMG (which corresponds to the classical appearance) and a "delicate" type (which the authors call a "curly" cortical ribbon).[214] It seems logical that these two different appearances would reflect different pathologies, especially as the curly (or "delicate") PMG seems not to be necessarily associated with aberrant sulcation (see **Fig. 24**D). As a consequence, the authors classify PMG as:

- Classical, idiopathic PMG
- PMG syndromes
- PMG-like malformations.

Classical (idiopathic) PMG

Classical idiopathic PMG is typically found in the perisylvian regions (**Figs. 53** and **54**). The sylvian fissure itself often is exceedingly oblique and extends posterosuperiorly into what apparently is the parietal lobe (given the abnormal sulcation, a precise lobar identification is uncertain). In roughly half the cases PMG is unilateral (see **Fig. 53**) and in half it is bilateral; when it is bilateral, it is not strictly symmetric (see **Fig. 54**). It may be restricted to the opercular region or may extend further, even over the vertex toward the medial wall of the hemisphere; however, it seems never to affect the limbic structures.

The cortex appears irregular. Although it may appear thick on 4- to 5-mm cuts, use of thin 3D-T1 acquisition has shown that the cortical ribbon itself is thin, and the apparent thickening results from juxtaposition of the folds.[215] The molecular layer is difficult to identify on MR images. The cortical-subcortical junction appears well demarcated, if irregular. The sulcation is aberrant, without any recognizable pattern; this may extend even beyond the recognizable area of PMG, presumably because of a distorted connectivity (see **Figs. 53** and **54**).[215] The sulci may be shallow or, on the contrary, indent deeply in the parenchyma. The white matter is decreased in volume, with a corresponding ventriculomegaly and thin interhemispheric commissures. This hypoplasia extends to the cerebral peduncles, pons, and medullary pyramids, resulting in a striking asymmetry when the malformation is unilateral. There may be some delay in myelination; however,

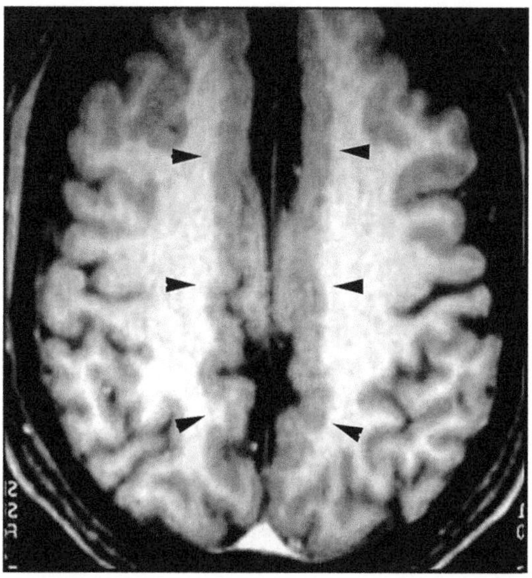

Fig. 55. Bilateral medial frontal polymicrogyria (*arrowheads*).

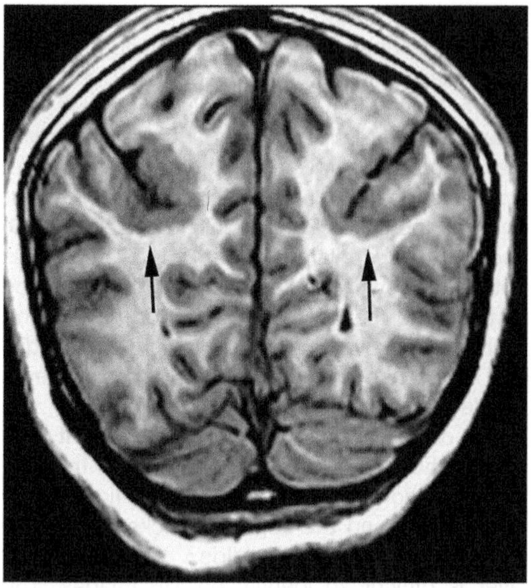

Fig. 56. Bilateral parietal polymicrogyria (*arrows*).

significant bright T2/FLAIR changes in the white matter, especially when organized in subcortical and periventricular layers,[215] are highly suggestive of PMG secondary to cytomegalovirus infection (see **Fig. 51**).[216] Over the brain surface dysplastic vessels, mostly veins, are common and correlate well with the pathologic finding of leptomeningeal vascular dysplasia.

Secondary and possibly secondary PMG

CMV has for a long time been shown to be associated with PMG.[217,218] The PMG features may be severe, associating PMG and schizencephalic clefts supratentorially as well as infratentorially, and with microcephaly (see **Fig. 51**). In other instances the lesions may be milder. As mentioned

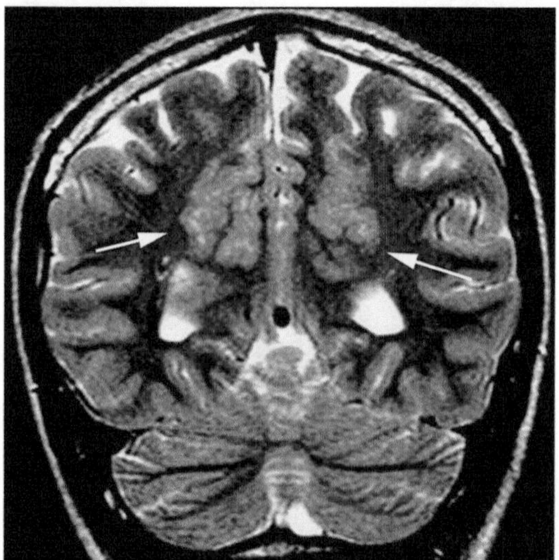

Fig. 57. Bilateral parieto-occipital polymicrogyria (*arrows*).

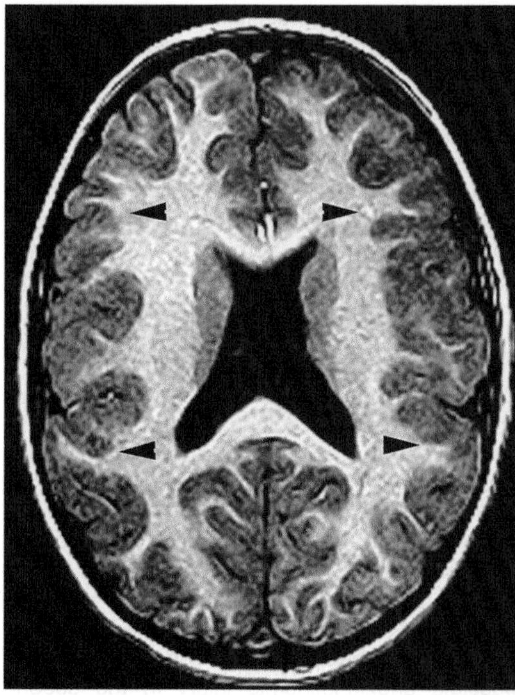

Fig. 58. Bilateral perisylvian polymicrogyria with septal agenesis (*arrowheads*).

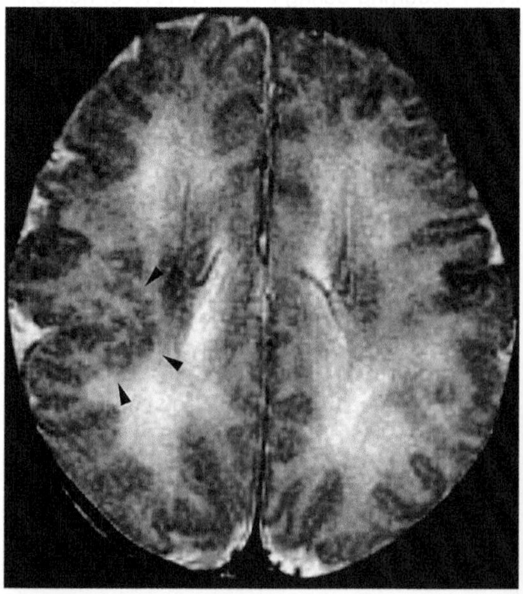

Fig. 59. Zellweger disease. The PMG-like cortical abnormality is typically located in the posterior insular/opercular area (*arrowheads*).

earlier, the presence of large areas of unmyelinated white matter often organized in two separate layers is very suggestive of the etiology.

PMG may be associated with meningeal dysplasia. The association is common in commissural agenesis with dysplastic interhemispheric meningeal cysts, often in association with SCNHs (see earlier discussion). It may be observed in cases of meningeal angiomatosis[219] or meningeal lipoma.[3,220]

Bilateral symmetric PMG

Not all presumably genetic PMG are bilateral, and there are familial instances of unilateral PMG,[221,222] not necessarily on the same side, in different family members (Charles Raybaud,

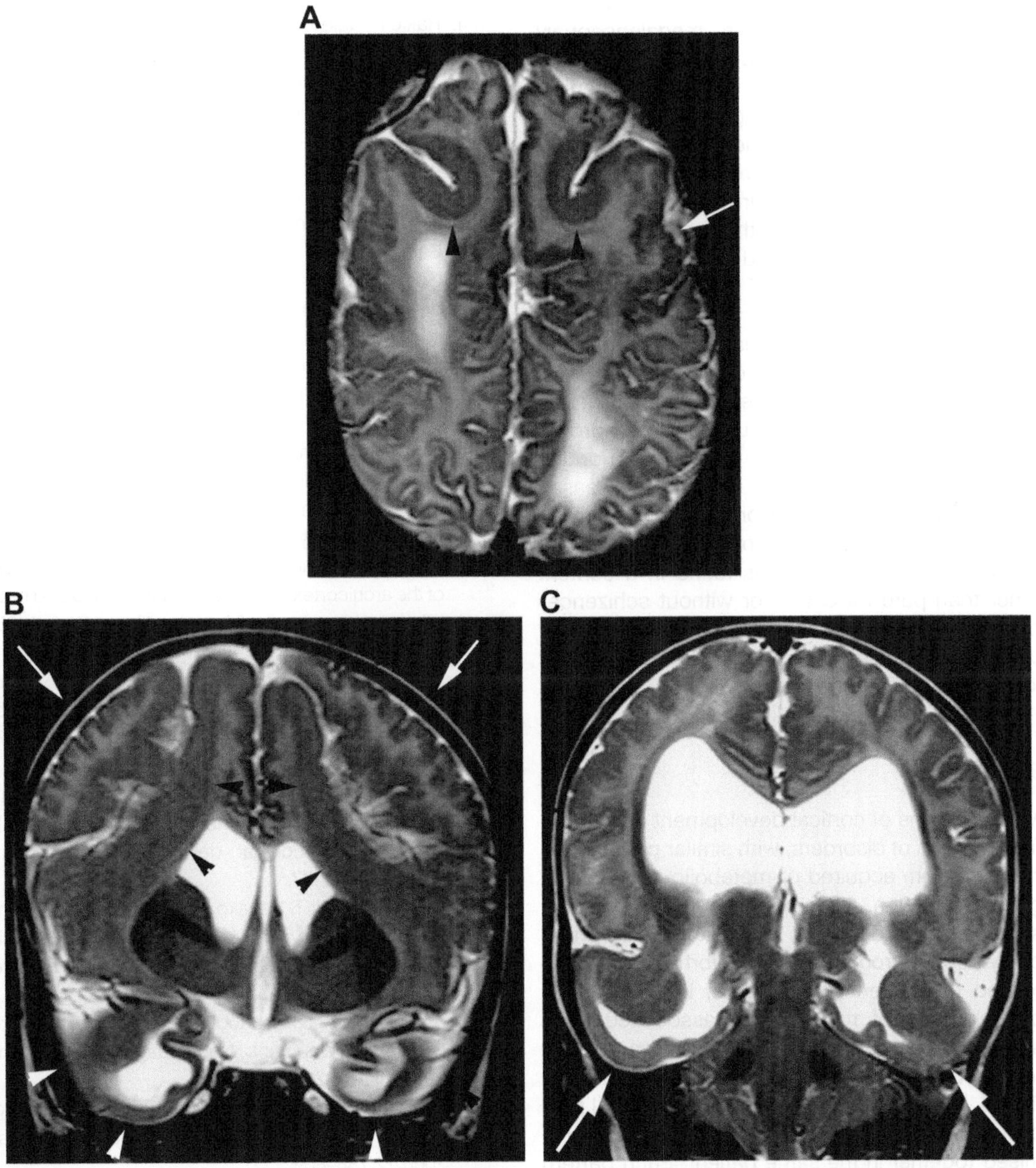

Fig. 60. Undetermined complex cortical malformative syndrome. (*A*) Axial T2. Bilateral symmetric deep frontal clefts (*arrow*) lined with thick dysgenetic cortex (*arrowheads*) associated with diffuse medial and lateral frontal polymicrogyria; the posterior parts of the hemispheres appear normal. (*B*) Coronal T2. The deep bilateral frontal clefts are associated with thick cortex (*black arrowheads*) and polymicrogyria (*white arrows*); anterior temporal agyria (*white arrowheads*). (*C*) Coronal T2. Marked ventriculomegaly. The anterior temporal cortex is smooth (agyric) with dysplastic hippocampi. (*Courtesy of* Dr Xin-Chang Wei, Calgary, AB.)

personal data). Yet most cases of genetic PMG are bilateral and symmetric (**Figs. 55–58**). In contrast to the idiopathic form of PMG, bilateral symmetric PMG may also involve the cortex that lines abnormally deep but normally located sulci. Such PMG syndromes are: the bilateral perisylvian polymicrogyria syndromes (Xq21.33–q23/SRPX2; 22q11.2; Xq28)[223]; the BFPP, better identified now as a pial basement membrane disease (GPR56) (see earlier); the bilateral symmetric frontal polymicrogyria[224]; the bilateral medial parietal-occipital polymicrogyria[225]; a megalencephaly with polymicrogyria and hydrocephalus, or with polymicrogyria, polydactyly, and hydrocephalus[226]; and a syndrome of mega-corpus callosum, polymicrogyria, and psychomotor retardation.[227] It is likely that more will be recognized over the years. Finally, the rare occurrence of a bilateral, symmetric polymicrogyria with absent septum pellucidum is more likely related to an inborn defect than to a forme fruste of porencephaly (see **Fig. 58**).[228]

PMG-like cortical malformations are common and have been described in different contexts of MCD: microcephaly, hemimegalencephaly, bilateral frontoparietal PMG, Fukuyama syndrome (see earlier), and massive subcortical nodular heterotopia,[229] but also in metabolic diseases such as the peroxisomal disorders (**Fig. 59**), mitochondrial disorders, and glycogenosis type III.[230] It is felt that when the PMG is found in a context other than pure PMG with or without schizencephaly, the descriptive term "PMG-like" should be used to differentiate it from the true PMG, either idiopathic, disruptive, or inborn.

SUMMARY

Malformations of cortical development are a confusing group of disorders, with similar phenotypes resulting from acquired or metabolic disorders or genetic mutation. Although the main morphologic subtypes (microcephaly, heterotopia, lissencephaly, polymicrogyria, and so forth) have been related to different mechanisms, the findings of different types of malformations associated in the same brain (eg, cortical dysplasia, agyria, heterotopia, polymicrogyria, schizencephaly) (see **Figs. 24, 26**, and **47**; **Fig. 60**) suggest that several processes of corticogenesis are commonly compromised together in the same patient. Each pattern is a malformative feature only, and together these features may form various combinations, which depend on the etiopathogenetic process involved (genetic mutation, metabolic disease, infection, syndromic association and so forth).

REFERENCES

1. Taylor DC, Falconer MA, Brutton CJ, et al. Focal dysplasia of the cerebral cortex in epilepsy. J Neurol Neurosurg Psychiatr 1971;34:369–87.
2. Friede RL. Disturbance in the bulk growth of nervous tissue. In: Friede RL, editor. Developmental neuropathology. Springer; 1975. p. 271–9.
3. Friede RL. Dysplasias of cerebral cortex. In Friede RL, editor. Developmental neuropathology. Springer; 1975. p. 297–313.
4. Rakic P. Guidance of neurons migrating to the fetal monkey neocortex. Brain Res 1971;33:471–6.
5. Sidman RL, Rakic P. Neuronal migration, with special reference to developing human brain: a review. Brain Res 1973;62:1–35.
6. Smith AS, Ross JS, Blaser SI, et al. Magnetic resonance imaging of disturbances in neuronal migration: illustration of an embryologic process. Radiographics 1989;9:509–22.
7. Guerrini R, Dobyns WB, Barkovich AJ. Abnormal development of the human cerebral cortex: genetics, functional consequences and treatment options. Trends Neurosci 2008;31:154–62.
8. Barkovich AJ, Kuzniecky RI, Dobyns WB, et al. A classification scheme for malformations of cortical development. Neuropediatrics 1996;27:59–63.
9. Raymond AA, Fish DR, Sisodiya SM, et al. Abnormalities of gyration, heterotopias, tuberous sclerosis, focal cortical dysplasia, microdysgenesis, dysembryoplastic neuroepithelial tumor and dysgenesis of the archicortex in epilepsy. Clinical, EEG and neuroimaging features in 100 adult patients. Brain 1995; 118:629–60.
10. Barkovich AJ, Kuzniechy RI, Jackson GD, et al. Classification system for malformations of cortical development. Update 2001. Neurology 2001;57: 2168–78.
11. Barkovich AJ, Kuzniecky RI, Jackson GD, et al. A developmental and genetic classification for malformations of cortical development. Neurology 2005;65:1873–87.
12. Kaido T, Otsuki T, Kaneko Y, et al. Anterior striatum with dysmorphic neurons associated with the epileptogenesis of focal cortical dysplasia. Seizure 2010;19:256–9.
13. Barkovich AJ, Raybaud CA. Malformations of cortical development. Neuroimaging Clin N Am 2004;14:401–23.
14. Raybaud C, Shroff M, Rutka JT, et al. Imaging surgical epilepsy in children. Childs Nerv Syst 2006;22:786–809.
15. Deblaere K, Achten E. Structural magnetic resonance imaging in epilepsy. Eur Radiol 2008;18:119–29.
16. Widjaja E, Raybaud C. Advances in neuroimaging in patients with epilepsy. Neurosurg Focus 2008; 25:E3.

17. Gaillard WD, Chiron C, Cross JH, et al. Guidelines for imaging infants and children with recent-onset epilepsy. Epilepsia 2009;50:2147–53.
18. Woermann FG, Vollmar C. Clinical MRI in children and adults with focal epilepsy: a critical review. Epilepsy Behav 2009;15:40–9.
19. Bernasconi A, Bernasconi N, Bernhardt BC, et al. Advances in MRI for cryptogenic epilepsies. Nat Rev Neurol 2011;7:99–108.
20. Saini J, Singh A, Kesavadas C. Role of three-dimensional fluid-attenuated inversion recovery (3D FLAIR) and proton density imaging for the detection and evaluation of lesion extent of focal cortical dysplasia in patients with refractory epilepsy. Acta Radiol 2010;51:218–25.
21. Sankar R, Curran JG, Kevill JW, et al. Microscopic cortical dysplasia in infantile spasms: evolution of the white matter abnormalities. AJNR Am J Neuroradiol 1995;16:1265–72.
22. Yagishita A, Arai N, Maehara T, et al. Focal cortical dysplasia: appearance on MR images. Radiology 1997;203:553–9.
23. Lee BC, Schmitt RE, Hatfield GA, et al. MRI of focal cortical dysplasia. Neuroradiology 1998;40:675–83.
24. Mackay MT, Becker LE, Chuang SH, et al. Malformations of cortical development with balloon cells. Clinical and radiological correlates. Neurology 2003;60:580–7.
25. Eltze CM, Chong WK, Bhate S, et al. Taylor-type focal cortical dysplasia in infants: some MRI lesions almost disappear with maturation of myelination. Epilepsia 2005;46:1988–92.
26. Duprez T, Ghariani S, Grandin C, et al. Focal seizure induce premature myelination: speculation from serial MRI. Neuroradiology 1998;40:580–2.
27. Demerens C, Stankoff B, Logak M, et al. Induction of myelination in the central nervous system by electrical activity. Proc Natl Acad Sci U S A 1996; 93:9887–92.
28. Ishibashi T, Dakin KA, Stevens B, et al. Astrocytes promote myelination in response to electrical impulses. Neuron 2006;49:823–32.
29. Jacoby CG, Yuh WTC, Afifi AK, et al. Accelerated myelination in early Sturge-Weber syndrome demonstrated by MR imaging. J Comput Assist Tomogr 1987;11:226–31.
30. Eriksson SH, Free SL, Thom M, et al. Correlation of quantitative MRI and neuropathology in epilepsy surgical resection specimens—T2 correlates with neuronal tissue in gray matter. Neuroimage 2007; 37:48–55.
31. Sisodiya SM, Free SL. Disproportion of cerebral surface areas and volumes in cerebral dysgenesis. MRI-based evidence for connectional abnormalities. Brain 1997;120:271–81.
32. Diehl B, Symms MR, Boulby P, et al. Postictal diffusion tensor imaging. Epilepsy Res 2005;65:137–46.
33. Guye M, Ranjeva JP, Bartolomei F, et al. What is the significance of interictal water diffusion changes in frontal lobe epilepsies? Neuroimage 2007;35:28–37.
34. Chen Q, Lui S, Li CX, et al. MRI-negative refractory partial epilepsy: role for diffusion tensor imaging in high field MRI. Epilepsy Res 2008;80:83–9.
35. Eriksson SH, Rugg-Gunn FJ, Symms MR, et al. Diffusion tensor imaging in patients with epilepsy and malformations of cortical development. Brain 2001;124:617–26.
36. Wieshmann UC, Krakow K, Symms GJM, et al. Combined functional magnetic resonance imaging and diffusion tensor imaging demonstrates widespread modified organisation in malformation of cortical development. J Neurol Neurosurg Psychiatr 2001;70:521–3.
37. Briellmann RS, Mitchell LA, Waites AB, et al. Correlation between language organization and diffusion tensor abnormalities in refractory partial epilepsy. Epilepsia 2003;44:1541–5.
38. Dumas de la Roque A, Oppenheim C, Chassoux F, et al. Diffusion tensor imaging of partial intractable epilepsy. Eur Radiol 2005;15:279–85.
39. Widjaja E, Blaser S, Miller E, et al. Evaluation of subcortical white matter and deep white matter tracts in malformations of cortical development. Epilepsia 2007;48:1460–9.
40. Li L, Cendes F, Bastos A, et al. Neuronal metabolic dysfunction in patients with cortical developmental malformations: a proton magnetic resonance spectroscopic imaging study. Neurology 1998;50:755–9.
41. Widjaja E, Griffiths PD, Wilkinson ID. Proton MR spectroscopy of polymicrogyria and heterotopia. AJNR Am J Neuroradiol 2003;24:2077–81.
42. Simister RJ, McLean MA, Barker GJ, et al. Proton magnetic resonance spectroscopy of malformations of cortical development causing epilepsy. Epilepsy Res 2007;74:107–15.
43. Vuori K, Kankaanranta L, Häkkinen AM, et al. Low-grade gliomas and focal cortical developmental malformations: differentiation with proton MR spectroscopy. Radiology 2004;230:703–8.
44. Widjaja E, Wilkinson ID, Griffiths PD. Magnetic resonance perfusion imaging in malformations of cortical development. Acta Radiol 2007;46:907–17.
45. Jeong MG, Chung TS, Coe CJ, et al. Application of magnetization transfer imaging for intracranial lesions of tuberous sclerosis. J Comput Assist Tomogr 1997;21:8–14.
46. Girard N, Zimmerman RA, Schnur RE, et al. Magnetization transfer in the investigation of patients with tuberous sclerosis. Neuroradiology 1997;39:523–8.
47. Zikou A, Ioannidou MC, Tzoufi M, et al. Magnetization transfer ratio measurements of the brain in children with tuberous sclerosis complex. Pediatr Radiol 2005;35:1071–4.

48. Rugg-Gunn FJ, Eriksson SH, Boulby PA, et al. Magnetization transfer imaging in focal epilepsy. Neurology 2003;60:1638–45.
49. Widjaja E, Mahmoodabadi SZ, Otsubo H, et al. Subcortical alterations in tissue microstructure adjacent to focal cortical dysplasia: detection at diffusion-tensor MR imaging by using magnetoencephalic dipole cluster localization. Radiology 2009;251:206–15.
50. Janszky J, Ebner A, Kruse B, et al. Functional organization of the brain with malformations of cortical development. Ann Neurol 2003;53:759–67.
51. Detre JA. fMRI: applications in epilepsy. Epilepsia 2004;45(Suppl 4):26–31.
52. Duncan JS. Imaging in the surgical treatment of epilepsy. Nat Rev Neurol 2010;6:537–50.
53. Anderson DP, Harvey AS, Saling MM, et al. fMRI localization of expressive language in children with cerebral lesions. Epilepsia 2006;47:998–1008.
54. Gaillard WD, Berl MM, Moore EN, et al. Atypical language in lesional and nonlesional complex partial epilepsy. Neurology 2007;69:1761–71.
55. Govindan RM, Chugani HT, Luat AF, et al. Presurgical prediction of motor functional loss using tractography. Pediatr Neurol 2010;43:70–2.
56. Nilsson D, Starck G, Ljundberg M, et al. Intersubject variability in the anterior extent of the optic radiation assessed by tractography. Epilepsy Res 2007;77:11–6.
57. Otsubo H, Snead OC III. Magnetoencephalography and magnetic source imaging in children. J Child Neurol 2001;16:227–35.
58. O'Brien TJ, So EL, Mullan BP, et al. Subtraction SPECT co-registered to MRI improves postictal SPECT localization of seizure foci. Neurology 1999;52:137–46.
59. Salamon N, Kung J, Shaw SJ, et al. FDG-PET/MRI coregistration improves detection of cortical dysplasia in patients with epilepsy. Neurology 2008;71:1594–601.
60. Thornton R, Laufs H, Rodionov R, et al. EEG correlated functional MRI and postoperative outcome in focal epilepsy. J Neurol Neurosurg Psychiatry 2010;81:922–7.
61. Marin-Padilla M. Prenatal and early postnatal ontogenesis of the human motor cortex: a Golgi study. I. The sequential development of the cortical layers. Brain Res 1970;33:167–83.
62. Supèr H, Soriano E, Uylings HB. The functions of the preplate in development and evolution of the neocortex and hippocampus. Brain Res Bull 1998;27:40–64.
63. Nadarajah B, Parnavelas JG. Modes of neuronal migration in the developing cerebral cortex. Nat Rev Neurosci 2002;3:423–32.
64. Kriegstein AR, Noctor SC. Pattern of neuronal migration in the embryonic cortex. Trends Neurosci 2004;27:392–9.
65. Kriegstein AR. Constructing circuits: neurogenesis and migration in the developing cortex. Epilepsia 2005;46(Suppl 7):15–21.
66. Rakic P. A century of progress in corticoneurogenesis: from silver impregnation to genetic engineering. Cereb Cortex 2006;16:i3–17.
67. Bystron I, Blakemore C, Rakic P. Development of the human cerebral cortex: Boulder Committee revisited. Nat Rev Neurosci 2008;9:110–22.
68. Clowry G, Molnár Z, Rakic P. Renewed focus on the developing human neocortex. J Anat 2010;217:276–88.
69. Stiles J, Jernigan TL. The basics of brain development. Neuropsychol Rev 2010;20:237–48.
70. Bayer SS, Altman J. The human brain during the early first trimester. Boca Raton (FL); London; New York: CRC Press/Taylor and Francis Group; 2008.
71. Marin-Padilla M. Early prenatal ontogenesis of the cerebral cortex (neocortex) of the *Felix domestica*. A Golgi study. I. The primordial neocortical organization. Z Anat Entwicklungsgesch 1971;134:117–42 (quoted by [Super]).
72. Tau GZ, Peterson BS. Normal development of brain circuits. Neuropsychopharmacology 2010;35:147–68.
73. McKinstry RC, Mathur A, Miller JH, et al. Radial organization of developing preterm human cerebral cortex revealed by non-invasive water diffusion anisotropy MRI. Cereb Cortex 2002;12:1237–43.
74. Smart IH, McSherry GM. Gyrus formation in the cerebral cortex of the ferret. II. Description of the internal histological changes. J Anat 1986;147:27–43.
75. Ferrer I, Hernández-Martí M, Bernet E, et al. Formation and growth of the cerebral convolutions. I. Development of the median-suprasylvian gyrus and adjoining sulci in the cat. J Anat 1988;160:89–100.
76. Ferrer I, Hernández-Martí M, Bernet E, et al. Formation and growth of the cerebral convolutions. I. Cell death in the suprasylvius gyrus and adjoining sulci in the cat. Dev Brain Res 1989;45:303–8.
77. Kostović I, Jovanov-Milošević N. The development of cerebral connections during the first 20–45 weeks' gestation. Semin Fetal Neonatal Med 2006;11:415–22.
78. López-Bendito G, Molnár Z. Thalamocortical development: how are we going to get there? Nat Rev Neurosci 2003;4:276–89.
79. Ten Donkelaar HJ, Lammens M, Wesseling P, et al. Development and malformations of the human pyramidal tract. J Neurol 2004;251:1429–42.
80. Stanfield BB. The development of the corticospinal projection. Prog Neurobiol 1992;38:169–202.
81. Hevner RE. Development of connections in the human visual system during fetal mid-gestation. A DiI-tracing study. J Neuropathol Exp Neurol 2000;59:385–92.

82. Raybaud C. Normal and abnormal embryology and development of the intracranial vascular system. Neurosurg Clin N Am 2010;21:399–426.
83. Klosovskii BN. Fundamental facts concerning the stages and principles of development of the brain and its response to noxious agents. In: Klosovskii BN, editor. The development of the brain and its disturbance by harmful factors. London: Pergamon Press; 1963. p. 3–43 [Translated from Russian and edited by B Haigh]. Chapter 1.
84. Encha-Razavi F, Sonigo P. Features of the developing brain. Childs Nerv Syst 2003;16:426–8.
85. Volpe JJ. Hypoxic ischemic encephalopathy: biochemical and physiological aspects. In: Volpe JJ, editor. Neurology of the newborn. 4th edition. Saunders; 2001. p. 217–76.
86. Chiron C, Raynaud C, Maziere B, et al. Changes in regional cerebral blood flow during brain maturation in children and adolescent. J Nucl Med 1992; 33:696–703.
87. Kehrer M, Schöning M. A longitudinal study of cerebral blood flow over the first 30 months. Pediatr Res 2009;66:560–4.
88. Kehrer M, Blumenstock G, Ehehalt S, et al. Development of cerebral blood flow volume in preterm neonates during the first two weeks of life. Pediatr Res 2005;58:927–30.
89. Krsek P, Maton B, Korman B, et al. Different features of histopathological subtypes of pediatric focal cortical dysplasia. Ann Neurol 2008;63:758–69.
90. Colombo N, Tassi L, Galli C, et al. Focal cortical dysplasias: MR imaging, histopathologic, and clinical correlations in surgically treated patients with epilepsy. AJNR Am J Neuroradiol 2003;24:724–33.
91. Francione S, Vigliano P, Tassi L, et al. Surgery for drug resistant partial epilepsy in children with focal cortical dysplasia: anatomical-clinical correlations and neurophysiological data in 10 patients. J Neurol Neurosurg Psychiatr 2003;74:1493–501.
92. Fauser S, Schultze-Bonhage A, Honegger J, et al. Focal cortical dysplasias: surgical outcome in 67 patients in relation to histological subtypes and dual pathology. Brain 2004;127:2406–18.
93. Hildebrandt M, Pieper T, Winkler P, et al. Neuropathological spectrum of cortical dysplasia in children with severe focal epilepsies. Acta Neuropathol 2005;110:1–11.
94. Mischel PS, Nguyen LP, Vinters HV. Cerebral cortical dysplasia associated with pediatric epilepsy. Review of neuropathologic features and proposal for a grading system. J Neuropathol Exp Neurol 1995;54:137–53.
95. Palmini A, Najm I, Avanzini G, et al. Terminology and classification of the cortical dysplasias. Neurology 2004;62(Suppl 3):S2–8.
96. Spreafico R, Blümcke I. Focal cortical dysplasia: clinical implication of neuropathological classification systems. Acta Neuropathol 2010;120:359–67.
97. Chamberlain WA, Cohen ML, Gyure KA, et al. Interobserver and intraobserver reproducibility in focal cortical dysplasia (malformations of cortical development). Epilepsia 2009;50:2593–8.
98. Marin-Padilla M. Developmental neuropathology and impact of perinatal brain damage. I: hemorrhagic lesions of neocortex. J Neuropathol Exp Neurol 1996;55:758–73.
99. Marin-Padilla M. Developmental neuropathology and impact of perinatal brain damage. II: white matter lesions of the neocortex. J Neuropathol Exp Neurol 1997;56:219–35.
100. Marin-Padilla M. Developmental neuropathology and impact of perinatal brain damage. III: gray matter lesions of the neocortex. J Neuropathol Exp Neurol 1999;58:407–29.
101. Lombroso CT. Can early postnatal closed head injury induce cortical dysplasia? Epilepsia 2000; 41:245–53.
102. Marin-Padilla M, Parisi JE, Armstrong DL, et al. Shaken infant syndrome: developmental neuropathology, progressive cortical dysplasia, and epilepsy. Acta Neuropathol 2002;103:321–32.
103. Kremer S, de Saint-Martin A, Minotti L, et al. Focal cortical dysplasia possibly related to a probable prenatal ischemic injury. J Neuroradiol 2002;29: 200–3.
104. Govaert P, Lequin M, Korsten A, et al. Postnatal onset cortical dysplasia associated with infarction of white matter. Brain Res 2006;1121:250–5.
105. Blümcke I, Thom M, Aronica E, et al. The clinicopathologic spectrum of focal cortical dysplasia: a consensus classification proposed by an ad hoc Task Force of the ILAE Diagnostic Methods Commission. Epilepsia 2011;52:158–74.
106. Cepeda C, Andre VM, Flores-Hernandez J, et al. Pediatric cortical dysplasia: correlation between neuroimaging, electrophysiology and location of cytomegalic neurons and balloon-cells and glutamate/GABA synaptic circuits. Dev Neurosci 2005;27:59–76.
107. Adamsbaum C, Robain O, Cohen PA, et al. Focal cortical dysplasia and hemimegalencephaly: histological and neuroimaging correlations. Pediatr Radiol 1998;28:583–90.
108. Andres M, Andre VM, Nguyen S, et al. Human cortical dysplasia and epilepsy: an ontogenetic hypothesis based on volumetric MRI and NeuN neuronal density and size measurements. Cereb Cortex 2005;15:194–210.
109. Huppertz HJ, Grimm C, Fauser C, et al. Enhanced visualization of blurred gray-white matter junctions in focal cortical dysplasia by voxel-based 3D MRI analysis. Epilepsy Res 2005;67:35–50.
110. Bonilha L, Montenegro MA, Rorden C, et al. Voxel-based morphometry reveals excess gray matter concentration in patients with focal cortical dysplasia. Epilepsia 2006;47:901–15.

111. Widdess-Walsh P, Diehl B, Najm I. Neuroimaging of focal cortical dysplasia. J Neuroimaging 2006;16:185–95.
112. Widjaja E, Otsubo H, Raybaud C, et al. Characteristics of MEG and MRI between Taylor's focal cortical dysplasia (type II) and other cortical dysplasia: surgical outcome after complete resection of MEG spike source and MR lesion in pediatric cortical dysplasia. Epilepsy Res 2008;82:147–55.
113. Focke NK, Bonelly SB, Yogarajah M, et al. Automated normalized FLAIR imaging in MRI-negative patients with refractory focal epilepsy. Epilepsia 2009;50:1484–90.
114. Madan N, Grant PE. New directions in clinical imaging of cortical dysplasias. Epilepsia 2009;50(Suppl 9):9–18.
115. Colombo N, Salamon N, Raybaud C, et al. Imaging of malformations of cortical development. Epileptic Disord 2009;11:194–205.
116. Krsek P, Pieper T, Karlmeier A, et al. Different presurgical characteristics and seizure outcomes in children with focal cortical dysplasia type I or II. Epilepsia 2009;50:125–37.
117. Barkovich AL, Kuzniecky RI, Bollen AW, et al. Focal transmantle dysplasia: a specific malformation of cortical development. Neurology 1997;49:1148–52.
118. Besson P, Andermann F, Dubeau F, et al. Small focal cortical dysplasia lesions are located at the bottom of a deep sulcus. Brain 2008;131:3246–55.
119. Fauser S, Sisodiya SM, Martinian L, et al. Multifocal occurrence of cortical dysplasia in epileptic patients. Brain 2009;132:2079–90.
120. Diehl B, Tkach J, Piao Z, et al. Diffusion tensor imaging in patients with focal epilepsy due to cortical dysplasia in the temporo-occipital region: electro-clinico-pathological correlation. Epilepsy Res 2010;90:178–87.
121. Komori T, Arai N, Shimizu H, et al. Cortical perivascular satellitosis in intractable epilepsy; a form of cortical dysplasia? Acta Neuropathol 2002;104:149–54.
122. Kasper BS, Paulus W. Perivascular clustering in temporal lobe epilepsy: oligodendroglial cells of unknown function. Acta Neuropathol 2004;108:471–5.
123. Hazrati LN, Kleinschmidt-DeMasters BK, Handler MH, et al. Astrocytic inclusions in epilepsy: expanding the concept of filaminopathies. J Neuropathol Exp Neurol 2008;67:669–76.
124. Van den Veyver IB, Panichkul PP, Antalffy BA, et al. Presence of Filamin in the astrocytic inclusions of Aicardi syndrome. Pediatr Neurol 2004;30:7–15.
125. Hamilton BE, Nesbit GM. MR imaging identification of oligodendroglial hyperplasia. AJNR Am J Neuroradiol 2009;30:1412–3.
126. Sasaki M, Hashimoto T, Furushima W, et al. Clinical aspects of hemimegalencephaly by means of a nationwide survey. J Child Neurol 2005;20:337–41.
127. Flores-Sarnat L. Hemimegalencephaly: part 1. Genetic, clinical and imaging aspects. J Child Neurol 2002;17:373–84.
128. Di Rocco C, Battaglia D, Pietrini D, et al. Hemimegalencephaly: clinical implications and surgical treatment. Childs Nerv Syst 2006;22:852–66.
129. Di Rocco F, Novegno F, Tamburrini G, et al. Hemimegalencephaly involving the cerebellum. Pediatr Neurosurg 2001;35:274–6.
130. Tinkle BT, Schorry EK, Franz DN, et al. Epidemiology of hemimegalencephaly. Am J Med Genet 2005;139:204–11.
131. Robain O, Gelot A. Neuropathology of hemimegalencephaly. In: Guerrini R, Andermann F, Canapicchi R, et al, editors. Dysplasia of cerebral cortex and epilepsy. Philadelphia: Lippincott-Raven; 1996. p. 89–92.
132. Flores-Sarnat L, Sarnat HB, Dávilla-Gutiérrez G, et al. Hemimegalencephaly: part 2. Neuropathology suggests a disorder of cellular lineage. J Child Neurol 2003;18:776–85.
133. Salamon N, Andres M, Chute DJ, et al. Contralateral hemimicrencephaly and clinical-pathological correlations in children with hemimegalencephaly. Brain 2006;129:352–65.
134. D'Agostino MD, Bastos A, Piras C, et al. Posterior quadrantic dysplasia or hemi-hemimegalencephaly: a characteristic brain malformation. Neurology 2004;62:2214–20.
135. Wolpert SM, Cohen A, Libenson MH. Hemimegalencephaly: a longitudinal MR study. AJNR Am J Neuroradiol 1994;15:1479–82.
136. Yagishita A, Arai N, Tamagawa K, et al. Hemimegalencephaly: signal changes suggesting abnormal myelination on MRI. Neuroradiology 1998;40:734–8.
137. Sato N, Ota M, Yagishita A, et al. Aberrant midsagittal fiber tracts in patients with hemimegalencephaly. AJNR Am J Neuroradiol 2008;29:823–7.
138. Takahashi T, Sato N, Ota M, et al. Asymmetric interhemispheric fiber tracts in patients with hemimegalencephaly on diffusion tensor magnetic resonance imaging. J Neuroradiol 2009;36:249–54.
139. Sato N, Yagishita A, Oba H, et al. Hemimegalencephaly: a study of abnormalities occurring outside the involved hemisphere. AJNR Am J Neuroradiol 2007;28:678–82.
140. Abuello D. Microcephaly syndromes. Semin Pediatr Neurol 2007;14:118–27.
141. Jones KL. Smith's recognizable patterns of human malformation. 6th edition. Philadelphia (PA): Elsevier-Saunders; 2006.
142. Woods CG, Bond J, Enard W. Autosomal recessive microcephaly (MCPH): a review of clinical, molecular and evolutionary findings. Am J Hum Genet 2005;76:717–28.
143. Thornton GK, Woods CG. Primary microcephaly: do all roads lead to Rome? Trends Genet 2009;25:501–10.

144. Adachi Y, Poduri A, Kawaguch A, et al. Congenital microcephaly with a simplified gyral pattern: associated findings and their significance. AJNR Am J Neuroradiol 2011;32(6):1123–9.
145. Widjaja E, Nilsson D, Blaser S, et al. White matter abnormalities in children with developmental delay. Acta Radiol 2008;49:589–95.
146. Olney AH. Macrocephaly syndromes. Semin Pediatr Neurol 2007;14:128–35.
147. Schaefer GB, Bodensteiner JB, Buehler BA, et al. The neuroimaging findings in Sotos syndrome. Am J Med Genet 1997;68:462–5.
148. Thom M, Martinian L, Parnavelas JG, et al. Distribution of cortical interneurons in gray matter heterotopia in patients with epilepsy. Epilepsia 2004;45:916–23.
149. Hevner RF. Layer specific markers as probes for neuron type identity in human neocortex and malformations of cortical development. J Neuropathol Exp Neurol 2007;66:101–9.
150. Garbelli R, Rossini L, Moroni RF, et al. Layer-specific genes reveal a rudimentary laminar pattern in human nodular heterotopia. Neurology 2009;73:746–53.
151. Hatazawa J, Sasajima E, Fujita H, et al. Regional cerebral blood flow response in gray matter heterotopia during finger tapping: an activation study with positron emission tomography. AJNR Am J Neuroradiol 1996;17:479–82.
152. Pinard JM, Feydy A, Carlier R, et al. Functional MRI in double cortex: functionality of heterotopias. Neurology 2000;54:1531–3.
153. Valton L, Guye M, McGonigal A, et al. Functional interaction in brain networks underlying epileptic seizures in bilateral diffuse periventricular heterotopia. Clin Neurophysiol 2008;119:212–23.
154. Vitali P, Minati L, D'Incerti L, et al. Functional MRI in malformations of cortical development: activation of dysplastic tissue and functional reorganization. J Neuroimaging 2008;18:296–305.
155. Meroni A, Galli C, Bramerio M, et al. Nodular heterotopia: a neuropathological study in 24 patients undergoing surgery for drug-resistant epilepsy. Epilepsia 2009;50:116–24.
156. Jaglin XH, Chelly J. Tubulin-related cortical dysgeneses: microtubule dysfunction underlying neuronal migration defects. Trends Genet 2009;25:555–66.
157. Dobyns WB, Reiner O, Carozzo R, et al. Lissencephaly: a human brain malformation associated with deletion of the LIS1 gene located at chromosome 17p13. JAMA 1993;270:2838–42.
158. des Portes V, Pinard JM, Billuart P, et al. A novel CNS gene required for neuronal migration and involved in X-linked subcortical laminar heterotopia and lissencephaly syndrome. Cell 1998;92:51–61.
159. Gleeson JG, Allen KM, Fox JW, et al. *doublecortin*, a brain-specific gene mutated in human X-linked lissencephaly and double cortex syndrome, encodes a putative signaling protein. Cell 1998;92:63–72.
160. Dobyns JW. The clinical patterns and molecular genetics of lissencephaly and subcortical band heterotopia. Epilepsia 2010;51(Suppl 1):5–9.
161. Fitzgerald MP, Covio M, Lee KS. Disturbances in the positioning, proliferation and apoptosis of neural progenitors contribute to subcortical band heterotopia formation. Neuroscience 2011;176:455–71.
162. Forman MS, Squier W, Dobyns WB, et al. Genotypically defined lissencephalies show distinct pathologies. J Neuropathol Exp Neurol 2005;64:847–57.
163. Kappeler C, Dhenain M, Phan Dinh Tuy F, et al. Magnetic resonance imaging and histological studies of corpus callosal and hippocampal abnormalities linked to doublecortin deficiency. J Comp Neurol 2007;500:239–54.
164. Saillour Y, Carion N, Quelin C, et al. *LIS1*-related isolated lissencephaly. Arch Neurol 2009;66:1007–15.
165. Koizumi H, Tanaka T, Gleeson JG. *doublecortin-like kinase* functions with *doublecortin* to mediate fiber tract decussation and neuronal migration. Neuron 2006;49:55–66.
166. Ross ME, Swanson K, Dobys WB. Lissencephaly with cerebellar hypoplasia (LCH): a heterogeneous group of cortical malformations. Neuropediatrics 2001;32:256–63.
167. Jissendi-Tchofo P, Kara S, Barkovich AJ. Midbrain-hindbrain involvement in lissencephalies. Neurology 2009;72:410–8.
168. Dobyns WB, Truwit CL, Ross ME, et al. Differences in the gyral pattern distinguish chromosome 17-linked and X-linked lissencephaly. Neurology 1999;53:270–7.
169. D' Agostino MD, Bernasconi A, Das S, et al. Subcortical band heterotopia (SBH) in males: clinical, imaging and genetic findings in comparison with females. Brain 2002;125:2507–22.
170. Mai R, Tassi L, Cossu M, et al. A neuropathological, stereo-EEG, and MRI study of subcortical band heterotopia. Neurology 2003;60:1834–8.
171. Viot G, Sonigo P, Simon I, et al. Neocortical neuronal arrangement in LIS1 and DCX lissencephaly may be different. Am J Med Genet 2004;126:123–8.
172. Cardoso C, Leventer RJ, Dowling JJ, et al. Clinical and molecular basis of classical lissencephaly: mutations in the *LIS1* gene (*PAFAH1B1*). Hum Mutat 2002;19:4–15.
173. Poirier K, Keays DA, Francis F, et al. Large spectrum of lissencephaly and pachygyria phenotypes resulting from de novo missense mutations in Tubulin Alpha 1A (TUBA1A). Hum Mutat 2007;28:1055–64.
174. Fallet-Bianco C, Loeuillet L, Poirier K, et al. Neuropathological phenotype of a distinct form of

lissencephaly associated with mutations in TUBA1A. Brain 2008;131:2304–20.
175. Kumar RA, Pilz DT, Babatz TD, et al. TUBA1A mutations cause wide spectrum lissencephaly (smooth brain) and suggest that multiple neuronal migration pathways converge on alpha tubulins. Hum Mol Genet 2010;19:2817–27.
176. Dobyns WB, Berry-Kravis E, Havernik NJ, et al. X-linked lissencephaly with absent corpus callosum and ambiguous genitalia. Am J Med Genet 1999; 86:331–7.
177. Kato M, Dobyns WB. X-linked lissencephaly with abnormal genitalia as a tangential migration disorder causing intractable epilepsy: proposal for a new term "interneuronopathy". J Child Neurol 2005;20:392–7.
178. Kitamura K, Yanazawa M, Sugiyama N, et al. Mutation of ARX causes abnormal development of forebrain and testes in mice and X-linked lissencephaly with abnormal genitalia in humans. Nat Genet 2002;32:359–69.
179. Colombo E, Collombat P, Colasante G, et al. Inactivation of Arx, the murine ortholog of the X-linked lissencephaly with ambiguous genitalia gene, leads to severe disorganization of the ventral telencephalon with impaired neuronal migration and differentiation. J Neurosci 2007;27:4786–98.
180. Miyata R, Hayashi M, Miyai K, et al. Analysis of the hypothalamus in a case of X-linked lissencephaly with abnormal genitalia (XLAG). Brain Dev 2009; 31:456–60.
181. Zhang G, Assadi AH, McNeil RS, et al. The Pafah1b complex interacts with the reelin receptor VLDLR. PLoS One 2007;2:e252.
182. Conti Reed U. Congenital muscular dystrophy. Part I. A review of phenotypical and diagnostic aspects. Arq Neuropsiquiatr 2009;67:144–68.
183. Conti Reed U. Congenital muscular dystrophy. Part II. A review of pathogenesis and therapeutic perspectives. Arq Neuropsiquiatr 2009;67:343–62.
184. Clement E, Mercuri E, Godfrey C, et al. Brain involvement in muscular dystrophies with defective dystroglycan glycosylation. Ann Neurol 2008;64: 573–82.
185. Bahi-Buisson N, Poirier K, Boddaert N, et al. *GPR56*-related bilateral frontoparietal polymicrogyria: further evidence for an overlap with the cobblestone complex. Brain 2010;133:3194–209.
186. Li S, Jin Z, Koraila S, et al. *GPR56* regulates pial basement membrane integrity and cortical lamination. J Neurosci 2008;28:5817–26.
187. Raymond AA, Fish DR, Stevens JM, et al. Subependymal heterotopia: a distinct neuronal migration disorder associated with epilepsy. J Neurol Neurosurg Psychiatry 1994;57:1195–202.
188. Dubeau F, Tampieri D, Lee N, et al. Periventricular and subcortical nodular heterotopia. A study of 33 patients. Brain 1995;118:1273–87.
189. Oda T, Nagai Y, Fujimoto S, et al. Hereditary nodular heterotopia accompanied by mega cisterna magna. Am J Med Genet 1993;47:268–71.
190. Walker LM, Katzir T, Liu T, et al. Gray matter volumes and cognitive ability in the epileptogenic brain malformation of periventricular nodular heterotopia. Epilepsy Behav 2009;15:456–60.
191. Ekşioğlu YZ, Scheffer IE, Cardenas P, et al. Periventricular heterotopia: an X-linked dominant epilepsy locus causing aberrant cerebral cortical development. Neuron 1996;16:77–87.
192. Fox JW, Lamperti ED, EkşioğluYZ, et al. Mutations in *filamin 1* prevent migration of cerebral cortical neurons in human periventricular heterotopia. Neuron 1998;21:1315–25.
193. Parrini E, Ramazzotti A, Dobyns WB, et al. Periventricular heterotopia: phenotypic heterogeneity and correlation with Filamin A mutation. Brain 2006; 129:1892–906.
194. Barkovich AJ. Morphologic characteristics of subcortical heterotopias: MR imaging study. AJNR Am J Neuroradiol 2000;21:290–5.
195. Raybaud C. The corpus callosum, the other great brain commissures and the septum pellucidum: anatomy, development and malformation. Neuroradiology 2010;52:447–77.
196. Poduri A, Golja A, Riviello JJ, et al. A distinct asymmetrical pattern of cortical malformation: large unilateral malformation of cortical development with contralateral periventricular nodular heterotopia in three pediatric cases. Epilepsia 2005;46:1317–21.
197. Novegno F, Battaglia D, Chieffo D, et al. Giant subcortical heterotopia involving the temporo-parieto-occipital region: a challenging cause of drug-resistant epilepsy. Epilepsy Res 2009;87:88–94.
198. Levine DN, Fisher MA, Caviness VS Jr. Porencephaly with microgyria: a pathologic study. Acta Neuropathol (Berl) 1974;29:99–113.
199. Yakovlev PI, Wadworth RC. Schizencephalies. A study of congenital clefts in the cerebral mantle. I. Clefts with fused lips. J Neuropathol Exp Neurol 1946;5:116–30.
200. Yakovlev PI, Wadworth RC. Schizencephalies. A study of congenital clefts in the cerebral mantle. II. Clefts with hydrocephalus and lips separated. J Neuropathol Exp Neurol 1946;5:169–206.
201. Dekaban A. large defects in cerebral hemispheres associated with cortical dysgenesis. J Neuropathol Exp Neurol 1965;24:512–30.
202. Raybaud C. Destructive lesions of the brain. Neuroradiology 1983;25:265–91.
203. Takano T, Takikita S, Shimada M. Experimental schizencephaly induced by Kilham strain of mumps virus. Pathogenesis of cleft formation. Neuroreport 1999;10:3149–54.
204. Robinson RO. Familial schizencephaly. Dev Med Child Neurol 1991;33:1010–4.

205. Hilburger A, Willis JK, Bouldin E, et al. Familial schizencephaly. Brain Dev 1993;15:234–6.
206. Brunelli S, Faiella A, Capra V, et al. Germline mutation in the homeobox gene *EMX2* in patients with severe schizencephaly. Nat Genet 1996;12:94–6.
207. Hayashi N, Tsutsumi Y, Barkovich AJ. Morphological features and associated anomalies of schizencephaly in the clinical population: detailed analysis of MR images. Neuroradiology 2002;44:418–27.
208. Raybaud C, Girard N, Levrier O, et al. Schizencephaly: correlation between the lobar topography of the cleft(s) and absence of the septum pellucidum. Childs Nerv Syst 2001;17:217–22.
209. Barkovich AJ, Fram EK, Norman D. Septo-optic dysplasia: MR imaging. Radiology 1989;171:189–92.
210. Squier W, Jansen A. Abnormal development of the human cerebral cortex. J Anat 2010;217:312–23.
211. Eriksson SH, Thom M, Hefferman J, et al. Persistent reelin-expressing Cajal-Retzius cells in polymicrogyria. Brain 2001;124:1350–61.
212. Jansen A, Anderman E. Genetics of the polymictogyria syndromes. J Med Genet 2005;42:369–78.
213. Barkovich AJ. Current concepts of polymicrogyria. Neuroradiology 2010;52:479–87.
214. Barkovich AJ. MRI analysis of sulcation morphology in polymicrogyria. Epilepsia 2010;51(Suppl 1):17–22.
215. Raybaud C, Girard N, Canto-Moreira N, et al. High-definition magnetic resonance imaging identification of cortical dysplasias: micropolygyria versus lissencephaly. In: Guerrini R, Andermann F, Canapicchi R, et al, editors. Dysplasias of cerebral cortex and epilepsy. Philadelphia: Lippincott-Raven; 1996. p. 131–43.
216. van der Knaap MS, Vermeulen G, Barkhof F, et al. Pattern of white matter abnormalities at MR imaging: use of polymerase chain reaction testing of Guthrie cards to link pattern with congenital cytomegalovirus infection. Radiology 2004;230:529–36.
217. Crome RL, France NE. Microgyria and cytomegalic inclusion disease in infancy. J Clin Pathol 1959;12:427–34.
218. Friede RL, Mikolasek J. Postencephalitic porencephaly, hydranencephaly or polymicrogyria. A review. Acta Neuropathol (Berl) 1978;43:161–8.
219. Maton B, Kršek P, Jayakar P, et al. Medically intractable epilepsy in Sturge-Weber syndrome is associated with cortical malformation: implication for surgical therapy. Epilepsia 2010;51:257–67.
220. Guye M, Gastaut JL, Bartolomei F. Epilepsy and perisylvian lipoma/cortical dysplasia complex. Epileptic Disord 1999;1:69–73.
221. Chang BS, Apse KA, Caraballo, et al. A familial syndrome of unilateral polymicrogyria affecting the right hemisphere. Neurology 2006;66:133–5.
222. Jaglin XH, Poirier K, Saillour Y, et al. Mutations in the beta-tubulin gene TUBB2B result in asymmetrical polymicrogyria. Nat Genet 2009;41:746–52.
223. Borgatti R, Triulzi F, Zucca C, et al. Bilateral perisylvian polymicrogyria in three generations. Neurology 1999;52:1910–3.
224. Guerrini R, Barkovich AJ, Sztriha L, et al. Bilateral frontal polymicrogyria: a newly recognized brain malformation syndrome. Neurology 2000;54:909–13.
225. Guerrini R, Dubeau F, Dulac O, et al. Bilateral parasagittal parietooccipital polymicrogyria and epilepsy. Ann Neurol 1997;41:65–73.
226. Mirzaa G, Dodge NN, Glass I, et al. Megalencephaly and perisylvian polymicrogyria with postaxial polydactyly and hydrocephalus: a rare brain malformation syndrome associated with mental retardation and seizures. Neuropediatrics 2004;35:353–9.
227. Pierson TM, Zimmerman RA, Tennekoon GI, et al. Mega-corpus callosum, polymicrogyria, and psychomotor retardation: confirmation of a syndromic entity. Neuropediatrics 2008;39:123–7.
228. Siejka S, Strefling AM, Urich H. Absence of septum pellucidum and polymicrogyria: a forme frusta of the porencephalic syndrome. Clin Neuropathol 1989;8:174–8.
229. Wieck G, Leventer RJ, Squier WM, et al. Periventricular nodular heterotopia with overlying polymicrogyria. Brain 2005;128:2811–21.
230. Vincentiis S, Valente KD, Valente M. Polymicrogyria in glycogenosis type III: an incidental finding? Pediatr Neurol 2004;31:143–5.

Congenital Arterial and Venous Anomalies of the Brain and Skull Base

Sudhir Kathuria, MD[a,b], James Chen, BS[a],
Lydia Gregg, MA, CMI[a], Hemant A. Parmar, MD[c],
Dheeraj Gandhi, MBBS, MD[a,b,d,e,*]

KEYWORDS

- Congenital arterial anomalies • Venous anomalies
- Brain • Skull base

Congenital arterial and venous anomalies of the brain and skull base comprise diverse abnormalities that result from early disturbances in cerebrovascular development. Broadly, these conditions may result in one or more of the following structural abnormalities: absence or hypoplasia of normal vessels, persistence of transient embryonic vessels, vessels with abnormal morphology, and pathologic intracerebral shunts (arteriovenous malformations [AVM] and arteriovenous fistulae [AVF]). Some of these anomalies are hemodynamically compensated and lack clinically significant symptoms. These abnormalities often go unrecognized or are only detected incidentally on imaging studies. Others can cause significant morbidity and mortality from hemorrhagic or ischemic sequelae and warrant appropriate identification and management. Knowledge of the underlying etiology and associated imaging findings is essential in properly differentiating lesions with benign nature from those that have significant clinical implications and may need management. Full description of complex embryologic processes is beyond the scope of this article and the reader is referred to the works of Streeter[1] and Padget.[2] The authors' aim is to provide a brief overview of normal cerebrovascular development and embryologic pathogenesis of common, congenital arterial and venous anomalies of the cerebral vasculature and highlight key imaging characteristics that should be considered for their diagnosis.

OVERVIEW OF NORMAL CEREBROVASCULAR DEVELOPMENT

Vascular development of the brain is driven at the molecular level by angiogenic signaling cascades and at the morphologic level by the metabolic demands of the growing central nervous system. At 2 to 4 weeks of gestation, the neural plate is still primarily fed by free diffusion of nutrients from the amniotic fluid. By 4 weeks, the neural tube has closed and the neuroectoderm begins to derive nutrients from the surrounding meninx primitiva, a mesodermal structure that will give rise to the future calvarium, dura, and leptomeninges. Although primordial cerebral vessels can be seen within the meninx primitiva at this early stage, the channels are largely arranged in an indistinct network and have limited arterial or venous

[a] Department of Radiology, Johns Hopkins Hospital, 600 North Wolfe Street, Baltimore, MD 21287, USA
[b] Department of Neurosurgery, Johns Hopkins Hospital, 600 North Wolfe Street, Baltimore, MD 21287, USA
[c] Department of Radiology, University of Michigan Health System, 1500 East Medical Center Drive, Ann Arbor, MI 48109, USA
[d] Department of Neurology, Johns Hopkins Hospital, 600 North Wolfe Street, Baltimore, MD 21287, USA
[e] Johns Hopkins Bayview Program, Interventional Neuroradiology, Johns Hopkins School of Medicine, 600 North Wolfe Street/Radiology B-100, Baltimore, MD 21287, USA
* Corresponding author. Interventional Neuroradiology, Johns Hopkins Bayview Program, Johns Hopkins School of Medicine, 600 North Wolfe Street/Radiology B-100, Baltimore, MD 21287.
E-mail address: dgandhi2@jhmi.edu

Neuroimag Clin N Am 21 (2011) 545–562
doi:10.1016/j.nic.2011.05.002
1052-5149/11/$ – see front matter

differentiation.[1] The mature framework of the proximal cerebral arterial system is laid out by 8 weeks of gestation and that of the venous system is laid out by 12 weeks.[2] Distal vessel development and remodeling continue until birth for the arterial system and continues postnatally for the venous system. Details of arterial and venous morphogenesis and their implications in the development of anomalous vessel anatomy are discussed in subsequent sections.

ARTERIAL SYSTEM

Internal Carotid Arteries

Development

The internal carotid arteries (ICA) play an essential role in supplying the vesicles of the developing brain and appear early in gestation, before closure of the neural tube. These paired structures can first be seen arising from the dorsal aorta and third aortic arch at the 3- to 5-mm embryonic stage.[2] By the 4- to 5-mm (28–29 day) stage, the primitive ICA lies within the vascular meshwork of the meninx primitiva and provides blood supply to the forebrain, midbrain, and hindbrain vesicles.[2] A more mature ICA can be seen by 6 weeks, although its branches continue to develop beyond that point.[2]

The widely accepted system proposed by Lasjuanias and Santoyo-Vazquez,[3] divides the ICA into 7 segments, each bordered by an embryonic precursor vessel. The cervical segment (first) of the ICA starts at the common carotid artery bifurcation and ends at its entrance into the skull base. The ascending petrous segment (second) begins as the ICA enters the skull base through the carotid foramen and extends to the apex of the anterior-medial curvature within the petrous bone, marked by the caroticotympanic artery distally. The horizontal petrous segment (third) traverses the carotid canal from the caroticotympanic artery to the vidian artery where the ICA emerges from the skull base through the foramen lacerum. The ascending cavernous segment (fourth) enters the cavernous sinus (CS) and ends at the meningohypophyseal trunk (MHT) where the ICA assumes an anterior-inferior course within the CS. The MHT is likely an adult derivative of the primitive trigeminal artery (TA),[3] whereas the inferior hypophyseal artery, which branches from the ICA medial and distal to the MHT, is speculated to be a derivative of the medial branch of the primitive maxillary artery.[2] The horizontal cavernous segment (fifth) extends from the MHT to the inferolateral trunk (ILT) within the CS. The clinoidal segment of the ICA (sixth) is bordered proximally by the ILT and distally by the adult ophthalmic artery (OA).[3,4] The terminal segment (seventh) of the ICA lies between the primitive OA and anterior cerebral artery.[3]

Carotid artery agenesis and hypoplasia

Congenital absence of the ICA is a rare developmental abnormality with incidence reported at approximately 0.01% and is often discovered incidentally on head and neck imaging.[5–7] ICA hypoplasia is more common, with an incidence of 0.079%.[7] Improper development of one or more of the 7 different embryologic segment branches that form the ICA can lead to poor formation of the carotid system.

Unilateral absence of the ICA is generally asymptomatic, because sufficient collateral pathways usually exist via the circle of Willis, intracavernous anastomoses, and persistent embryologic arteries. Occasionally, in the presence of insufficient collaterals, symptoms related to cerebral ischemia from uncompensated blood flow can occur.[7] Absence of one ICA can result in excessive shear stress from increased flow in contralateral ICA or other associated collaterals. These hemodynamic changes can lead to the development of intracranial aneurysms.[7,8] Congenital absence of an ICA can sometimes be confused with acquired occlusions. Similarly, congenital hypoplasia can be mistaken as acquired stenosis. It is important to understand the presentation, imaging features, and clinical implications of these entities because improper diagnosis caused by associated symptoms may lead to unnecessary and risky interventions.

The typical morphology of a hypoplastic ICA is an artery of small caliber that becomes diminutive at, or shortly after, its origin. Commencement of the hypoplasia 1 to 2 cm past the bifurcation is a common finding.[8,9] It remains small throughout its course and may either continue intracranially or become completely occluded. The key-imaging finding is the absence of petrous bony carotid canal in ICA agenesis and smaller canal size in ICA hypoplasia (**Fig. 1**). The bony carotid canals normally develop at the fifth and sixth embryonic weeks following the completion of ICA development at the fourth week. ICA development serves as a stimulus without which carotid canals do not develop. Demonstration of a small or absent carotid canal by computed tomography (CT) helps to differentiate from acquired stenosis or occlusion.[5]

Aberrant internal carotid artery

The ICA normally ascends in the neck and enters into the temporal bone via the carotid canal. As it courses through the carotid canal, a thin plate of bone, the carotid ridge, separates it from the

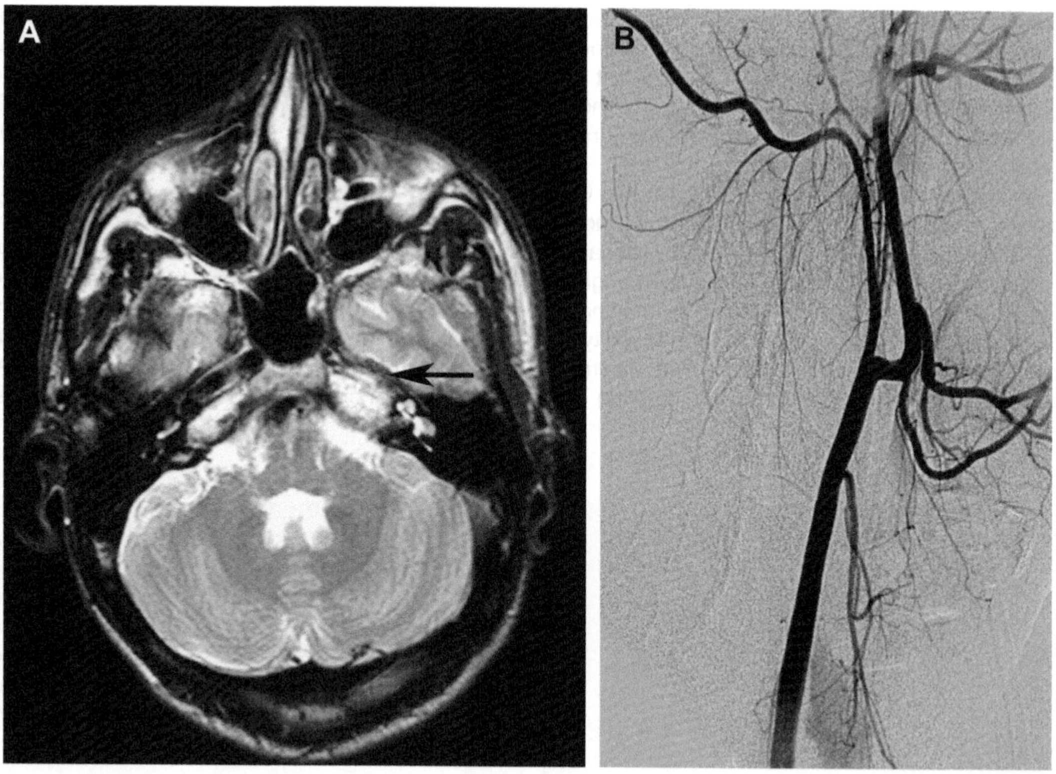

Fig. 1. A young boy with multiple congenital anomalies and temporal region arteriovenous fistula underwent an MR imaging brain study (*A*) and DSA (*B*). (*A*) Axial T2-weighted MR shows a lack of normal expected left ICA flow void in carotid canal (*arrow*) on axial T2-weighted MR image, suggesting a possible left carotid agenesis. (*B*) Lateral digital subtraction angiogram image from left common carotid artery catheterization confirms a complete lack of development of left internal carotid artery. The common carotid artery is continuing entirely into left external carotid artery.

posteriorly located internal jugular vein. The artery then runs superiorly to form the initial vertical segment, anterior to the cochlea, and is separated from the tympanic cavity by a thin plate of bone. The ICA then turns anteriorly (inferoposterior and medial to the eustachian tube), traverses the foramen lacerum, and enters the middle cranial fossa.[10] An aberrant ICA, on the other hand, enters the floor of the middle ear, turns forward, and then passes through the middle-ear instead of staying anterior to this space before entering the foramen lacerum. Although termed aberrant ICA, the basic pathology in this condition is thought to be hypoplasia or agenesis of the ICA. In the setting of ICA agenesis, the inferior tympanic artery does not undergo normal regression and instead hypertrophies. It is this hypertrophied inferior tympanic artery that appears as aberrant ICA and anastomoses with the caroticotympanic artery to carry the blood to the carotid siphon.[11]

An aberrant ICA can present at any age and is more commonly seen in women, on right side.[12] Clinical diagnosis of aberrant ICA can be difficult because of the lack of any pathognomonic symptoms. Patients may be completely asymptomatic or can present with nonspecific signs and symptoms, such as conductive hearing loss, pulsatile tinnitus, ear fullness, otalgia, and vertigo. Pulsatile tinnitus and hearing loss are caused by contact between the malleus handle and the exposed carotid artery.[13] The pulsatile bruit can often be heard with a stethoscope in the ear canal or around the ear. The presentation of an asymptomatic middle-ear mass is common. It can also present as a vascular mass behind the tympanic membrane on otoscopic examination. An aberrant ICA can be confused with a glomus tumor, dehiscent jugular bulb, cholesterol granuloma, or petrous carotid aneurysm.[14]

It is important to recognize aberrant ICAs because misdiagnosis of this entity may subject the patients to potentially life-threatening iatrogenic ear bleeding. There are several reported cases when aberrant ICA was first recognized during middle-ear surgery or myringotomy. Hemorrhage can occur from surgical manipulation, biopsy, or myringotomy.[15] If an aberrant ICA is suspected within the middle ear on imaging, it is crucial to inform the clinician to avoid any inappropriate surgical intervention.

An aberrant carotid artery can be evaluated with several available radiologic techniques, including CT, CT angiography (CTA), magnetic resonance angiography (MRA), or digital subtraction angiography (DSA). CT with high-resolution imaging is the study of choice because of its capability to provide exquisite bony details. The aberrant carotid artery can easily be seen entering the middle ear through an enlarged inferior tympanic canal that lies posterior to the normal carotid canal. This entrance point of ICA into the tympanic canal can also be seen as a focal narrowing (**Fig. 2**) on angiography.[16]

Intracranial Arterial Vasculature: Embryology and Variations

The arterial vasculature of the brain can be described in the context of anterior circulation, supplied primarily by the ICAs, along with contributions from the external carotid artery (ECA) and posterior circulation, supplied by the vertebral

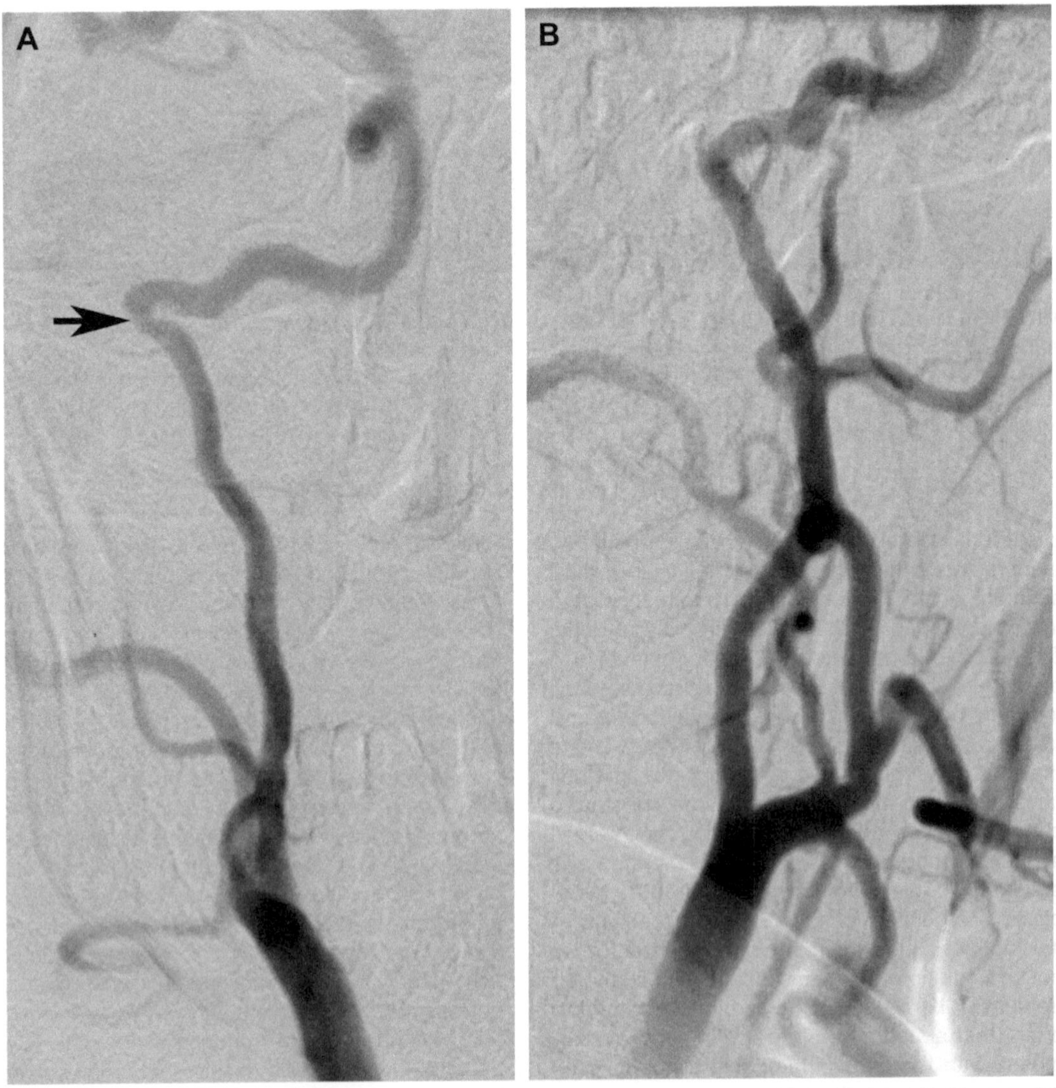

Fig. 2. Frontal (*A*) and lateral (*B*) projection of common carotid artery angiogram demonstrates findings typical of an aberrant ICA. Note a characteristic, smaller caliber vessel with abnormal posterior and lateral course at the level of skull base. Also note a focal narrowing (*arrow*) of this vessel where it enters into the tympanic canal.

arteries (VA). The development of the cerebral arterial system mirrors the corresponding metabolic demands of the growing cephalic vesicles.[1] The formation of the circle of Willis occurs progressively with staggered development of the anterior and posterior circulation. The primitive anterior circulation can be well recognized by 35 days of gestation, with anterior cerebral artery (ACA) and middle cerebral artery (MCA) branches from the rostral ICA. The primitive posterior circulation is completed later in development (6–7 weeks), with capture of the hindbrain vascular territory by the vertebrobasilar system. Although the posterior communicating artery (PCOM) forms at the 29-day stage, the posterior circulation continues to be maintained by the proatlantal artery (ProA) until 6 weeks of gestation. The circle of Willis is finalized by 6 to 7 weeks of gestation, with formation of the posterior cerebral arteries and cerebellar arteries.

Distal vessels are generally less variable in morphology because the final vascular architecture is restricted by the parenchymal metabolic requirements, but the proximal vessels (ie, at the circle of Willis) can vary far more, depending on early hemodynamic factors.[17] A complete discussion of congenital variations of the circle of Willis is outside the scope of this article, but it is important to mention that anatomic variations here are the rule rather than the exception. Remodeling continues throughout life depending on individual hemodynamic factors, so the ultimate adult morphology can be further altered from the immediate postnatal appearance.[18]

Many of the cerebral vessels develop from initial plexiform networks and rely on proper fusion of branching segments to form a single adult channel. Interruptions to this process can cause fenestrations, which are characterized by division of the artery lumen into 2 distinct, parallel, endothelium-lined channels. Specific locations and etiologies of these anomalies are subsequently discussed for each cerebral artery. The overall angiographic incidence of fenestrations ranges from 0.03% to 1.0%, and the postmortem incidence is 1.3% to 5.3%,[8,19–21] suggesting that many of these lesions can be missed on imaging studies. These lesions are generally asymptomatic, but similar to arterial bifurcations, they may have a propensity for aneurysm formation.[20] On conventional DSA, fenestrations can be obscured depending on the viewing angle and because of overlapping structures. However, modern 3-dimensional rotational angiography[22] and CT/MR angiography with multiplanar reconstructions and rotational capabilities have allowed for better detection of these abnormalities.

Anterior cerebral artery

The ACA is the first cerebral artery visible in development. It emerges from a vascular meshwork as a distinct trunk by 32 days and extends rostrally around the growing hemispheric vesicle.[2] At 35 days, the paired ACAs approach the midline to form the anterior communicating artery (ACOM), which is plexiform at this stage and continues to remodel until full development of the cerebrovascular system.[2] Improper fusion of these branches into a single channel can result in arterial fenestration. The ACOM is among the more common locations for fenestrations in the cerebral circulation. At day 40, important modifications to the A2 and distal ACA segments produce the classic paired ACA anatomy; insults during this period can result in anomalous morphologies, such as bihemispheric or azygous ACAs.

A bihemispheric ACA describes the presence of a dominant A1 segment that gives supply to the distal paired ACA segments for both hemispheres. The contralateral A1 segment is typically hypoplastic or has an early termination.[23] Bihemispheric ACAs are more common than azygous ACAs in which the paired ACA pattern is replaced by a fused midline vessel. The azygous or undivided ACA is a single, midline vessel arising from the confluence of the two A1 segments. It supplies the medial aspects of the frontal and parietal lobes of both hemispheres. Compression of the contralateral carotid artery during DSA can help differentiate the presence of an azygous ACA from the more common bihemispheric ACA. Azygous ACAs can be well demonstrated on CTA, MRA, and DSA. An azygous ACA can be associated with midline central nervous system malformations, such as agenesis of corpus callosum, holoprosencephaly, intracranial arteriovenous malformation, and aneurysm.[24,25] Both saccular and nonsaccular aneurysms have been described in relation to azygous ACA (**Fig. 3**). A complex branching pattern of the distal azygous ACA often contributes to the unusual morphology of these aneurysms.[24,26] Such aneurysms are often challenging for both clipping and endovascular repair because of their nonsaccular morphology and difficult visualization of the efferent arterial branches.

Middle cerebral artery

The MCA forms as a basal striatal branch of the primitive ACA starting at 35 days of development, although its stem can be visible as early as 32 days.[2] It typically forms a single channel from the coalescence of 2 or 3 initial vessel stems. Full maturation of the MCA continues until 7 to 8 weeks, when the proximal framework of the

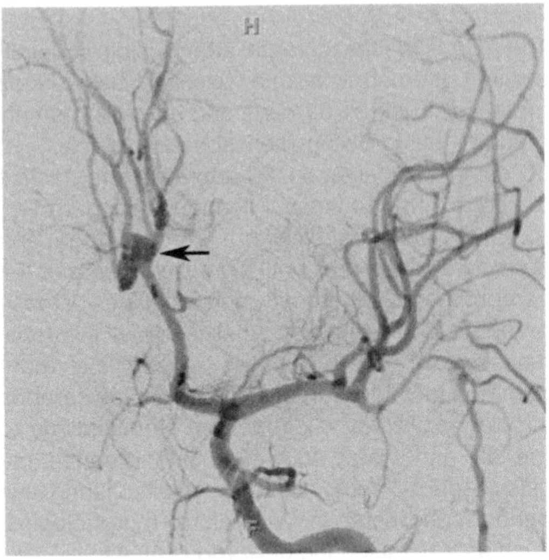

Fig. 3. A young female child with multiple congenital anomalies, blindness, and multiple nerve sheath neoplasms underwent an angiogram because of a suspicious aneurysm demonstrated on MR imaging study. The DSA demonstrates findings of an azygos ACA. Frontal projection of left ICA DSA demonstrates the left A1 segment providing supply to the distal paired ACA segments for both hemispheres. Please note a complex fusiform aneurysm (*arrow*) at the branching point where all distal ACA vessels originate.

cerebral arterial system is fully established.[2] Various mechanisms have been proposed for development of different fenestrations. Early branching of the temporopolar artery could possibly interrupt the normal coalescence of the primordial MCA branches and can lead to the appearance of fenestrations in postnatal artery (**Fig. 4**).

MCA duplication refers to the early origin of the MCA from the distal ICA.[27] This anomaly can be observed on angiographic and anatomic studies at a frequency of 0.2% to 2.9%.[28] The duplicated MCA is typically a small vessel that supplies the anterior temporal lobes and has little clinical significance.[28]

An accessory MCA refers to the origin of the MCA from the proximal or distal A1 segment.[29] The frequency of this anomaly has been reported between 0.3% and 4.0% on angiographic and anatomic studies.[28] Because the MCA is a phylogenetic branch of the ACA, investigators have suggested that the accessory MCA is a vestigial remnant of this embryonic anastomosis. Others have proposed that this morphology is in fact a medial extension of the artery of Heubner into the territory of the MCA.[28] Increased hemodynamic turbulence at the accessory MCA origin has been also proposed to be associated with increased risk of aneurysm formation.[30]

Posterior cerebral and anterior choroidal arteries

The development of the posterior cerebral artery (PCA) in the fetal brain occurs late and arises from the fusion of several embryonic vessels near the caudal end of the PCOM. The PCA begins as a continuation of the PCOM in the majority of cases, with the remainder of the PCAs originating from the basilar artery (BA). In adults, it has the most variable morphology of all the cerebral arteries.[17] It can be supplied by the ICA with the prominent P1 segment and persistent embryonic anastomoses or relegate its territory to the anterior choroidal artery (AchA). Depending on the relative contribution, the PCA can be classified as adult type when the P1 segment of the PCA is larger than the ipsilateral PCOM artery, transitional type when the P1 segment is of the same size as the PCOM artery, and fetal type when the P1 segment is smaller (or absent) than the PCOM artery.[31] The anterior choroidal artery is one of the most prominent arteries in the developing brain. At 32 days of gestation, it is the largest branch of the ICA and supplies much of the primitive diencephalon. It maintains this region until 7 to 8 weeks, at which point the growing posterior cerebral artery overtakes much of this territory.[2] By birth, the territory of the AchA is normally limited to only small regions of its original embryonic territory.[17]

In rare cases, the postnatal anterior choroidal artery can become hypertrophic and supply the entire hemispheric territory that is typically vascularized by the posterior cerebral artery. Embryologically, this is most likely caused by errors at the 7- to 8-week period when the developing PCA should assume dominance in these regions.

Vertebrobasilar arterial system

The developing hindbrain is initially fed by paired longitudinal neural arteries (LNAs) and transient anastomoses from the ICAs. At 29 gestational days, the LNAs begin as a craniocaudal, midline fusion to form the primitive BA, and at 32 gestational days, the vertebral arteries begin to form from longitudinal anastomoses between cervical intersegmental arteries.[2] Although the vertebrobasilar framework is established at this point, it is not until 7 to 8 weeks that the rhombencephalic and mesencephalic vascular territories of the PCA are taken over by the vertebrobasilar system from the ICAs.

Fusion of the basilar artery occurs in longitudinal and axial planes,[32] and failure of these normal processes on either axis can lead to abnormal

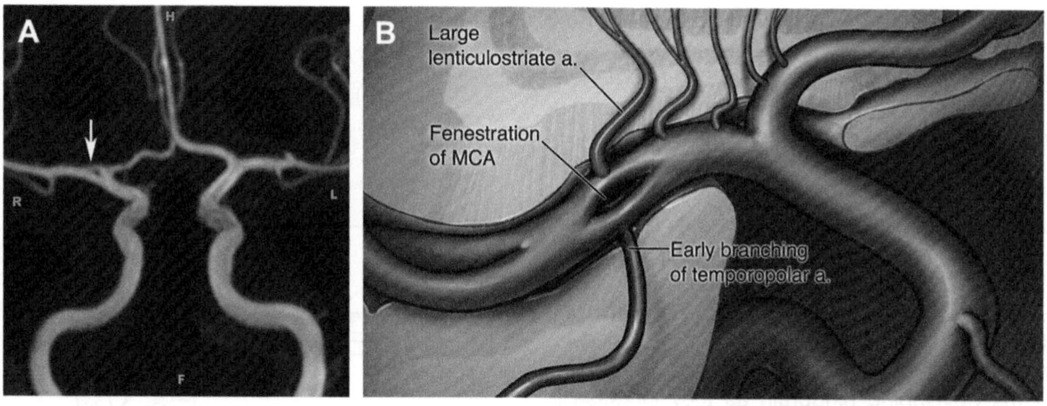

Fig. 4. MCA fenestration. (*A*) MR angiogram image showing fenestration of right M1 segment (*arrow*) of MCA. (*B*) MCA fenestration illustrating the early branching of the temporopolar artery that could interrupt the normal coalescence of primordial MCA branches. This is one of the proposed mechanisms for development of MCA fenestration.

vessel morphologies. Longitudinal fusion typically begins in a disparate fashion, with segmented unfused regions that only secondarily become a unified channel. Failure of this secondary fusion can leave residual fenestrations in the vessel, which is seen most commonly in the caudal BA.[17] Axial nonfusion occurs by a similar mechanism and results in discontinuities within the BA. This discontinuity can result in a segmented vertebrobasilar architecture that is fed by collateral paths from other anomalous vessels, like a persistent trigeminal artery, discussed later.[32] If a fenestration is visualized, careful attention should be given to look for any associated aneurysm.

Persistent Carotid-Basilar Anastomoses

By the time the human embryo is 4 to 5 mm long, the groundwork of anterior circulation is established as the primitive ICAs reach the developing forebrain. The paired LNA, precursors of the BA, also form on the medial edges of the bilateral vascular networks on the ventral surface of the hindbrain.[2,33] The first few small branches to be sent out from the ICA are responsible for delivering blood to the LNA to feed the developing hindbrain while the vertebrobasilar system is under construction. These branches include 3 transient presegmental arteries (carotid-basilar anastomoses), 1 permanent presegmental artery, and the first intersegmental artery.[2,33,34] These arteries also likely contribute to the formation of the LNA by anastomosis.[2,35]

The 3 presegmental arteries include the TA, the otic artery (OA), and the hypoglossal artery (HA), named for their associations with the fifth, eighth, and twelfth cranial nerves, respectively. All 3 of these arteries are present in embryos of 4 to 5 mm in length.[2] The trigeminal artery can be observed, at a 3-mm embryo length, branching from the ICA to the LNA directly opposite to the first arch at the level of the trigeminal ganglion. This branch remains the chief supply to the developing LNAs at a 4-mm embryo length, augmented caudally by the OA, the HA, and the ProA.[2]

The OA has been reported in 4-mm embryos opposite the second arch travelling with the vestibulocochlear nerve and the otic vesicle. It regresses concurrently with the second branchial arch artery.[2] Although definitive case reports of persistent TAs, HAs, and first intersegmental arteries can be found within the medical literature,[16,36] there are only a few reported cases of a persistent OA with angiographic documentation.[37,38] These cases better meet the criteria of a low-originating persistent primitive trigeminal artery, and true existence of the OA is under debate.

The HA originates from the ICA, following the course of the developing hypoglossal nerve and connecting to the LNA. It becomes visible at roughly a 4-mm embryo size as the second arch starts to regress, and remains patent for only a short period of time, dwindling as the LNA start to fuse into the BA.[2]

By a 5- to 7-mm embryo length, the primitive posterior communicating artery (PcomA) forms a permanent connection from the ICA to the LNAs, and TAs consequently begin to diminish in caliber. Few investigators have proposed that the PcomA most likely represents the cranial-most presegmental artery and refer to the PcomA as the first presegmental artery in addition to the 3 previously described presegmental arteries. Of these presegmental arteries, only the PcomA normally persists into adulthood, whereas the remaining 3 regress early on in development.[2,39]

The involution of the trigeminal artery is also dependent on the establishment of the first intersegmental artery, termed the proatlantal artery.[40] By the time the embryo is 4 to 5 mm in length, the ProA is the primary caudal source of blood for LNAs. The paired LNAs begin to merge around the time that the embryo is 5 mm.[2] Rather than shifting medially, the LNAs coalesce along the midline of the developing hindbrain as they increase in diameter. The fused LNA of a 12- to 14-mm embryo now represent the freshly formed BA.[2,41]

Bilateral channels form between the cervical segmental arteries that connect the developing subclavian arteries to the ProA once the embryo is 7 to 12 mm. It is not until this longitudinal paravertebral anastomosis, representing the future V1 segment of the VA, is complete that the proximal segment of the ProA regresses and its remaining portion is incorporated into the VA.[2] Like every intersegmental artery, the ProA provides a dorsospinal division with a radicular artery. The radicular artery of the ProA becomes the final segment of the adult VA. The anterior and posterior radicular branches of the ProA divide just before crossing the dura so that the anterior radicular artery serves as the V4 segment of the VA and the posterior radicular artery forms the posterior spinal artery.

The carotid-basilar anastomoses normally disappear during fetal development, but may persist in adult life with overall incidence of 0.1% to 1.0%.[42] Among all persistent carotid-basilar anastomosis (**Fig. 5**), the persistent trigeminal artery (PTA) is the most common and is the most cephalic in location. PTA arises from the posterior genu of the cavernous segment of ICA and joins the cephalic end of the BA adjacent to the clivus. It can either have a parasellar course when it passes lateral to the dorsum sellae or an intrasellar course when it passes medially and actually perforates the dorsum sellae. It can predominantly be seen in 3 types of patterns. In the Saltzman type I, it joins the BA between the superior cerebellar arteries and anterior inferior cerebellar arteries. The BA proximal to the junction is usually hypoplastic and the posterior communicating arteries are absent or poorly opacified. PTA supplies the entire vertebrobasilar system distal to the anastomosis. In Saltzman type II, it also joins the BA between the superior cerebellar arteries and the anterior inferior cerebellar arteries, but the posterior communicating arteries are present and supply the posterior cerebral arteries. The Saltzman type

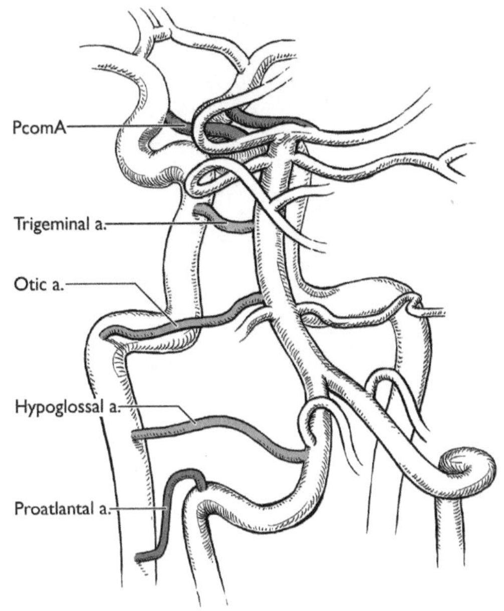

Fig. 5. The location of persistent carotid-basilar anastomoses at various levels.

III refers to the trigeminal artery variant when it directly joins to the cerebellar artery.[42,43]

As previously discussed, the persistent OA has been rarely reported with only a handful of cases published and many question its very existence. To be labeled as OA, it must originate from the lateral-most portion of the petrous segment of the ICA and then traverse through the internal auditory meatus before joining the caudal end of the BA. None of the reported cases have shown this detail in a convincing manner.[37]

The persistent hypoglossal artery (PHA) is the second most common after the PTA. This vestigial vessel normally regresses during week 5 of embryogenesis. The persistent vessel comes off ICA at the C1 to C3 level, enters the skull through the anterior condylar or hypoglossal canal and courses posteromedial to continue as the terminal segment of the vertebral artery and the BA (**Fig. 6**). The contralateral vertebral artery, if present, generally terminates in the posterior inferior cerebellar artery (PICA).[44,45]

The primitive proatlantal intersegmental artery generally disappears during week 6, at the time when the vertebral artery becomes functional. The persistent artery is the proximal segment of this artery, whereby the vertebrobasilar circulation derives supply either from the internal or external carotid arteries. A persistent proatlantal intersegmental artery type I usually originates from the extracranial ICA to join the vertebral artery between the occipital bone and C1. The type I vessel does

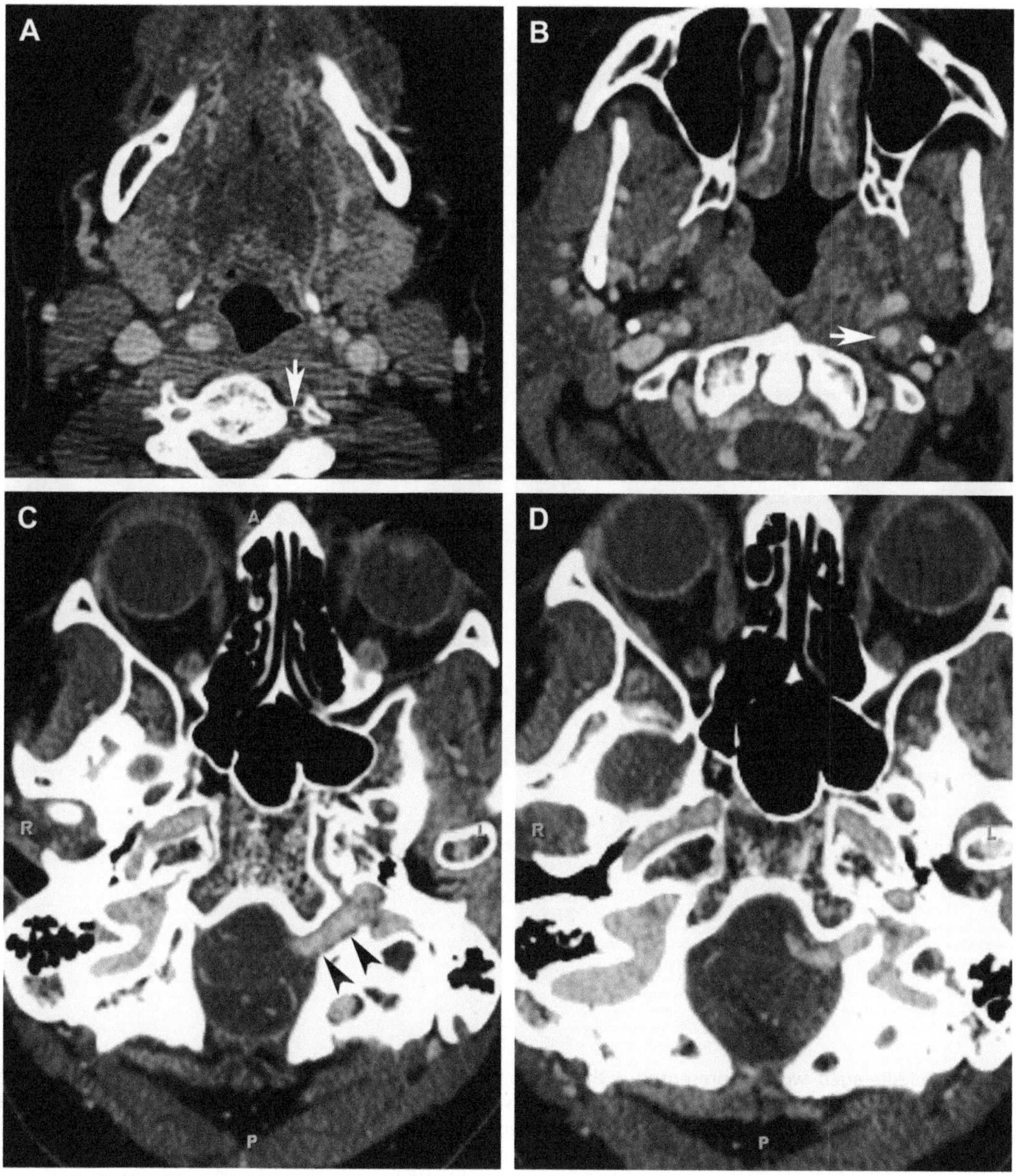

Fig. 6. Axial CTA images of PHA. (*A*) There is lack of visualization of left vertebral artery normally seen in foramen transversarium (*arrow*). (*B*) A vascular structure (PHA) is seen branching off from the internal carotid artery (*arrow*). This vessel subsequently courses posteriorly, traverses through the hypoglossal canal (*double arrowheads*), (*C*) and supplies the basilar artery (*D*).

not traverse a foramen transversarium. A type II persistent proatlantal intersegmental artery, on the other hand, originates from the external carotid artery and joins the normal course of the vertebral artery at the C1-C2 interspace.[46]

The clinical significance of various persistent carotid-basilar anastomoses lies in understanding and recognizing associated anatomic variations and vascular disorders. These persistent vestigial arteries are often noticed incidentally and probably have a low incidence of direct clinical impact. The reports of various clinical presentations are likely biased by the fact that the suggested associated disorders often lead to vascular investigations. Nevertheless, PTA has been associated with various vascular anomalies in up to 25% of the cases.[43] These anomalies include carotid-cavernous fistula (**Fig. 7**), aneurysms, Sturge-Weber syndrome,

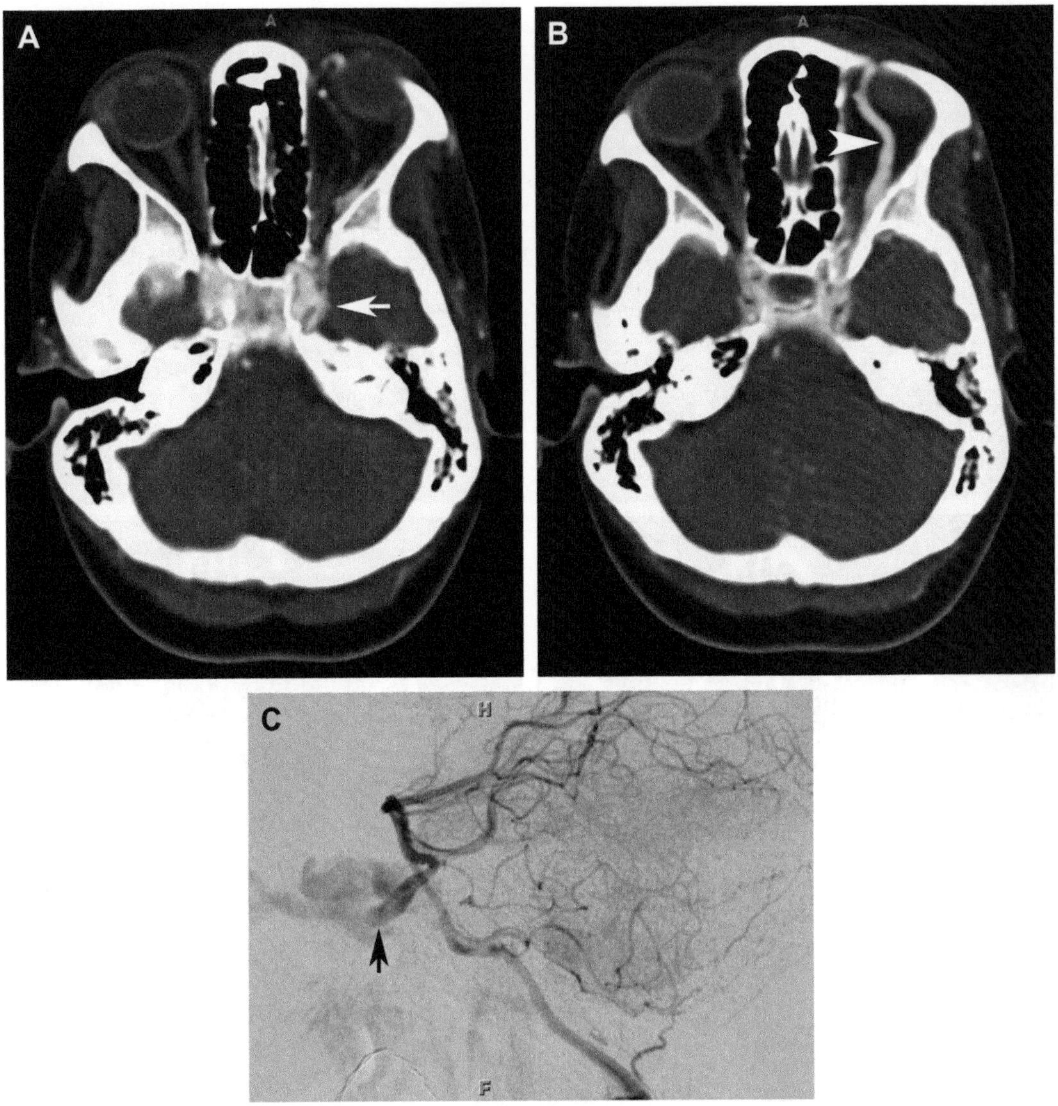

Fig. 7. A middle-aged woman presented with sudden onset of acute congestion of left eye, proptosis, and complete left-sided ophthalmoplegia. Imaging findings suggested a rupture of left-sided primitive trigeminal artery into the cavernous sinus. This rupture was treated with endovascular shunt occlusion and the trigeminal artery was preserved. (*A*) Axial CTA images show the presence of PTA (*arrow*) traversing toward the Meckel cave (*arrow*). (*B*) Marked enlargement of left superior ophthalmic vein (*arrowhead*) is consistent with left-sided carotid-cavernous fistula. (*C*) Lateral DSA image from vertebral artery injection confirms the site of rupture in the PTA (*arrow*) with high-flow fistula to the cavernous sinus.

hemangioma of the head and neck, cerebral AVM, and other arterial anomalies.[47–52] Other persistent anastomoses have been shown to be associated with similar anomalies.

It is important to understand these anatomic variations along with associated vascular disorders because they warrant appropriate modifications of interventional neuroradiology procedures. Recognizing the trigeminal artery is critical during the Wada test to avoid infusion of barbiturates into the posterior fossa. While treating lesions associated with a trigeminal artery and mid-basilar atresia or hypoplasia, it is vitally important to preserve the trigeminal artery, which is the main source of flow to the posterior circulation. Similarly, appropriate modifications are important to safely perform endovascular balloon occlusion tests and open surgical procedures when such lesions are present.

VENOUS SYSTEM

Cerebral venous drainage can be divided between 2 systems: a superficial cortical system that drains the superficial white matter and cortex toward the pial veins, cortical veins, and finally the dural venous sinuses; and a deep subependymal venous system that drains the deep white matter toward the vein of Galen and the straight sinus.[53]

Development and Abnormalities of Dural Venous Sinuses

Formation of the dural venous sinuses is influenced by both expansion of the brain vesicles and maturation of the cranial vault. The sinuses develop from primitive venous plexuses that are gradually reduced to a single channel by pressure from the surrounding anatomy and cerebrospinal fluid. In early embryogenesis, the brain is drained by a pair of ventrolateral channels, the primary head sinuses, which are continuous with the cardinal veins. By week 5, the primary head sinuses drain 3 large venous plexuses (anterior, middle, and posterior) around the dorsolateral aspect of the brain. Subsequent growth and anastomoses between these plexuses lay the framework for the major dural venous sinuses of the mature brain.

The precursors to the transverse sinuses develop at week 6 as the anterior plexus expands and forms dorsal anastomoses with the middle plexus. By 7 to 8 gestational weeks, the sagittal plexus, precursor to the superior sagittal sinus and straight sinus, is formed from the anterior plexus between the growing cerebral hemispheres. By week 9, the superior sagittal sinus can be detected as a concentration of the sagittal plexus. The mature straight sinus later forms from the confluence of the internal cerebral vein, posterior thalamic veins, and basal veins during the third gestational month and communicates with the superior sagittal sinus at the torcula. During the fifth gestational month, a transient falcine sinus is visible between the leaves of the falx cerebri.[54] It originates near the junction of the straight sinus and vein of Galen to join with the posterior third of the superior sagittal sinus.[55] This channel normally regresses by birth, but its persistence can be seen in association with certain congenital anomalies,[56] particularly vein of Galen malformations.[55] It is thought to provide a collateral drainage route for an absent or hypoplastic straight sinus in many of these cases.

Rapid enlargement of the sinuses occurs between the fourth and sixth gestational months.[57] Abnormalities during this period are common and an asymmetric course and caliber of the transverse sinuses can be frequently observed postnatally on angiographic studies.

Several occipital sinuses begin to be visible during the third gestational month as a series of plexiform channels from the primitive torcula. Between four and five months of development, these sinuses undergo dramatic growth and form connections between the torcula as well as medial transverse sinuses and the marginal sinuses around the foramen magnum.[58] By the sixth to seventh gestational months, many of these channels decrease in caliber or fuse with 1 or more prominent, remaining occipital sinuses. Variable or incomplete fusion within this period is thought to lead to diverse connection patterns and paired occipital sinuses.[59,60] In the adult, this sinus generally provides a minor drainage pathway from the torcula to the marginal sinuses and vertebral venous plexuses. When the sigmoid or transverse sinuses are occluded or hypoplastic, the occipital sinus can serve as an important collateral route for cerebral venous drainage.[61] This sinus can be delineated on angiographic studies and is particularly important to consider in patients who will undergo posterior fossa surgeries.

Dural sinus malformations

Dural sinus malformations are an extremely rare congenital abnormality that is characterized by abnormal dilatation of a physiologic or embryonic dural venous sinus, which is often termed a giant dural lake. It most commonly involves the torcula and associated portions of the superior sagittal and transverse sinuses. This dilated venous sinus has slow flow communication with other sinuses and rarely has pial venous reflux, but can be secondarily associated with arteriovenous shunts.

The developmental etiology of these lesions is uncertain. Some groups have suggested that dural sinus malformations may be the result of abnormal persistence of physiologic sinus ballooning that occurs between 4 and 7 gestational months.[58] Others have theorized that these dilatations are the result of excessive development of the sinuses, secondary to a local developmental insult.

The clinical course of these lesions is commonly marked by antenatal and perinatal thrombosis, which can result in focal hemorrhage, pial venous congestion, diffuse venous ischemia, hydrocephalus, and elevated intracranial pressure (ICP).[62] In some patients, the existence of alternative venous outflow paths may allow for better prognosis with conservative management[63] and as the malformation self-involutes over time,[64] but our current prognostic insight still remains limited.

On routine fetal ultrasound examinations, dural sinus malformations can be seen as a dilated hypoechoic lesion, most often involving the torcula. Thrombus within the lesion can cause a heterogeneous appearance. It is appropriate to follow these lesions with ultrasound through pregnancy with attention to signs of cerebral tissue damage or ventricular enlargement. The delivery process can aggravate the venous hypertension caused by these malformations, therefore, at birth, children should be evaluated by MR imaging for hemorrhagic infarcts.[63] MR angiography or DSA may be necessary to better delineate associated arteriovenous fistulas and decide appropriate management.

Craniosynostosis and dural sinus development

Given the intimate developmental relationship between the dural venous sinuses and cranial vault, it is not unexpected that abnormalities of the skull anatomy could influence cerebral venous drainage. Craniosynostosis is a rare condition of premature suture fusion that can either present as part of a branchial arch syndrome or as an isolated finding.[65,66] Developmentally, the premature fusion of the cranial sutures in craniosynostosis can impact the development of dural sinuses and result in stenosis of the sigmoid-jugular sinus complex (**Fig. 8**). Often, the venous outflow from the intracranial compartment in these patients occurs via enlarged transosseous channels, suboccipital venous plexus, and enlarged scalp and facial veins. This phenomenon is more commonly observed in syndromic forms of craniosynostosis, where multiple suture involvement is more common. The precise etiologic insult remains unknown.

Clinically, these abnormalities have been correlated with venous hypertension and elevated ICPs.[65,66] This anomaly should thus be considered during the imaging workup of patients with craniosynostosis with elevated ICPs, particularly when other common etiologies are ruled out. Taylor and colleagues,[65] in their angiographic series, demonstrated severe unilateral and bilateral stenosis of the sigmoid-jugular sinus complex in 18 of 23 pediatric patients with craniosynostosis. In cases of bilateral stenosis, prominent collateral circulation was seen through the stylomastoid emissary venous plexus.[65]

Sinus pericranii

Sinus pericranii is a rare and minimally symptomatic anomaly characterized by abnormal communication between the intracranial and extracranial venous drainage pathways. It is typically detected as a nonpulsatile mass in the midline of the frontal skull region. This mass represents an underlying venous varix, which connects the pericranial veins and superior sagittal sinus through a bony defect.[67] Gandolfo and colleagues[67] characterized these anomalies into dominant and accessory types depending on whether the varix served as the primary venous outflow tract of the superior sagittal sinus (dominant) or not (accessory).

The etiology of this disorder can be multifactorial, including congenital, posttraumatic, and spontaneous. An embryologic origin of sinus pericranii was postulated because of its frequent association with developmental venous anomalies and other

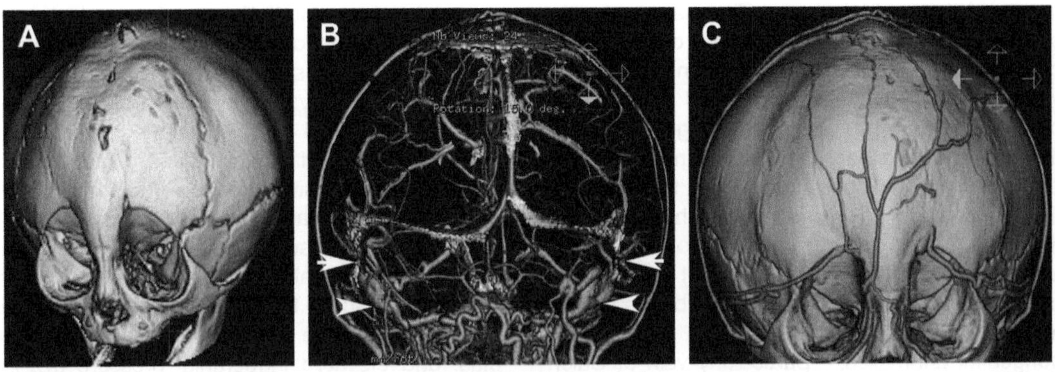

Fig. 8. Craniosynostosis with venous sinus stenosis/occlusion. CT images of an infant who presented with abnormal skull shape and hypotelorism. Corrective surgery was being considered, but incidental finding of many visible dilated facial veins on physical examination led to further imaging. (*A*) Note the fusion of metopic and sagittal skull sutures as seen on 3-dimensional reconstructed CT image. (*B*) CT venogram (CTV) shows complete occlusion of bilateral distal sigmoid sinuses (*arrows*) and absence of bilateral internal jugular veins. Instead, extensive collaterals are seen at skull base, including bilateral dilated suboccipital venous plexus pouches (*arrowheads*) and emissary veins as bypass channels. (*C*) Surface-rendered CTV image demonstrates the prominent scalp, and periorbital and facial veins that are serving as venous bypass channels to drain the intracranial venous system. Because of these findings, corrective surgery was cancelled because inadvertent injury of these by channels during surgery could result in excessive bleeding or venous infarction of the brain.

vascular anomalies.[67–70] It has been proposed that transient venous hypertension during development may increase the size of the superior sagittal sinus and prevent its normal caudal migration after gestational week 9.[68,69] The resulting venous pouch could erode through the primitive anterior skull and lead to the persistence of an epicranial varix postnatally.

The diagnosis of sinus pericranii can often be performed through physical examination of the lesion and confirmed with Doppler ultrasonography. Contrast-enhanced MR imaging and MR angiography can delineate the anatomy and drainage pattern within the dilated varix.[67] CT can be used to demonstrate the bony defect, but it is typically not the primary diagnostic modality. DSA can most precisely demonstrate the hemodynamic and anatomic details of the sinus, but it is typically only used before therapeutic planning.[67]

Development and Abnormalities of Cerebral Veins

Like the arterial system, development of the cerebral venous system is heavily dictated by increasing metabolic demands of the growing brain. The venous system, however, develops after corresponding portions of the arterial system have developed and refinement continues after birth. Before the maturation of either superficial or deep venous systems, transcerebral veins provide the first drainage to the developing parenchyma. These early vessels are followed by development of the meningeal system and then by the subependymal system. As the hemispheres expand, the transcerebral veins gradually become discontinuous and the adult venous drainage patterns become apparent.[17] The venous system is also generally more variable in its final morphology. Congenital anomalies involving the veins are thus more common.

Developmental venous anomaly

Developmental venous anomalies (DVAs) are the most common congenital cerebral vascular anomaly with an incidence of 2.6%.[71] These lesions are characterized by abnormal drainage of superficial veins toward the subependymal venous system or, alternatively, of deep veins toward the meningeal venous system. Their anatomy includes a radial complex of venous radicals that converge into a dilated collecting vein, forming a characteristic caput medusa appearance. The collecting vein can then drain into the deep veins or into the dural sinus. The size of the DVA can range from small to an entire hemisphere. They can be observed anywhere in the brain, but have a greater prevalence in the frontal lobes and posterior fossa. Although etiology of these anomalies remains to be fully understood, several investigators have postulated that these lesions form in early development because of arrested formation or thrombosis of the normal venous drainage to a parenchymal region.[72] This insult is followed by a compensatory persistence of early transcerebral venules, which cluster to form a large draining vein.[73–76]

These lesions are generally clinically benign and provide sufficient drainage to the involved brain territory. Occasional focal neurologic deficits, hemorrhage, and seizures have been reported,[77,78] but conservative management is appropriate for most patients.[79] Importantly, DVAs have been associated with other vascular malformations, including cavernomas, capillary telangiectasias, and arteriovenous malformations.[72,80,81] These related pathologies should be considered during the diagnostic process.

Because DVAs are most often asymptomatic, they typically appear as incidental findings on imaging studies. Although it can be detected on both CT and MR studies, MR is preferred for its ability to evaluate related parenchymal abnormalities.[80] The addition of hemosiderin sensitive or susceptibility-weighted images further aids detection of associated cavernous malformations. DSA is still the preferred method for the hemodynamic evaluation of DVAs and is appropriate for cases that present with ischemic or hemorrhagic infarction (**Fig. 9**) or when an associated vascular malformation is suspected.[72]

PATHOLOGIC CEREBRAL SHUNTS (COMBINED ARTERIAL-VENOUS MALFORMATIONS)

Pial Arteriovenous Malformations and Fistulae

Pial AVM and AVF are abnormal connections between arteries and veins in the subpial space.[82] Although much less common than vein of Galen malformations (VGMs), these lesions comprise approximately 25% of neonatal cerebral vascular malformations.[82] A single lesion can have multiple feeding arteries, but usually has only 1, dominant ectatic draining vein. These malformations are seen more commonly in the supratentorial space,[83] but can also be found infratentorially.[84] Although the fistulae (AVFs) consist of direct connections between the artery and the veins (**Fig. 10**), an intervening nidus is the hallmark of true arteriovenous malformations. Sometimes, the distinction between these entities may be difficult. On the other hand, in some cases the two types of shunts may coexist in the same lesion.

During development, a radial network of pial veins can be found below the cortical surface from approximately 9 to 11 gestational weeks,

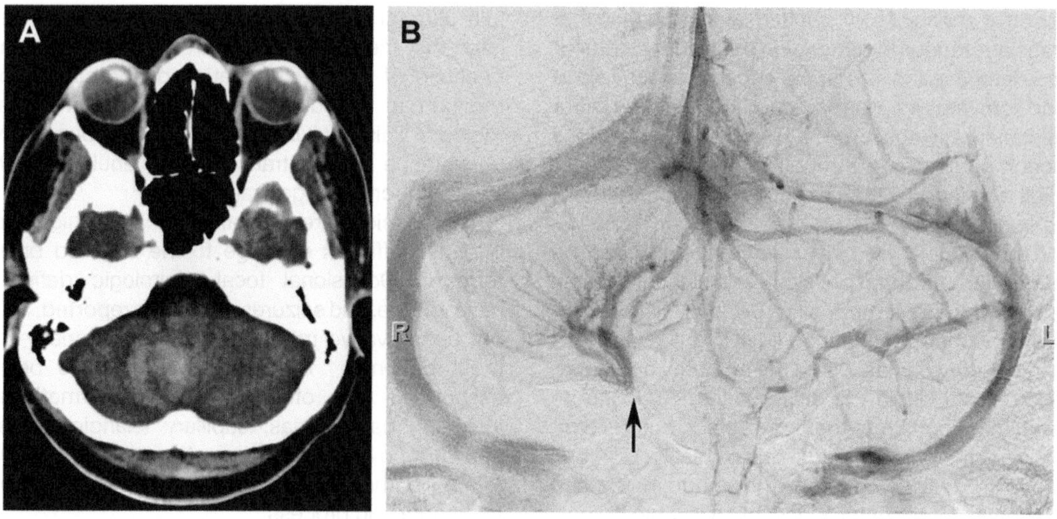

Fig. 9. DVA presenting with venous hypertension and cerebellar hemorrhage. (*A*) Axial noncontrast CT image shows acute hemorrhage in right cerebellar hemisphere. (*B*) DSA image in venous phase shows characteristic caput medusa appearance of multiple radial complex venous radicals converging into a dilated collecting vein with severe focal stenosis (*arrow*). No associated cavernous malformation was seen on MR imaging studies (not shown). The hemorrhage was thought to be a result of venous hypertension induced by DVA.

with normal involution occurring after that period.[53] It has been hypothesized that some of these pial veins may persist beyond that point, when the corresponding cortical venous segment is disrupted or fails to develop appropriately. Subsequent thrombosis in these pial vessels may promote arterial fistulization and formation of a pial AVF, in a similar mechanism to dural arteriovenous fistulas (DAVFs).[85]

The clinical presentation of pial AVMs/AVFs can be similar to that of VGMs; affected neonates can suffer cardiomegaly as a result of high-output

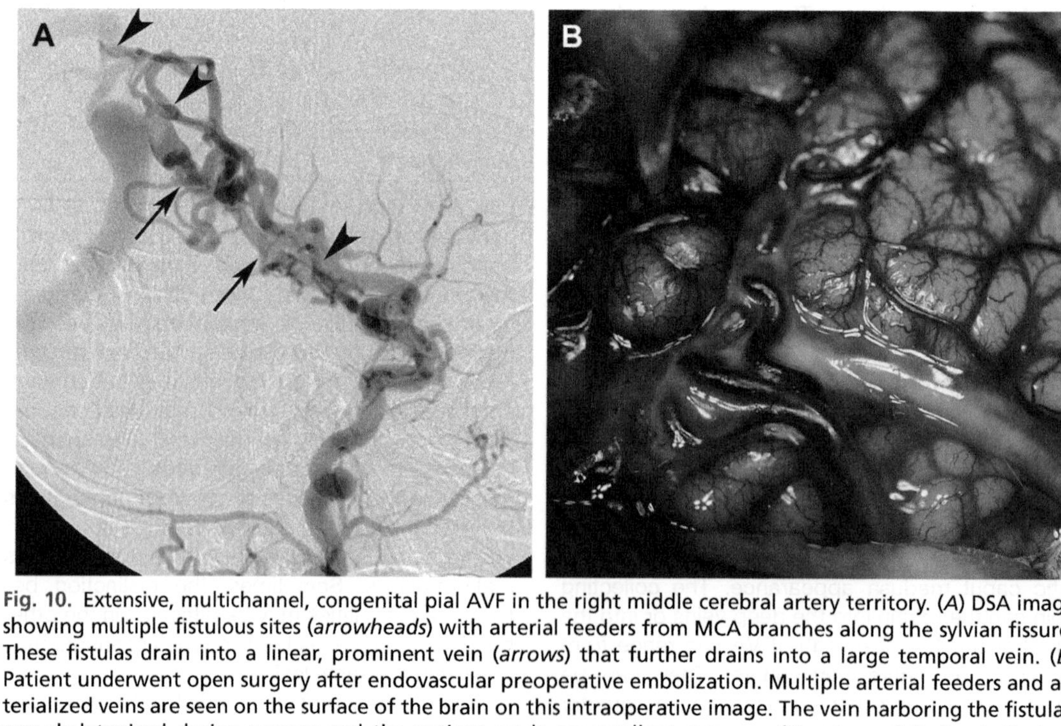

Fig. 10. Extensive, multichannel, congenital pial AVF in the right middle cerebral artery territory. (*A*) DSA image showing multiple fistulous sites (*arrowheads*) with arterial feeders from MCA branches along the sylvian fissure. These fistulas drain into a linear, prominent vein (*arrows*) that further drains into a large temporal vein. (*B*) Patient underwent open surgery after endovascular preoperative embolization. Multiple arterial feeders and arterialized veins are seen on the surface of the brain on this intraoperative image. The vein harboring the fistulae was skeletonized during surgery and the patient made an excellent recovery. (*Courtesy of* Dr Hugh Garton, Department of Neurosurgery, University of Michigan, Ann Arbor, MI.)

congestive heart failure or have spontaneous intracerebral hemorrhages. It is important to note that even asymptomatic neonates are at high risk of ischemic injury to cerebral tissues. Intervention to address the fistula should be instituted as early as possible to preserve neurocognitive function.[82,86]

Routine fetal ultrasound can sometimes detect a pial AVF, but the diagnosis is made more frequently during the perinatal period. If there is suspicion of a vascular malformation on ultrasonography, fetal MR imaging should be conducted because it offers a superior view of the feeding and draining vessels. In cases where the malformation drains into the vein of Galen, MR imaging can also better differentiate the pial AVF from a VGM, which is an important distinction for subsequent therapeutic planning.

Vein of Galen Malformations

VGMs are rare anomalies characterized by the presence of 1 or more arteriovenous shunts draining into a dilated, persistent median prosencephalic vein of Markowski (MProsV). The feedings vessels can include the choroidal arteries, distal pericallosal artery, and transmesencephalic branches from the basilar tip or proximal posterior cerebellar arteries. The venous drainage is usually through a persistent falcine sinus but can also occur through the straight sinus or a combination of both. Variations are common and include hypoplastic or absent straight sinuses, multiple or sinuous falcine sinuses, and prominent occipital and marginal sinuses.

In normal development, the MProsV serves as the primary venous drainage for the brain between 6 and 11 gestational weeks, when a choroidal vascular pattern dominates the brain circulation. After that point, the subependymal venous system takes over the deep drainage, and the MProsV concurrently regresses and is partially assimilated into the vein of Galen.[87] Persistence of the vessel and formation of the VGAM is thought to be caused by anomalous connections between the MProsV and choroidal arteries around 8 gestational weeks.[88] This process causes progressive enlargement of the MProsV under the abnormal hemodynamic stresses from high inflow of choroidal feeders and prevents its normal regression.[89]

Clinical symptoms can emerge in the neonatal, pediatric, or adult age groups, with earlier, more severe presentations correlating to lesions with greater degrees of arteriovenous shunting.[90]

Prenatal imaging diagnosis of VGMs may be accomplished with prenatal ultrasound and fetal MR imaging. Sufficient dilatation of the MProsV is required before it can be detected on first- or even second-trimester ultrasound. Therefore, most diagnoses by ultrasound occur in the third trimester.[91] Fetal MR imaging has been used increasingly to confirm the initial diagnosis and better delineate the size and configuration of the venous sac as well as the anatomy of the arterial feeders.[89] It can also provide a concurrent evaluation of the brain parenchyma (**Fig. 11**) and investigate other associated prognostic factors.[91,92] The most important predictors of poor outcome are the presence of brain parenchymal changes, including focal encephalomalacia and diffuse brain volume loss, and calcifications.[47] DSA is the gold standard for evaluating hemodynamic and anatomic details of the malformation and is conducted to assist planning for potential endovascular therapy.

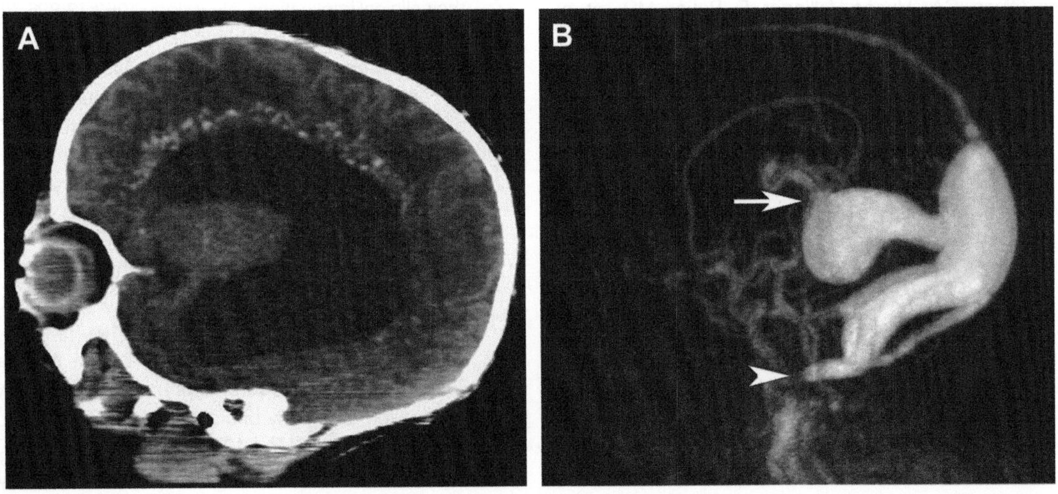

Fig. 11. Vein of Galen malformation. (*A*) Sagittal CT image showing dilated ventricular system with foci of periventricular calcifications. (*B*) MR angiography image demonstrates the site of shunt (*arrow*), markedly dilated straight sinus and bilateral transverse sinuses with severe focal stenosis in distal sigmoid sinuses (*arrowhead*).

SUMMARY

Congenital cerebral vascular anomalies include a spectrum of conditions that result from perturbation of normal developmental processes. Although some of these conditions are asymptomatic and well compensated by collateral circulation, others can cause significant morbidity for affected patients. Knowledge of the underlying developmental etiologies and associated imaging characteristics is essential for understanding the morphologic and hemodynamic details of these lesions and determining the necessity for any intervention.

REFERENCES

1. Streeter G. The developmental alterations in the vascular system of the brain of the human embryo. Contrib Embryol 1918;271(24):5–38.
2. Padget DH. The development of the cranial arteries in the human embryo. Contrib Embryol 1948;212(32):205–71.
3. Lasjaunias P, Santoyo-Vazquez A. Segmental agenesis of the internal carotid artery: angiographic aspects with embryological discussion. Anat Clin 1984;6(2):133–41.
4. Lasjaunias P, Santoyo-Vazquez A. Surgical neuroangiography. Part 1: clinical vascular anatomy and variations. 2nd edition. Berlin: Springer-Verlag; 2001.
5. Quint D, Silbergleit R, Young W. Absence of the carotid canals at skull base CT. Radiology 1992;182:477–81.
6. Pilleul F, Guibaud L, Badinand N, et al. Bilateral internal carotid agenesis: value of CT angiography and correlation to embryogenesis. Eur Radiol 2001;11(5):858–60.
7. Given CA, Huang-Hellinger F, Baker MD, et al. Congenital absence of the internal carotid artery: case reports and review of the collateral circulation. AJNR Am J Neuroradiol 2001;22(10):1953–9.
8. Takahashi M, Tamakawa Y, Kishikawa T, et al. Fenestration of the basilar artery. Report of three cases and review of the literature. Radiology 1973;109(1):79–82.
9. Heth JA, Loftus CM, Piper JG, et al. Hypoplastic internal carotid artery mimicking a classic angiographic "string sign". Case report. J Neurosurg 1997;86(3):567–70.
10. Swartz J, Harnsberger H. Imaging of the temporal bone. 2nd edition. New York: Thieme Medical; 1992.
11. Jacobsson M, Davidsson A, Hugosson S, et al. Aberrant intratympanic internal carotid artery: a potentially hazardous anomaly. J Laryngol Otol 1989;103(12):1202–5.
12. Goldman NC, Singleton GT, Holly EH. Aberrant internal carotid artery presenting as a mass in the middle ear. Arch Otolaryngol 1971;94(3):269–73.
13. Anand VK, Casano PJ, Flaiz RA. Diagnosis and treatment of the carotid artery in the middle ear. Otolaryngol Head Neck Surg 1991;105(5):743–7.
14. Moret J, Delvert J, Bretonneau C, et al. Vascularization of the middle ear. Normal-variations-glomus tumors. J Neuroradiol 1982;9:209–60.
15. Oates JW, McAuliffe W, Coates HL. Management of pseudo-aneurysm of a lateral aberrant internal carotid artery. Int J Pediatr Otorhinolaryngol 1997;42(1):73–9.
16. Brismar J. Persistent hypoglossal artery, diagnostic criteria. Report of a case. Acta Radiol Diagn (Stockh) 1976;17(2):160–6.
17. Raybaud C. Normal and abnormal embryology and development of the intracranial vascular system. Neurosurg Clin N Am 2010;21(3):399–426.
18. Lazorthes G, Gouaze A. Modeling of the diameter of segments of Willis' polygon (circulus arteriosus cerebri). Role of the movements of the head. C R Acad Sci Hebd Seances Acad Sci D 1970;271(19):1682–5 [in French].
19. Hoffman WF, Wilson CB. Fenestrated basilar artery with an associated saccular aneurysm. Case report. J Neurosurg 1979;50(2):262–4.
20. Sanders WP, Sorek PA, Mehta BA. Fenestration of intracranial arteries with special attention to associated aneurysms and other anomalies. AJNR Am J Neuroradiol 1993;14(3):675–80.
21. Teal JS, Rumbaugh CL, Bergeron RT, et al. Angiographic demonstration of fenestrations of the intradural intracranial arteries. Radiology 1973;106(1):123–6.
22. van Rooij SB, van Rooij WJ, Sluzewski M, et al. Fenestrations of intracranial arteries detected with 3D rotational angiography. AJNR Am J Neuroradiol 2009;30(7):1347–50.
23. Baptista AG. Studies on the arteries of the brain. II. The anterior cerebral artery: some anatomic features and their clinical implications. Neurology 1963;13:825–35.
24. Preul M, Tampieri D, Leblanc R. Giant aneurysm of the distal anterior cerebral artery: associated with an anterior communicating artery aneurysm and a dural arteriovenous fistula. Surg Neurol 1992;38(5):347–52.
25. Niizuma H, Kwak R, Uchida K, et al. Aneurysms of the azygos anterior cerebral artery. Surg Neurol 1981;15(3):225–8.
26. LeMay M, Gooding C. The clinical significance of the azygous anterior cerebral artery. Am J Roentgenol Radium Ther Nucl Med 1966;98:602–10.
27. Teal JS, Rumbaugh CL, Bergeron RT, et al. Anomalies of the middle cerebral artery: accessory artery, duplication, and early bifurcation. Am J Roentgenol Radium Ther Nucl Med 1973;118(3):567–75.
28. Komiyama M, Nakajima H, Nishikawa M, et al. Middle cerebral artery variations: duplicated and accessory arteries. AJNR Am J Neuroradiol 1998;19(1):45–9.

29. Crompton MR. The pathology of ruptured middle-cerebral aneurysms with special reference to the differences between the sexes. Lancet 1962;2(7253):421–5.
30. Yasargil MG, Smith RD. Association of middle cerebral artery anomalies with saccular aneurysms and moyamoya disease. Surg Neurol 1976;6(1):39–43.
31. Malamateniou C, Adams ME, Srinivasan L, et al. The anatomic variations of the circle of Willis in preterm-at-term and term-born infants: an MR angiography study at 3T. AJNR Am J Neuroradiol 2009;30(10): 1955–62.
32. Hoh BL, Rabinov JD, Pryor JC, et al. Persistent nonfused segments of the basilar artery: longitudinal versus axial nonfusion. AJNR Am J Neuroradiol 2004;25(7):1194–6.
33. Sabin F. Origin and development of the primitive vessels of the chick and of the pig. Contributions to Embryology 1917;6(18):63–124.
34. Moffat D. Development of anterior cerebral artery and its related vessels in rat. Am J Anat 1961; 108(1):17.
35. Congdon ED. Transformation of the branchial-arch system during the development of the human embryo. Contrib Embryol 1922;68:47–110.
36. Hutchinson NA, Miller JD. Persistent proatlantal artery. J Neurol Neurosurg Psychiatry 1970;33(4):524–7.
37. Reynolds AF Jr, Stovring J, Turner PT. Persistent otic artery. Surg Neurol 1980;13(2):115–7.
38. Matsushita A, Yanaka K, Hyodo A, et al. Persistent primitive otic artery with IC-cavernous aneurysm. J Clin Neurosci 2003;10(1):113–5.
39. Gailloud P, Clatterbuck RE, Fasel JH, et al. Segmental agenesis of the internal carotid artery distal to the posterior communicating artery leading to the definition of a new embryologic segment. AJNR Am J Neuroradiol 2004;25(7):1189–93.
40. Padget DH. Designation of the embryonic intersegmental arteries in reference to the vertebral artery and subclavian stem. Anat Rec 1954;119(3):349–56.
41. Moffat DB. The development of the hind-brain arteries in the rat. J Anat 1957;91(1):25–39.
42. Yilmaz E, Ilgit E, Taner D. Primitive persistent carotid-basilar and carotid-vertebral anastomoses: a report of seven cases and a review of the literature. Clin Anat 1995;8(1):36–43.
43. Okahara M, Kiyosue A, Mori H. Anatomic variations of the cerebral arteries and their embryology: a pictorial review. Eur Radiol 2002;12:2548–61.
44. Oelerich M, Schuierer G. Primitive hypoglossal artery: demonstration with digital subtraction-, MR- and CT angiography. Eur Radiol 1997;7(9):1492–4.
45. Basekim CC, Silit E, Mutlu H, et al. Type I proatlantal artery with bilateral absence of the external carotid arteries. AJNR Am J Neuroradiol 2004;25(9): 1619–21.
46. Guglielmi G, Vinuela F, Dion J, et al. Persistent primitive trigeminal artery-cavernous sinus fistulas: report of two cases. Neurosurgery 1990;27(5):805–8 [discussion: 808–9].
47. McKenzie JD, Dean BL, Flom RA. Trigeminal-cavernous fistula: Saltzman anatomy revisited. AJNR Am J Neuroradiol 1996;17(2):280–2.
48. Kwak R, Kadoya S. Moyamoya disease associated with persistent primitive trigeminal artery. Report of two cases. J Neurosurg 1983;59(1):166–71.
49. Suzuki S, Morioka T, Matsushima T, et al. Moyamoya disease associated with persistent primitive trigeminal artery variant in identical twins. Surg Neurol 1996; 45(3):236–40.
50. Tomsick TA, Lukin RR, Chambers AA. Persistent trigeminal artery: unusual associated abnormalities. Neuroradiology 1979;17(5):253–7.
51. Fortner AA, Smoker WR. Persistent primitive trigeminal artery aneurysm evaluated by MR imaging and angiography. J Comput Assist Tomogr 1988;12(5):847–50.
52. Loevner L, Quint DJ. Persistent trigeminal artery in a patient with Sturge-Weber syndrome. AJR Am J Roentgenol 1992;158(4):872–4.
53. Padget DH. The cranial venous system in man in reference to development, adult configuration, and relation to the arteries. Am J Anat 1956;98(3):307–55.
54. Yokota A, Oota T, Matsukado Y, et al. Structures and development of the venous system in congenital malformations of the brain. Neuroradiology 1978; 16:26–30.
55. Raybaud CA, Strother CM, Hald JK. Aneurysms of the vein of Galen: embryonic considerations and anatomical features relating to the pathogenesis of the malformation. Neuroradiology 1989;31(2):109–28.
56. Sener RN. Association of persistent falcine sinus with different clinicoradiologic conditions: MR imaging and MR angiography. Comput Med Imaging Graph 2000;24(6):343–8.
57. Widjaja E, Griffiths PD. Intracranial MR venography in children: normal anatomy and variations. AJNR Am J Neuroradiol 2004;25(9):1557–62.
58. Okudera T, Huang YP, Ohta T, et al. Development of posterior fossa dural sinuses, emissary veins, and jugular bulb: morphological and radiologic study. AJNR Am J Neuroradiol 1994;15(10):1871–83.
59. Kobayashi K, Suzuki M, Ueda F, et al. Anatomical study of the occipital sinus using contrast-enhanced magnetic resonance venography. Neuroradiology 2006;48(6):373–9.
60. Balak N, Ersoy G, Uslu U, et al. Microsurgical and histomorphometric study of the occipital sinus: quantitative measurements using a novel approach of stereology. Clin Anat 2010;23(4):386–93.
61. Dora F, Zileli T. Common variations of the lateral and occipital sinuses at the confluens sinuum. Neuroradiology 1980;20(1):23–7.
62. Lasjaunias P. Vascular diseases in neonates, infants and children: interventional neuroradiology management. Berlin: Springer; 1997.

63. Merzoug V, Flunker S, Drissi C, et al. Dural sinus malformation (DSM) in fetuses. Diagnostic value of prenatal MRI and follow-up. Eur Radiol 2008;18(4):692–9.
64. Jenny B, Zerah M, Swift D, et al. Giant dural venous sinus ectasia in neonates. J Neurosurg Pediatr 2010; 5(5):523–8.
65. Taylor WJ, Hayward RD, Lasjaunias P, et al. Enigma of raised intracranial pressure in patients with complex craniosynostosis: the role of abnormal intracranial venous drainage. J Neurosurg 2001; 94(3):377–85.
66. Kurosu A, Wachi A, Bando K, et al. Craniosynostosis in the presence of a sinus pericranii: case report. Neurosurgery 1994;34(6):1090–2 [discussion: 1092–3].
67. Gandolfo C, Krings T, Alvarez H, et al. Sinus pericranii: diagnostic and therapeutic considerations in 15 patients. Neuroradiology 2007;49(6):505–14.
68. Sakai K, Namba K, Meguro T, et al. Sinus pericranii associated with a cerebellar venous angioma–case report. Neurol Med Chir (Tokyo) 1997;37(6):464–7.
69. Nomura S, Kato S, Ishihara H, et al. Association of intra- and extradural developmental venous anomalies, so-called venous angioma and sinus pericranii. Childs Nerv Syst 2006;22(4):428–31.
70. Nakasu Y, Nakasu S, Minouchi K, et al. Multiple sinus pericranii with systemic angiomas: case report. Surg Neurol 1993;39(1):41–5.
71. Sarwar M, McCormick WF. Intracerebral venous angioma. Case report and review. Arch Neurol 1978; 35(5):323–5.
72. Ruiz DS, Yilmaz H, Gailloud P. Cerebral developmental venous anomalies: current concepts. Ann Neurol 2009;66(3):271–83.
73. Hammoud D, Beauchamp N, Wityk R, et al. Ischemic complication of a cerebral developmental venous anomaly: case report and review of the literature. J Comput Assist Tomogr 2002;26(4): 633–6.
74. Ostertun B, Solymosi L. Magnetic resonance angiography of cerebral developmental venous anomalies: its role in differential diagnosis. Neuroradiology 1993; 35(2):97–104.
75. Oran I, Kiroglu Y, Yurt A, et al. Developmental venous anomaly (DVA) with arterial component: a rare cause of intracranial haemorrhage. Neuroradiology 2009;51(1):25–32.
76. Lee C, Pennington MA, Kenney CM 3rd. MR evaluation of developmental venous anomalies: medullary venous anatomy of venous angiomas. AJNR Am J Neuroradiol 1996;17(1):61–70.
77. Topper R, Jurgens E, Reul J, et al. Clinical significance of intracranial developmental venous anomalies. J Neurol Neurosurg Psychiatry 1999;67(2):234–8.
78. Garner TB, Del Curling O Jr, Kelly DL Jr, et al. The natural history of intracranial venous angiomas J Neurosurg 1991;75(5):715–22.
79. Kondziolka D, Dempsey PK, Lunsford LD. The case for conservative management of venous angiomas. Can J Neurol Sci 1991;18(3):295–9.
80. San Millan Ruiz D, Delavelle J, Yilmaz H, et al. Parenchymal abnormalities associated with developmental venous anomalies. Neuroradiology 2007; 49(12):987–95.
81. Rigamonti D, Spetzler RF, Drayer BP, et al. Appearance of venous malformations on magnetic resonance imaging. J Neurosurg 1988;69(4):535–9.
82. Rodesch G, Malherbe V, Alvarez H, et al. Nongalenic cerebral arteriovenous malformations in neonates and infants. Review of 26 consecutive cases (1982–1992). Childs Nerv Syst 1995;11(4):231–41.
83. Weon YC, Yoshida Y, Sachet M, et al. Supratentorial cerebral arteriovenous fistulas (AVFs) in children: review of 41 cases with 63 non choroidal single-hole AVFs. Acta Neurochir (Wien) 2005;147(1):17–31 [discussion: 31].
84. Yoshida Y, Weon YC, Sachet M, et al. Posterior cranial fossa single-hole arteriovenous fistulae in children: 14 consecutive cases. Neuroradiology 2004;46(6): 474–81.
85. Mullan S, Mojtahedi S, Johnson DL, et al. Embryological basis of some aspects of cerebral vascular fistulas and malformations. J Neurosurg 1996;85(1):1–8.
86. Garel C, Azarian M, Lasjaunias P, et al. Pial arteriovenous fistulas: dilemmas in prenatal diagnosis, counseling and postnatal treatment. Report of three cases. Ultrasound Obstet Gynecol 2005;26(3): 293–6.
87. Streeter GL. The developmental alterations in the vascular system of the brain of the human embryo. Washington, DC: Carnegie Institution; 1918.
88. Raybaud CA, Strother CM. Persisting abnormal embryonic vessels in intracranial arteriovenous malformations. Acta Radiol Suppl 1986;369:136–8.
89. Gailloud P, O'Riordan DP, Burger I, et al. Diagnosis and management of vein of Galen aneurysmal malformations. J Perinatol 2005;25(8):542–51.
90. Gold AP, Ransohoff J, Carter S. Vein of Galen malformation. Acta Neurol Scand Suppl 1964; 40(Suppl 11):1–31.
91. Geibprasert S, Krings T, Armstrong D, et al. Predicting factors for the follow-up outcome and management decisions in vein of Galen aneurysmal malformations. Childs Nerv Syst 2010;26(1):35–46.
92. Brunelle F. Brain vascular malformations in the fetus: diagnosis and prognosis. Childs Nerv Syst 2003; 19(7–8):524–8.

Congenital Midface Abnormalities

Daniel J.G. Baxter, MD CM, FRCPC[a],
Manohar Shroff, MD, FRCPC[b,*]

KEYWORDS

- Congenital anomaly • Midface • Pharyngeal arch
- Embryogenesis

DEVELOPMENT OF THE FACE

Congenital anomalies of the midface originate during transformation of the first pair of pharyngeal arches into adult structures. The first stage of facial development occurs during the fourth week of gestation around the primordial mouth or stomodeum. The first pair of pharyngeal arches gives rise to 5 facial prominences: a single frontonasal prominence, paired maxillary prominences, and paired mandibular prominences.[1] These 5 facial prominences form the boundaries of the stomodeum, as illustrated in **Fig. 1**. The facial prominences are the result of migration and proliferation of neural crest cells into the first pair of pharyngeal arches. Neural crest cells are the predominant source of facial connective tissue components including bone, cartilage, and ligaments.

Facial development mainly takes place between the fourth and eighth week of gestation. The frontal part of the frontonasal prominence forms the forehead and dorsum of the nose. The nasal part of the frontonasal prominence gives rise to bilateral nasal placodes. A nasal placode is composed of an oval thickening of surface ectoderm. The margins of a nasal placode proliferate to form a ridge with a medial and lateral nasal prominence. The central depression in a nasal placode between the nasal prominences is the nasal pit. The developing nasal pits deepen to become the anterior nares (nostrils), and nasal cavity.[2]

The lateral nasal prominences are separated from the maxillary prominences by clefts called the nasolacrimal grooves. Medial growth of the maxillary prominences causes the medial nasal prominences to move toward each other and fuse. The fused medial nasal prominences give rise to the medial upper lip, philtrum (infranasal depression), primary palate, incisor teeth, and nasal septum. The lateral nasal prominences form the nasal alae (sides of the nose). The maxillary prominences form the lateral upper lip, most of the maxilla, and secondary palate.

CHOANAL ATRESIA AND STENOSIS

The developing nasal pits deepen to form the primitive nasal cavity. At first, the posterior aspect of the nasal cavity is separated from the oral cavity by the oronasal membrane. In the sixth week of gestation, the oronasal membrane normally ruptures. The site of continuity between the posterior nasal and oral cavities are the choanae. Later, after the development of the secondary palate, the choanae are located between the nasal cavity and nasopharynx. Cells that line the nasal cavity proliferate to form a temporary epithelial plug that is subsequently resorbed.

Choanal atresia is the most common cause of neonatal nasal obstruction, occurring in up to 1 in 5000 newborns. Bilateral choanal atresia causes respiratory distress in newborns who are obligate nose breathers. The diagnosis can be suggested by the inability to advance a nasal catheter. Computed tomography (CT) examination is the imaging modality of choice in neonates with suspected choanal atresia. CT should be performed immediately after suctioning of nasal secretions.[3]

[a] Diagnostic Imaging, University of Toronto, 555 University Avenue, Toronto, Ontario, Canada, M5G 1X8
[b] Diagnostic Imaging, The Hospital for Sick Children, University of Toronto, 555 University Avenue, Toronto, Ontario, Canada, M5G 1X8
* Corresponding author.
E-mail address: manohar.shroff@sickkids.ca

Neuroimag Clin N Am 21 (2011) 563–584
doi:10.1016/j.nic.2011.05.003
1052-5149/11/$ – see front matter

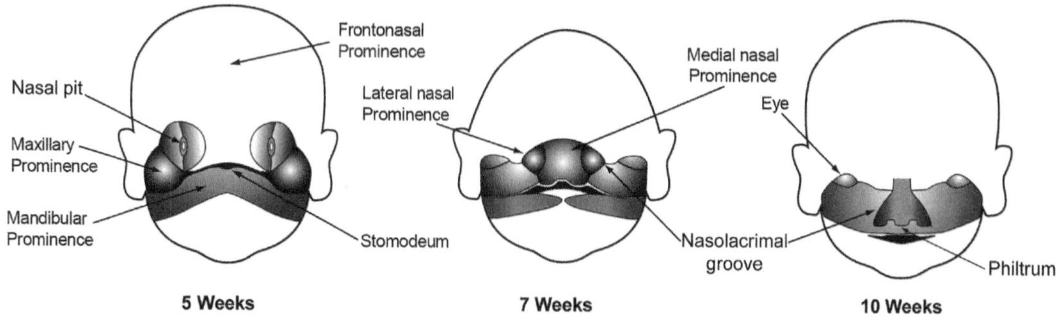

Fig. 1. Development of the face. Five facial prominences are arranged around the stomodeum.

It can identify whether the obstruction is osseous (85%) or membranous (15%). Osseous choanal atresia is related to failure of rupture of the oronasal membrane. Membranous choanal atresia is caused by incomplete resorption of the nasal epithelial plugs.

Choanal atresia is commonly associated with other congenital anomalies (50%–70%). Common associations include coloboma, heart defects, choanal atresia, retarded growth and development, genital malformations and ear anomalies (CHARGE) syndrome, Apert syndrome, Crouzon syndrome, Treacher Collins syndrome, and bowel malrotation. Individuals with CHARGE syndrome have various combinations of the abnormalities listed in the acronym, as shown in **Figs. 2** and **3**.

CT examination may show a bony or soft tissue septum extending across the posterior choanae.

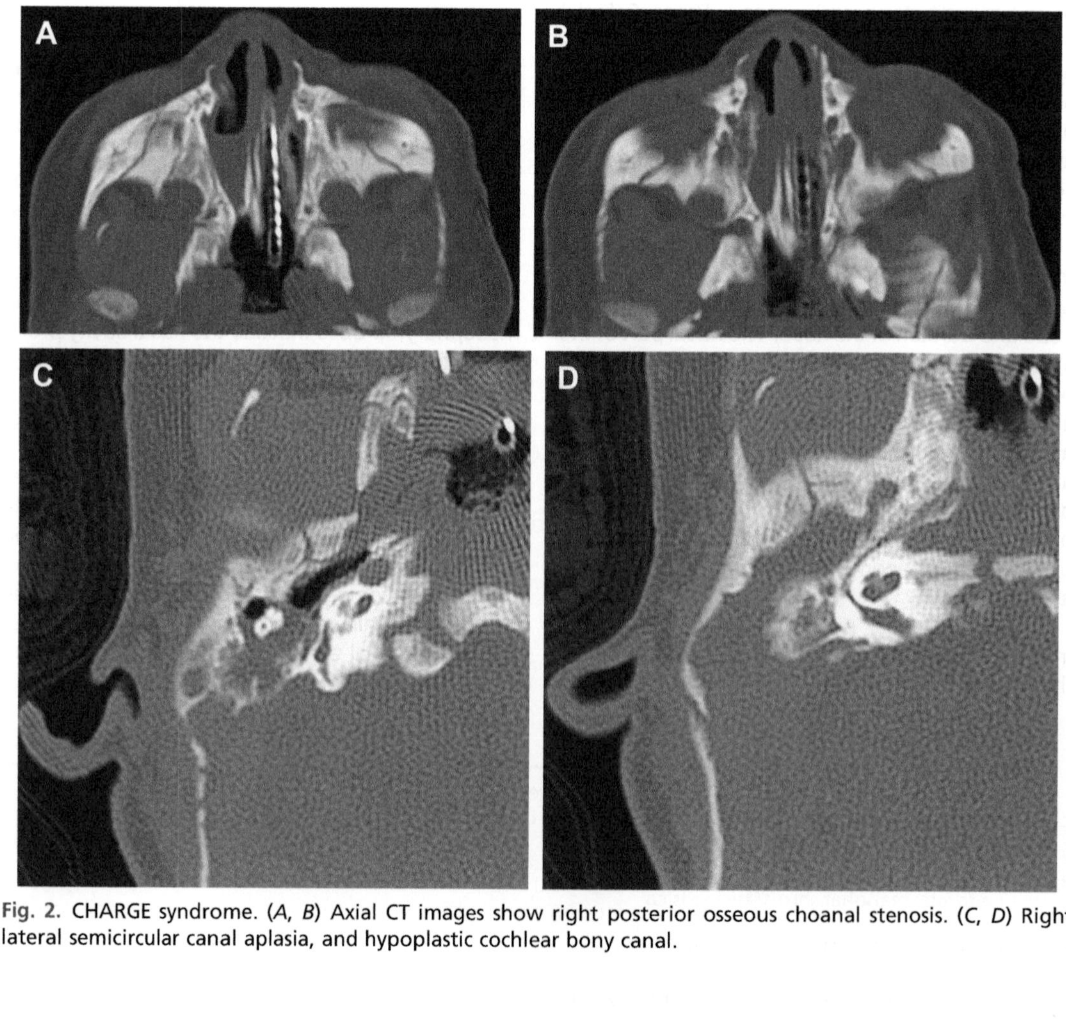

Fig. 2. CHARGE syndrome. (*A, B*) Axial CT images show right posterior osseous choanal stenosis. (*C, D*) Right lateral semicircular canal aplasia, and hypoplastic cochlear bony canal.

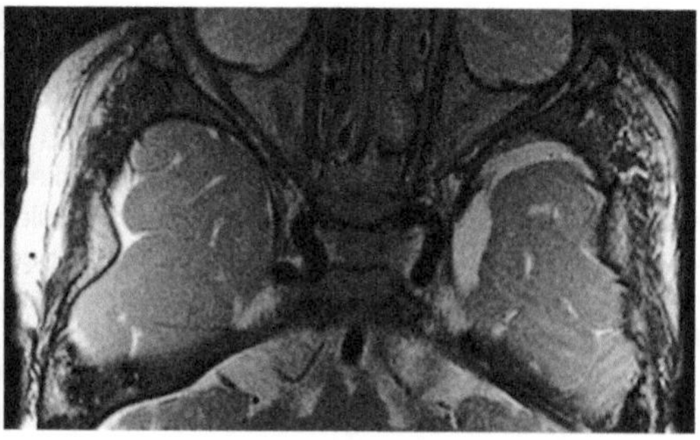

Fig. 3. CHARGE syndrome. An axial T2 MR image in the same patient shows bilateral colobomas.

Associated imaging features in bony choanal atresia include inward bowing of the posterior maxilla, and fusion or thickening of the vomer.[5] In children younger than 2 years old, narrowing of the posterior choanal opening less than 0.34 cm is defined as choanal stenosis. The current treatment of choanal atresia causing neonatal nasal obstruction is endoscopic perforation or choanal reconstruction.[6]

CONGENITAL NASAL PIRIFORM APERTURE STENOSIS

Congenital nasal piriform aperture stenosis is an infrequent cause of nasal obstruction in neonates and infants. It can mimic choanal atresia, including the inability to easily advance a nasal catheter. This condition is exacerbated by upper respiratory tract infections that further compromise the narrow nasal aperture.

CT examination is the imaging modality of choice to accurately measure the piriform aperture width. A width less than 11 mm in a term infant is diagnostic. Associated imaging features include an abnormal dentition with a central megaincisor, and a triangular configuration of the palate (**Fig. 4**). The underside of the palate often has a midline bone ridge.[7] Magnetic resonance (MR)

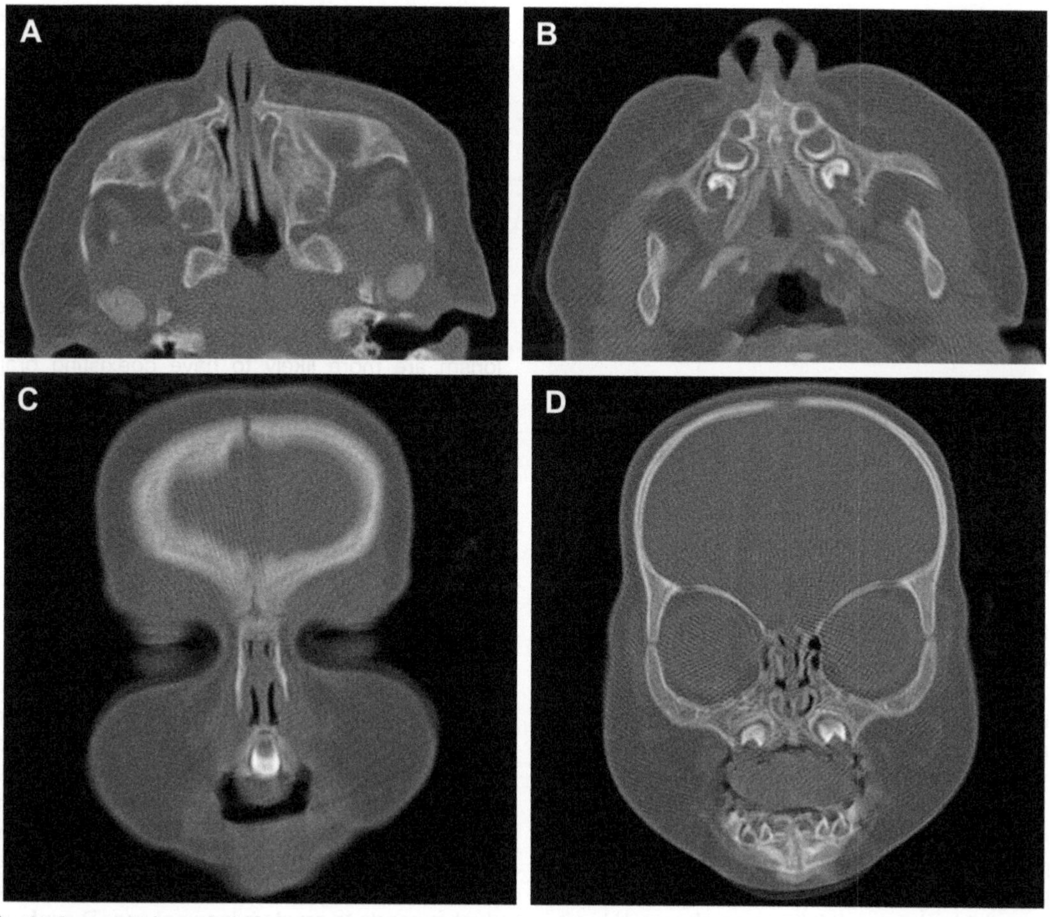

Fig. 4. Congenital nasal piriform aperture stenosis. Axial and coronal CT images show (*A*) nasal piriform aperture stenosis, (*B*) triangular configuration of the palate, (*C*) central megaincisor, and (*D*) a midline bone ridge on the underside of the palate.

imaging is helpful to evaluate for associated intracranial anomalies including holoprosencephaly and pituitary abnormalities.

One theory about the pathogenesis of nasal piriform aperture stenosis is faulty development of the palate. The palate is the floor of the nasal cavity and roof of the mouth. It develops from 3 structures: the primary palate and 2 lateral palatal shelves. The primary palate constitutes the small part of the adult hard palate anterior to the incisive fossa. The 2 lateral palatal shelves form the remainder of the adult hard palate and soft palate. Normally, the primary palate is formed by the fused medial nasal prominences in the sixth week of gestation. The secondary palate develops as 2 lateral palatal shelves extend from the inner maxillary prominences. Following a sequence of intricately timed events, the 2 lateral palatal shelves fuse to each other, the primary palate, and nasal septum.

Nasal piriform aperture stenosis can be explained by a deficiency of the fused medial nasal prominences, with subsequent development of a small triangular primary palate, abnormal incisors, and narrow anterior nasal cavity.[8] The midline bony ridge along the underside of the palate may be related to abnormal overlap and adhesive contact of the palatal shelves during formation of the secondary palate. Most patients with congenital nasal piriform aperture stenosis have an excellent prognosis. These patients are usually treated conservatively with special feeding techniques until the obstruction is relieved by growth of the nasal cavity. Severe cases may require surgical reconstruction.

CLEFT LIP, CLEFT PALATE, AND FACIAL CLEFTS

Cleft lip is the most common craniofacial malformation. The incidence of cleft lip varies between ethnic groups (white population 1:1000 live births). It results from failure of fusion of the maxillary prominence on the affected side with the medial nasal prominence. The least severe form of a cleft lip involves only the superficial vermilion border of the lip. Increasingly severe clefts extend through the maxillary alveolar arch between the lateral incisor and cuspid tooth. If epithelium is entrapped between the globular portion of the medial nasal process and the maxillary process, a globulomaxillary (fissural) cyst can develop between the maxillary lateral incisor and cuspid. Cleft lip may occur with or without a cleft palate. Cleft lip is bilateral in 20% of cases. Prenatal ultrasound can reliably show a cleft lip as an abnormal hypoechoic line extending from the upper lip into the nostril.[9]

Cleft palate is caused by incomplete fusion of the lateral palatal shelves with each other, the nasal septum, and the primary palate. It can be unilateral or bilateral. The least severe form of a cleft palate is a bifid uvula. More severe clefts extend anteriorly along the expected lines of fusion of the lateral palatal shelves and posterior aspect of the primary palate. The nasal septum may fuse with the left or right palatal shelf or neither. An isolated cleft palate may be missed on prenatal ultrasound. In the setting of bilateral cleft lip and palate, the infranasal soft tissue, alveolar ridge, and dental structures between the clefts can cause a conspicuous premaxillary protrusion.

The development of the face may be disrupted by multiple toxic substances, nutritional imbalance, and genetic factors. There are several different classifications used to describe rare facial clefts, including the Tessier, DeMeyer, and Sedano systems. The Tessier system numbers the topographic location of facial clefts from 1 to 14.[10] Clefts 1 to 7 are below the orbit, and 8 to 14 are above. Rare facial clefts can be predicted based on the expected embryologic fusion lines of the 5 facial prominences (**Fig. 5**). For example, incomplete fusion of the paired mandibular prominences leads to a midline mandibular cleft. Failure to merge a maxillary and lateral nasal prominence causes an oblique facial cleft (orbitofacial fissure) extending from the nasal ala to the medial canthus. Within the oblique facial cleft, the nasolacrimal duct remains as an open groove. Facial clefts that do not respect embryologic fusion lines are most likely secondary to amniotic band syndrome.

Rare facial clefts with hypotelorism or hypertelorism are more likely to have coexisting brain anomalies. Facial clefts with hypotelorism have been described with ventral induction malformations ranging from alobar holoprosencephaly to septo-optic dysplasia. Facial clefts with hypertelorism can have associated dysgenesis of the corpus callosum, and pituitary gland anomalies.

NASOLACRIMAL DUCT STENOSIS AND ATRESIA

The nasolacrimal duct develops from an ectodermal thickening in the floor of the nasolacrimal groove at 1 month gestational age. This ectodermal thickening makes a solid cord that separates from the surface ectoderm and is enveloped by the underlying mesenchyme. The solid cord becomes canalized to form the nasolacrimal duct. The superior end of the nasolacrimal duct expands to create a lacrimal sac. The inferior end of the duct empties into the inferior meatus via the Hasner membrane. Spontaneous rupture of the

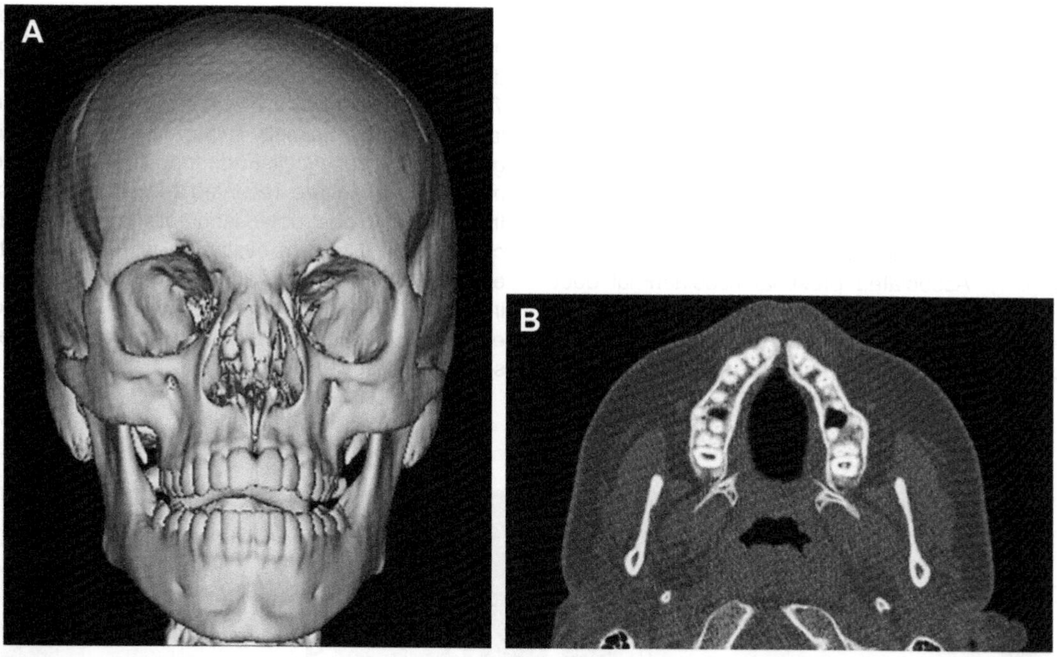

Fig. 5. Median facial cleft. (*A*) Three-dimensional (3D) surface rendered CT, and (*B*) axial CT image show a rare median facial cleft caused by failure of fusion of the 2 median nasal prominences.

Hasner membrane with production of a mucosal fold called the Hasner valve is required for nasolacrimal duct patency. Rupture of the Hasner membrane likely occurs after birth when a newborn first attempts to breathe and cry.

Nasolacrimal duct stenosis is common in neonates. It is caused by partial persistence of the Hasner membrane. CT is the imaging modality of choice in suspected nasolacrimal duct anomalies. Imaging findings can include an asymmetrically enlarged opacified nasolacrimal canal (**Fig. 6**). However, nasolacrimal duct stenosis can also appear normal.[11] Nasolacrimal stenosis resolves spontaneously in 90% of infants within the first year of life with conservative management. Prophylactic antibiotics may be administered during this period to prevent periorbital cellulitis. In selected cases, canalicular probing and intubation are widely accepted treatment options.[12]

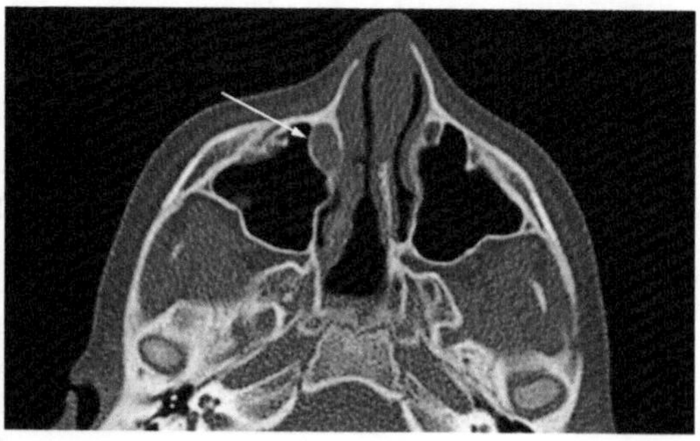

Fig. 6. Right nasolacrimal duct stenosis. Axial CT image shows enlargement and opacification of the right nasolacrimal canal (*arrow*). Note the normal appearance of the left nasolacrimal canal.

Nasolacrimal duct atresia is an uncommon congenital anomaly. It is caused by failure to canalize the epithelial cord that is the precursor of the nasolacrimal duct. Usually atresia of the nasolacrimal duct occurs at its inferior aspect. Congenital atresia of the lacrimal drainage system can also occur superiorly at the lacrimal puncta and canaliculi.

Nasolabial cysts are briefly described in this article because their origin is most likely related to aberrant nasolacrimal duct development. If an embryonic nasolacrimal epithelial rest becomes entrapped within the nasal alar region, it can form a benign cystic lesion called a nasolabial cyst. These rare cysts may encroach on the nasal aperture. Their characteristic extraosseous location should prevent confusion with maxillary cysts.

DACRYOCYSTOCELES

Dacryocystoceles are a frequent cause of neonatal nasal obstruction. A dacryocystocele is caused by obstruction of the lacrimal drainage system above and below the lacrimal sac. Subsequently the lacrimal sac becomes distended with accumulated secretions and prone to infection. The distal obstruction is often an imperforate Hasner membrane. The proximal obstruction is most likely at the Rosenmuller valve near the entrance of the common canaliculus into the lacrimal sac. CT is the imaging modality of choice to diagnose a dacryocystocele and exclude other nasal masses.[13] The imaging features include a round cystic mass at the medial canthus with a thin peripheral wall (**Fig. 7**). Associated proximal nasolacrimal duct dilatation with bony remodeling can produce elevation of the adjacent inferior turbinate and contralateral shift of the nasal septum.[14]

Dacryocystoceles require expedient management to decrease the risk of superimposed infection and scarring of the lacrimal drainage system. Treatment ranges from manual pressure on the lacrimal sac to minimally invasive probing and irrigation of the canaliculi. Endoscopic resection and marsupialization are reserved for severe cases. Infection of an obstructed lacrimal sac is called dacryocystitis. It is best evaluated with a contrast-enhanced CT examination. Imaging features include a distended lacrimal sac with associated enhancing thickened walls, and surrounding preseptal soft tissue swelling (**Fig. 8**).

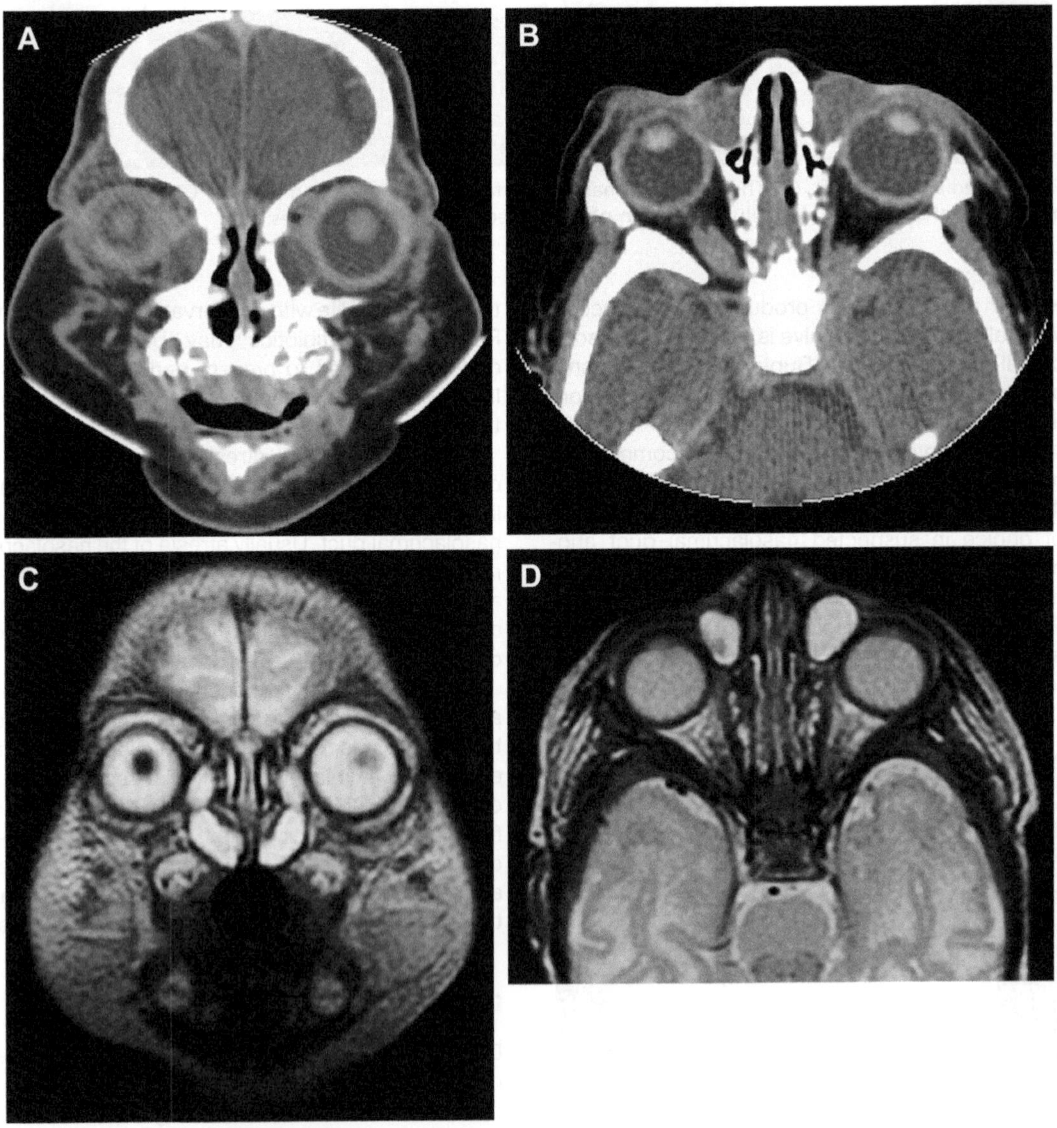

Fig. 7. Bilateral dacryocystoceles. (*A, B*) Coronal and axial CT images and corresponding (*C, D*) coronal and axial T2-weighted MR images of bilateral dacryocystoceles.

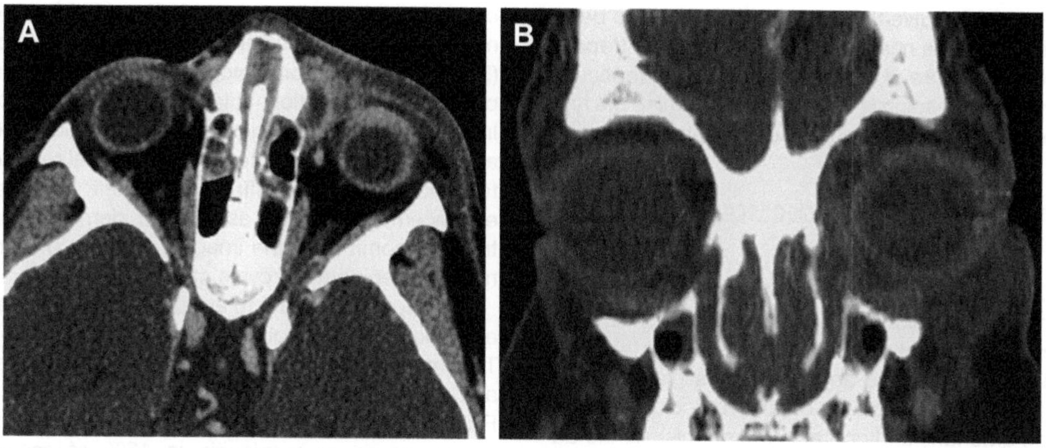

Fig. 8. Left dacryocystitis. (*A*) Axial contrast-enhanced CT shows a left dacryocystitis and preseptal cellulitis. (*B*) Coronal CT shows enlarged opacified nasolacrimal ducts greater on the left side.

CONGENITAL MIDLINE NASAL MASSES

The frontonasal region forms by a complex mechanism. A small fontanelle called the fonticulus frontalis temporarily separates the frontal and nasal bones. Progressive growth of the frontal and nasal bones obliterates this small fontanelle, leaving behind the frontonasal suture. In addition, a transient space called the prenasal space separates the nasal bones and underlying cartilaginous nasal capsule (**Fig. 9**).

An embryonic dural diverticulum extends from the anterior cranial fossa through the foramen cecum into the prenasal space. This dural diverticulum normally reaches to the tip of the nose before it regresses back into the cranium. The prenasal space eventually becomes obliterated by growth of the nasal bones.

Congenital midline nasal masses are related to faulty regression or abnormal location of the embryonic dural diverticulum.[15] These lesions are rare, with an incidence of 1:20,000 live births. There are 3 major categories of congenital midline nasal masses: dermoid and epidermoid cysts, sincipital encephaloceles, and nasal gliomas.

Dermoid and epidermoid cysts occur when skin elements are pulled into the prenasal space by the regressing dural diverticulum. Encephaloceles are produced by persistent herniation of dural diverticulum through the foramen cecum and/or fonticulus frontalis. Nasal gliomas are caused by sequestered neurogenic tissue along the course

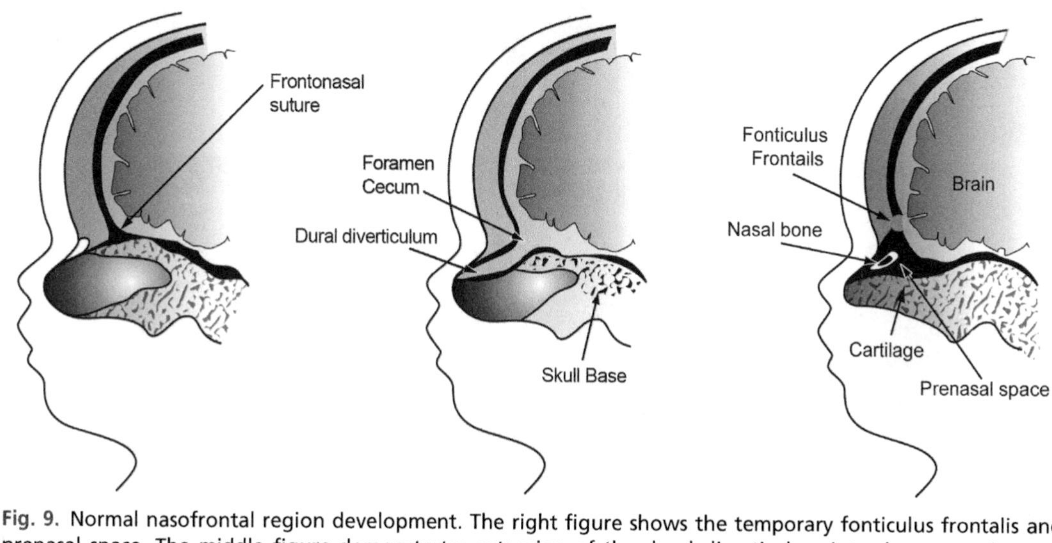

Fig. 9. Normal nasofrontal region development. The right figure shows the temporary fonticulus frontalis and prenasal space. The middle figure demonstrates extension of the dural diverticulum into the prenasal space. The left figure shows complete closure of the fonticulus frontalis and prenasal space.

of the dural diverticulum. Nasal gliomas are better described as nasal cerebral heterotopias trapped by the closure of the foramen cecum or fonticulus frontalis. Imaging is essential to determine the type of lesion and appropriate surgical approach.

DERMOID CYSTS, EPIDERMOID CYSTS, AND DERMAL SINUS TRACTS

Dermoid and epidermoid cysts are congenital inclusion cysts. Both contain ectodermal elements, but only dermoids contain skin appendages (hair follicles and sebaceous glands). Both lesions occur when the dural diverticulum extends too anteriorly and contacts the dermis. As the dural diverticulum regresses, it pulls dermal elements into the prenasal space. Dermoid and epidermoid cysts can form anywhere along the course of the regressing dural diverticulum from anterior cranial fossa to columella.[16] An associated intracranial connection is present in 57% of cases. A coexisting sinus tract opening on the skin surface can occur in up to 84% of cases.

Dermoid cysts are more common than epidermoid cysts. Usually, a dermoid cyst is located in the midline near the glabella. Important imaging features of dermoid cysts are fat attenuation on CT, intrinsic hyperintense T1 signal (liquefied cholesterol contents), absent contrast enhancement, and an associated dermal sinus tract (**Figs. 10** and **11**). Epidermoid cysts are most often paramidline in location, adjacent to the columella. Imaging features of epidermoid cysts include fluid attenuation on CT, isointense T1/T2 signal relative to fluid, restricted diffusion, absent contrast enhancement, and an associated dermal sinus tract. Uncommonly, the imaging features of dermoid and epidermoid cysts can overlap.

Imaging is necessary to evaluate for intracranial extension and surgical planning (**Figs. 12** and **13**). Treatment of dermoid cysts, epidermoid cysts, and dermal sinus tracts is complete resection. Failure to achieve complete resection can lead to recurrence or meningitis in 15% of cases. Therefore, any intracranial extension requires a combined intracranial and extracranial surgical approach.

SINCIPITAL ENCEPHALOCELES

An encephalocele is a term that describes herniation of intracranial contents through a skull defect. A meningocele specifically refers to herniation of meninges and cerebrospinal fluid. A meningoencephalocele designates herniation of brain, meninges, and cerebrospinal fluid. Encephaloceles

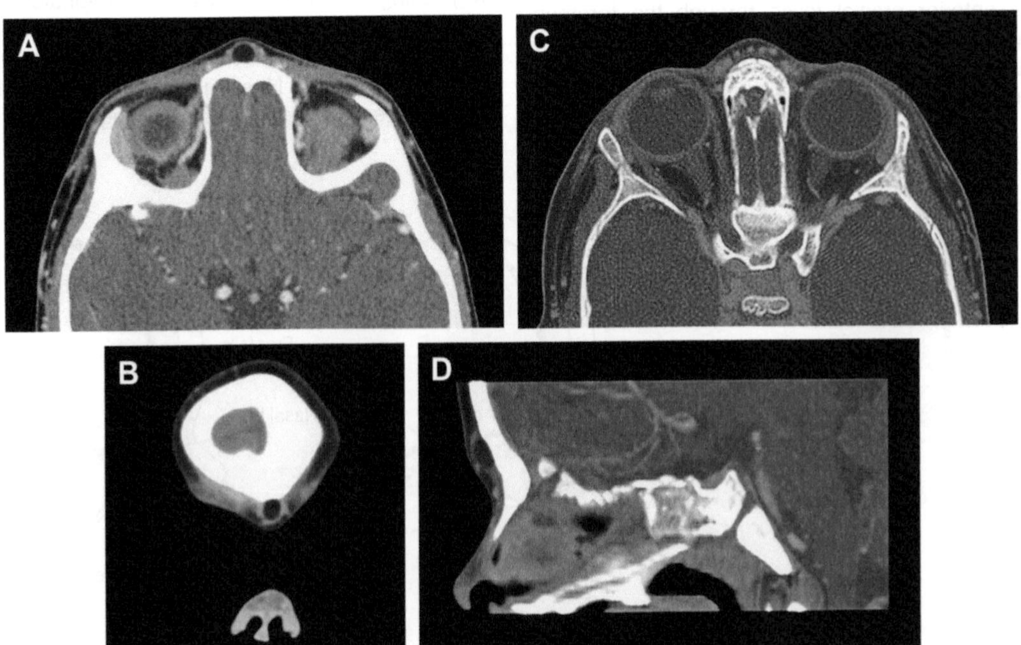

Fig. 10. Dermoid cyst. (*A*) CT axial and (*B*) coronal soft tissue algorithm images show a small fat attenuation midline mass adjacent to the glabella, typical of a dermoid cyst. (*C*) CT axial and (*D*) sagittal bone algorithm images show the appearance of an enlarged foramen cecum; however, there is no definite intracranial connection.

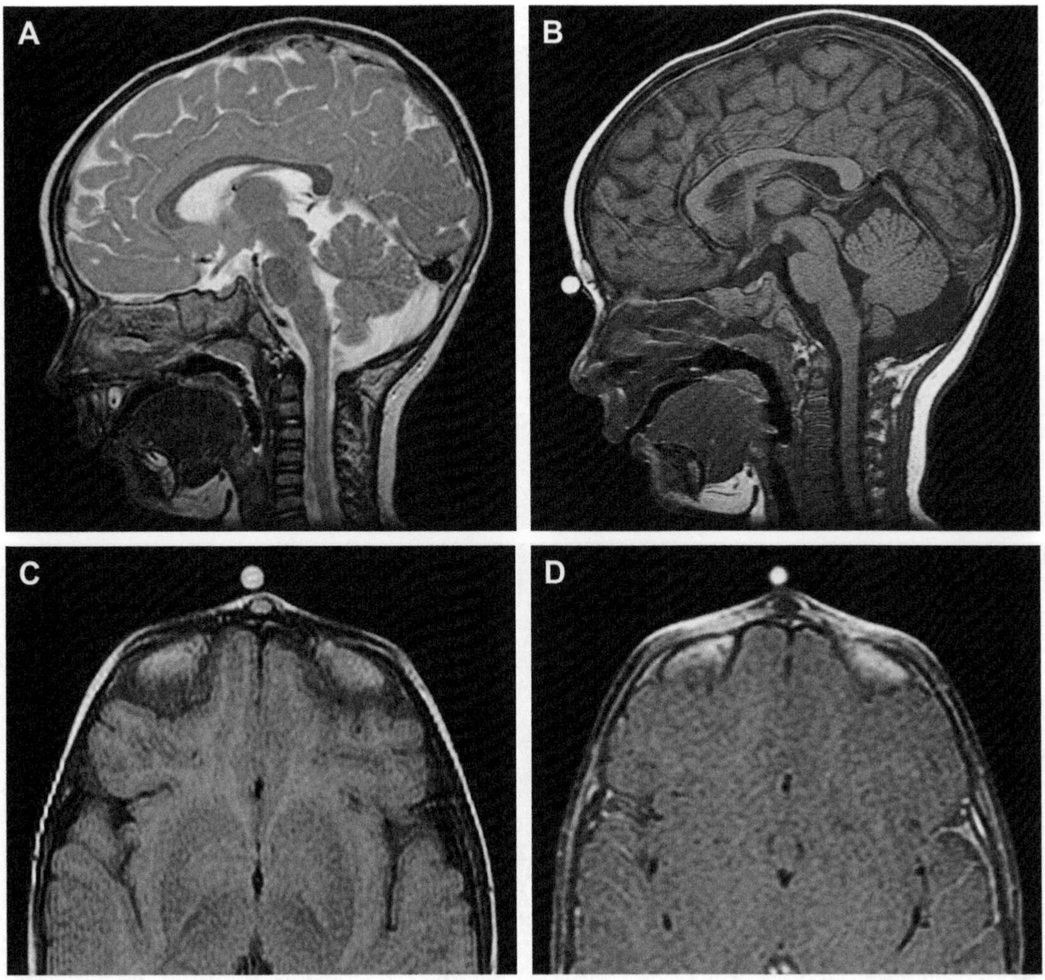

Fig. 11. Dermoid cyst. In the same child, (*A*) sagittal T2 and (*B*) T1 images show intrinsic hyperintense T1 signal of the small dermoid cyst. Note the overlying vitamin E capsule. Axial T1 (*C*) and (*D*) postcontrast fat-saturated images illustrate fat saturation of the lesion with no contrast enhancement. The MR imaging study confirms that there is no intracranial extension.

are classified by location, including occipital (75%), sincipital (15%), and basal (10%). In addition, encephaloceles are named based on the bony roof and floor of the skull defect. For example, the roof and floor of frontonasal encephaloceles are the frontal and nasal bones respectively.[17]

Sincipital encephaloceles involve the midface about the forehead, orbits, and dorsum of the nose. This variety of encephalocele is most common in southeast Asia, occurring in 1:40,000 live births. There are 3 major types of sincipital encephaloceles: frontonasal (40%–60%), nasoethmoidal (30%), and naso-orbital (10%). Frontonasal encephaloceles are caused by persistent herniation of dura through the fonticulus frontalis and foramen cecum into the glabellar region. Nasoethmoidal encephaloceles are produced by persistent herniation of dura through the foramen cecum into the prenasal space.

Frontonasal encephaloceles can present as an obvious nasal mass, broad nasal root, or hypertelorism. Skin-covered frontonasal encephaloceles have a bluish coloration. Encephaloceles not covered by skin are red and moist. Clinical examination shows a compressible nasal mass that transilluminates. An encephalocele with an intracranial connection of sufficient size changes in size with crying. Enlargement of the mass with compression of the internal jugular veins is a characteristic positive finding called a positive Furstenberg test.[8]

Nasoethmoidal encephaloceles present as an intranasal mass that extends downward from the

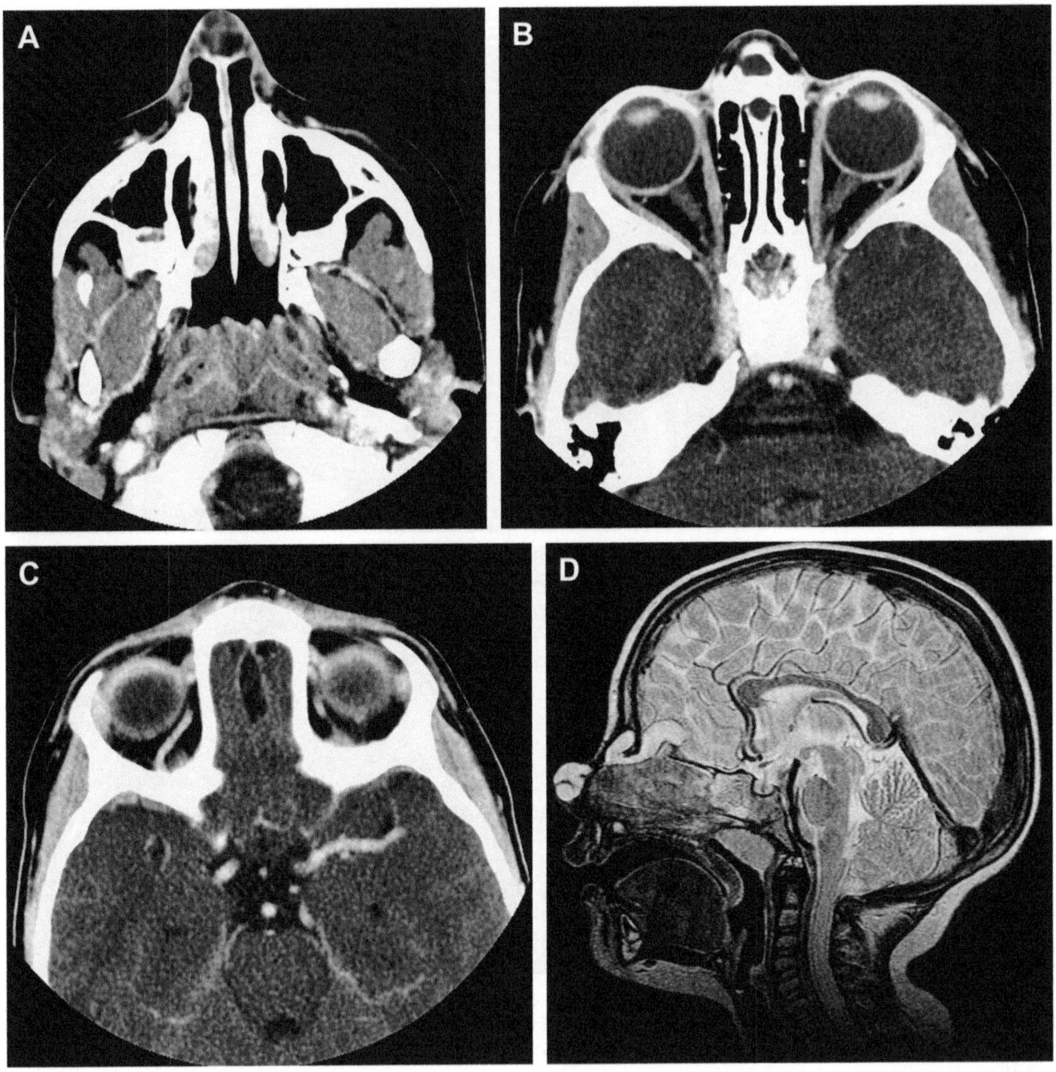

Fig. 12. Dermoid cyst with intracranial extension. (*A–C*) Contiguous axial CT images from inferior to superior show a midline nasal fatty mass extending intracranially via an enlarged foramen cecum. (*D*) The corresponding sagittal T2-weighted image shows the intracranial extension of the dermoid cyst.

superior nasal cavity. Lateral advancement of a nasal catheter can help differentiate midline nasoethmoidal encephaloceles from other, more common nasal masses like dacryocystoceles. Biopsy of encephaloceles is contraindicated because of the high risk of cerebrospinal fluid leak and meningitis.

MR imaging is the initial modality of choice to evaluate sincipital encephaloceles because it facilitates evaluation of the herniated contents, skull defect, and associated intracranial anomalies (**Fig. 14**). Reported associations include dysgenesis of the corpus callosum, interhemispheric lipomas, neural migration anomalies, and facial clefting. Herniated brain within encephaloceles is usually isointense to normal brain parenchyma, although it may be slightly hyperintense on T2-weighted images because of gliosis.

CT examination is complementary to MR imaging. CT is especially useful in evaluating the location and morphology of the skull defect. CT imaging findings that are highly suggestive of intracranial extension include widening of the foramen cecum, a bifid crista galli, or a frontal bone defect. Three-dimensional (3D) CT reconstruction is often performed for surgical planning (**Fig. 15**). Encephaloceles are treated with complete surgical resection and dural repair to decrease the risk of accidental trauma, cerebrospinal fluid leakage, and meningitis. No new neurologic deficit is

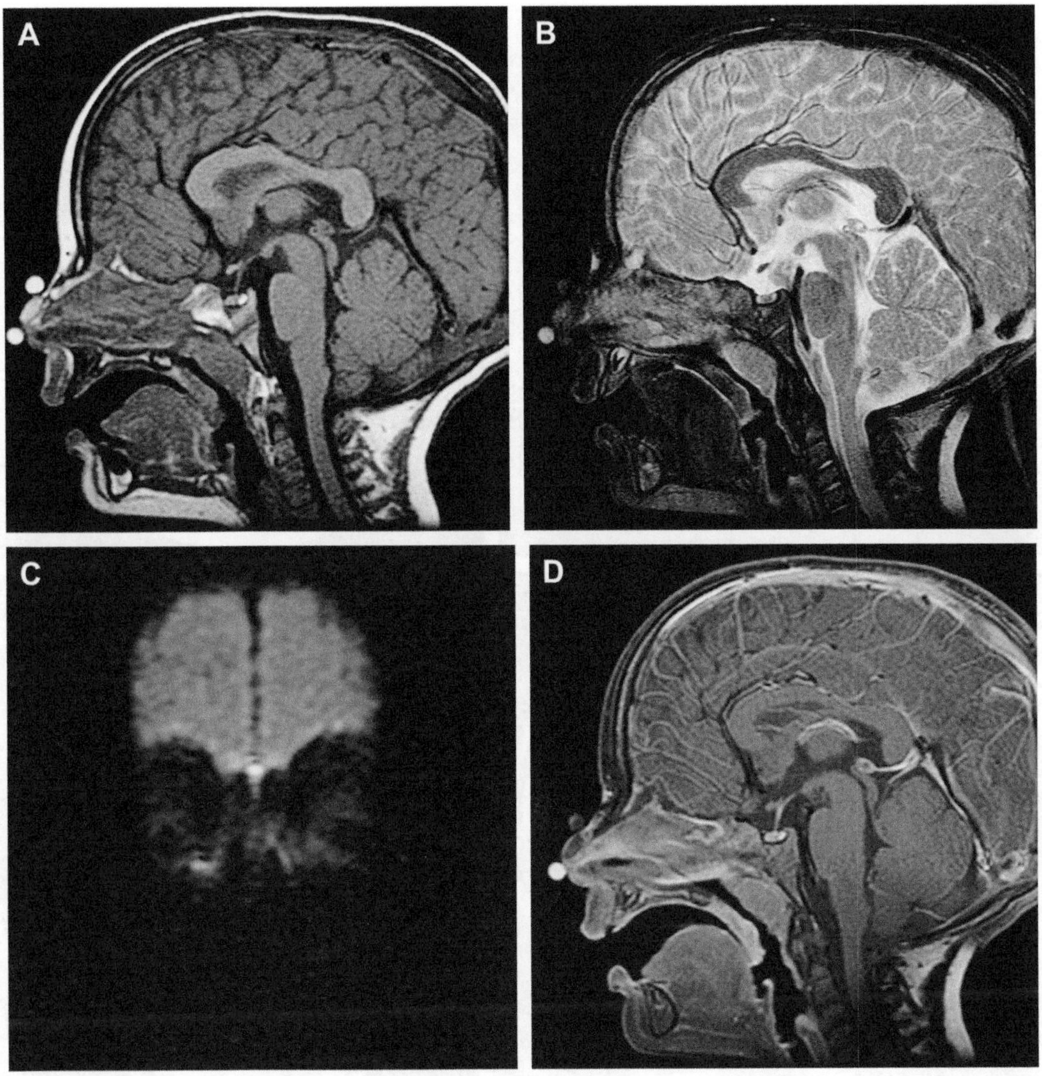

Fig. 13. Dermal sinus tract with intracranial epidermoid cyst. (*A, B*) Sagittal T1-weighted and T2-weighted images show a dermal sinus tract with an intracranial epidermoid cyst. (*C*) Coronal diffusion-weighted image shows restricted diffusion within the epidermoid cyst. (*D*) A sagittal postcontrast T1-weighted image does not show associated thickened meningeal enhancement to suggest meningitis.

incurred by resection of herniated brain tissue because of its abnormal function.

NASAL GLIOMA

The term nasal glioma is a misnomer that should be replaced by nasal cerebral heterotopia. It refers to a rare developmental mass consisting of dysplastic sequestered neuroglial tissue without any neoplastic features.[18] Nasal cerebral heterotopias may have an intracranial connection by a fibrous stalk in up to 30% of cases. The mass can be extranasal (60%), intranasal (30%), or mixed extranasal and intranasal (10%).

Extranasal cerebral heterotopias occur because of herniation of the embryonic dural diverticulum through the fonticulus frontalis. Subsequent faulty regression of the dural diverticulum causes neurogenic tissue to be sequestered external to the frontonasal suture. Imaging features of an extranasal cerebral heterotopia include a soft tissue intensity mass superficial to the glabella. Classically, the lesion is described as hyperintense to gray matter on T2-weighted, and hypointense to isointense on T1-weighted MR images (**Fig. 16**). It is isodense on CT studies often with remodeling of the subjacent nasal bones.

Intranasal cerebral heterotopias are caused by faulty regression of the embryonic dural diverticulum

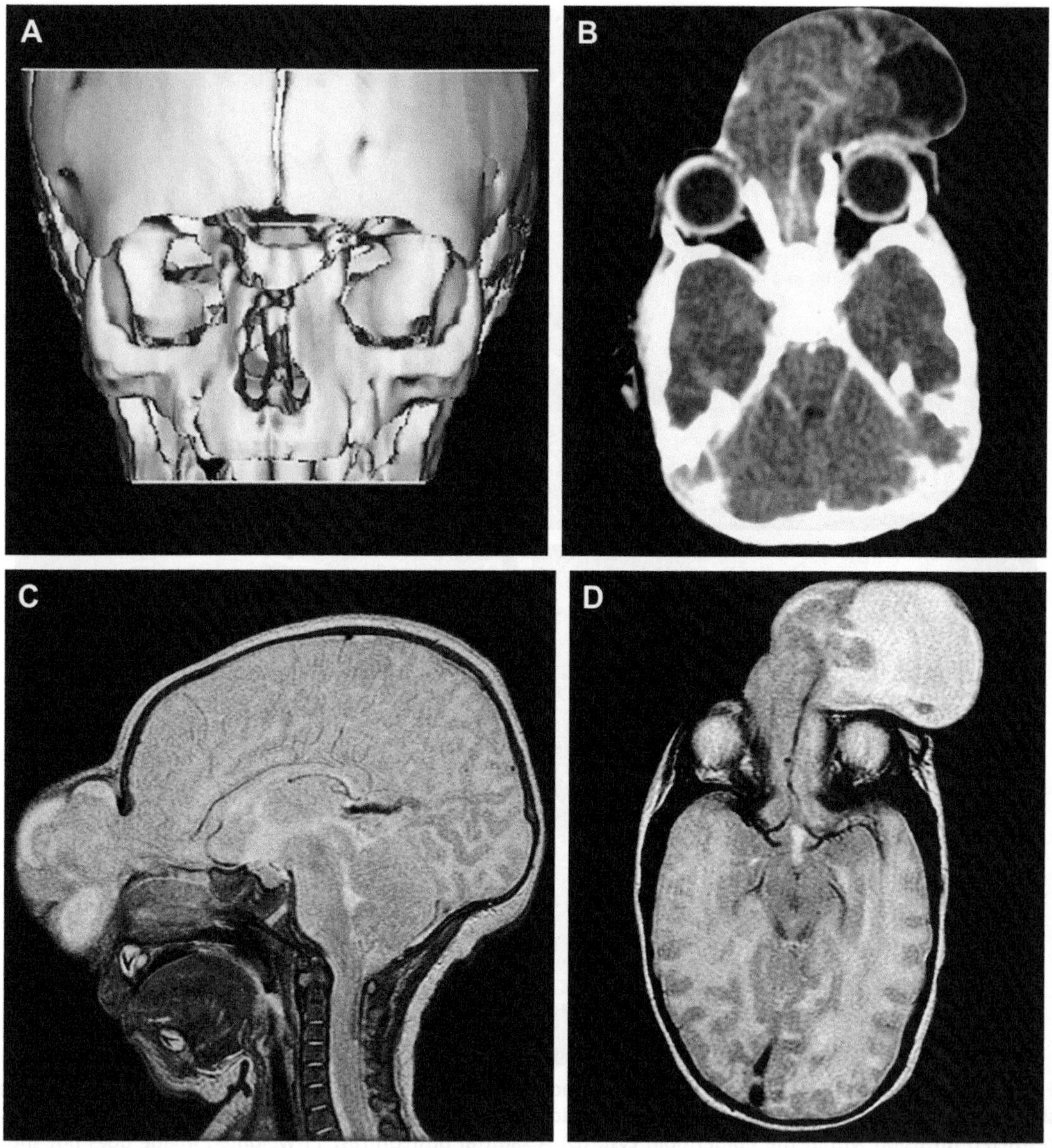

Fig. 14. Large frontonasal encephalocele. (*A*) 3D CT facial bone shows a large frontonasal bone defect. (*B*) Axial contrast-enhanced CT, (*C*) sagittal T2, and (*D*) axial T2-weighted images show the large frontonasal encephalocele. Note the anterior cerebral arteries extending through the skull defect with the herniated brain.

with sequestered neurogenic tissue in the prenasal space. Intranasal cerebral heterotopias are usually attached to the anterior nasal septum or adjacent middle turbinate. Mixed extranasal and intranasal cerebral heterotopias have components in each location that are continuous through a defect in the nasal bones.

IMAGING APPROACH TO CONGENITAL MIDLINE NASAL MASSES

Imaging is indicated before biopsy when a congenital midline nasal mass is suspected. Imaging permits a robust evaluation for lesions with a potential intracranial connection. Following the proper diagnostic work-up prevents inadvertent biopsy of encephaloceles and associated iatrogenic complications. CT and MR imaging facilitate complementary assessment of the bone, brain, and congenital mass.

Axial and coronal CT scans obtained with 1 mm section thickness on bone algorithm provide exquisite detail of frontonasal bone defects. Three-dimensional CT reconstructions give an excellent overview of bone structures for surgical planning. CT findings suggestive of intracranial

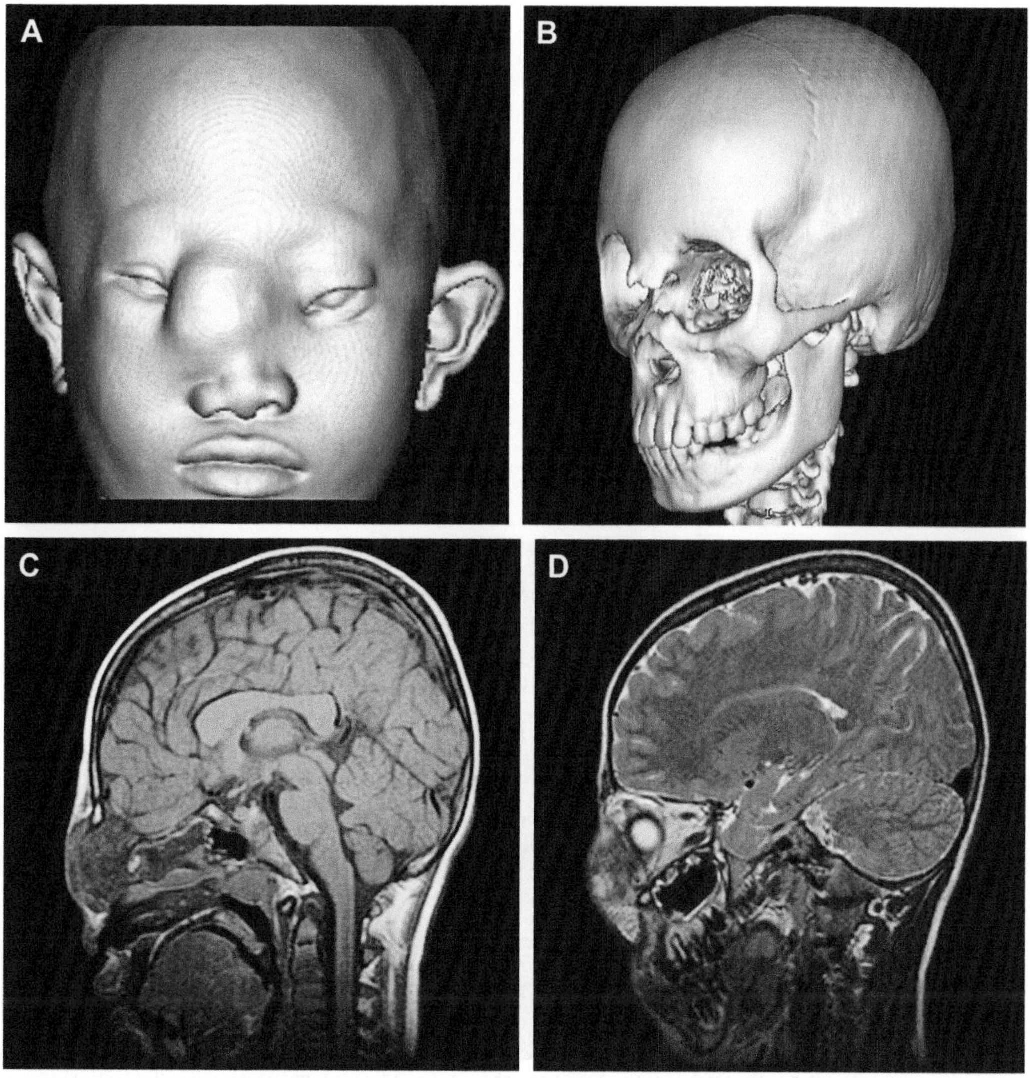

Fig. 15. Frontonasal encephalocele. (*A, B*) 3D CT soft tissue and bone algorithm images show a large nasal root mass with associated bone defect. (*C, D*) Sagittal T1-weighted and T2-weighted images show a frontonasal encephalocele encroaching on the right medial orbit.

extension include an enlarged foramen cecum or bifid crista galli. The absence of these CT findings is fairly reliable in excluding intracranial extension at this site. However, the presence of these CT findings in isolation is inconclusive. False positives have been reported related to the normal appearance of a nonossified cribriform plate.

MR imaging including high-resolution axial, coronal, and sagittal T1-weighted and T2-weighted images is valuable to evaluate congenital midline nasal masses for potential intracranial connection and associated brain anomalies. A T1-weighted spin echo with and without fat saturation can confirm fat signal within a dermoid cyst. Diffusion-weighted images and apparent diffusion coefficient maps can show restricted diffusion in an epidermoid cyst or abscess. Contrast-enhanced, fat-suppressed T1-weighted MR images are needed when a neoplasm or infection is a possibility. Because of the risk of additional anesthesia and extra health care expense for performing 2 imaging investigations, the initial modality of choice is MR imaging.[1]

CRANIOSYNOSTOSIS

Craniosynostosis refers to premature closure of 1 or more cranial sutures, often resulting in an abnormal head shape.[19] Primary craniosynostosis results from a defect of ossification. Secondary

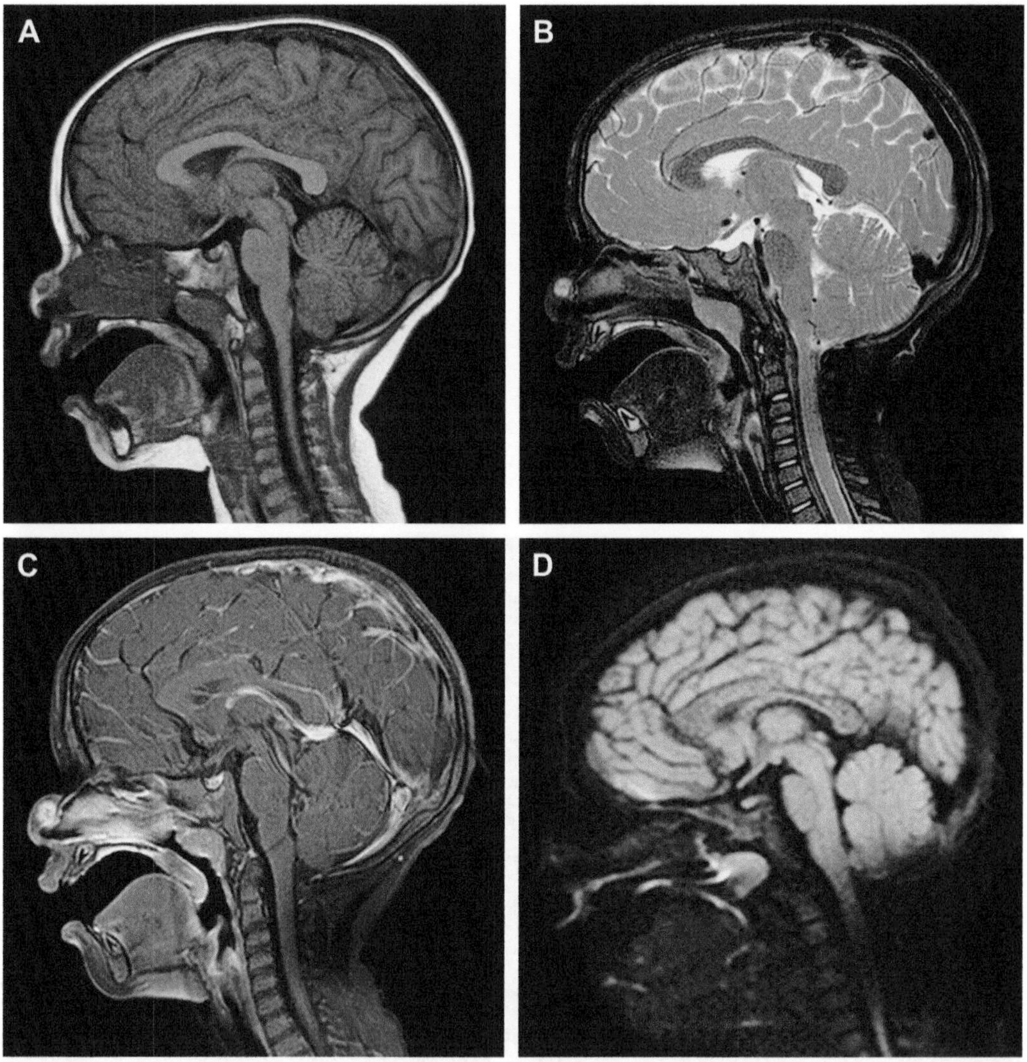

Fig. 16. Nasal glioma. (*A*) Sagittal T1-weighted and (*B*) T2-weighted images illustrate a small nasal glioma with isointense T1 and hyperintense T2 signal. (*C*) A sagittal postcontrast fat-saturated T1-weighted image shows mild enhancement of the lesion. (*D*) Diffusion-weighted images show no associated restricted diffusion.

craniosynostosis is caused by several systemic disorders, including endocrine abnormalities, hematologic conditions, inadequate brain growth, and following shunted hydrocephalus.[20]

Primary craniosynostosis is subdivided into nonsyndromic (85%) and syndromic (15%) forms. Nonsyndromic craniosynostosis usually manifests as a single prematurely fused suture. Syndromic craniosynostoses often have multiple prematurely fused sutures, facial malformations, and associated brain anomalies. Apert syndrome is commonly recognized as craniosynostosis and syndactyly. Crouzon syndrome involves craniosynostosis, maxillary hypoplasia, and shallow orbits. Several syndromic craniosynostoses result from genetic mutations responsible for fibroblast growth factor receptors that promote the number osteogenic precursor cells.

Secondary craniosynostosis typically result from endocrine abnormalities such as renal osteodystrophy and hyperthyroidism that disrupt normal bone remodeling and turnover. Hematologic disorders including sickle cell disease and thalassemia can cause bone marrow hyperplasia with subsequent narrowing and closure of cranial sutures. Inadequate brain growth and shunted hydrocephalus can cause diminished expansile forces on the calvarium, leading to sutural closure.

The imaging work-up of suspected craniosynostosis frequently begins with skull radiographs including anterior-posterior, lateral, and Waters views. Prematurely fused sutures can appear sclerotic with indistinct suture margins. The fused suture often shows ridging along the suture line. The altered head shape is often diagnostic. Careful evaluation is needed because the synostosis does not always involve the entire length or depth of the suture. The definite imaging modality is CT examination with 3D reconstruction. The 3D CT study is useful for surgical planning. MR evaluation is usually not required, with the exception of syndromic craniosynostoses with associated brain anomalies.

NONSYNDROMIC CRANIOSYNOSTOSIS

Sagittal Craniosynostosis

Normal skull growth occurs in a direction perpendicular to the axis of an open suture. The skull grows in a direction parallel to a closed suture. Sagittal craniosynostosis is caused by premature fusion of the sagittal suture. It produces elongation of the calvarium in the anteroposterior diameter, and reduction in the biparietal diameter (**Fig. 17**). The appearance of the skull is called dolichocephaly (dolicho meaning long) or scaphocephaly (scapho meaning boat shaped). Sagittal craniosynostosis is the most common type of primary synostosis. A well-defined ridge of bone is often seen at the site of fused suture.

Coronal Craniosynostosis

Coronal craniosynostosis is caused by premature fusion of the coronal suture. It can be unilateral or bilateral. Unilateral coronal craniosynostosis produces ipsilateral flattening of the frontal bone and elevation of the superolateral orbital rim resulting in a harlequin eye. Bilateral coronal craniosynostosis gives rise to elongation of the calvarium in the biparietal diameter, and reduction in the anteroposterior diameter (**Fig. 18**). The appearance of the skull is called brachycephaly (brachy meaning short). The coronal suture develops in conjunction with the sutures at the skull base. Bilateral coronal craniosynostosis is often syndromic and associated with midface hypoplasia.

Metopic Craniosynostosis

The metopic suture usually closes by the second year of life. Metopic craniosynostosis is caused by premature closure of the metopic suture. It produces the appearance of a pointed forehead or trigonocephaly (trigono meaning triangle). The bifrontal diameter is decreased. Metopic craniosynostosis often gives rise to hypotelorism (**Fig. 19**).

Lambdoid Craniosynostosis

Lambdoid craniosynostosis is caused by premature fusion of the lambdoid suture. It can be unilateral or bilateral. It is the least common type of simple craniosynostosis (**Fig. 20**). Unilateral lambdoid fusion produces ipsilateral occipital flattening and contralateral frontal bossing. The appearance is called posterior plagiocephaly (plagio meaning oblique). The calvarium has a trapezoid shape. The pinna, external auditory canal, and petrous

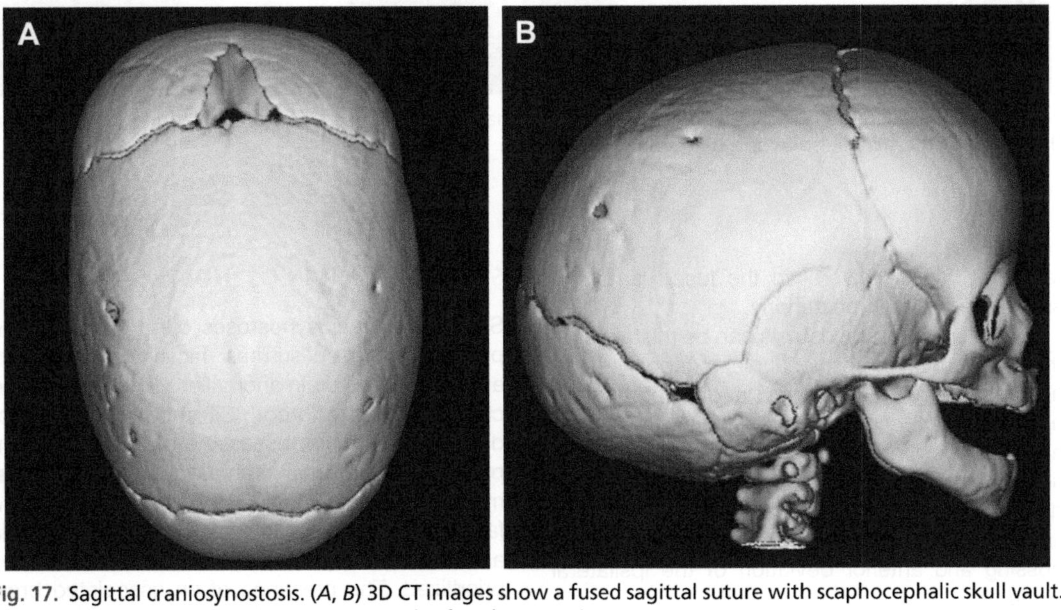

Fig. 17. Sagittal craniosynostosis. (*A, B*) 3D CT images show a fused sagittal suture with scaphocephalic skull vault. A well-defined ridge of bone is present at the fused suture site.

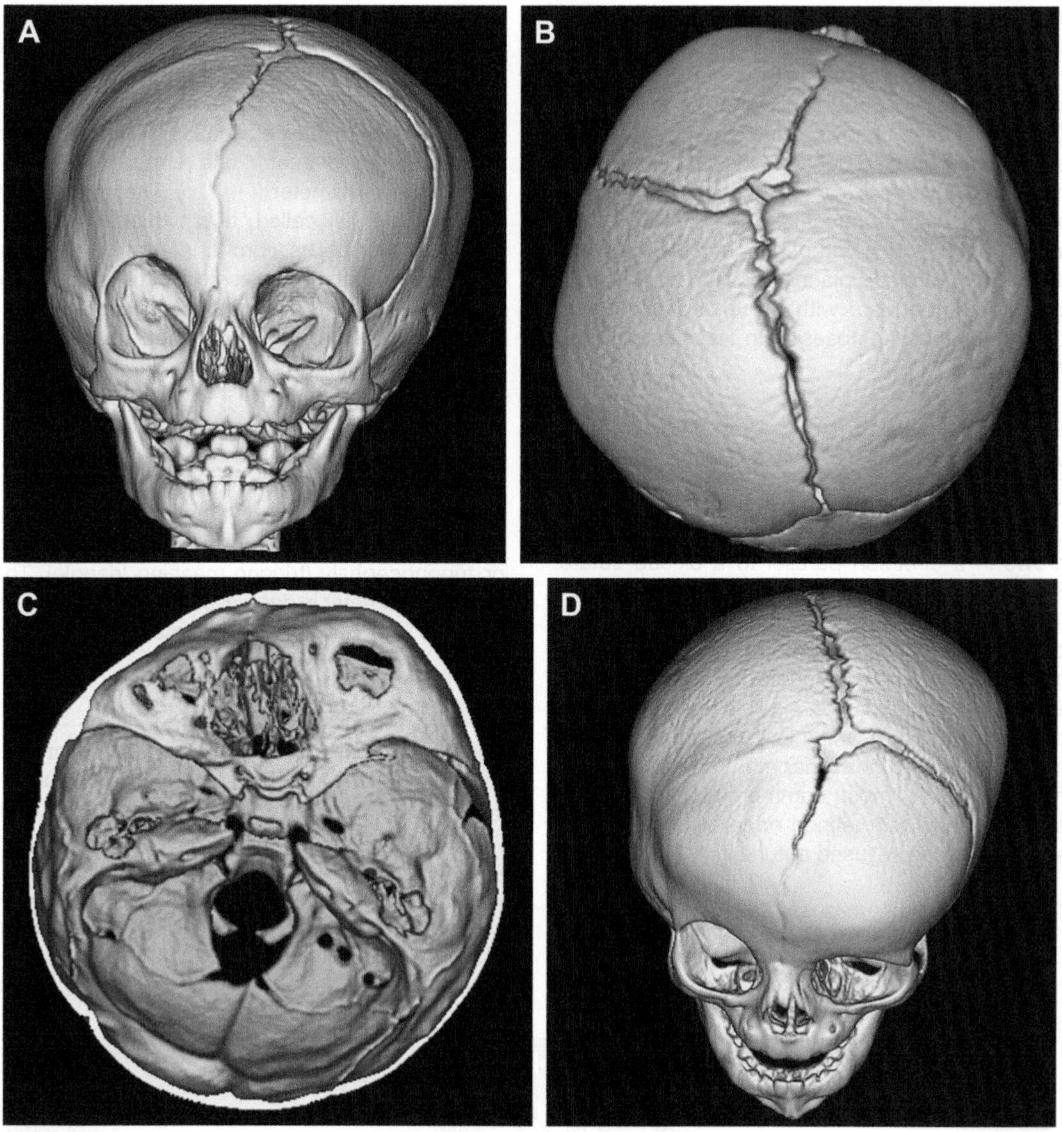

Fig. 18. Unilateral coronal craniosynostosis. (*A–D*) 3D CT images show a fused left coronal suture with ipsilateral flattening of the frontal bone and harlequin eye.

temporal bone ipsilateral to the fused lambdoid suture are deviated posteriorly.

Lambdoid craniosynostosis can be mistaken for the more common positional plagiocephaly. Positional plagiocephaly occurs in developmentally normal infants who preferentially sleep with their head in 1 position for long periods of time. Positional craniocephaly is differentiated from lambdoid craniosynostosis because occipital bone flattening is associated with ipsilateral frontal bossing and anterior deviation of the ipsilateral pinna.

SYNDROMIC CRANIOSYNOSTOSIS

Syndromic craniosynostoses often have multiple prematurely fused sutures, facial malformations, and associated brain anomalies. Patients are typically evaluated with both CT and MR imaging for detailed anatomic assessment and treatment planning. Syndromic craniosynostoses are best managed by a multidisciplinary team with a family-centered approach. Each organ system is addressed independently and medical issues prioritized. The presence of an associated brain anomaly is important because of its significant

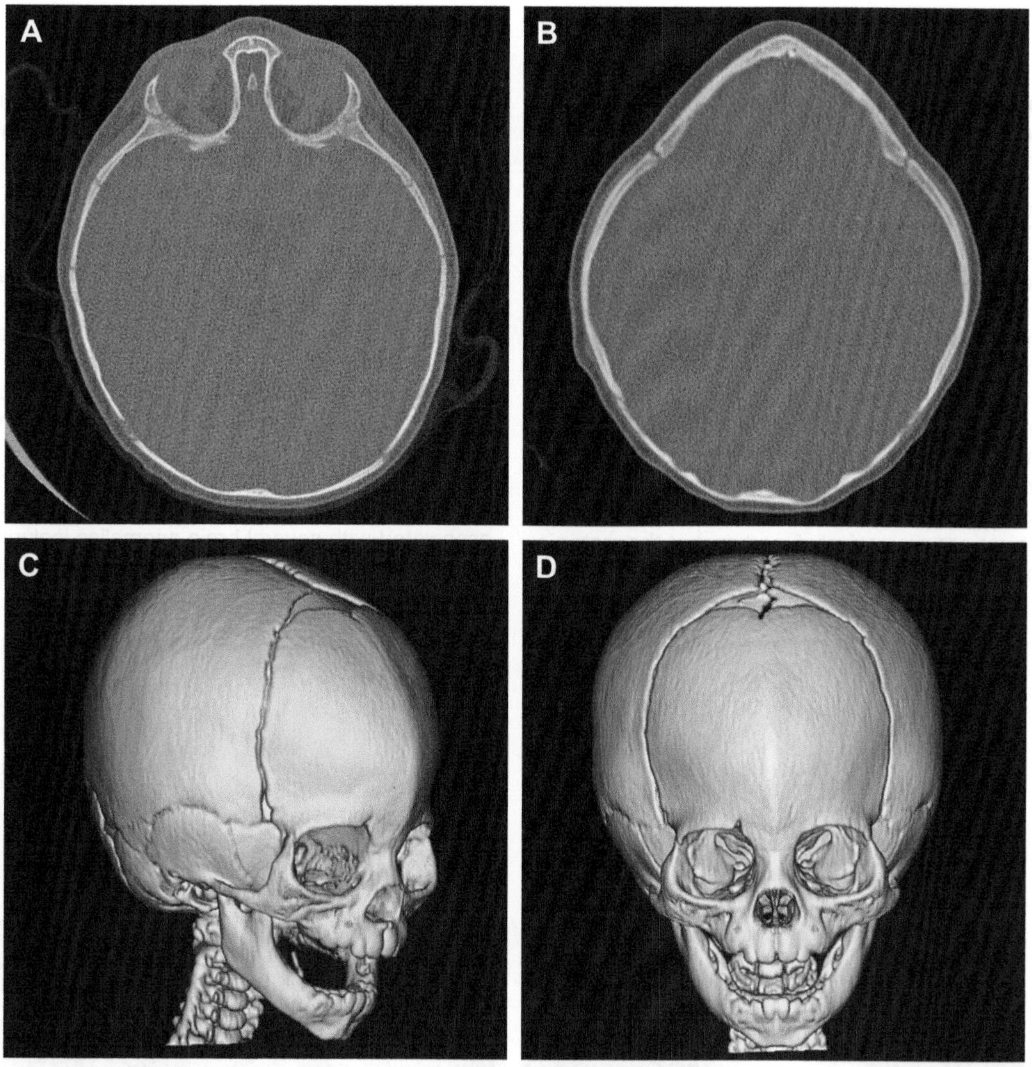

Fig. 19. Metopic craniosynostosis. (*A, B*) Axial CT, and (*C, D*) 3D CT reconstructions showing hypotelorism, fusion of the metopic suture, and trigonocephaly.

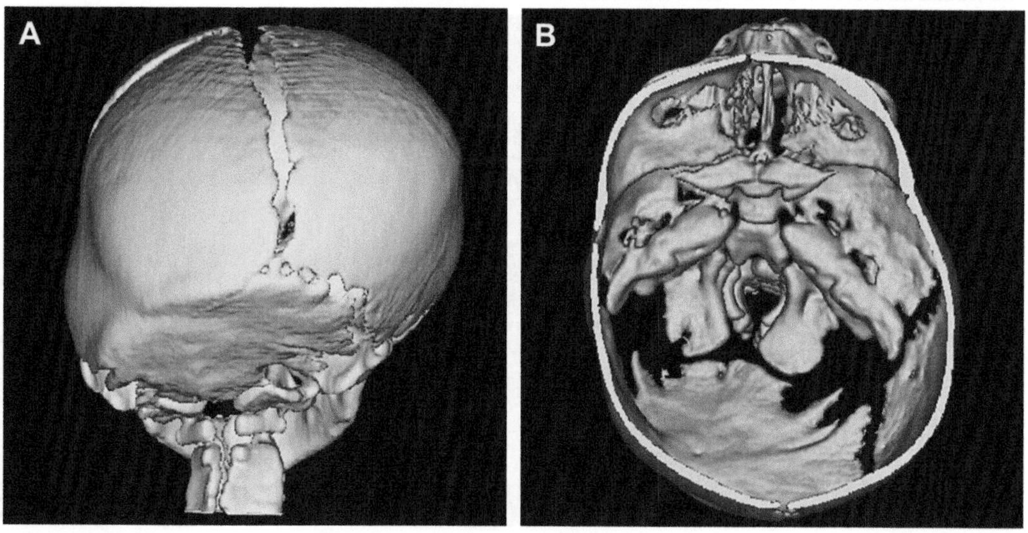

Fig. 20. Unilateral lambdoid craniosynostosis. (*A, B*) 3D CT images show fusion of the right lambdoid suture. The calvarium has a trapezoid shape.

impact on general prognosis and treatment outcome.

Apert Syndrome

Apert syndrome is the most common syndromic craniosynostosis. It is also referred to as acrocephalosyndactyly (type I). The major diagnostic criteria are craniosynostosis and syndactyly (**Fig. 21**). The craniosynostosis typically involves the coronal sutures producing brachycephaly with a flat appearance of the occiput. Sagittal and metopic sutures are often widened. Apert syndrome may also cause a cloverleaf-shaped skull (kleeblattschadel), where all the cranial sutures are prematurely fused except the metopic and squamosal sutures. The syndactyly is severe and symmetric. It often affects the hands and feet. Fusion of the second, third, and fourth digits creates a mid-digital mass.

Apert syndrome has an estimated incidence of 1:200,000 live births and accounts for about 5% of all craniosynostosis cases. The syndrome can be inherited in an autosomal dominant pattern but most cases are sporadic. Apert syndrome is the result of specific mutations in the fibroblast growth factor receptor 2 (FGFR2) gene.[21] Fibroblast growth factor receptors have a central role in the complex regulation of cranial and limb morphogenesis.

Normal intelligence is present in 70% of patients with Apert syndrome. However, the syndrome is associated with several brain anomalies including agenesis of the corpus callosum, neural migration

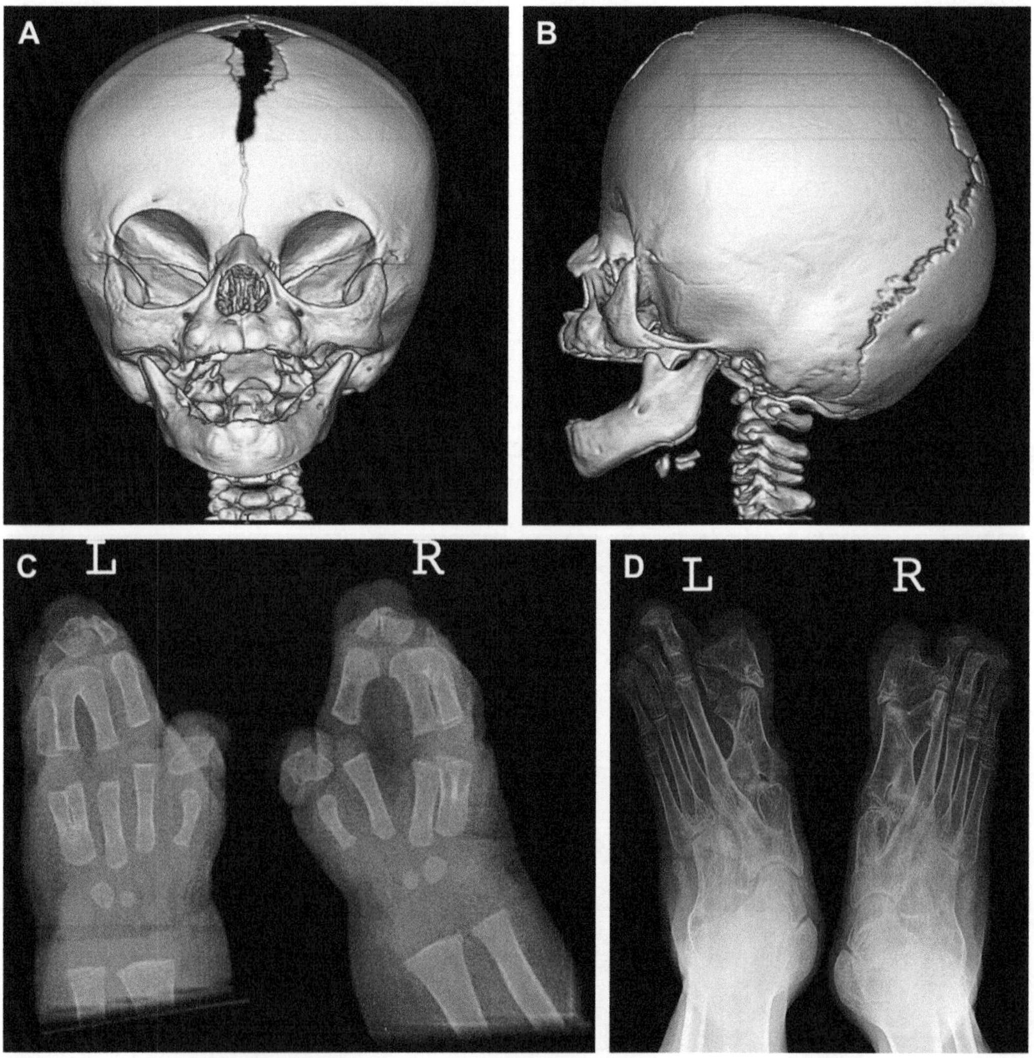

Fig. 21. Apert syndrome. (*A, B*) 3D CT images show bilateral coronal craniosynostosis with brachycephaly. (*C, D*) Hand and foot radiographs show bilateral symmetric syndactyly.

disorders, and sincipital encephaloceles. Secondary anomalies such as midface hypoplasia and choanal stenosis often respond well to facial advancement surgery. Up to 70% of patients have cervical spine fusion anomalies. Genitourinary and cardiovascular abnormalities occur in 10% of patients.

Crouzon Syndrome

Crouzon syndrome is the second most common syndromic craniosynostosis. It is also referred to as craniofacial synostosis. The syndrome is an autosomal dominant disorder caused by specific mutations in the FGFR2 gene. Crouzon syndrome is characterized by craniosynostosis, maxillary hypoplasia, and shallow orbits (**Fig. 22**).[22] The type of craniosynostosis can include brachycephaly, scaphocephaly, trigonocephaly, or kleeblattschadel deformity. Crouzon syndrome is not associated with syndactyly. There is no associated distinctive limb deformity.

Maxillary hypoplasia is an important feature of Crouzon syndrome. Secondary facial anomalies include a parrot-beak nose, cleft palate, dental abnormalities, and mandibular prognathism. Shallow orbits are problematic because exophthalmos can lead to exposure keratitis. Secondary orbital abnormalities are hypertelorism and strabismus. Crouzon syndrome is associated with significant intracranial abnormalities including anomalous venous drainage and progressive hydrocephalus.

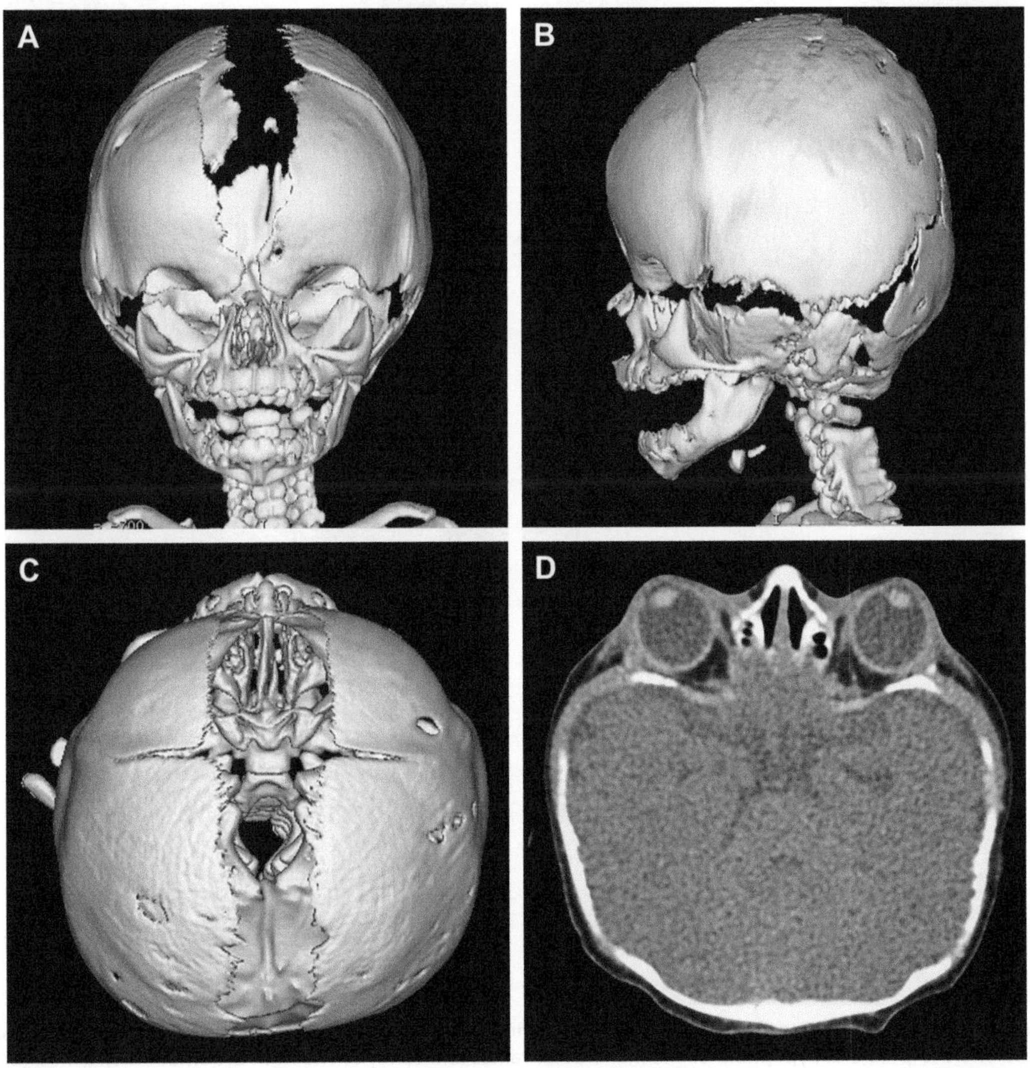

Fig. 22. Crouzon syndrome. (*A–C*) 3D CT images show partial bilateral coronal craniosynostosis with brachycephaly. Sagittal and metopic sutures are widened. The maxilla appears hypoplastic. (*D*) Axial CT image shows shallow orbits and exophthalmos.

Up to 70% of patients have a Chiari I malformation, which may be related to premature lambdoid suture closure. Cervical spine fusion anomalies occur in approximately 40% of cases. Acanthosis nigrans is a reported skin manifestation.

FIRST PHARYNGEAL ARCH SYNDROMES

Abnormal development of the first pair of pharyngeal arches during the fourth to eighth week of gestation can produce complex patterns of midface anomalies. Several systems of classification have been proposed to describe the wide spectrum of observed abnormalities. Each first pharyngeal arch syndrome can have an extremely variable expression. Two unique conditions merit further consideration: Goldenhar syndrome, and Treacher Collins syndrome.

Goldenhar Syndrome

Goldenhar syndrome is predominantly a unilateral malformation of structures derived from the first pharyngeal arch. It is also referred to as oculo-auriculo-vertebral spectrum.[23] Goldenhar syndrome results from a deficiency in the developing frontonasal and maxillary prominences. This deficiency is probably caused by a local ischemic insult or abnormal neural crest cell migration during the fourth week of gestation.

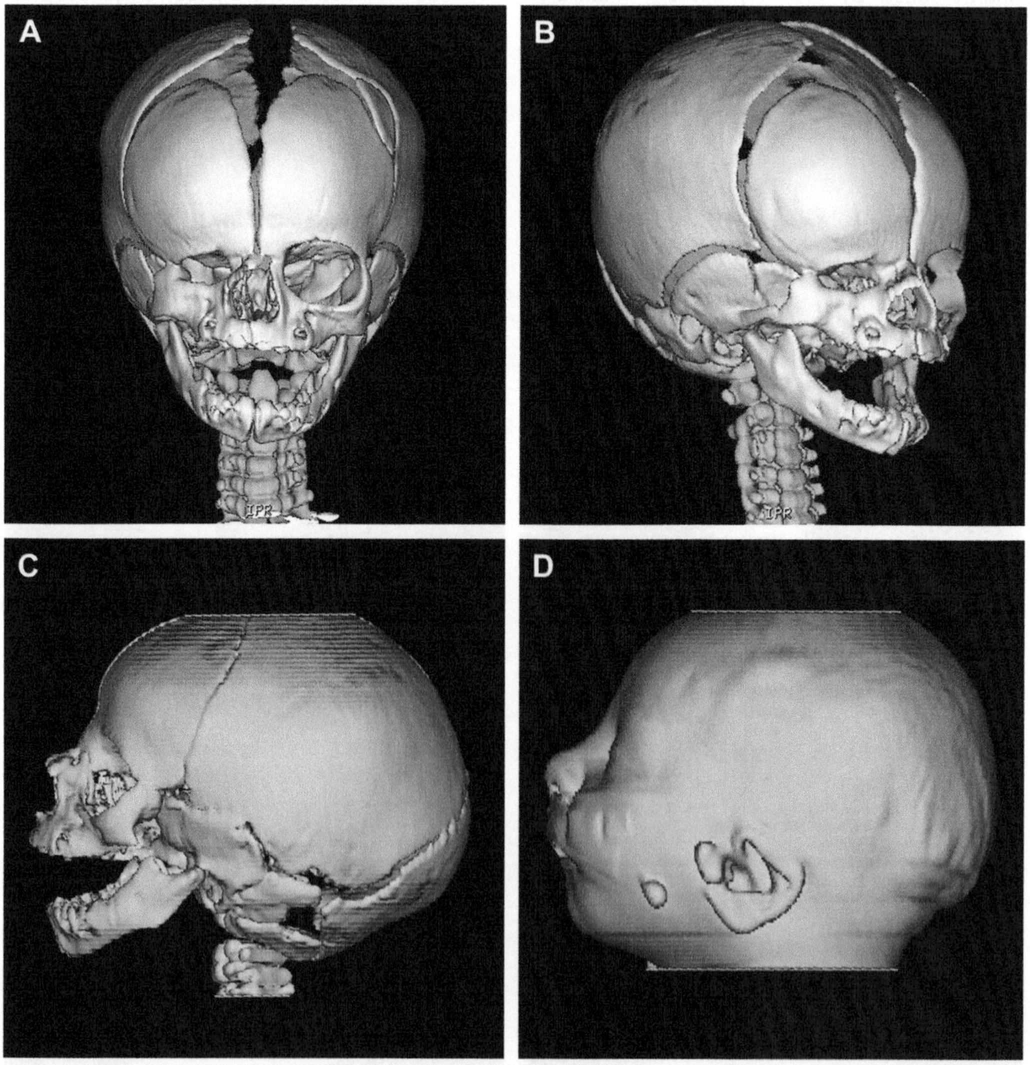

Fig. 23. Goldenhar syndrome. (*A, B*) 3D CT bone algorithm images show right hemifacial microsomia with a small orbit. There is ipsilateral hypoplasia of the mandibular ramus and condyle. The right zygomatic arch is flat. (*C*) In a second patient, a 3D CT bone algorithm image illustrates a hypoplastic left mandibular ramus, and absent zygomatic arch. (*D*) The corresponding 3D CT soft tissue algorithm image shows a deformed pinna and preauricular skin tag.

There are no minimal diagnostic criteria for Goldenhar syndrome. However, the facial phenotype is usually characteristic. The classic facial defects are hemifacial microsomia with associated ipsilateral micrognathia and macrostomia (**Fig. 23**). The mandibular ramus and condyle are often hypoplastic. The zygomatic arch is flat or absent. The most common ocular manifestation is an epibulbar dermoid occurring in up to 92% of patients. Secondary ocular abnormalities include colobomas, and micro-ophthalmia.

External and middle ear anomalies are diverse. The classic appearance is microtia with a preauricular skin tag. External auditory canal and ossicular atresia are frequent imaging findings. Up to 50% of patients have conductive hearing loss. Cervical vertebral fusions occur in up to 60% of cases. Several intracranial anomalies have been reported, including sincipital encephaloceles, holoprosencephaly, and dysgenesis of the corpus callosum.

Treacher Collins Syndrome

Treacher Collins syndrome causes a bilaterally symmetric malformation of structures derived from the first pharyngeal arch. This syndrome is also referred to as mandibulofacial dysostosis. It is an autosomal dominant disorder with variable penetrance. Treacher Collins syndrome results from mutations in the Treacher Collins–Franceschetti syndrome 1 (*TCOF1*) gene located on chromosome

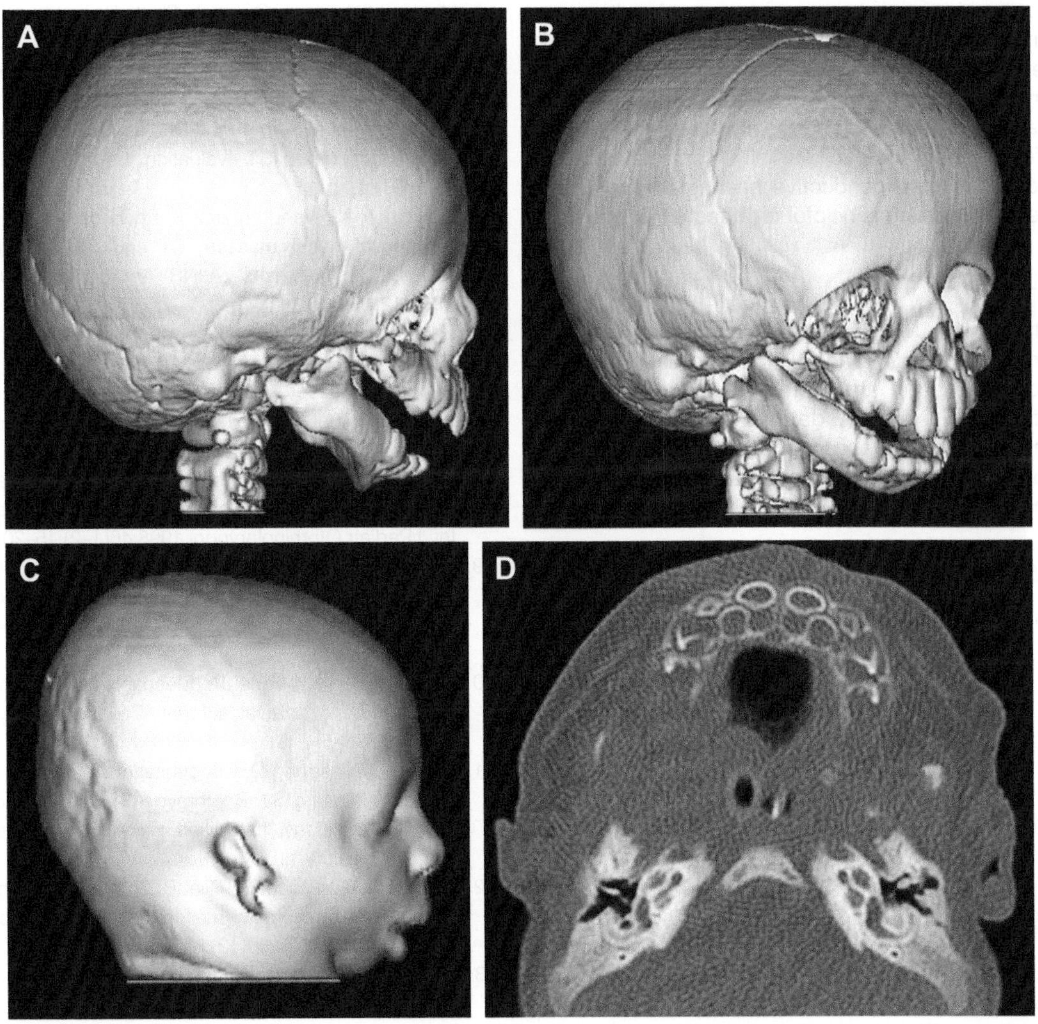

Fig. 24. Treacher Collins syndrome. (*A, B*) 3D CT bone algorithm images show an absent right zygoma, and hypoplastic mandible (the abnormality was bilaterally symmetric). (*C*) 3D CT soft tissue algorithm image shows a small deformed pinna and retrognathia. (*D*) Axial CT image illustrates bilateral external auditory canal atresia, and pinna deformity.

5q.[24] Deficient function of the gene product, named Treacle, leads to apoptosis of neural crest cells during early midface development.

Treacher Collins syndrome is characterized by a bilaterally symmetric facial bone hypoplasia, especially the mandible, maxillae, and zygomatic arches (**Fig. 24**). The mandibular rami are often absent, causing retrognathia. Ocular abnormalities include downward slanting of the palpebral fissures, lower lid colobomas, and absent eyelashes. Ear anomalies consist of pinnae deformity, external auditory canal atresia, and ossicular hypoplasia/aplasia. Approximately 50% of patients have bilateral conductive hearing loss. Cleft palate is also reported. Most patients with Treacher Collins are of normal intelligence.

Management of Treacher Collins syndrome requires a multidisciplinary approach. The primary concern is airway compromise secondary to retrognathia and maxillary hypoplasia. Treatment may require maxillary and mandibular advancement and reconstruction. Lower lid colobomas and cleft palate are addressed surgically in the first year of life. Hearing loss is partially correctable with bone-anchored conductive hearing devices. Genetic counseling is helpful for affected parents.

SUMMARY

There are a wide variety of congenital midface abnormalities. CT and MR imaging are important components in the comprehensive evaluation of these lesions. A detailed understanding of midface embryogenesis and developmental anatomy is important in directing appropriate patient management.

REFERENCES

1. Shroff M. Congenital midface and sinus abnormalities. In: Shankar L, Evans K, editors. An atlas of imaging of the paranasal sinuses. 2nd edition. Abingdon, Oxon: Informa Healthcare; 2006. p. 189–207.
2. Castillo M. Congenital abnormalities of the nose: CT and MR findings. AJR Am J Roentgenol 1994;162:1211–7.
3. Harris J, Robert E, Kallen B. Epidemiology of choanal atresia with special reference to the CHARGE association. Pediatrics 1997;99:363–7.
4. Black CM, Dungan D, Fram E, et al. Potential pitfalls in the work-up and diagnosis of choanal atresia. AJNR Am J Neuroradiol 1998;19:326–9.
5. Slovis TL, Renfro B, Watts FB, et al. Choanal atresia: precise CT evaluation. Radiology 1985;155:345–8.
6. Corrales CE, Koltai PJ. Choanal atresia: current concepts and controversies. Curr Opin Otolaryngol Head Neck Surg 2009;17(6):466–70.
7. Belden CJ, Mancuso AA, Schmalfuss IM. CT features of congenital nasal piriform aperture stenosis: initial experience. Radiology 1999;213:495–501.
8. Lowe LH, Booth TN, Joglar JM, et al. Midface anomalies in children. Radiographics 2000;20:907–22.
9. Nyberg DA, Sickler GK, Hegge FN, et al. Fetal cleft lip with and without cleft palate: US classification and correlation with outcome. Radiology 1995;195:677–84.
10. Tessier P. Anatomical classification of facial, cranio-facial and latero-facial clefts. J Maxillofac Surg 1976;4:69–92.
11. Janssen AG, Mansour K, Bos JJ, et al. Diameter of the bony lacrimal canal: normal values and values related to nasolacrimal duct obstruction: assessment with CT. AJNR Am J Neuroradiol 2001;22:845–50.
12. Casady DR, Meyer DR, Simon JW, et al. Stepwise treatment paradigm for congenital nasolacrimal duct obstruction. Ophthal Plast Reconstr Surg 2006;22:243–7.
13. Koch BL. Case 73: nasolacrimal duct mucocele. Radiology 2004;232:370–2.
14. Rand PK, Ball WS Jr, Kulwin DR. Congenital nasolacrimal mucoceles: CT evaluation. Radiology 1989;173:691–4.
15. Barkovich AJ, Vandermarck P, Edwards MS, et al. Congenital nasal masses: CT and MR imaging features in 16 cases. AJNR Am J Neuroradiol 1991;12:105–16.
16. Zapata S, Kearns DB. Nasal dermoids. Curr Opin Otolaryngol Head Neck Surg 2006;14(6):406–11.
17. Songur E, Mutluer S, Gurler T, et al. Management of frontoethmoidal (Sincipital) encephalocele. J Craniofac Surg 1999;10(2):135–9.
18. Claros P, Bandos R, Claros A, et al. Nasal gliomas: main features, management and report of five cases. Int J Pediatr Otorhinolaryngol 1998;46(1–2):15–20.
19. Behrman RE, Kuelman R, Jenson H. Craniosynostosis. In: Kliegman R, editor. Nelson textbook of pediatrics. 16th edition. Philadelphia: WB Saunders; 2000. p. 1831–2.
20. Alden TD, Lin KY, Jane JA. Mechanisms of premature closure of cranial sutures. Childs Nerv Syst 1999;15:670–5.
21. Blaser S, Armstrong D. Congenital malformations of the face. In: King SJ, Boothroyd AE, editors. Pediatric ENT radiology. 1st edition. Berlin: Springer-Verlag; 2002. p. 99–118.
22. Binaghi S, Gudinchet F, Rilliet B. Three-dimensional spiral CT of craniofacial malformations in children. Pediatr Radiol 2000;30(12):856–60.
23. Santos DT, Miyazaki O, Cavalcanti MG. Clinical-embryological and radiological correlations of oculo-auriculo-vertebral spectrum using 3D-CT. Dentomaxillofac Radiol 2003;32(1):8–14.
24. Dixon MJ. Treacher Collins syndrome. J Med Genet 1995;32:806–8.

Congenital Malformations of the Orbit

Sachin K. Gujar, MBBS, MD[a,*],
Dheeraj Gandhi, MBBS, MD[b,c,d,e]

KEYWORDS

• Orbit • Optic • Eye • Embryology
• Congenital malformations

The eye forms directly from the brain early in the embryonic life by means of an outgrowth from the anterolateral portion of the embryonic neural tube.[1] Malformations of the eye therefore may occur in isolation, accompany other complex malformations of the nervous system or may be a part of multisystem developmental abnormalities. Several genes linked with growth and development of the eye, as well as some specific embryologic defects have been identified. Developmental anomalies affecting vision, as well as those that cause visually obvious manifestations can be detected by clinical examination. However, many of the ocular and orbital anomalies require careful radiologic assessment to establish a definite diagnosis.

This article provides a brief discussion of pertinent embryology of the orbit as well as a review of the commonly encountered congenital malformations of the orbit.

EMBRYOLOGY

Development of the Ocular Globe

That the optic vesicle is derived from the forebrain was first established in 1817 by Pander.[2] During the fourth week of development, on approximately day 22, the future eyes first appear as a pair of shallow linear grooves on either side of the developing forebrain.[2] These optic sulci or optic grooves evaginating from the forebrain neural folds enlarge rapidly to form outpouchings called the optic vesicles and grow toward the surface ectoderm. As the expanded optic vesicle approximates the surface ectoderm (approximately on day 28), the distal surface of the optic vesicle called the retinal disc starts to invaginate, transforming into a goblet shaped optic cup.

Between day 31 and day 33 of development, the adjacent surface ectoderm starts to thicken to form the lens placode, which then invaginates and pinches off from the surface ectoderm during the fifth week to form the lens vesicle.[2,3] The lens vesicle is a precursor to the solid lens of the eye. The double walled optic cup is connected to the forebrain vesicle by a narrow, hollow optic stalk. The invagination of the optic cup is see in the central portion and also a part of the inferior surface that forms a longitudinal groove called the choroidal fissure (also called the choroid fissure, the optic fissure and the retinal fissure). Eventually, the lips of the choroidal fissure fuse and the mouth of the optic cup becomes a round opening - the site of the future pupil.[4]

The inner and the outer layers of the optic cup are initially separated by a lumen, the intra-retinal space, which will soon disappear with apposition

The authors have nothing to disclose.
[a] Division of Neuroradiology, Johns Hopkins University School of Medicine, 600 North Wolfe Street, Phipps B-100, Baltimore, MD 21287, USA
[b] Johns Hopkins Bayview Program, Interventional Neuroradiology, Johns Hopkins School of Medicine, 600 North Wolfe Street/Radiology B-100, Baltimore, MD 21287, USA
[c] Department of Radiology, Johns Hopkins Hospital, 600 North Wolfe Street, Baltimore, MD 21287, USA
[d] Department of Neurosurgery, Johns Hopkins Hospital, 600 North Wolfe Street, Baltimore, MD 21287, USA
[e] Department of Neurology, Johns Hopkins Hospital, 600 North Wolfe Street, Baltimore, MD 21287, USA
* Corresponding author.
E-mail address: sgujar1@jhmi.edu

Neuroimag Clin N Am 21 (2011) 585–602
doi:10.1016/j.nic.2011.05.004

of the 2 layers.[3,4] The inner wall of the 2-layered optic cup develops into the neural retina, whereas/although the outer layer of the optic cup forms the melanin containing pigment layer of the retina. It has been suggested that a sheath of neural crest cells that envelop the optic vesicle receive contribution from the optic evagination and develop into the uveal pigment cells.[2] The neural retina differentiates between the sixth week and the eighth month of fetal life.[3] Axons from the neurons developing in the retina extend to the brain through the optic stalk, converting it to the optic nerve (**Fig. 1**).

At the end of the fifth week, the primordial eye is surrounded by loose mesenchymal tissue that is derived in part from the neural crest. This sheath of mesenchymal tissue differentiates to form the inner choroid and outer sclera (comparable to the inner pia mater and outer dura mater of the brain). The sclera remains contiguous with the dura mater around the optic nerve.[4] The pupillary muscles develop within this tissue from the underlying ectoderm of the optic cup. The pigment containing external layer of the optic cup forms the anterior surface of the iris. The anterior portion of the inner layer of the optic cup forms the inner layer of the iris and participates in the formation of the ciliary body as well.[4] The pupillary muscles also form in this mesenchymal tissue. Anteriorly, the mesenchymal tissue splits into 2 layers, including a space that develops into the anterior chamber of the globe. The anterior layer of mesenchyme, along with the surface ectoderm forms the cornea, whereas/although the inner wall of the anterior chamber forms the pupillary membrane, which later disappears completely to form the pupil.

The mesenchymal tissue that enters the optic cup via the choroidal fissure gives increase to the hyaloid vessels during intrauterine life and also forms a network of delicate fibers between the lens and the retina, which later fills with a transparent gelatinous substance forming the vitreous body.[4] The hyaloid artery provides the blood

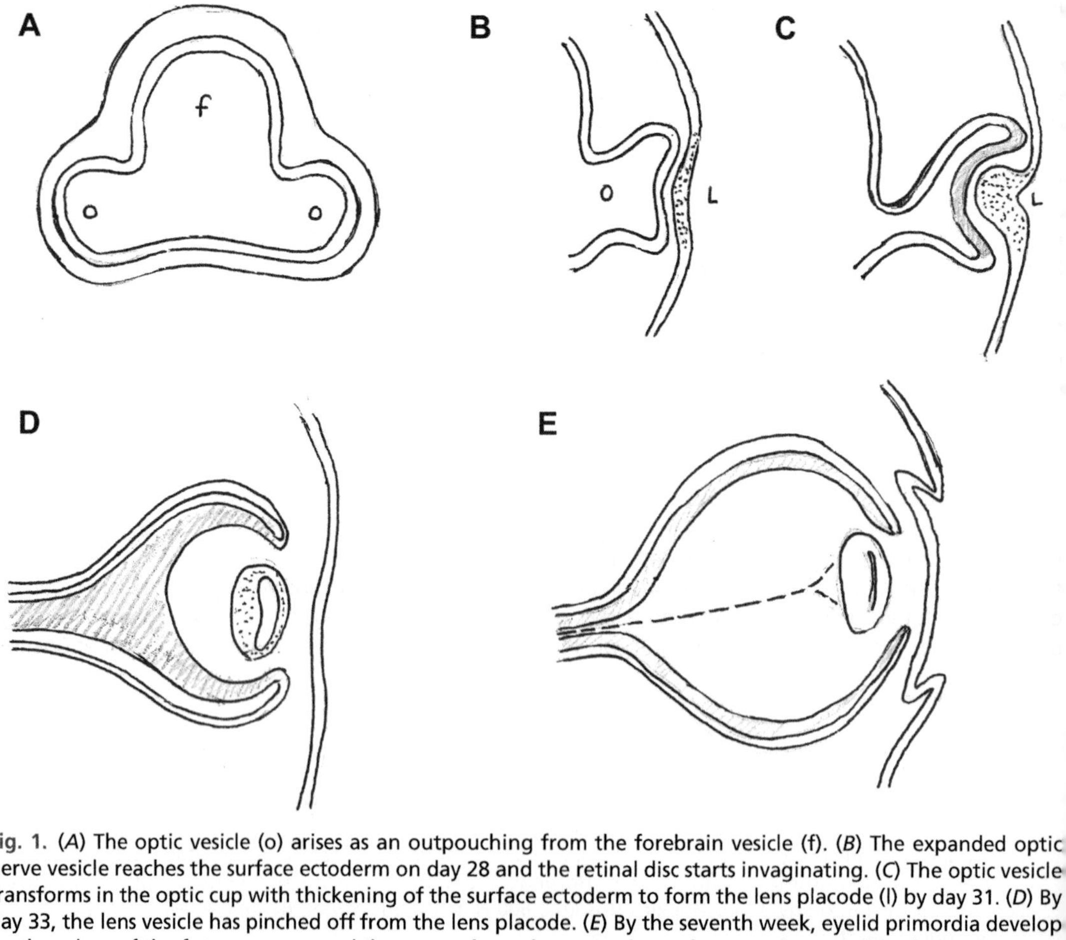

Fig. 1. (*A*) The optic vesicle (o) arises as an outpouching from the forebrain vesicle (f). (*B*) The expanded optic nerve vesicle reaches the surface ectoderm on day 28 and the retinal disc starts invaginating. (*C*) The optic vesicle transforms in the optic cup with thickening of the surface ectoderm to form the lens placode (l) by day 31. (*D*) By day 33, the lens vesicle has pinched off from the lens placode. (*E*) By the seventh week, eyelid primordia develop on the edges of the future cornea, and the mesenchyme between the surface ectoderm and the future lens start differentiating into the structures of the anterior chamber. (*Adapted from* Miller SJ. Parson's diseases of the eye. 18th edition. London: Churchill Livingstone; 1990; with permission.)

supply to the developing lens as well as the retina, and is a branch of the ophthalmic artery which reaches the inner chamber of the optic globe via the choroidal fissure on the ventral surface of the optic cup and the optic stalk. The portion of the hyaloid artery that traverses the vitreous region to the lens degenerates in fetal life as the lens matures. As the hyaloid vessels in this segment are obliterated, a hyaloid canal is left behind. The remainder of this artery remains as the central artery of the retina[3] as the lips of the choroidal (retinal) fissure fuse during the sixth and the seventh week (**Fig. 2**).[2]

Development of the Other Orbital Structures

The extraocular muscles develop from the mesenchyme surrounding the optic vesicle. It is believed that the connective tissue associated with the extrinsic ocular muscles is derived from the neural crest.[3] The primordia of the first of the extraocular muscles appear as early as day 28, and the primordia of all muscles appear by the sixth week.

The oculomotor nerve is the first to develop followed by the trochlear and the abducent nerves appear during the fifth week of the fetal life, on days 32 and 33.[2]

Eyelid grooves first appear on day 37.[2] Small folds of the surface ectoderm with a mesenchymal core appear on the cranial and caudal aspects of the developing cornea, representing the primordia of the upper and lower eyelids during the seventh week. These folds grow toward each other and fuse. The space between the fused eyelids and cornea develops into the conjunctival sac. The eyelids separate between the fifth and seventh months of development.[3]

The neurocranium (part of the head that houses the brain) is divided into 2 parts – the chondrocranium made up of bones that ossify in cartilage forming the structures of the skull base, and the desmocranium consisting of the flat bones that form the calvarial vault and ossify in membrane. The body of the sphenoid develops from the hypophyseal cartilages of the prechordal chondrocranium, with the lesser and greater wings developing from the adjacent mesenchymal condensations called the ala orbitalis and the ala temporalis respectively.[3,4] The mesenchyme for the development of the face including the nasal and lacrimal bones is derived from the neural crest cells. The ossification of these bones starts between the sixth and 16th week. In the fetus, the neurocranium far exceeds the size of the viscerocranium (facial skeleton), and the fetal orbit is represented mainly by the frontal bone.[5]

In the 1970s, working on a doctoral thesis, deHaan described the development of the orbit in great detail, although the thesis remained incomplete at the time.[6] In the embryonic and early fetal stages, the primordium of the eye is present; however, the other tissues of the eye socket cannot be identified. Only vague condensations of the mesenchymal connective tissue are seen. The author refers to the region as the primordial orbit during the early part of the fourth month (days 95–105 after ovulation) when the connective tissue structures can be clearly distinguished.[6] The face of the fetus acquires more human features during the third month as the eyes, which are oriented laterally until then, move to the anterior aspect of the face. The optic nerves are at an angle of 180 degrees in embryonic stage 16 (day 37), 84 degrees in stage 23 (day 57), and 55

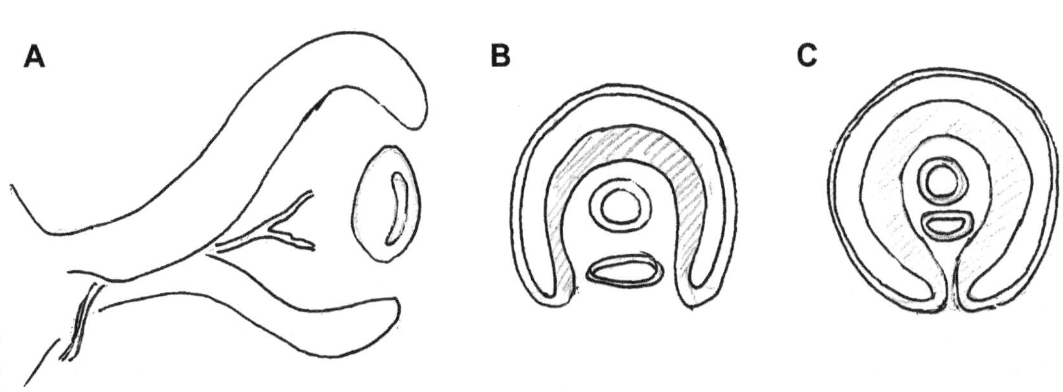

Fig. 2. (*A*) The optic vesicle invaginates in the central portion to form the optic cup and, inferiorly, to form the choroidal fissure. The hyaloid vessels develop in the mesenchymal tissue in the choroidal fissure of the optic stalk. (*B*) The choroidal fissure and the hyaloid vessels in cross section. (*C*) As the lips of the choroidal fissure fuse between the sixth and seventh week of development, the hyaloid artery gets enclosed in the region of the optic stalk and persists as the central artery of the retina. (*Adapted from* Larsen WJ. Human embryology. 2nd edition. London: Churchill Livingstone; 1997; with permission.)

degrees from a fetus of 65 mm crown breech length (CBL) (third month) until term. Further maturation and rotation of the axis of the ocular globe occurs until adulthood.[6]

Genetic Factors in the Early Development of the Eye

The PAX6 gene is considered the master regulator or master selector of eye development.[7] This transcription factor is expressed in the anterior neural ridge of the neural plate before neurulation begins. At this stage, a single eye field exists that later separates into 2 optic primordia under the influence of the sonic hedgehog (SHH) expressed in the prechordal plate, by upregulation of the PAX2 gene and downregulation of PAX6 gene in the center of the single eye field. Later in development, the PAX2 gene is expressed in the optic stalks, whereas the PAX6 gene is expressed in the optic cup and the overlying surface ectoderm where it is considered essential for the lens development.[2,8] After the induction of the lens, bone morphometric protein (BMP) 7 is necessary to maintain eye development. Other genes that have been associated with early eye development include the SOX2 gene (expressed in the optic cup along with PAX6), the OTX2 gene, and the fibroblast growth factor (FGF), signals from which overlap with the BMP7 gene[2,7,9] along with other members of the BMP family[10] and the retinal homeodomain transcription factor (Rx/RAX).[11,12]

CONGENITAL/DEVELOPMENTAL MALFORMATIONS OF THE OCULAR GLOBE

Anomalies of Number and Size

Anophthalmia and microphthalmia

Anophthalmia and microphthalmia are among the most common ocular birth defects and a significant cause of congenital blindness.[11,13] Either of these defects can occur in isolation or as part of a syndrome. Anophthalmia (or anophthalmos) refers to the absence of the ocular globe, whereas microphthalmia refers to a small size of the ocular globe. The mean maximum axial length of the neonatal human eye is approximately 17 mm (compared with 23.8 mm of the adult eye).[13]

Primary anophthalmia is a sporadic anomaly unassociated with a systemic defect, where the ocular primordia never form,[14,15] with failure of outpouching of the wall of the forebrain. Seventy-five percent of the cases may be bilateral.[14] The defect occurs early in development, at about 22 to 27 gestational days (3 mm embryo stage).[16] Secondary anophthalmia results from degeneration or failure of development of the entire neural tube.[14] Consecutive anophthalmos refers to degeneration of the optic vesicle after evagination and, consequently, some neuroectodermal elements may be present.[13,14,16] There have been observations of extraocular muscles inserting into a fibrous nodule in an apparently or clinically anophthalmic socket that might represent an aborted eye (**Fig. 3**).[13,16] A similar situation may be inferred if portion of the optic nerve or chiasm is formed. The size of the orbit and the conjunctival sac are reduced in anophthalmia. Disorganized mesodermal and surface ectodermal elements may be present, although neuroectodermal elements are absent in true anophthalmia. However, this is often difficult to confirm, and many cases may represent a severe microphthalmia.

Microphthalmia can be unilateral or bilateral, and may represent a primary ocular developmental abnormality, be associated with a craniofacial dysplasia, or be part of larger syndrome, such as with chromosomal anomalies including trisomy 13 and trisomy 18.[13,15,17] It can also occur with other ocular processes including congenital infections (rubella), septo-optic dysplasia, or retinopathy of prematurity.[15,18] Most common ocular malformations associated with microphthalmia include persistent hyperplastic primary vitreous, nuclear cataract, and coloboma.[17]

Several genetic mutations have been linked to anophthalmia and microphthalmia. The first gene to be identified was the PAX6 gene,[9,16,18] although SOX2 is a major causative gene.[13] Other reported genetic associations include RAX gene leading to anophthalmia in humans,[11,12] abnormalities of SOX2 gene,[9,16,19] and loss of function mutation in the OTX2[20] and CHX10 genes related to microphthalmia.[13]

Cyclops and synophthalmia

Both refer to a clinical state in which only 1 eye is present. Cyclops, or cyclophthalmia, refers to a complete fusion or a single median eye that is associated with holoprosencephaly. Synophthalmia represents partial fusion of optic vesicles, resulting in duplication of some anterior structures.[14,21]

Cryptophthalmos

As discussed earlier in the article, the eyelid folds appear during the seventh week, grow toward each other, and fuse. The eyelids later separate between the fifth and seventh months of development.[3] Cryptophthalmos is a result of failure of development of the eyelid folds. The eyelids, eyebrows, and the cornea are absent, and skin is continuous from the forehead to the cheeks. Absence of the eyelashes, meibomian glands, and the lacrimal apparatus is noted.

Cryptophthalmos is often a part of a systemic syndrome. Imaging studies are needed to show

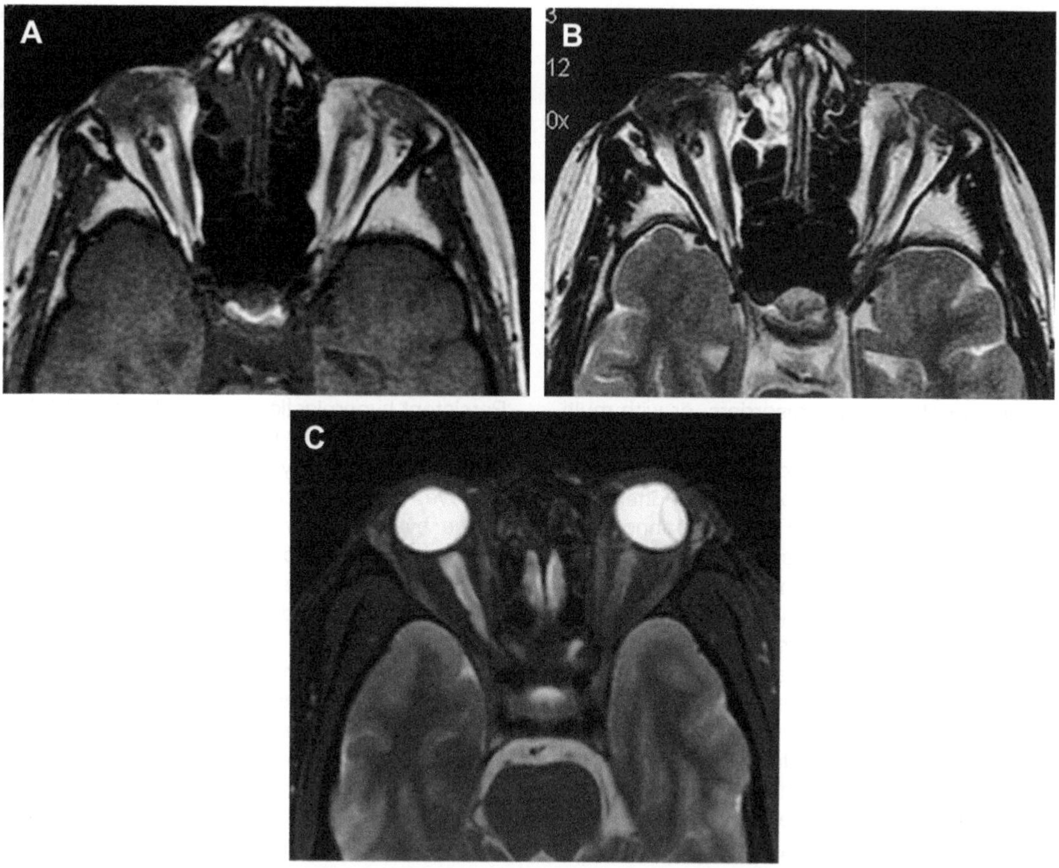

Fig. 3. Anophthalmia and microphthalmia. (*A, B*) Anophthalmia. The T1-weighted and T2-weighted axial images of the orbit show complete absence of the ocular globes, with presence of undifferentiated tissue at the site. Extraocular muscles are seen within the small underdeveloped orbit. (*C*) Microphthalmia. Reduced axial diameter of the globes in an adult patient with Nance-Horan syndrome. ([*A, B*] *Courtesy of* Dr Leonardo Macedo, MD, Cedimagem Clinic, Juiz de Fora, Brazil.)

the underlying ocular globes and the other orbital structures before surgical intervention.[22]

Buphthalmos

Buphthalmos (also called hydrophthalmos) refers to an enlarged eye caused by congenital or infantile glaucoma. It can be an isolated finding and bilateral in up to 80% of cases.[15] The corneal diameter is increased.[1] This may occur in conjunction with systemic disorders such as Marfan syndrome.

Enlargement of ocular globe from buphthalmos must be differentiated from other conditions resulting in uniform or focal enlargement of the eye. In buphthalmos, the globe is generally enlarged uniformly, but it may occasionally have oval or bizarre configurations. Imaging is helpful in excluding an underlying ocular mass such as retinoblastoma. In the absence of an intraocular mass, an enlarged ocular globe occurring early in life may also be associated with neurofibromatosis type I or Sturge-Weber syndrome.

An enlarged ocular globe can also be a feature of axial myopia with an elongated anteroposterior dimension, but with a normal cornea. In cases of severe myopia, a posterior outpouching/ posterior staphyloma may be present, occurring as a result of thinning of the posterior sclera.[23]

Congenital Cystic Eye

This is a rare anomaly that results from the failure of invagination of the optic vesicle during embryogenesis.[13,14,24] This condition presents at birth as a complex cyst lined by cells derived from undifferentiated retina and retinal pigment epithelium, or may present clinically following postnatal expansion.

The neuroglial tissue consists of dystrophic calcified bodies and degenerated primitive nerve fibers. The cyst may enlarge because of the fluid produced by glial tissue. The main differential considerations for cystic anomalies include microphthalmia with cyst, microphthalmia with cystic teratoma, ectopic brain tissue, and meningoencephalocele.

Coloboma

This is a developmental abnormality that occurs as a result of failure of closure of the embryonic choroidal fissure, and presents as a cleft in the inferonasal quadrant. Depending on the extent of involvement, colobomas may affect the iris, ciliary body, retina, choroid, and sclera, and may even involve the optic nerve.[14,15,24] The developmental insult occurs during the period of gestational days 35 to 41.[16] Colobomas can be seen in isolation or with other ocular disorders, or with multisystem abnormalities.

Colobomas may be present with normal or with small size of the ocular globes and are often bilateral. Sometimes there may be a mild abnormality with unremarkable findings on imaging.[15] In the mildest form, an optic nerve coloboma may present as a visually insignificant enlargement of the optic disc with a large optic cup.[17] The globe may be misshapen, with a very deep optic cup, extending along the optic nerve (**Fig. 4**).[15] In the morning glory syndrome, the disc is posteriorly displaced in a posterior staphylomatous excavation at the optic nerve head.[1,15] The retina in the coloboma is at risk for spontaneous detachment.[1,17]

A more severe abnormality is microphthalmia associated with a colobomatous cyst. The relative sizes of the ocular globe and the cyst are variable and, on occasion, the cyst may be much larger than the ocular globe (**Fig. 5**). In these cases, the defect in the sclera allows for an extraocular herniation of the intraocular neural ectoderm and the vitreous body to form a cyst with a tunnel-like connection to the globe. The ocular globe may be distinguished from the cyst by the presence of the other intraocular contents, such as the lens.[15,24]

Colobomas can be an isolated abnormality in autosomal dominant coloboma-microphthalmos.[17,25] Colobomas can occur in several multisystem syndromes, the most notable being the CHARGE (coloboma, heart defects, choanal atresia, retarded growth and development, genital malformations and ear anomalies) association.[17,24] Genetic disorders and associations include focal dermal hypoplasia, Aicardi syndrome, brachi-oculo-facial syndrome, and trisomies 13 and 18,[24] and have also been reported with fetal alcohol syndrome.

Persistent Hyperplastic Primary Vitreous

Persistent hyperplastic primary vitreous (PHPV) is a congenital, usually unilateral, abnormality clinically characterized by leukokoria in a microphthalmic eye.[15,26,27] This condition results if the portion of the hyaloid artery that traverses the vitreous region from the optic nerve head to the lens and the fibrovascular tissue of the primary vitreous fail to degenerate and resorb, with a resultant vascularized plaque on the posterior aspect of the ocular lens. The term persistent fetal circulation has also been suggested for this entity.[17]

There is generalized increased density of the vitreous on computed tomography (CT), which may show enhancement following contrast administration.[26] Microphthalmia and visualization of portions of a septum extending from the optic nerve head to the site of the primary vitreous behind the lens is diagnostic.[15] Tubular, cylindrical, triangular, or other intravitreal densities suggest persistence of fetal tissue in the Cloquet canal or congenital nonattachment of the retina.[26] There may be a generalized increase in the density of the vitreous chamber,[27] but calcification is absent, allowing differentiation from retinoblastoma.[15] Similarly, magnetic resonance (MR) imaging may show abnormal hyperintensity of the vitreous

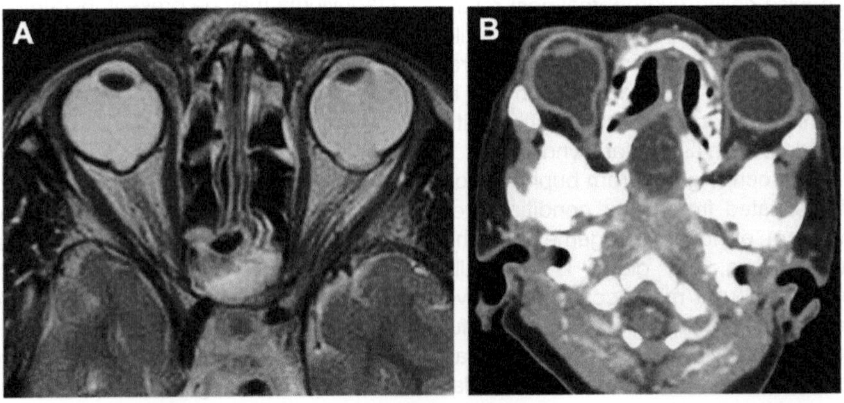

Fig. 4. (*A*) Coloboma. Small defects seen bilaterally at the optic nerve heads. (*B*) A more pronounced coloboma on the right extending farther along the optic nerve with basal sphenoid meningoencephalocele seen in a different patient. ([*A*] *Courtesy of* Dr Leonardo Macedo, MD, Cedimagem Clinic, Juiz de Fora, Brazil.)

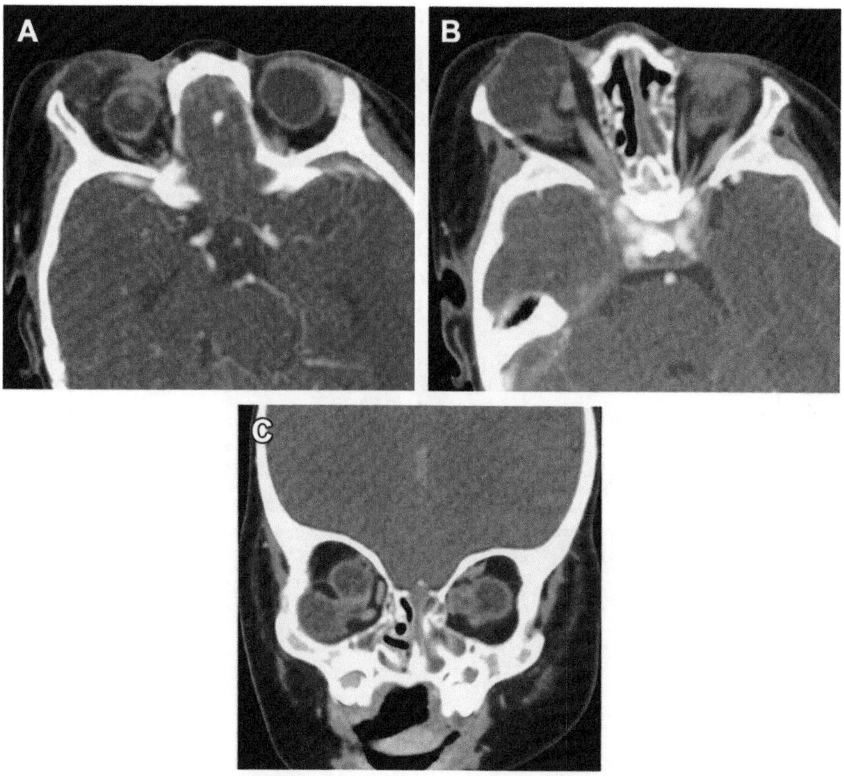

Fig. 5. (*A–C*) Microphthalmia with a colobomatous cyst, seen along the inferior aspect. This is a more severe deformity and occasionally the cyst is larger than the microphthalmic eye.

related to the blood products.[27] The lens may also appear abnormal and MR imaging may show abnormal enhancement in the fibrovascular mass posterior to the lens (**Fig. 6**).[26,27]

Bilateral PHPV may be present in a congenital syndrome such as Warburg disease, and similar bilateral findings of a retrolental mass and hyperdense retinal detachment have been described with an X-linked recessive condition called Norrie disease (oculoacoustic cerebral degeneration) (**Fig. 7**).[23,26,27] When microphthalmia is present, it may also aid differentiation from Coats disease and retinoblastoma, although differentiation of PHPV from a noncalcified retinoblastoma in a normal-sized globe may be difficult.[23] The other clinical condition in the differential diagnosis of leukokoria associated with microphthalmia in the neonatal age group is retinopathy of prematurity.[26,27] Many of these conditions eventually lead to phthisis bulbi and may show calcification.

Retinopathy of Prematurity

Retinopathy of prematurity (ROP: previously called retrolental fibroplasia) is a condition seen in premature infants who have required prolonged oxygen therapy for respiratory distress syndrome/hyaline membrane disease.[15,18] This is a condition limited to the immature retinal vasculature, and the involvement is usually bilateral. There is vasoconstriction and chronic retinal ischemia that induces abnormal vascular proliferation and neovascularization of the retina that extends into the vitreous. Vitreous hemorrhage and tractional retinal detachment[15,23,26] may occur. CT and MR findings are relevant to the stage of blood products. Imaging is usually not performed. At an early stage, there may be no specific signs on CT or MR imaging, except that the eye may be micro-ophthalmic. In advanced cases, the differential considerations include PHPV, retinoblastoma, endophthalmitis, and other conditions that result in retinal detachment. Calcification is rarely present in ROP, helping differentiation from retinoblastoma.[15,23]

Coats' Disease

This is an idiopathic primary retinal vascular disease, characterized by telangiectasias, neovascularization, and beading and tortuosity of retinal vessels, with progressive accumulation of lipoproteinaceous exudate leading to retinal detachment.[15,23,26] Although this is a developmental abnormality, patients (more frequently boys) often present later in childhood, between 4 and 6 years of age (rarely younger than 2 years), when the main

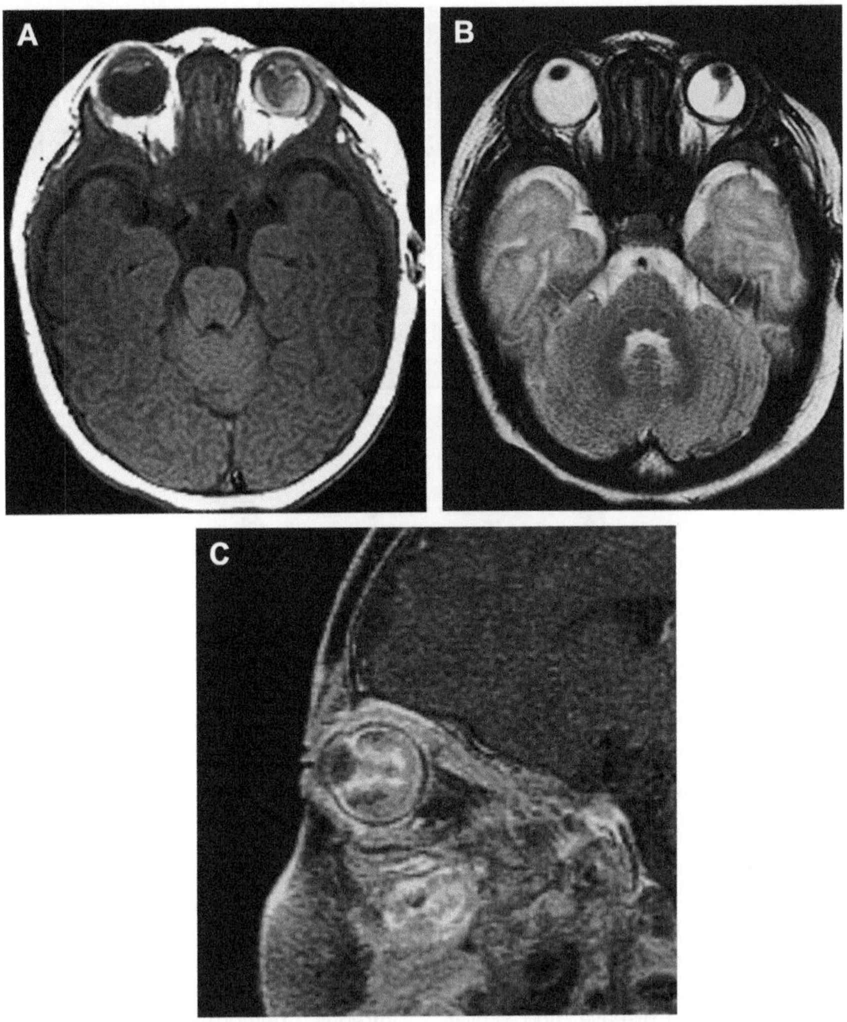

Fig. 6. PHPV. (*A, B*) Axial T1-weighted and T2-weighted images show abnormal soft tissue behind the lens with T1 hyperintensity related to vitreous hemorrhage. (*C*) Postcontrast sagittal T1 image shows enhancement in the retrolental soft tissue. (*Courtesy of* Dr Mohannad Ibrahim, University of Michigan, Ann Arbor, MI.)

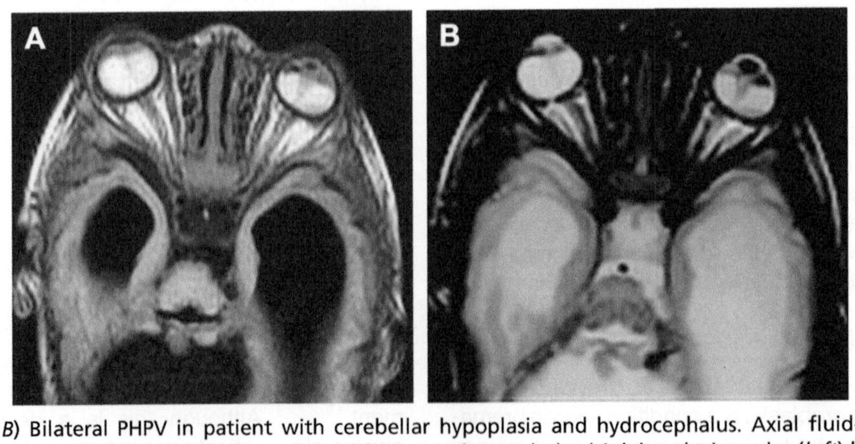

Fig. 7. (*A, B*) Bilateral PHPV in patient with cerebellar hypoplasia and hydrocephalus. Axial fluid-attenuated inversion-recovery (FLAIR) (*A*) and T2-weighted (*B*) images show tubular (*right*) and triangular (*left*) hypointense soft tissue behind the lens extending from the optic nerve heads, and abnormal FLAIR signal in the vitreous related to hemorrhage. (*Courtesy of* Dr Mohannad Ibrahim, University of Michigan, Ann Arbor, MI.)

ifferential diagnosis is retinoblastoma. Both can resent with a triad of retinal detachment, dilated etinal vessels, and appearance of a subretinal nass in a child presenting with leukokoria.

On CT, advanced Coats disease shows abormal density posterior to a contracted vitreous, vith infrequently reported calcification on pathoogic specimens.[26] There is no enhancement of he subretinal mass (unlike retinoblastoma), and here may be a slight linear enhancement at the oundary between the mass and the vitreous. The bnormal tissue is intraocular (unlike retinoblasoma, in which extraocular spread is possible) nd the eye is normal sized to slightly enlarged.[15] On MR imaging, the subretinal material appears yperintense on T1-weighted and T2-weighted mages, although the T2 signal can be varied ecause of areas of fibrosis and organized emorrhage.[26]

hakomatoses

s mentioned earlier, macrophthalmos (large eye) nay be associated with neurofibromatosis type I s well as Sturge-Weber syndrome. Hamartomas alled Lisch nodules are known to occur in the ris in neurofibromatosis, but are too small to be een on imaging.

In von Hippel-Lindau (VHL) disease, retinal angiomatosis or capillary hemangioblastomas are characteristic lesions that are often bilateral and multifocal, being the first manifestation in about 50% of patients with VHL.[28] The diagnosis is made on ophthalmoscopic examination, with a minor role for radiology, because most retinal lesions are too small. MR imaging may show signal abnormalities in the globe related to retinal detachment and rarely show the enhancing ocular lesions.[29] The patients are typically in the third decade of life.

In tuberous sclerosis, retinal hamartomas may occur that appear as smooth elevations that may calcify. Retinal giant cell astrocytomas have been reported.

Retinal arteriovenous malformations are known to occur in the Wyburn-Mason syndrome, along with lesions in the ipsilateral brain (**Fig. 8**) and, less frequently, the face.[30,31]

CONGENITAL/DEVELOPMENTAL ABNORMALITIES OF THE ORBIT

Inclusion Lesions: Epidermoid and Dermoid

These are also classified as developmental choristomas and are the most common space-occupying lesions of the orbit, representing about 30% to 46% of excised orbital tumors in

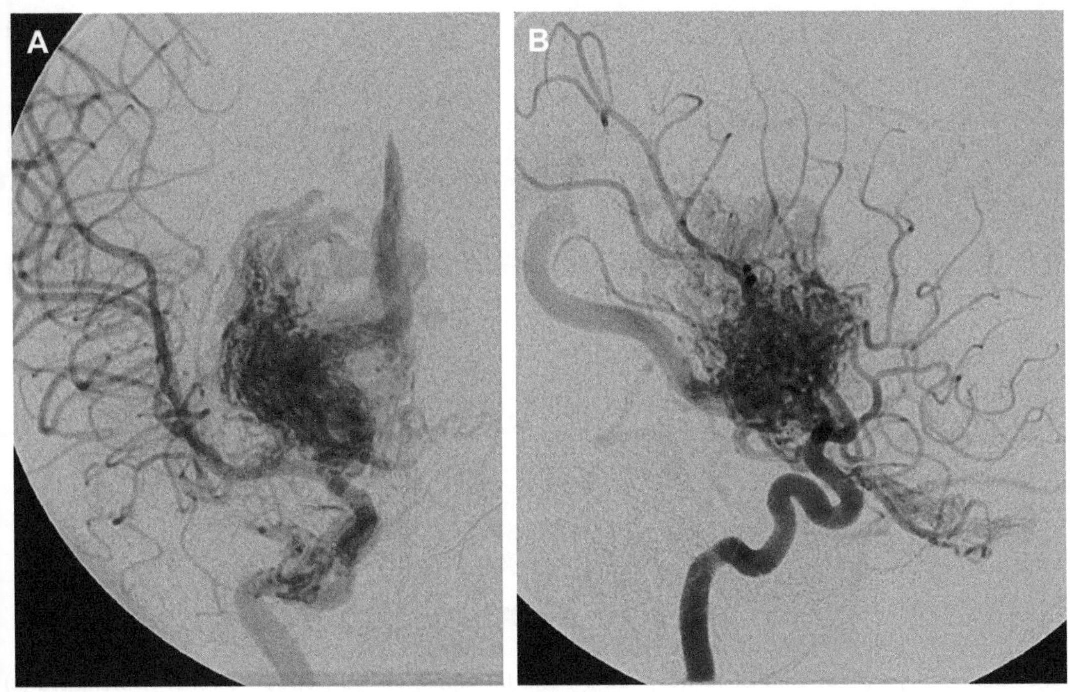

Fig. 8. Anteroposterior (*A*) and lateral (*B*) view of the right internal carotid artery injection shows a large, right basal ganglia arteriovenous malformation. Note that the ophthalmic artery is hypertrophied and there is a linear arteriovenous malformation involving the entire right optic nerve. In addition, there were small retinal arteriovenous malformations in the retina in this patient with Wyburn-Mason syndrome.

children.[24,32] These lesions likely arise from rests of epithelial cells (sequestered embryonic ectoderm) entrapped in the orbital bony sutures and can be superficial (subcutaneous) or intraorbital in location.[22,32] Both epidermoid and dermoid lesions are lined by keratinizing stratified squamous epithelium, with the dermoids also containing the skin adnexa including hair and sebaceous glands. Epidermoids contain cholesterol crystals.

Lesions are smoothly marginated and well circumscribed with nonenhancing, central, low-attenuation contents, and rarely show enhancement of the cyst wall. Because of their slow growth, larger lesions show evidence of remodeling and scalloping of the adjacent bone. The dermoid cysts may be homogeneous or heterogeneous, and some lesions may show a fat-fluid level or be diffusely fatty (**Fig. 9**). These dermoids with macroscopic fat can also be considered well-differentiated teratomas.[24] If a dermoid cyst ruptures, an intense inflammatory reaction ensues. On imaging studies, an ill-defined enhancing mass is noted that may even mask the underlying dermoid.[32]

Teratomas contain tissue from 2 or more embryonic remnants and, in the orbit, are usually benign.[22,24] The tumor may be cystic or solid, and present at birth or in infancy with proptosis. CT and MR imaging show heterogeneous mass with fatty and calcified or ossified contents (**Fig. 10**).[32]

Vascular Lesions and Malformations

Mulliken and Glowacki[33] proposed a classification of vascular abnormalities in their paper in 1982, which classified vascular lesions as tumors (hemangiomas) or malformations. Vascular malformations, in contrast with the neoplasms, are present (although occult) and more often recognized at birth, and grow commensurately (pari passu) with the child, show normal endothelial mitotic activity, and do not involute.

Hemangiomas

Hemangiomas (infantile or capillary hemangiomas, or benign hemangioendothelioma) are the most common orbital vascular tumor, appearing just

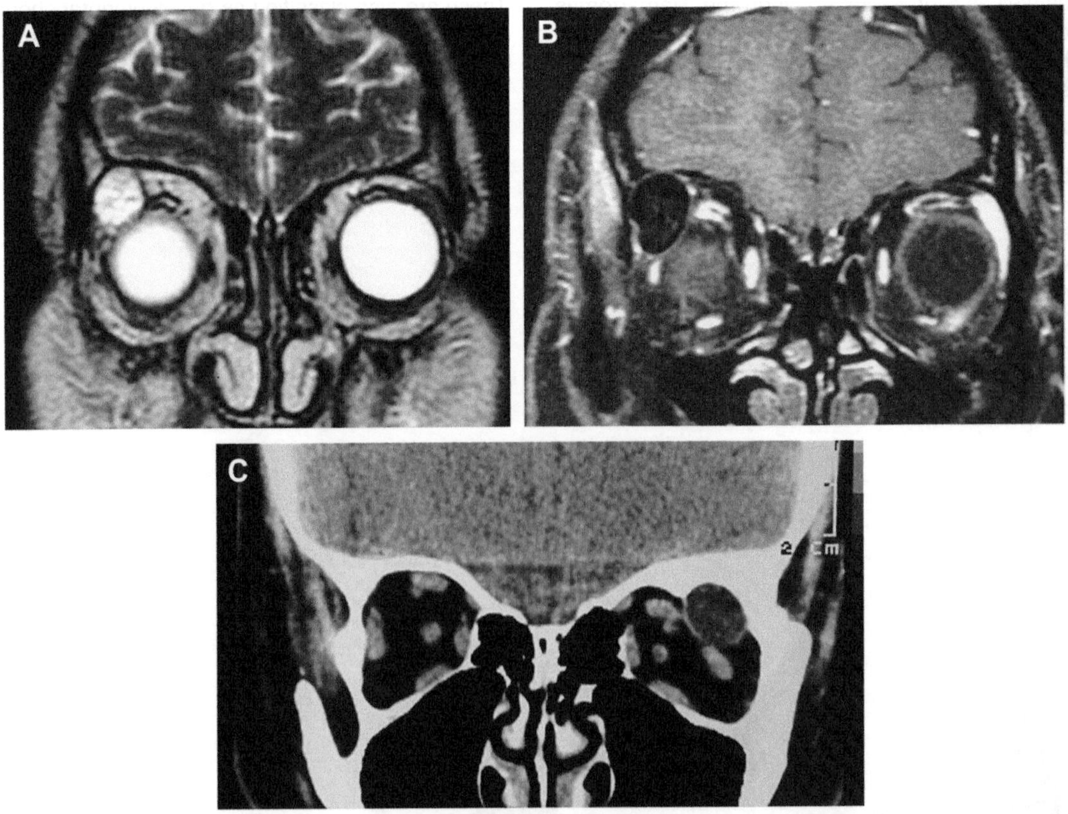

Fig. 9. Dermoid cyst (*A, B*) Coronal T2-weighted (*A*) and fat-suppressed postcontrast coronal T1-weighted (*B*) images of the orbit show a T2 hyperintense lesion in the superolateral quadrant of the right orbit that suppresses completely on the fat-suppressed T1 images. (*C*) Coronal reformatted images of a CT study in another patient shows bone remodeling related to a low-density mass in the superolateral quadrant. (*Courtesy of* Dr Leonardo Macedo, MD, Cedimagem Clinic, Juiz de Fora, Brazil.)

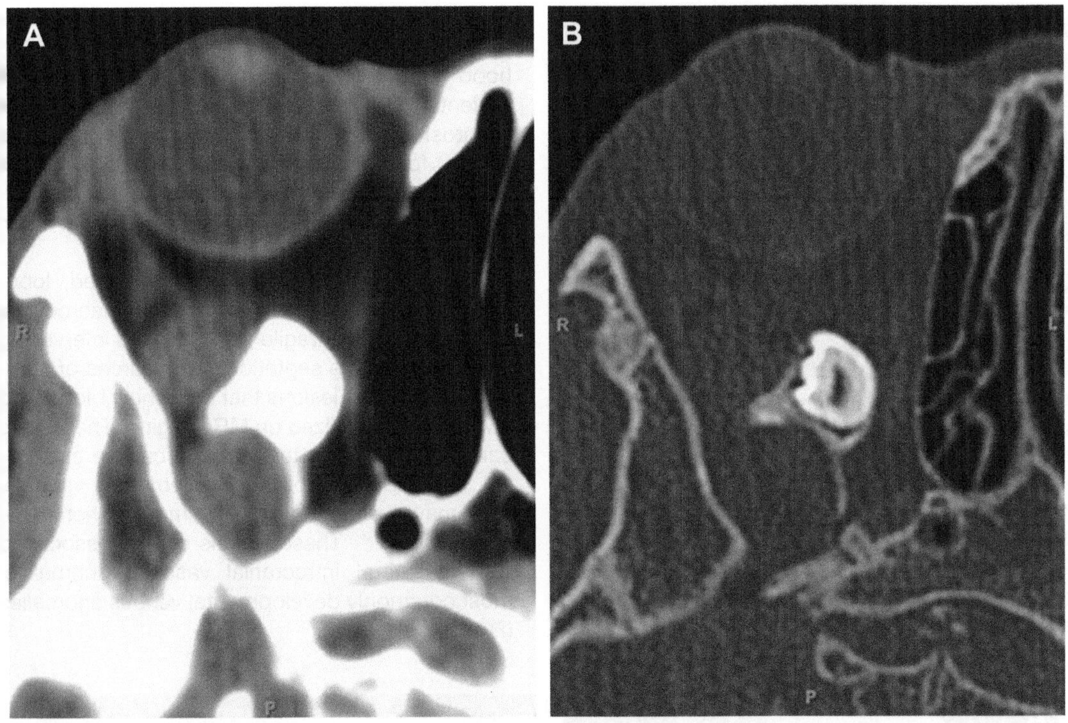

Fig. 10. (*A, B*) Orbital teratoma. Right orbital soft tissue mass with fat, a formed tooth, and bone seen in this 6-year-old patient with Pallister-Hall syndrome. (*Courtesy of* Dr Aylin Tekes, MD and Dr Ari Blitz, MD, Johns Hopkins University, Baltimore, MD.)

before, or shortly after, birth.[30,32–34] The lesion grows rapidly in infancy during the phase of endothelial proliferation and has an involutional phase with spontaneous regression of most lesions in childhood during the next 5 to 7 years.[30,33,35] These lesions can be isolated occurrences or may occur with syndromes such as posterior fossa malformations, hemangiomas, arterial anomalies, coarctation of the aorta and other cardiac defects, and eye abnormalities (PHACE) syndrome (discussed later). Treatment may be sought for orbital lesions that show complications such as ocular axis occlusion, astigmatism, amblyopia or tear duct obstruction, proptosis related to enlargement and risk of corneal ulceration, bone remodeling or optic nerve compression.[30,34,35]

In the orbit, most hemangiomas are entirely or largely extraconal in location and may rarely show intracranial extension.[30,32,34] In the proliferative phase, the tumor enhances promptly and markedly. Fatty replacement occurs in the involutional phase. Calcification is not seen. CT may also reveal orbital enlargement or bony scalloping (**Fig. 11**). MR imaging shows the lesion to be isointense to hyperintense to muscle on T1-weighted images, hyperintense on the T2-weighted images with flow voids of enlarged arterial feeders and draining veins in or around the lobulated lesion.[34]

Vascular malformations

Vascular malformations are subdivided into low-flow and high-flow types. The high-flow lesions include arterial lesions, arteriovenous malformations, and arteriovenous fistulae. The low-flow lesions are subdivided into venous, capillary, lymphatic, and mixed venolymphatic forms.[33,35]

The Orbital Society in 1999, seeking to reconcile terminology related with lymphangiomas, classified vascular malformations by their hemodynamic relationships as no-flow (including the so-called lymphangiomas), venous-flow, and arterial-flow lesions, to emphasize features that affect management decisions,[36] specifically excluding vascular lesions that expand by cellular proliferation (hemangiomas) from this system of classification.

Venous malformations

Venous malformations are well-circumscribed lesions that occur in the intraconal compartment, often present late in the fourth or fifth decade of life with a slight female predilection, and show the presence of phleboliths. Because of the slow flow, on multiphase imaging, poor enhancement

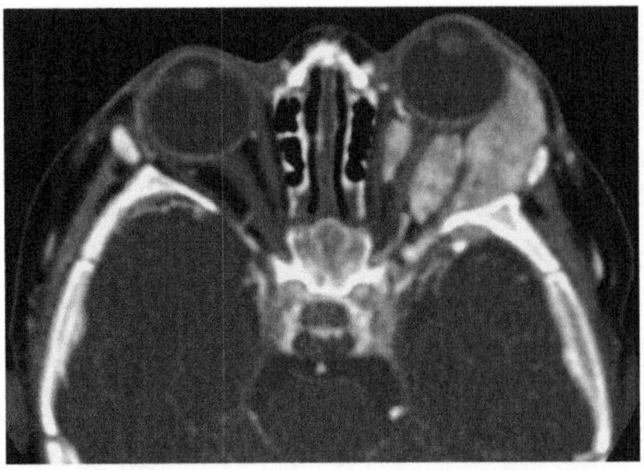

Fig. 11. Infantile hemangioma. Contrast-enhanced CT shows a large, intensely enhancing intraconal and extraconal lesion with proptosis and orbital remodeling.

is noted early, with the lesion filling in from the periphery.[30]

Venous-lymphatic (venolymphatic) malformations (previously called lymphangiomas) represent the no-flow or low-flow vascular malformations. These malformations are common and may be present at birth, although most present in childhood with no gender predilection.[30,34] Most patients with deep lesions present because of proptosis secondary to enlargement of the lesion following intralesional hemorrhage or following upper respiratory infection.[30,34] Acceleration of growth may occur at puberty or in pregnancy.

These are usually unilateral, ill-defined, lobulated lesions with microcystic and macrocystic components. The fragile vessels in the intervening connective tissue septations are sources of hemorrhage in these lesions that may show blood fluid levels, best visualized on MR imaging. The lesions can be multicompartmental and can be extraconal, intraconal, or both. Enhancement is variable, and may be absent or minimal to heterogeneous.[24,30,32,34] These lesions can be associated with ipsilateral intracranial vascular anomalies, most commonly developmental venous anomalies (**Figs. 12** and **13**).[34]

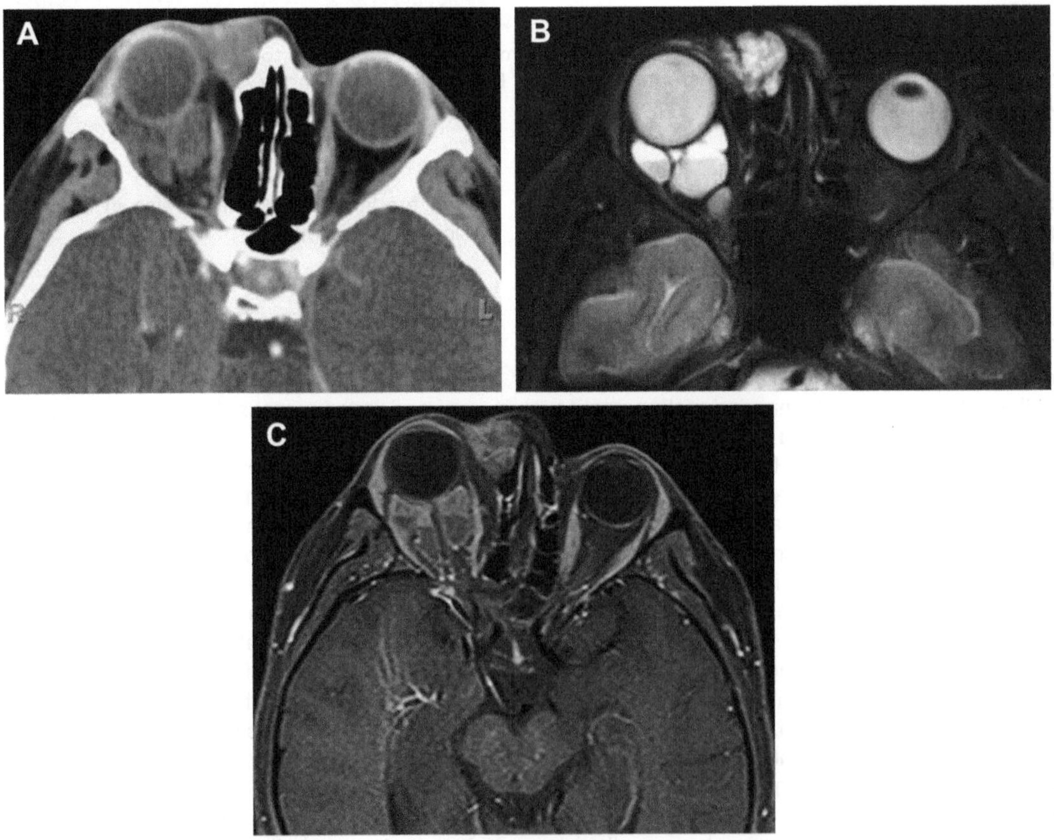

Fig. 12. Venolymphatic malformation. Axial contrast-enhanced CT (*A*), and axial fat-suppressed T2-weighted (*B*), and postcontrast fat-suppressed T1-weighted (*C*) images of the orbit show a low-density to intermediate-density lesion that appears hyperintense on T2 images with blood fluid levels. Note the developmental venous anomaly in the ipsilateral right temporal lobe. (*Case courtesy of* Dr Nafi Aygun, MD, Johns Hopkins University, Baltimore, MD.)

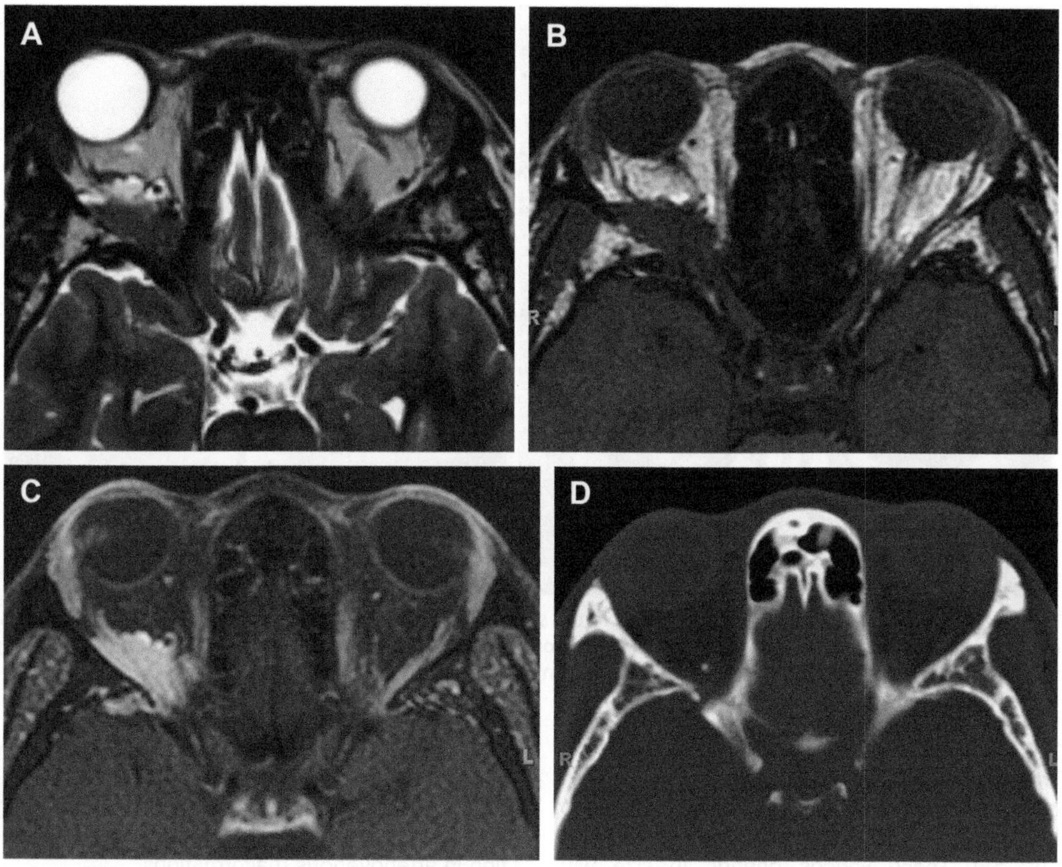

Fig. 13. Venolymphatic malformation. Axial T2-weighted (*A*), T1-weighted (*B*), and postcontrast fat-suppressed T1-weighted (*C*) images of the orbit in an older patient with proptosis show an enhancing malformation in the orbit that shows blood fluid levels and a small phlebolith seen as a focal T2 hypointensity and confirmed on the axial CT (*D*) images.

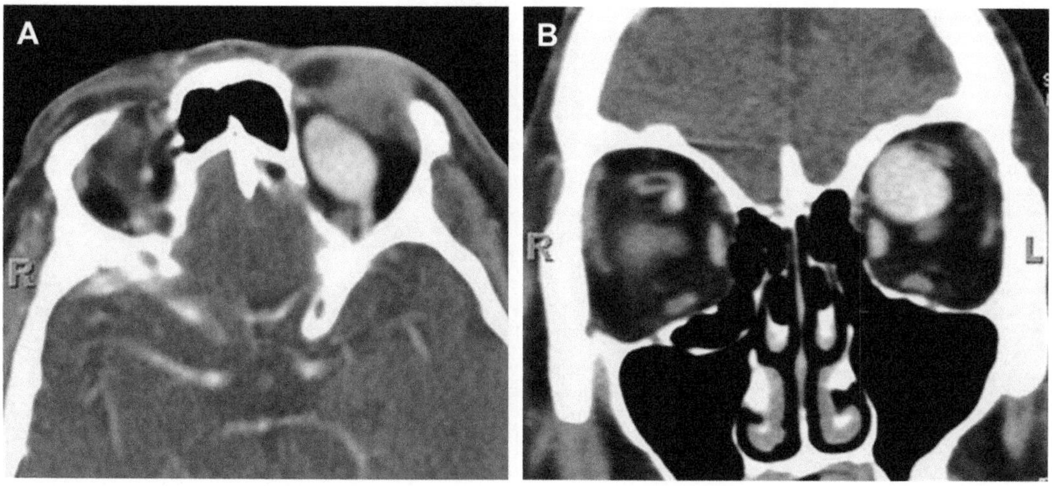

Fig. 14. (*A*, *B*) Axial and coronal contrast-enhanced CT images of the orbit show a focal dilatation of the superior ophthalmic vein.

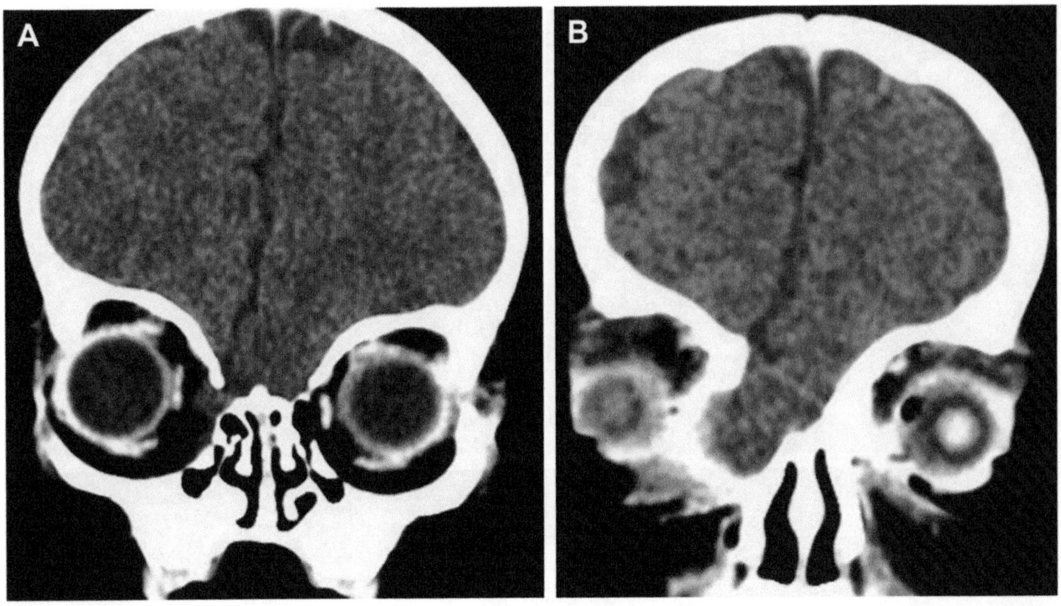

Fig. 15. (*A*, *B*) Coronal CT images show a defect in the superomedial orbital wall with a frontoethmoid encephalocele. The falx is eccentrically attached and the left frontal lobe herniates into the anterior right orbit. (*Courtesy of* Dr Mohannad Ibrahim, University of Michigan, Ann Arbor, MI.)

Orbital venous varices

Orbital venous varices (primary varices) refer to focal lesions related to weakened segments of the orbital venous system that are distensible (Fig. 14). These varices change in size with changes in venous pressure; for example, they enlarge in response to dependent posture, straining, and the Valsalva maneuver.[24,36] However, secondary varices refer to areas of venous dilatation in arteriovenous malformations.

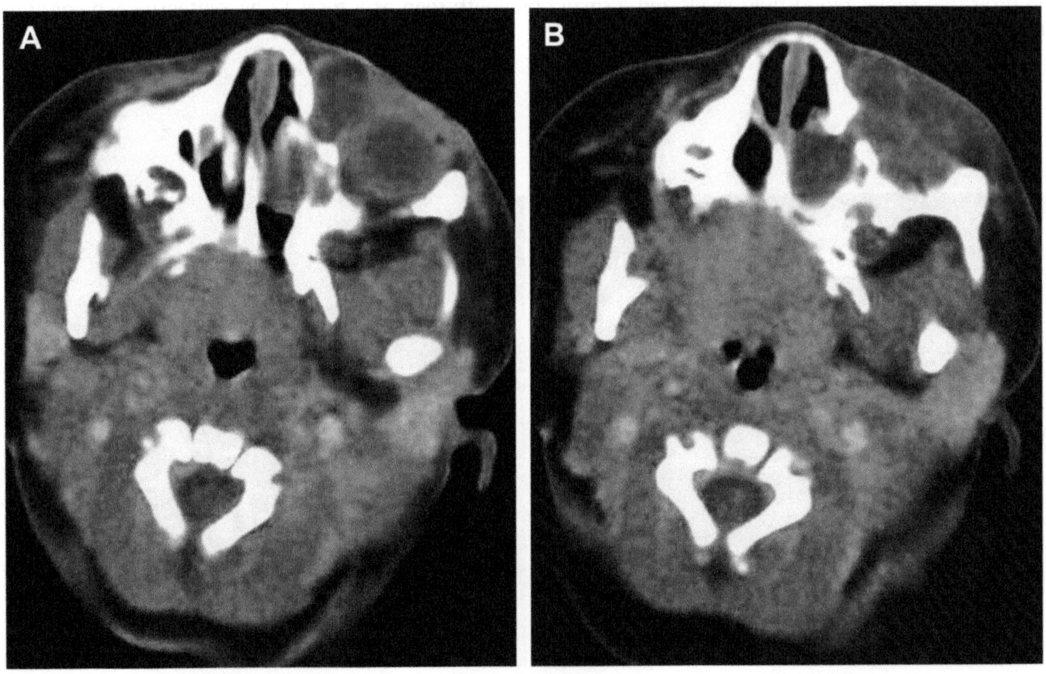

Fig. 16. (*A*, *B*) Nasolacrimal mucocele. The dilated lacrimal sac causes a medial canthal mass, and there is dilatation of the nasolacrimal duct and a nasal submucosal mass.

PHACE syndrome

This is an uncommon neurocutaneous syndrome related to large cervicofacial infantile hemangiomas, with a striking female preponderance.[37,38] The syndrome comprises posterior fossa malformations, hemangiomas, arterial malformations, coarctation of the aorta and other cardiac defects, and eye abnormalities. PHACE syndrome includes the presence of ventral defects including sternal cleft and supraumbilical raphe.[39] Patients present early, with most presenting younger than age 2 years. Posterior fossa malformations include a spectrum of developmental abnormalities, from hypoplastic or absent cerebellar vermis or cerebellar hypoplasia, rarely a Dandy-Walker malformation, and arachnoid cyst. Cerebral migrational anomalies, callosal dysgenesis, and extra-axial intracranial hemangiomas have been reported. The unilateral brain abnormalities tend to be ipsilateral to the cutaneous hemangioma. The arterial

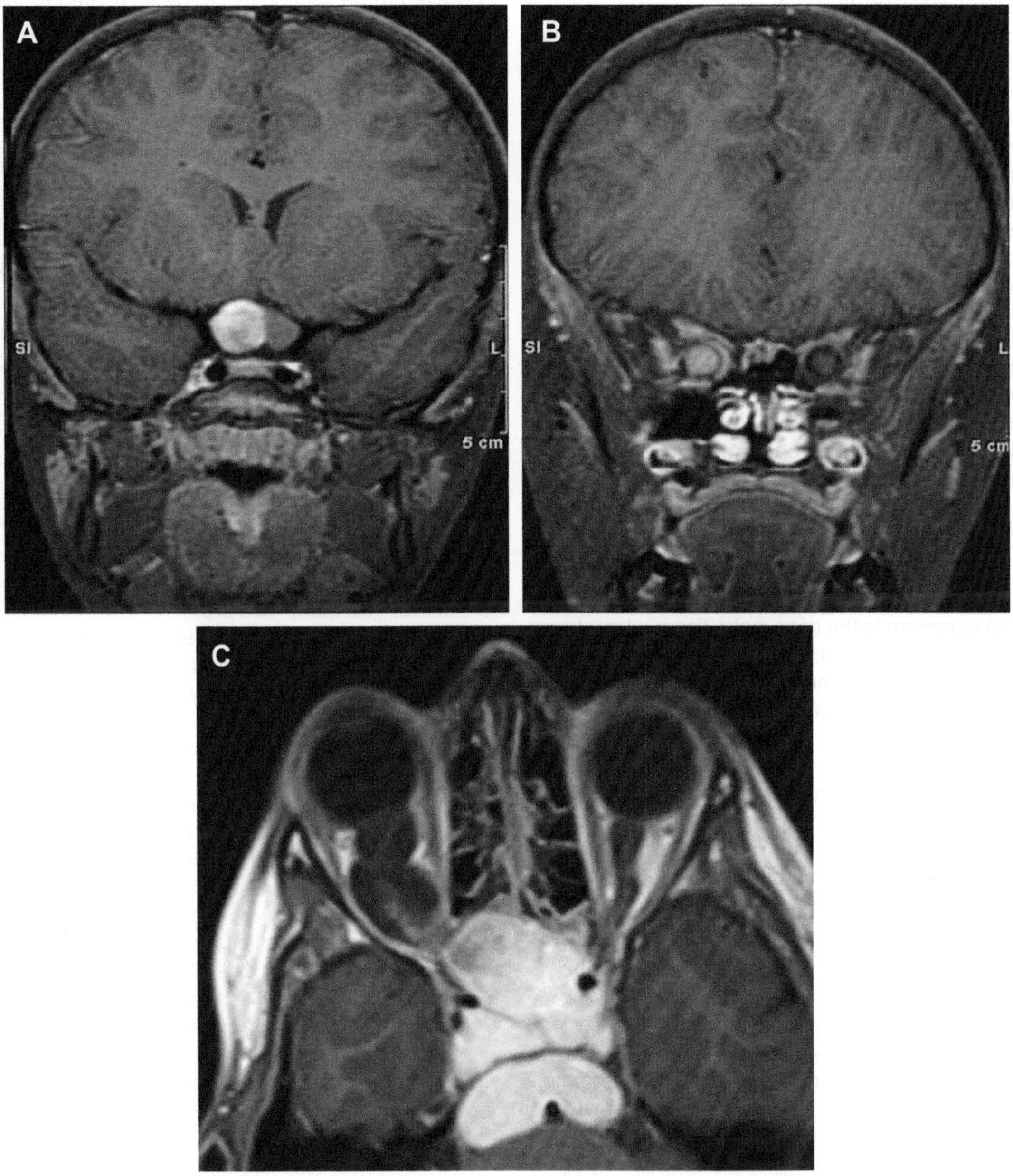

Fig. 17. (*A, B*) Enlarged optic nerves and chiasm in a patient with neurofibromatosis with enhancement only seen on the right. (*C*) Patient with a large chiasmatic hypothalamic mass and dilatation of the right optic nerve sheath.

complications include dysgenesis and malformations of the cerebral vasculature, segmental stenoses,[38] and, rarely, steno-occlusive moyamoya-like vasculopathy.[37] Infarcts may be present. Brain and arterial abnormalities typically are ipsilateral to the facial cutaneous hemangioma. The eye abnormalities are less common but include colobomas, microphthalmos, and optic nerve hypoplasia, and vascular anomalies including PHPV.[38]

Encephalocele

Sincipital (frontoethmoidal type) encephaloceles (meningoceles and meningoencephaloceles) represent herniation of meninges and brain toward the soft tissues of the forehead, external nose, and the orbit. These encephaloceles are particularly common in southeast Asia. The frontoethmoidal encephaloceles are further classified as nasofrontal, nasoethmoidal, and naso-orbital (anterior and posterior orbital),[40,41] named according to the bones at the superior and inferior margins of the defect.

Congenital/developmental meningoencephaloceles are believed to result from an abnormality of the closure of rostral neuropore. The herniating brain is often abnormal. The herniation presents as a subconjunctival mass or with proptosis (**Fig. 15**). An association between orbital varices and cranial defects, including midline or medial orbital encephaloceles, has been reported.[42] Rarely, posttraumatic orbital encephaloceles may also occur.

Nasolacrimal Mucocele

The nasolacrimal duct is formed by canalization of the caudal end of an epithelial cord derived from the ectoderm in the naso-optic fissure. Impatency of the nasolacrimal duct at birth is a frequent phenomenon, presenting with epiphora (tearing) in neonates and infants, resolving spontaneously in most. However, a nasolacrimal mucocele occurs in about 2% of these children, when there is obstruction distally (failure of perforation of the distal membrane) and proximally at the level of the common canaliculus proximal to the lacrimal sac. The presence of a cystic mass at the medial canthus with dilatation of the nasolacrimal duct and a contiguous nasal submucosal mass in the inferior meatus are features of a nasolacrimal mucocele (**Fig. 16**).[43]

Neurofibromatosis

Visual pathway gliomas are the most common orbital masses that occur in neurofibromatosis. The enlarged optic nerve is often accompanied by a dilated optic nerve sheath; however, optic nerve sheath ectasia (a form of dural ectasia) can also occur in the absence of a optic nerve gliomas (**Fig. 17**).[44,45] Occasionally, neurofibromas or a plexiform neurofibroma may arise from the first and second divisions of the trigeminal nerve, presenting as soft tissue masses in the orbit. A lesion that is rare but characteristic of neurofibromatosis is sphenoid wing dysplasia, allowing herniation of the temporal lobe into the orbit and presenting as unilateral pulsatile exophthalmos, although more commonly in older children.[45,46] The bony orbital dysplasias, including enlargement of the orbital rim, bony erosion, and decalcification and enlargement of cranial nerve foramina, are believed to be secondary dysplasia related to the presence of plexiform neurofibromas.[47]

SUMMARY

The development of the eye is complex and has been studied in detail in the past several decades. More recently, the genes involved or associated with development are being identified along with specific genetic defects that result in congenital anomalies. Numerous ocular anomalies can be recognized and diagnosed on clinical evaluation, whereas others may need radiologic differentiation.

REFERENCES

1. Apple DJ, Rabb MF. Introduction. In: Apple DJ, Rabb MF, editors. Ocular pathology, clinical applications and self assessment. 4th edition. St Louis (MO): Mosby-Year Book; 1991. p. 6.
2. O'Rahilly R. The timing and sequence of events in the development of the human eye and ear during the embryonic period proper. Anat Embryol 1983; 168:87–99.
3. Larsen WJ. Development of the eyes. In: Larsen WJ, editor. Human embryology. 2nd edition. Hong Kong (China): Churchill Livingstone; 1997. p. 375–84.
4. Sadler TW. Eye. In: Sadler TW, editor. Langman's medical embryology. 8th edition. Philadelphia: Lipincott Williams & Wilkins; 2000. p. 394–404.
5. Haas A, Weiglein A, Faschinger C, et al. Fetal development of the human orbit. Graefes Arch Clin Exp Ophthalmol 1993;231:217–20.
6. deHaan AB, Willekens B, Klooster J, et al. The prenatal development of the human orbit. Strabismus 2006;14:51–6.
7. Hever AM, Williamson KA, van Heyningen V. Developmental malformations of the eye: the role of PAX6, SOX2 and OTX2. Clin Genet 2006;69:459–70.
8. Grindley JC, Davidson DR, Hill RE. The role of Pax-6 in eye and nasal development. Development 1995; 121(5):1433–42.

9. Matsushima D, Heavner W, Pevny LH. Combinatorial regulation of optic cup progenitor cell fate by SOX2 and PAX6. Development 2011;138:443–54.
10. Muller F, Rohrer H, Vogel-Hopker A. Bone morphogenetic proteins specify the retinal pigment epithelium in the chick embryo. Development 2007; 134(19):3483–93.
11. Voronina VA, Kozhemyakina EA, O'Kernick CM, et al. Mutations in the human RAX homeobox gene in a patient with anophthalmia and sclerocornea. Hum Mol Genet 2004;13(3):315–22.
12. Fuhrmann S. Eye morphogenesis and patterning of the optic vesicle. Curr Top Dev Biol 2010;93: 61–84.
13. Verma AS, FitzPatrick DR. Anophthalmia and microphthalmia. Orphanet J Rare Dis 2007;26(2):47.
14. Smith CG, Gallie BL, Morin JD. Normal and abnormal development of the eye. In: Crawford JS, Morin JD, editors. The eye in childhood. New York: Grune & Stratton; 1982. p. 1–18.
15. Barkovich AJ. Congenital malformations of the brain and skull. In: Barkovich AJ, editor. Pediatric neuroimaging. 4th edition. Philadelphia: Lippincott Williams & Wilkins; 2005. p. 291–439.
16. Fitzpatrick DR, van Heyningen V. Developmental eye disorders. Curr Opin Genet Dev 2005;15:348–53.
17. Levin AV. Congenital eye anomalies. Pediatr Clin North Am 2003;50:55–76.
18. Hopper KD, Sherman JL, Boal DK, et al. CT and MR Imaging of the pediatric orbit. Radiographics 1992; 12:485–503.
19. Stark Z, Storen R, Bennetts B, et al. Isolated hypogonadotropic hypogonadism with SOX2 mutation and anophthalmia/microphthalmia in offspring. Eur J Hum Genet 2011;19(7):753–6.
20. Tajima T, Ohtake A, Hoshino M, et al. OTX2 loss of function mutation causes anophthalmia and combined pituitary hormone deficiency with a small anterior and ectopic posterior pituitary. J Clin Endocrinol Metab 2009;94(1):314–9.
21. Torczynski E, Jakobiec FA. Cyclopia and synophthalmia. In: Jakobiec FA, editor. Ocular anatomy, embryology and teratology. Philadelphia: Harper & Row; 1982. p. 143.
22. Bilaniuk LT, Farber M. Imaging of developmental anomalies of the eye and orbit. AJNR Am J Neuroradiol 1992;13:793–803.
23. Ball WS Jr, Kulwin DR. The eye and orbit. In: Ball WS Jr, editor. Pediatric neuroradiology. Philadelphia: Lippincott-Raven Publishers; 1997. p. 565–606.
24. Kaufman LM, Villablanca JP, Mafee MF. Diagnostic imaging of cystic lesions in the child's orbit. Radiol Clin North Am 1998;36(6):1149–63.
25. Warburg M. Classification of microphthalmos and colobomas. J Med Genet 1993;30:664–9.
26. Edward DP, Mafee MF, Garcia-Valenzuela E, et al. Coats' disease and persistent hyperplastic primary vitreous. Role of MR Imaging and CT. Radiol Clin North Am 1998;36(6):1119–31.
27. Smirniotopoulos JG, Bargalio N, Mafee MF. Differential diagnosis of leukokoria: radiologic-pathologic correlation. Radiographics 1994;14:1059–79.
28. Niemela M, Lemeta S, Sainio M, et al. Hemangioblastomas of the retina: impact of von Hipple Lindau disease. Invest Ophthalmol Vis Sci 2000;41(7):1909–15.
29. Sato Y, Waziri M, Smith W, et al. Hippel-Lindau disease: MR imaging. Radiology 1988;166:241–6.
30. Smoker WR, Gentry LR, Yee NK, et al. Vascular lesions of the orbit: more than meets the eye. Radiographics 2008;28:185–204.
31. Reck SD, Zacks DN, Eibschitz-Tsimhoni M. Retinal and intracranial arteriovenous malformations: Wyburn-Mason syndrome. J Neuroophthalmol 2005; 25(3):205–8.
32. Gorospe L, Royo A, Berrocal T, et al. Imaging of orbital disorders in pediatric patients. Eur Radiol 2003;13:2012–26.
33. Mulliken JB, Glowacki J. Hemangiomas and vascular malformations in infants and children: a classification based on endothelial characteristics. Plast Reconstr Surg 1982;69:412–22.
34. Chung EM, Smirniotopoulos JG, Specht CS, et al. Pediatric orbit tumors and tumorlike lesions: nonosseous lesions of the extraocular orbit. Radiographics 2007;27:1777–99.
35. Tucci FM, De Vincentiis GC, Sitzia E, et al. Head and neck vascular anomalies in children. Int J Pediatr Otorhinolaryngol 2009;73(Suppl 1):S71–6.
36. Harris GJ. Orbital vascular malformations: a consensus statement on terminology and its implications. Am J Ophthalmol 1999;127:453–5.
37. Heyer GL, Millar WS, Ghatah S, et al. The neurologic aspects of PHACE: case report and review of literature. Pediatr Neurol 2006;35(6):419–24.
38. Hess CP, Fullerton HJ, Metry DW, et al. Cervical and intracranial arterial anomalies in 70 patients with PHACE syndrome. AJNR Am J Neuroradiol 2010; 31:1980–6.
39. Puttgen KB, Lin DD. Neurocutaneous vascular syndromes. Childs Nerv Syst 2010;26:1407–15.
40. Suwanwela C, Suwanwelka N. A morphological classification of sincipital encephalomeningocoeles. J Neurosurg 1972;36:201–11.
41. Pellant A, Chrobok V, Mejzlik J. Anterior orbital meningoencephalocele. Eur Arch Otorhinolaryngol 2010;267:1475–6.
42. Islam N, Mireskandari K, Burton B. Orbital varices, cranial defects and encephaloceles. An unrecognised association. Ophthalmology 2004;111:1244–7.
43. Rand PK, Ball WS Jr, Kulwin DR. Congenital nasolacrimal mucoceles: CT evaluation. Radiology 1989; 173:691–4.
44. Lövblad KO, Remonda L, Ozdoba C, et al. Dural ectasia of the optic nerve sheath in neurofibromatosis

type I: CT and MR features. J Comput Assist Tomogr 1994;18(5):728–30.
45. Barkovich AJ. The phakomatoses. In: Barkovich AJ, editor. Pediatric neuroimaging. 4th edition. Philadelphia: Lippincott Williams & Wilkins; 2005. p. 440–505.
46. Binet EF, Kieffer SA, Martin SH, et al. Orbital dysplasia in neurofibromatosis. Radiology 1969;93:829–33.
47. Jacquemin C, Bosley TM, Svedberg H. Orbit deformities in craniofacial neurofibromatosis type 1. AJNR Am J Neuroradiol 2003;24:1678–82.

Congenital Malformations of the Temporal Bone

Shraddha S. Mukerji, MD[a,b], Hemant A. Parmar, MD[b,*], Mohannad Ibrahim, MD[b], Suresh K. Mukherji, MD[b]

KEYWORDS

- Congenital malformations • Temporal bone • Ear
- Hearing restoration

Cochlear implants have revolutionized the thinking and approach to congenitally deaf children. More and more otologists are now performing surgeries on the malformed ear, especially for malformed cochleae.[1] Faster, safer, and better imaging techniques have greatly contributed to understanding of the ear anatomy. Although bony abnormalities of the labyrinth account for only 20% of all cases of congenital deafness, such information is of practical importance to a dedicated cochlear implant team that is likely to encounter these uncommon cases.[2–4] Recognition of these malformations forewarns a surgeon to the possibility of potential complications and guides parental expectations during preoperative counseling. Similarly, imaging provides vital information about external and middle ear malformations to the surgeons. This article provides a common portal for both neurotologists and neuroradiologists to understand the wide spectrum of ear malformations, gain insight into their embryogenesis, formulate correct candidacy decisions, and also become equipped with the clinical knowledge of what to expect when encountering a malformed ear.

EMBRYOLOGY OF EAR STRUCTURES

The temporal bone has 2 separate precursors. The pars branchialis forms from the first and second branchial arches, the first branchial cleft, and the adjacent mesenchyme, and subsequently forms the external ear and middle ear structures. The pars otica develops from the otic vesicle and gives rise to the inner ear structures.[5–7] The development of the inner ear is therefore largely independent of the development of the external and middle ear.

The pinna or the auricle develops from the ectoderm of the first (mandibular) and second (hyoid) arches.[6,8,9] Development begins around the 40th to 45th day and is completed by fourth month of fetal life. The external auditory canal (EAC) arises as a shallow pit in the first branchial cleft. Development begins around the sixth fetal week and is completed by the seventh month. The invaginations of the first branchial cleft and the first branchial pouch with the associated mesenchyme result in the formation of the primitive tympanic membrane. The tubotympanic recess develops from the first branchial pouch between weeks 4 and 30 and gives rise to the eustachian tube, tympanic cavity, and mastoid antrum (**Fig. 1**). The middle ear ossicles, except stapes footplate, arise from the mesenchyme of the first and second branchial arches. The stapes footplate and annular ligament develop from the otic capsule.

The inner ear develops between the fourth and eighth week of gestation and ossifies as the temporal bone between the 16th and 24th weeks.[1,10] The membranous cochlea begins to develop at 22 days as the otic placode (see **Fig. 1**); this invaginates into the surrounding

[a] Department of Pediatric Otolaryngology, University of Texas Medical Branch, John Sealy Annex, 7.104, Galveston, TX 77555, USA
[b] Department of Radiology, University of Michigan Health System, 1500 East Medical Center Drive, Ann Arbor, MI 48109, USA
* Corresponding author. Department of Radiology, University of Michigan Health System, Taubman Center/B1/132 F, 1500 East Medical Center, Ann Arbor, MI 48109-0302.
E-mail address: hparmar@umich.edu

Neuroimag Clin N Am 21 (2011) 603–619
doi:10.1016/j.nic.2011.05.005
1052-5149/11/$ – see front matter

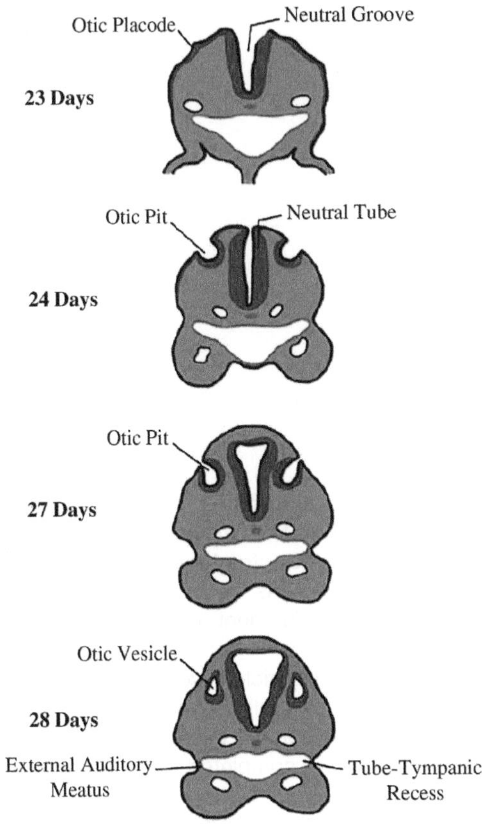

Fig. 1. Early development of the eustachian canal and inner ear.

mesenchyme and cochlear development (including bony and membranous coils) and is completed by the eighth week. The saccule and the utricle are completely formed by the 11th week of gestation (**Fig. 2**). The semicircular canals (SCCs) develop from the vestibular anlage between the sixth and eighth weeks and are completely formed by the

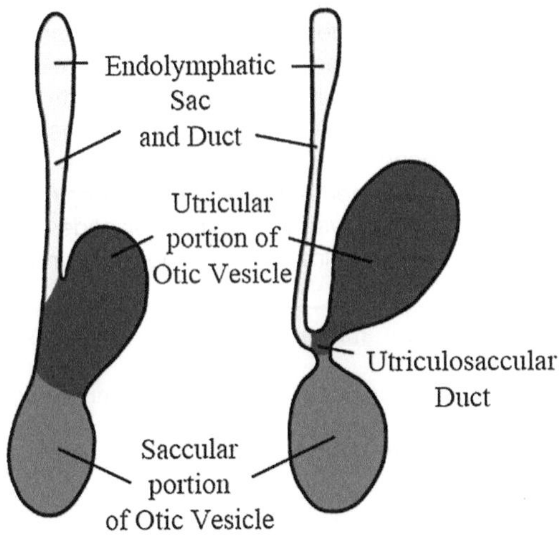

Fig. 2. Development of the utricle and saccule.

22nd week of gestation. The superior SCC develops first, followed by the posterior and the lateral SCC. Thus, developmental abnormalities before the eighth week may lead to various cochlear abnormalities depending on the stage of arrest of embryogenesis. Problems occurring between weeks 8 and 11 of gestation can affect the saccule, utricle, and/or the SCC with normal cochlea. Because the lateral SCC is the last to develop, it is most commonly affected.

INCIDENCE

Congenital malformations or dysplasias are distinct from anatomic variants because malformations have both abnormal anatomy and altered function. Malformations of the external ear are referred to as congenital aural dysplasias. Malformations of the auricle alone are called microtias. Congenital aural dysplasias have been reported to occur in 1:3000 to 1:10,000 births.[6,8,11] Most cases are unilateral, without other associated systemic abnormalities and without a known cause. In unilateral cases, the right side is most commonly affected (58%–61%).[8] Microtia has been reported to occur predominantly in boys, with a male/female ratio of 2:1. Congenital aural dysplasias may occur in association with genetic disorders, chromosomal anomalies, and intrauterine infections. Common syndromes associated include Treacher Collins, Goldenhar, and Klippel-Fiel syndromes.[6] Overall, combined congenital malformation of the external and middle ear occur more commonly than isolated middle ear anomalies. Associated inner ear malformations are less common (10%) because of the separate embryogenesis of the labyrinth.

A study by Westerhof and colleagues[12] revealed that most patients with inner ear anomalies had multiple abnormalities. The most common malformations of the inner ear include anomalies of the SCC (88%) followed by malformations of the vestibule (62%). Enlarged vestibular aqueduct is the most common isolated malformation. Among cochlear anomalies, the classic Mondini deformity accounts for nearly 55%, whereas common cavity malformations are seen in 25% of patients.[12] Syndromes such as CHARGE (coloboma, heart defects, choanal atresia, retarded growth and development, genital malformations and ear anomalies), Pendred, branchio-oto-renal (BOR), Phelps X-linked mixed deafness, Waardenburgh, and others are associated with inner ear malformations but are less common than nonsyndromic congenital bony abnormalities. **Table 1** summarizes the cochlear malformations, the gestational age of developmental arrest, and their frequency as reported in literature.

Table 1
Cochlear anomalies, gestational age at developmental arrest, and frequency of occurrence of some inner ear anomalies

Cochlear Deformities	Gestational Age at Arrest (wk)	Frequency
Michel deformity	Third	Very rare
Common cavity	Between fourth and fifth	25%
Cochlear aplasia	Fifth	Uncommon
Cochlear hypoplasia	Sixth	15%
IP I (pseudo-Mondini)	Between sixth and seventh	Uncommon
IP II (classic Mondini)	Seventh	55%

IMAGING TECHNIQUES FOR TEMPORAL BONE MALFORMATIONS

Computed tomography (CT) is the imaging method of choice to detect anomalies in congenital aural dysplasia. For best resolution, the slice thickness should be submillimeter with isovoxel imaging, bone algorithm, and a small field of view.[8,13] Multidetector CT is not only fast but also allows excellent coronal reconstruction, obviating the need to scan in a second plane.[2,10] Imaging for congenital aural dysplasia is not only important to confirm the presence or absence of malformations but is also required to grade the degree and severity of the malformation. This information is invaluable to a surgeon and serves as a basis for treatment decisions and outcomes. A surgical rating scale has been developed by Jahrsdoerfer and colleagues[14] from correlating clinical findings and CT images. The grading system is based on a possible score of 10. The stapes is assigned the highest rating (2 points) and the rest of the structures are awarded 1 point each. The higher the rating, the better are the chances of successful hearing restoration after surgery. Patients who have a score of 5/10 or less have been shown to not benefit from surgery. For children with congenital sensorineural deafness, both axial and coronal CT views and axial MR imaging views are the usual standard. CT enables simultaneous visualization of associated middle and external ear abnormalities. It provides knowledge of the thickness of the parietal bone, degree of pneumatization of mastoid air cells, and presence of retrocochlear and infracochlear air cells that may be mistaken for the round window niche.[15] MR imaging is performed to assess the membranous labyrinth, internal auditory canal (IAC), and cerebellopontine angle.[10] T2-weighted sequence or fluid-attenuated inversion recovery (FLAIR) for the brain to assess the auditory cortex is also required. Several thin gradient echo images are required, which can be achieved by T2 heavily weighted sequences like three-dimensional (3D) Fourier transform constructive interference in steady state (3DFT-CISS), true fast imaging with steady precession (FISP), or 3D driven enhancement (3D-T2 DRIVE).[2,10,12] Gadolinium is required to assess enhancement of the membranous labyrinth in case of postmeningitic or autoimmune labyrinthitis. Specific advantages of MR imaging include (1) detection of an existing cochlear nerve; (2) demarcation of cochlear and labyrinthine structures, which is essential to ensure correct insertion of the electrode array during surgery; (3) early detection of postmeningitis fibro-osseous change in the cochlea; and (4) evaluation of associated abnormalities within the brainstem and central auditory pathways. Plain radiographs do not have any role in the assessment of potential cochlear malformations, but are important after surgery in assessing the position and depth of electrode insertion.[1] A modified Stenver view shows the typical coiled appearance of a fully inserted electrode array. An intraoperative per orbital view using an image intensifier is required when there is doubt regarding correct placement of electrodes.

ANOMALIES OF THE EXTERNAL EAR

Auricle

Auricular malformations can affect the size, shape, position, and orientation of the pinna. Complete absence of the pinna (anotia) may occur. Various classification schemes have been proposed to grade the severity of deformity; however, Weerda's classification[8] is most widely used. This classification includes 3 grades of microtia with worsening severity. The important aspects of this classification have been summarized in **Table 2**.

EAC

Failure of recanalization of tissue of the first branchial cleft can lead to EAC malformations. The absence of a meatal opening under the tragus signifies complete aural atresia (**Fig. 3**). Incomplete atresia or stenosis should be suspected when the pinna is abnormal and the EAC diameter is less than 4 mm[16] or the tympanic membrane cannot be visualized. The stenosis can be fibrous, bony, or both. In the fibrous type, there is a soft tissue plug at the position of the tympanic membrane,

Table 2
Grades of auricular malformations

Grade of Dysplasia	Characteristics
Grade I (slight malformation)	Most structures of the normal pinna are recognizable. Surgery usually does not require use of additional skin or cartilage
Grade II (moderate malformation)	Some structures of a normal pinna are recognizable. Surgery involves use of additional skin or cartilage
Grade III (severe malformation)	None of the normal structures of the pinna are recognizable. Includes anotia. Total reconstruction is necessary, which requires much of the adjacent skin and cartilage

whereas the bony stenosis is characterized by the presence of a bony plate at the level of the tympanic membrane (**Fig. 4**A). Schuknecht[17] has classified EAC atresia into 4 types (A–D) and this classification is useful to both surgeons and the radiologists. Weerda has classified EAC malformations into 3 types (A–C) and these are described in **Table 3**. With abnormal EAC formation, the structures around the ear are also displaced from their normal position. The condylar fossa is higher than usual and posteriorly displaced, whereas the mastoid process is pushed anteriorly. The jugular bulb may be high and the tegmen tympani low. The facial nerve has an anomalous course in patients with congenital aural dysplasias. The tympanic and mastoid segments are most commonly affected. The tympanic segment is typically displaced inferiorly at the level of the round window, and may be dehiscent or displaced medially to overlie the oval window. The mastoid segment is shallow and displaced anterolaterally, exiting the temporal bone at the level of the round window (see **Fig. 4**B).[13,18]

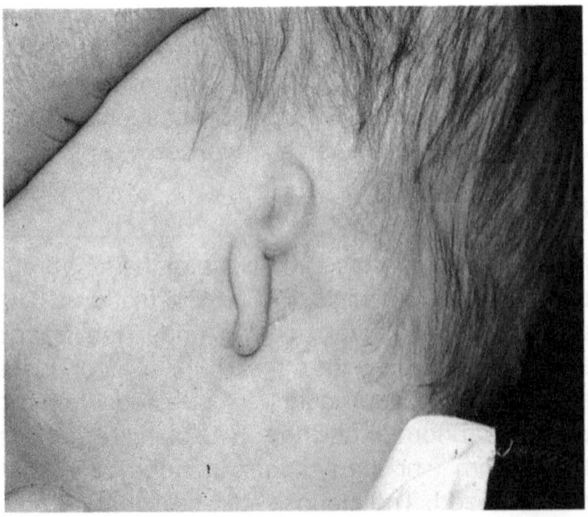

Fig. 3. Complete atresia of the left EAC in a 6-month-old infant. There is underdeveloped pinna as well.

First Branchial Cleft Anomalies

These occur as a result of abnormal ectodermal closure of the cleft. They typically occur along the line from the floor of the EAC to the submental area.[16] These anomalies may present as preauricular cyst, sinus, asymptomatic or infected parotid mass, or recurrent external otitis. Please refer to the article by Ibrahim and colleagues elsewhere in this issue for further details on this entity.

Congenital Cholesteatoma

Congenital cholesteatoma occurs more commonly in the middle ear and is also discussed later in this article. Children with atresia of the EAC may develop cholesteatomas (primary or secondary) at the site of the stenosis or deep to the atretic plate.

ANOMALIES OF THE MIDDLE EAR

It is generally known that the better developed the auricle and external ear the better developed the middle ear. A study by Ishimoto and colleagues[11] analyzing CT grading system for middle ear abnormalities versus severity of microtia suggested an inverse relationship between the two (ie, the better the CT score, the less the severity of microtia). Middle ear malformations can affect the normal development of the tympanic cavity, mastoid pneumatization, and ossicles. There are various classifications proposed, so it is important that the radiologist and the otologist use the same or similar classification to evaluate middle ear anatomy.

Anomalies of Ossicles and Related Structures

Malleus

These include aplasia, fixation of the incudomalleolar joint, bony fusion of the head of the malleus to the long process of the incus and stapes head (triple bony union), and deformed head.[9] A rare anomaly of the malleus is congenital fixation of the malleus head to the lateral epitympanic wall called the malleus bar (**Fig. 5**).

Incus

These include aplasia, deformity of the long process, fusion of short process of incus to lateral

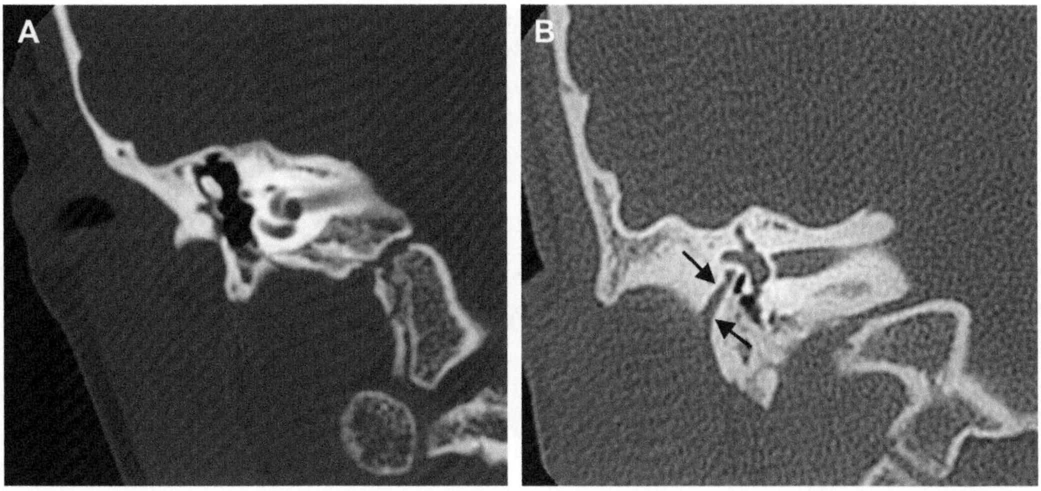

Fig. 4. EAC atresia. (*A*) Coronal CT image of the right temporal bone at the level of cochlea shows complete bony atresia of the external auditory canal. The ear ossicles are deformed and attached to the lateral bony wall. (*B*) A more posterior coronal CT image of the right temporal bone at the level of vestibule shows a shallow and foreshortened descending segment of the right facial nerve (*arrows*).

SCC, and fibrous union of the incudostapedial joint or absence of the joint.

Stapes
These include absence of the stapes suprastructure, aplasia, deformed head, monopod stapes (Fig. 6), fixation of head to promontory, and footplate fixation.

Other anomalies
These include persistence of stapedial artery (Fig. 7), absence of stapedius muscle, and absence or elongation of the pyramidal eminence. Congenital cholesteatomas are identified as a whitish mass behind an intact tympanic membrane (Fig. 8). They occur most commonly in the middle, but may also occur in the external ear and the petrous apex as well as at other sites.

Facial nerve anomalies
These anomalies are as described earlier.

Table 3
Types of EAC stenosis

Types of EAC Stenosis	Characteristics
Type A	Marked narrowing of the EAC with an intact skin layer
Type B	Partial development of the EAC with an atresia plate medially
Type C	Complete bony EAC stenosis

Tympanic cavity
May be hypoplastic, aplastic, or extracavitation,[8] which is an extra cavity in the wrong place.

Mastoid pneumatization
May be normal, reduced, or absent.

Principles of management of patients with congenital aural dysplasia
Surgery for congenital aural dysplasia is challenging and may be associated with a high complication rate. Treatment depends on the age of the child, the degree and nature of hearing loss, the presence of other anomalies, and unilateral versus bilateral microtia. Surgery for microtia is typically multistaged and may begin at 6 years of age after cartilage maturation and temporal bone pneumatization is complete.[19] Surgery for reconstruction of the EAC and hearing improvement may be performed at some stage after auricular reconstruction has begun. Predictors of good hearing outcomes after congenital aural dysplasia surgery include normal tympanic cavity, good mastoid pneumatization, and overall a low score on the CT grading system. Postoperative complications include facial nerve paralysis, failure to restore hearing, occurrence of sensorineural hearing loss, and restenosis of the EAC.

INNER EAR MALFORMATIONS

Classification of Inner Ear Malformations

Many classification schemes for congenital cochleovestibular anomalies have been suggested both in the radiology and otolaryngology literature.

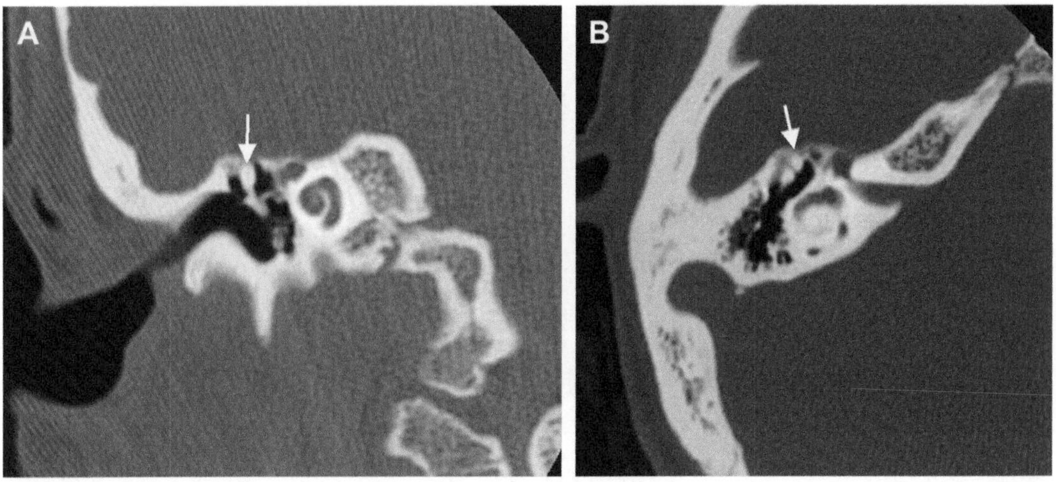

Fig. 5. Malleus fixation. Coronal (*A*) and axial (*B*) CT images of the right temporal bone shows bony fixation of the malleus to the superior and lateral epitympanic wall (*arrows*).

Inner ear malformations occur as a result of arrest at different stages of embryogenesis.[1] Smith and Harker[20] suggested a genetic basis for these malformations (ie, congenital inner ear anomalies may occur because of faulty expression of a patterning gene). A more recent classification has been proposed by Sennaroglu and colleagues[3] (**Fig. 9**). The basis of this classification is embryologic arrest, but it also distinguishes between classic Mondini and pseudo-Mondini deformities, which have been shown to have different clinical outcomes. This classification (**Table 4**) has been used as a basis for our manuscript.

Cochlear Abnormalities

- Michel deformity or labyrinthine aplasia
- Cochlear aplasia
- Common cavity deformity
- Incomplete partition (IP) type I: cystic cochleovestibular malformation
- Cochleovestibular or cochlear hypoplasia
- IP type II: classic Mondini deformity.

Michel deformity or labyrinthine aplasia

In this malformation there is complete labyrinthine aplasia and thus complete absence of all cochlear and vestibular elements. Because of failure of development of the otic vesicle, no further inner ear development occurs. CT imaging (**Fig. 10**) shows an absence of inner ear structures. Giesemann and colleagues[21] described a related anomaly called the otocyst deformity. This deformity occurs after formation of the otic vesicle and, because SCCs are the first structures to develop from the otic vesicle, the inner ear may

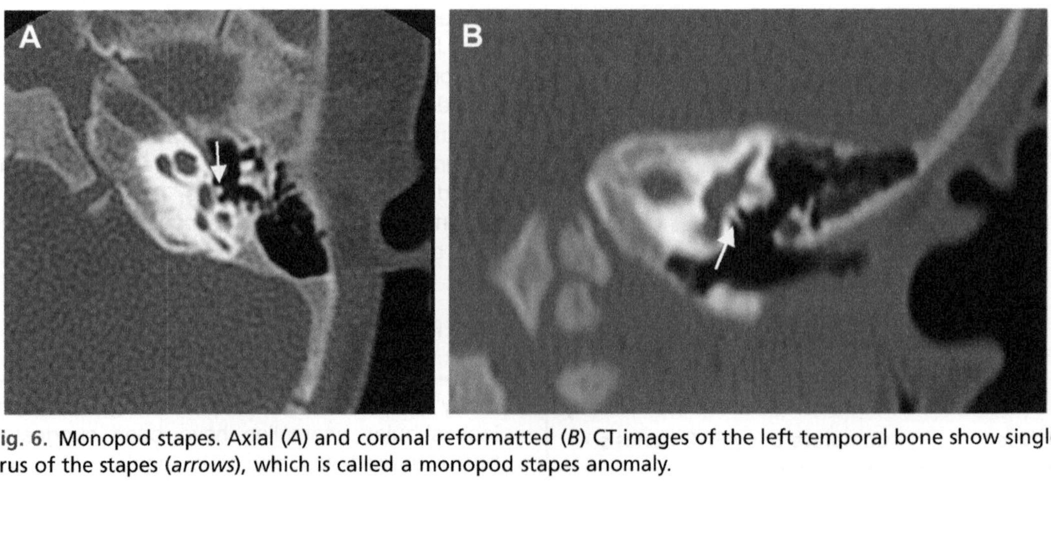

Fig. 6. Monopod stapes. Axial (*A*) and coronal reformatted (*B*) CT images of the left temporal bone show single crus of the stapes (*arrows*), which is called a monopod stapes anomaly.

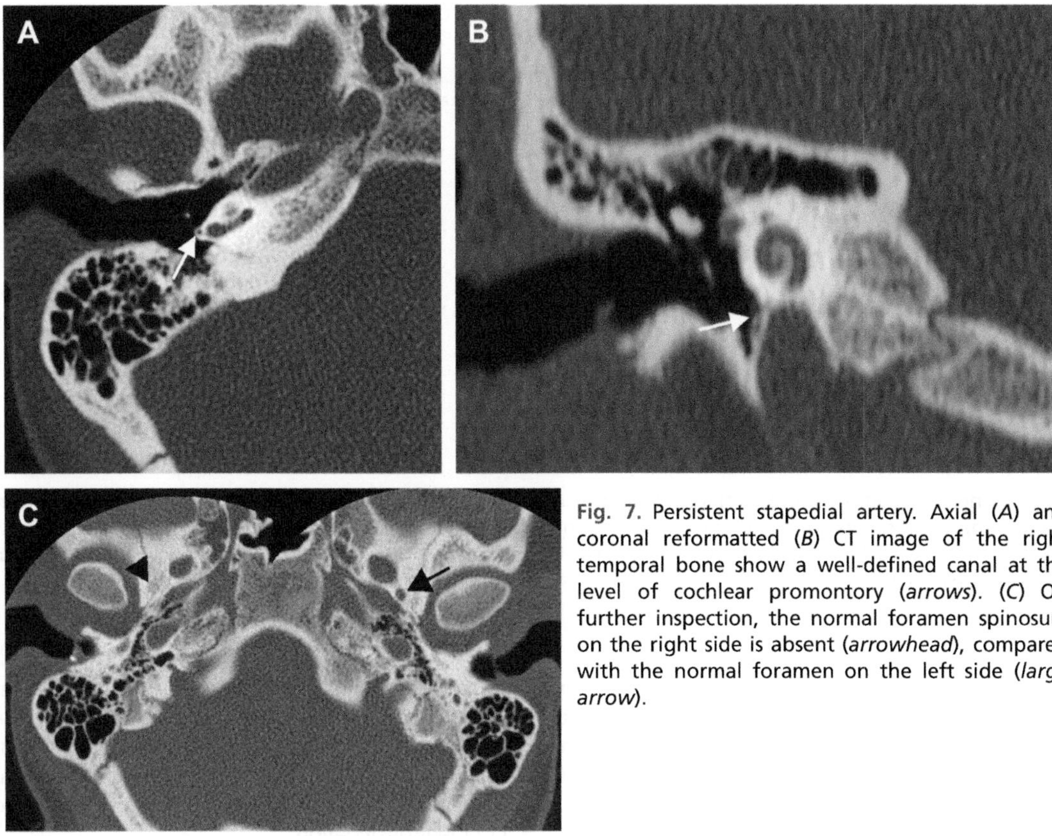

Fig. 7. Persistent stapedial artery. Axial (*A*) and coronal reformatted (*B*) CT image of the right temporal bone show a well-defined canal at the level of cochlear promontory (*arrows*). (*C*) On further inspection, the normal foramen spinosum on the right side is absent (*arrowhead*), compared with the normal foramen on the left side (*large arrow*).

be represented by some rudimentary SCC. No further inner ear characterization is seen. Both malformations may show middle ear abnormalities and hypoplastic petrous apex. The lack of cochlear promontory differentiates both these malformations from labyrinthitis ossificans (**Fig. 11**), an acquired condition often seen after meningitis, in which there is fibrous and bony replacement of the inner ear structures, including the cochlea.[12] However, the promontory bulge is

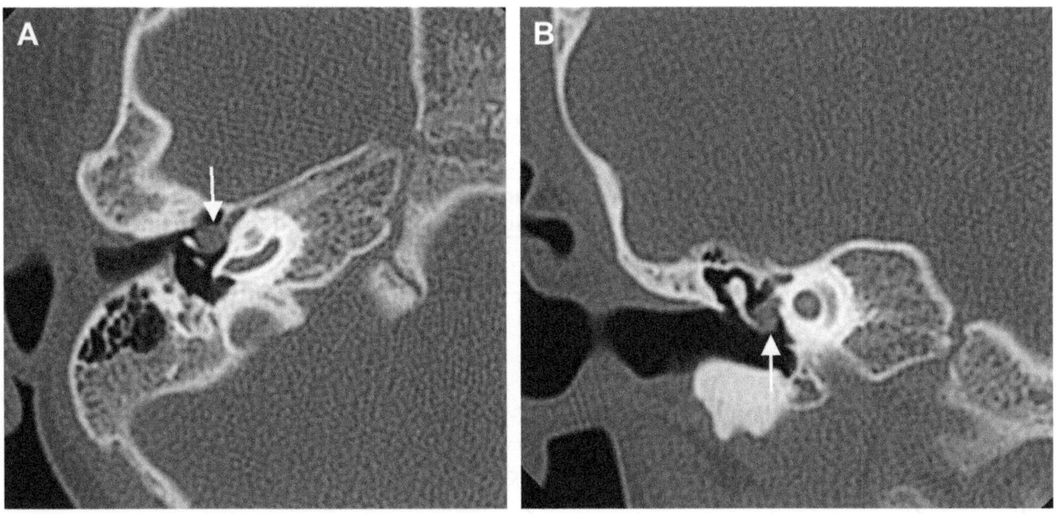

Fig. 8. Congenital cholesteatoma. Axial (*A*) and coronal (*B*) CT images of the right temporal bone show a well-defined rounded soft tissue within the middle ear cavity (*arrows*), which was operated on and found to be a congenital cholesteatoma.

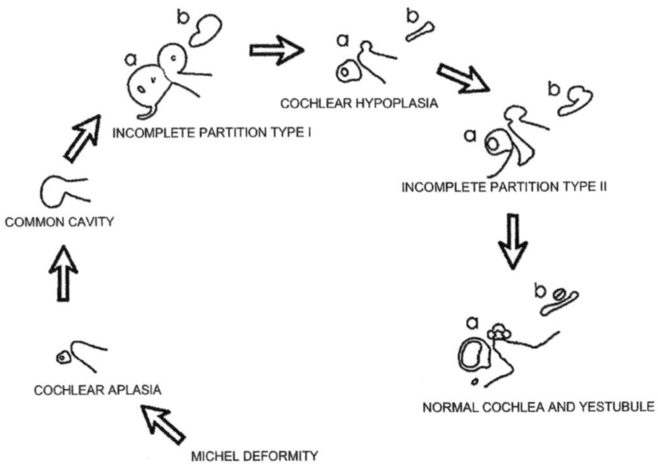

Fig. 9. Inner ear malformations. Different stages of developmental arrest in inner ear development. The letters a and b represent sections through the IAC and round window, respectively. (*From* Sennaroglu L, Saatci I. A new classification for cochleovestibular malformations. Laryngoscope 2002;112:2230–41; with permission of John Wiley & Sons, Inc.)

seen. This difference is important clinically because cochlear implantation is contraindicated in Michel anomaly, whereas implantation, although difficult, may be possible in patients with labyrinthitis ossificans.

Cochlear aplasia

In this malformation there is complete absence of the cochlea (**Fig. 12**). The vestibule, SCCs, and IACs are present and are either normal or hypoplastic. They can be differentiated from the cochlea by their position posterior to the IAC. As with labyrinthine aplasia, there is lack of cochlear promontory at the medial wall of the middle ear cavity. The labyrinthine segment of the facial nerve has a more posterior and lateral position than normal. Similar to labyrinthine aplasia, cochlear aplasia needs to be differentiated from complete cochlear ossification.

Common cavity deformity

In common cavity or cystic common cavity malformations, the cochlea, vestibule, and SCC fuse and form a common cavity of variable size (**Fig. 13**). This anomaly is commonly associated with either narrow or enlarged IAC and dysplasia of the

Table 4
Overview of various congenital inner anomalies based on the classification of Sennaroglu and Saatci[3]

Cochlear Abnormalities	Vestibular Malformations	Semicircular Canal Malformations	Internal Auditory Canal Malformations	Vestibular and Cochlear Aqueduct Anomalies
Michel deformity	Michel deformity	Absent	Absent	Enlarged
Cochlear aplasia	Common cavity deformity	Hypoplastic	Narrow	Narrow
Common cavity deformity	Absent vestibule	Enlarged	Enlarged	—
Cochlear hypoplasia	Hypoplastic vestibule	Lateral SCC-vestibule dysplasia	—	—
Incomplete partition type 1	—	Utriculosaccular anomaly	—	—
Incomplete partition type II	—	—	—	—

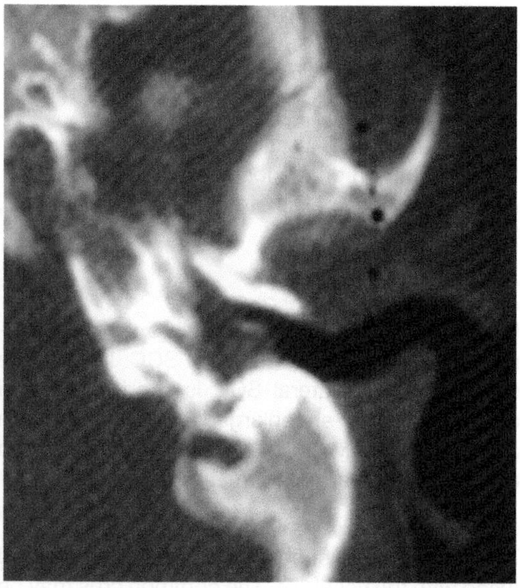

Fig. 10. Labyrinthine aplasia (Michel anomaly). Axial CT image of the left temporal bone shows complete absence of the left cochlea and vestibule, suggestive of labyrinthine aplasia or Michel anomaly.

SCC. Usually, the IAC communicates with the common cavity at its lateral end, and this may give rise to a gusher or perilymph leak during cochleostomy. The middle and external ears are well formed.

IP type I: cystic cochleovestibular malformation

Sennaroglu and colleagues[3] in 2002 suggested a classification to clearly distinguish between pseudo-Mondini (IP I) and classic Mondini (IP II) deformities. In IP I deformity, the cochlea and the vestibule have normal overall dimensions but lack internal architecture (**Fig. 14**). The cochlea is without a modiolus and appears cystic; the vestibule is also dilated without any internal structure, giving a figure-of-eight appearance. This deformity is distinct from IP II, which is discussed later. It is not associated with enlarged vestibular aqueduct. Slattery and Lungford[22] showed that the highest concentration of ganglion cells are found within the lower 1.5 turns of the cochlea. Because there are no cochlear characteristics in IP I deformity, hearing results after cochlear implantation are likely to be poorer than those seen after implantation of patients with IP II malformation. Phelps and colleagues[23] suggested a greater incidence of meningitis in IP I compared with IP II deformities.

Cochleovestibular or cochlear hypoplasia

This type of deformity (**Fig. 15**) represents an anomaly with clear differentiation of cochlea and vestibule; however, neither of these structures attains normal dimensions. The cochlea is usually hypoplastic and the vestibule may be hypoplastic or absent.

IP type II: classic mondini deformity

In this malformation there are 1.5 turns of the cochlea instead of the normal 2.75 turns. The interscalar defect is present between the middle and the apical turns, which are fused to form 1 cavity. Compared with IP I, IP II is more common, has a basal cochlear modiolus, minimal associated

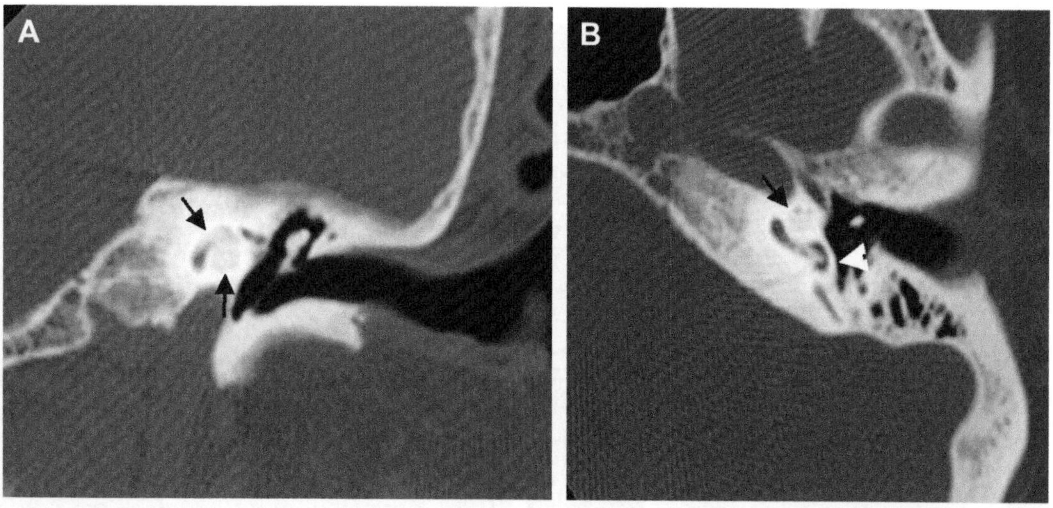

Fig. 11. Labyrinthitis ossificans. Coronal (*A*) and axial (*B*) CT images of the left temporal bone show marked ossification of the middle and apical turns (*black arrows*) of left cochlea from labyrinthitis ossificans. Note normal cochlear promontory (*arrowhead*).

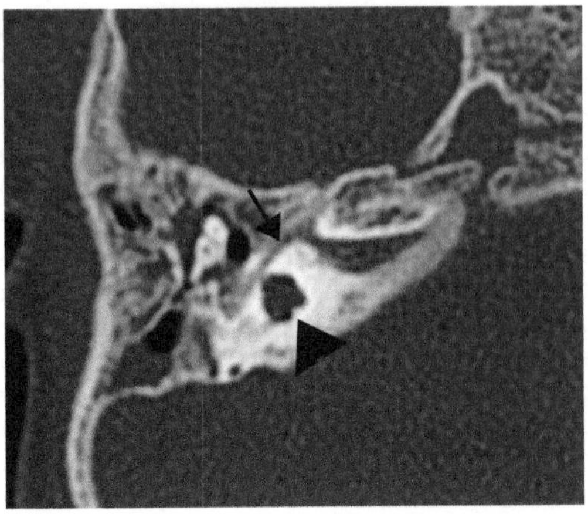

Fig. 12. Cochlear aplasia. Axial CT image of the right temporal bone shows absent cochlea. The right vestibule is dysplastic (*arrowhead*). There is a mildly anomalous course of the right facial nerve (*arrow*).

vestibular dilatation, and an enlarged vestibular aqueduct (**Fig. 16**). As discussed earlier, IP II has a lower incidence of meningitis and a better probability of hearing restoration after implantation. Association of this deformity with syndromic hearing loss such as Pendred syndrome (a common form of syndromic deafness characterized by sensorineural hearing loss and goiter) has also been reported.[24]

Vestibular Malformations

Isolated vestibular anomalies are rare. Vestibular malformations are usually associated with other anomalies such as IP I, IP II, and cochleovestibular hypoplasia.

Malformations of the SCC

- Lateral SCC-vestibule dysplasia
- Common crus anomalies
- Other anomalies of the SCC (eg, CHARGE, BOR).

Lateral SCC-vestibule dysplasia

Lateral SCC-vestibule dysplasia is one of the commonest anomalies affecting the SCC. In this type of anomaly, the lateral SCC is short and broad and fused with an enlarged vestibule to form a common cavity (**Fig. 17**A, B). The superior and posterior SCCs are of normal proportion.[10]

Common crus anomalies

The posterior and superior SCC may be broad and fused with the vestibule. The common crus may be dysplastic (see **Fig. 17**C, D).

Other anomalies of the SCC

Other subtle anomalies, such as wide, narrow, ectatic, or partial or complete absence of SCCs, have also been reported in the radiology literature.[10] Waardenburg and Alagille syndrome are associated with isolated posterior SCC aplasia.[25] Complete aplasia of all SCCs is characteristic of CHARGE anomaly (**Fig. 18**). BOR syndrome is an autosomal dominant disorder associated with abnormality of the EYA1 gene on chromosome 8 and characterized by branchial fistulae and cysts, ear abnormalities resulting in hearing loss, and renal malformations. Inner ear

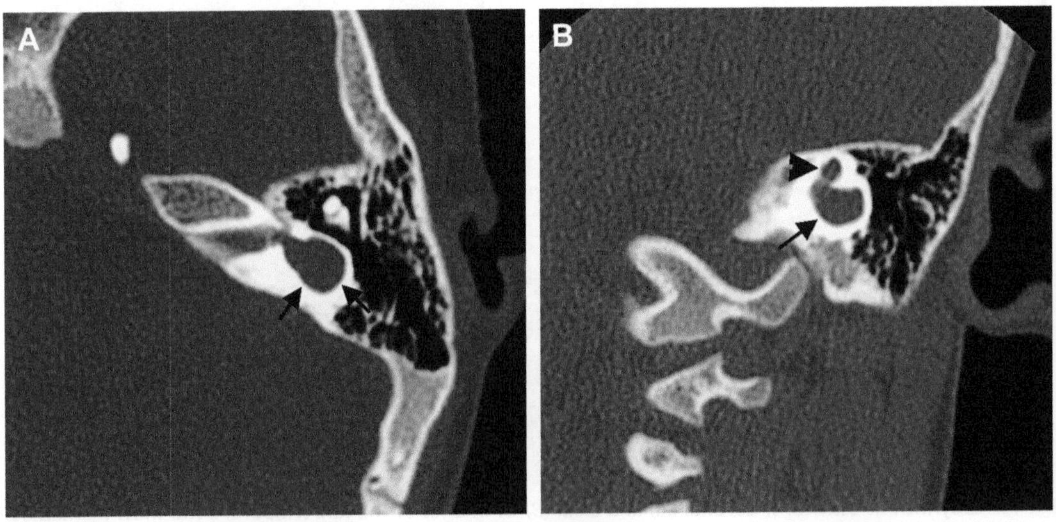

Fig. 13. Common cavity malformation. Axial (*A*) and coronal (*B*) CT images of right temporal bone shows featureless vestibule, cochlea suggestive of single cystic structure/CC (*arrows*). The SCCs are dysplastic (*arrowhead*).

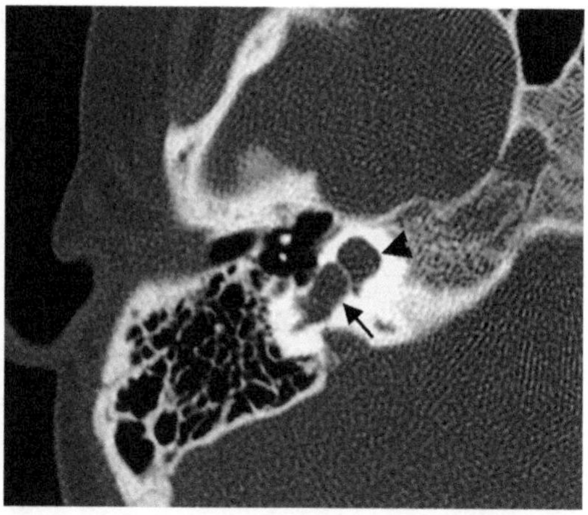

Fig. 14. IP type I (figure-of-eight malformation). Axial CT image of the right temporal bone shows cystic cochlea (*arrowhead*) and vestibule (*arrow*) with no internal structures, giving a figure-of-eight appearance. The middle ear cavity is well formed.

abnormalities include cochlear hypoplasia, hypoplasia of the lateral SCC, and enlargement of the cochlear and vestibular aqueduct (**Fig. 19**).[26]

Vestibular Aqueduct Anomalies

Enlarged vestibular aqueduct

This is one of the most frequently encountered inner ear malformations (**Fig. 20**). It may be isolated, unilateral, or bilateral. A study[10] has reported that enlarged vestibular aqueduct may be

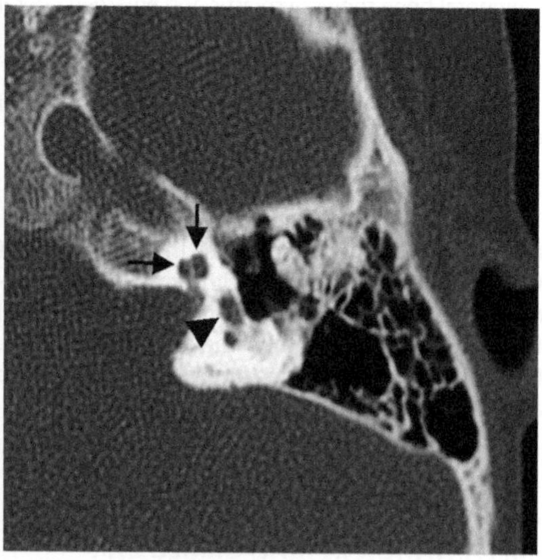

Fig. 15. Cochlear hypoplasia. Axial CT image of left temporal bone shows a small-appearing cochlea (*arrow*) and vestibule (*arrowhead*).

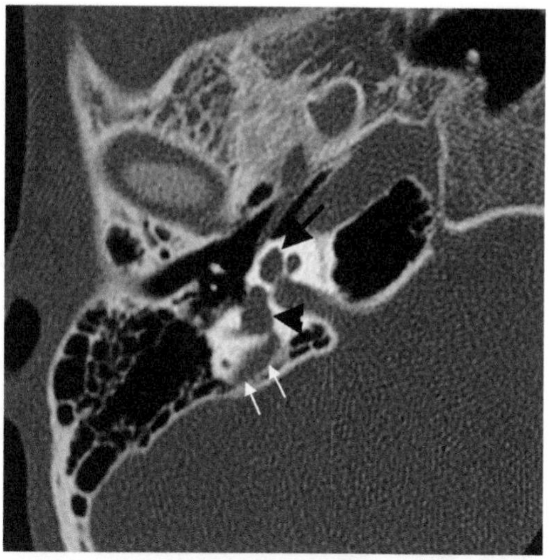

Fig. 16. IP type II (Mondini malformation). Axial CT image of the right temporal bone shows fused middle and apical turns of the cochlea (*black arrow*). The vestibule appears large (*arrowhead*) and there is an enlarged vestibular aqueduct (*white small arrows*).

associated with cochlear malformations in 76% and vestibular malformations in 40% of cases. Patients with enlarged vestibular aqueduct usually present with mixed hearing loss or progressive sensorineural deafness related to minor trauma or a minor illness, and these patients are advised to avoid contact sports.[3] This anomaly is easily identified on CT scans where the diameter of the vestibular aqueduct is compared with the diameter at the mid portion of the adjacent SCC. If the diameter of the vestibular aqueduct is larger than the SCC, a diagnosis of enlarged vestibular aqueduct is made.[3,10] Enlarged vestibular aqueduct is one of the important features of IP II[3] but is not seen in IP I malformations.

Cochlear Aqueduct Anomalies

This includes an enlarged cochlear aqueduct, but is rarely seen.[27]

Anomalies of the IAC

- Atretic IAC
- X-linked anomaly.

Atretic IAC

An atretic or stenotic IAC (<2 mm)[15] is an uncommon anomaly (**Fig. 21**). However, it is often associated with narrow or hypoplastic cochlear nerve canal and absent cochlear nerve. It therefore acquires great practical importance for surgical

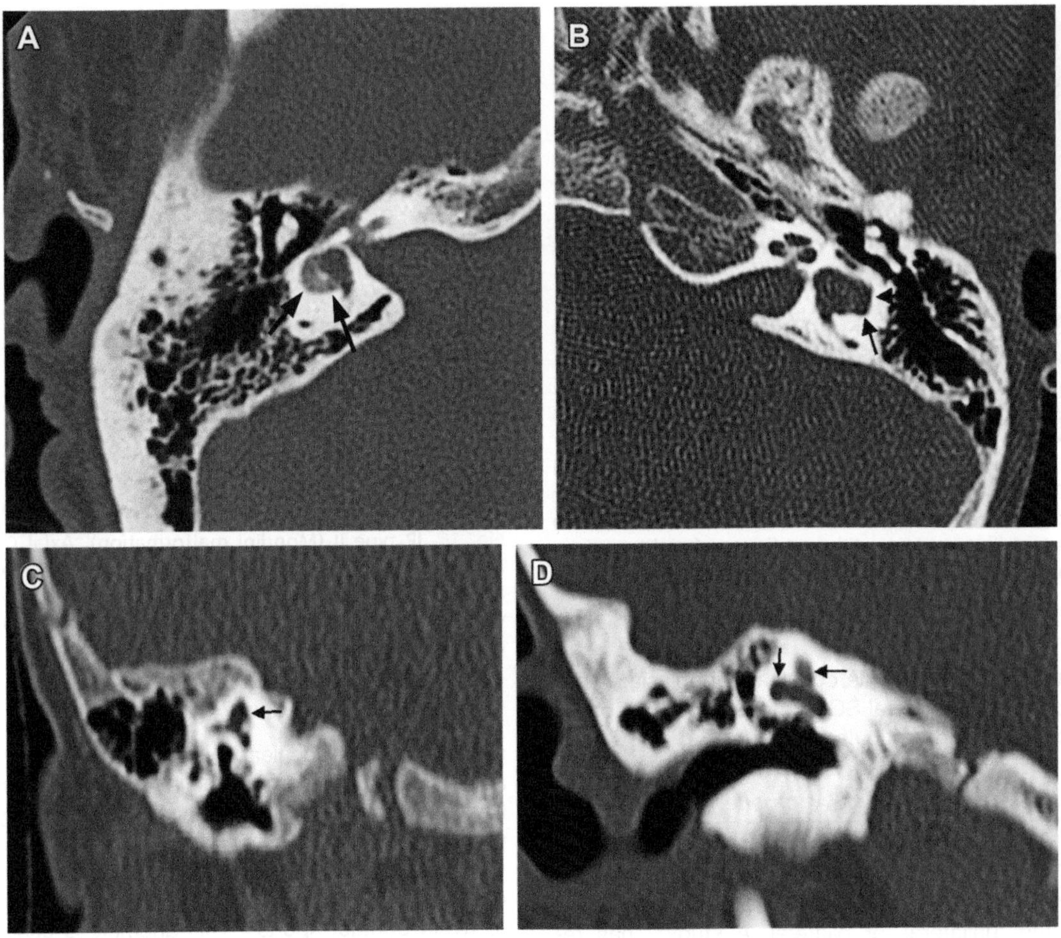

Fig. 17. Superior SCC dysplasia. (*A*) Axial CT image of the right temporal bone shows foreshortening of the lateral SCC (*arrows*), suggesting mild dysplasia. (*B*) Axial CT image of the left temporal bone in another patient shows dysplasia of the left vestibule and lateral SCC, which are fused to form a common cystic cavity (*arrows*). (*C*) Coronal CT image of the right temporal bone shows dysplastic and enlarged common crus of the right posterior and superior SCC (*arrow*). (*D*) Coronal CT image of the right temporal bone shows dysplastic and enlarged lateral SCC and the common crus of the posterior and superior SCC (*arrows*).

consideration. Both CT and T2-weighted gradient echo MR imaging can show the narrow IAC, but the VII and VIII nerves can only be evaluated by thin, heavily T2-weighted MR imaging, with sections perpendicular to the IAC (**Fig. 22**). Three different types of atretic IAC can be distinguished on imaging studies.[28] Each of the 3 anomalies has a different potential for cochlear implantation. Further, the facial nerve follows an aberrant course in each of these anomalies. Type 1 malformation has a stenotic IAC with absent VIII nerve. In type 2 malformation, a common VIII nerve is seen in addition to the stenotic IAC, but there is hypoplasia or aplasia of its cochlear division. When a type 2 anomaly is associated with other inner ear malformations, it is referred to as type 2A, and it is called type 2B when the inner ear is normal. Type 2 patients usually have residual hearing or unilateral involvement that usually precludes them from cochlear implantation surgery.

X-linked anomaly

This anomaly (**Fig. 23**) is a rare condition characterized by bulbous dilatation of the lateral end of the IAC.[29] It is associated with profound sensorineural deafness and there is a risk of cerebrospinal fluid (CSF) gusher at the time of cochleostomy. Flattening of the first genu of the facial canal is an additional finding in this condition.

SPECIFIC CONSIDERATIONS AND COMPLICATIONS OF COCHLEAR IMPLANTATION IN MALFORMED EAR

For experienced clinicians, malformed cochleae are no longer considered contraindications to

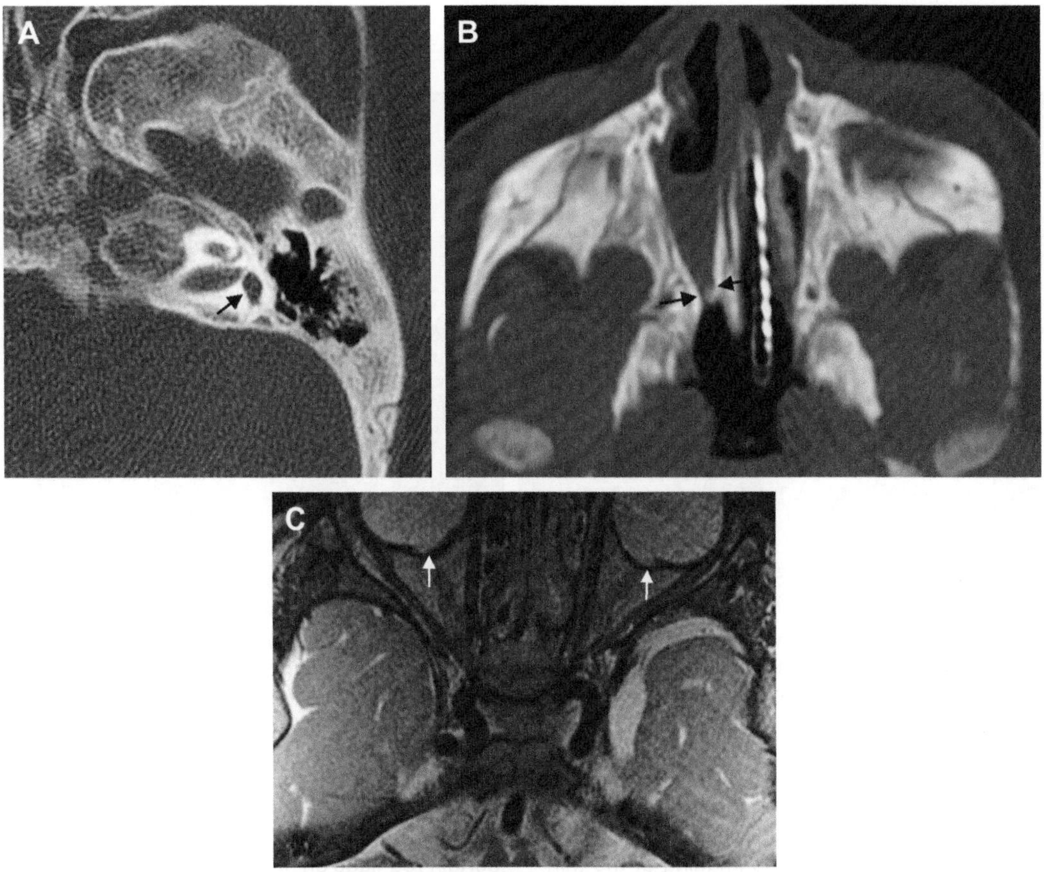

Fig. 18. CHARGE syndrome. (*A*) Axial CT image of the left temporal bone shows absence of all SCC with mild dysplasia of the left vestibule (*arrow*). (*B*) Axial CT image through the level of midface shows right posterior choanal atresia (*arrows*). (*C*) Axial T2-weighted MR imaging shows small colobomas along the posterior aspects of bilateral globes (*white arrows*).

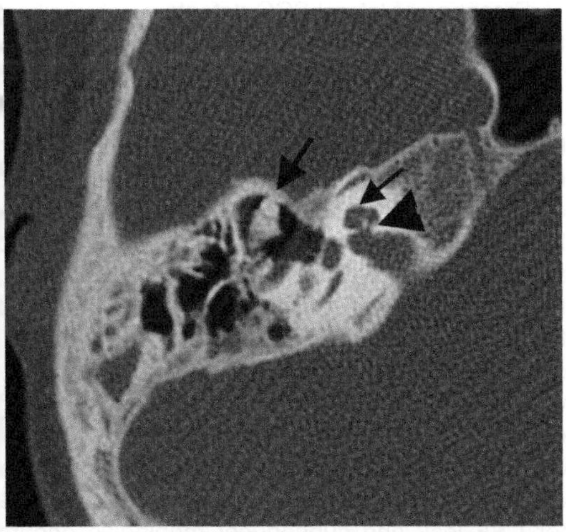

Fig. 19. Branchio-oto-renal syndrome. Axial CT image of the right temporal bone in a patient with branchio-oto-renal syndrome shows hypoplastic apical turn of the cochlea (*small arrow*). The cochlear modiolus does not appear like a square suggesting hypoplasia (*arrowhead*). Also note the short and calcified superior ligament with more anterior position of the middle ear ossicles than expected (*big arrow*).

cochlear implantation surgery. However caution is needed when certain anomalies are encountered. It may be necessary to distinguish between complete aplasia (Michel deformity) and postmeningitic labyrinthitis ossificans before attempting surgery. In patients with stenotic IAC, MR imaging is mandatory to assess integrity of the VIII nerve.[30] Perhaps the most important factor is the surgeon's skill to improvise on standard surgical approaches for cochlear implantation and the ability to deal with complications. It is possible to perform the standard mastoidectomy and facial recess approach for many patients with inner ear anomalies.[31,32] The use of alternate approaches is centered around the need for better exposure and avoidance of damage to a potentially abnormal facial nerve. Perilymph or CSF leaks are commonly (40%–50%) encountered in cochlear implantation surgery in children with malformed inner ears.[3] It is most commonly seen in children with common cavity deformity (37.5%).[10] The leak occurs because of a defect in the lateral bony end of the IAC allowing a clear communication between the CSF and the perilymph. In some common cavity ears, the defect

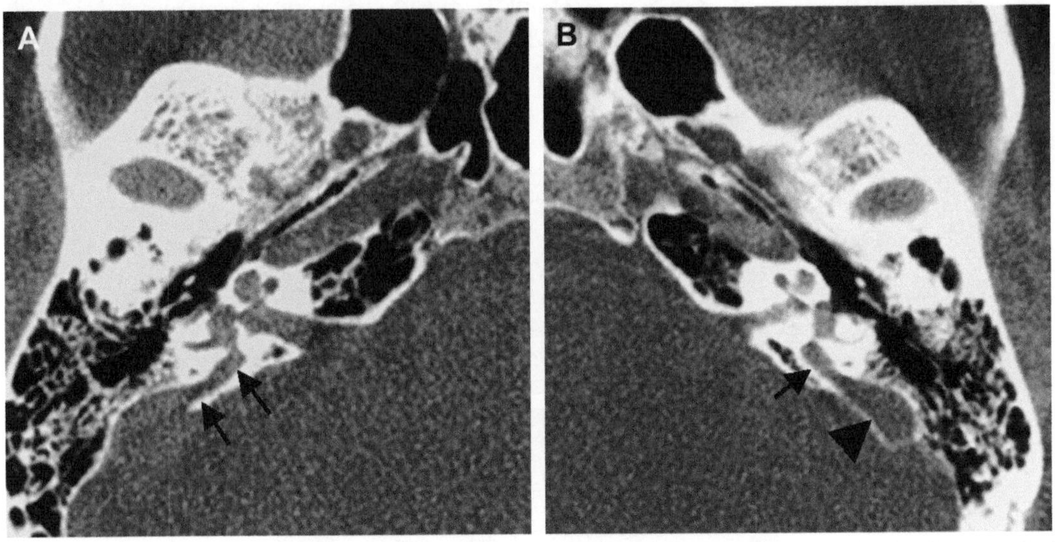

Fig. 20. Enlarged vestibular aqueduct syndrome. Axial CT images on the right (*A*) and left (*B*) side respectively show bilaterally enlarged vestibular aqueducts (*arrows*) and prominent endolymphatic sacs (*arrowhead*). Sudden hearing loss after head trauma is seen in these patients and they should be advised to avoid contact sports.

is wide enough to be picked up on CT scans. At present, it is difficult to identify small defects on CT because of partial volume imaging of the thin bony plate of the lateral fundus.[1] Patients with IP II deformity have apical modiolar defect and enlarged vestibular aqueduct. These patients may also have perilymph ooze during surgery related to abnormal endolymph pressures.[30] There are certain red flags on radiology that should raise the suspicion of a potential CSF leak:

1. Cochlear hypoplasia
2. Common cavity
3. Mondini deformity
4. Enlarged vestibular aqueduct
5. Presence of lateral SCC defects
6. Any case with modiolar deficiency.

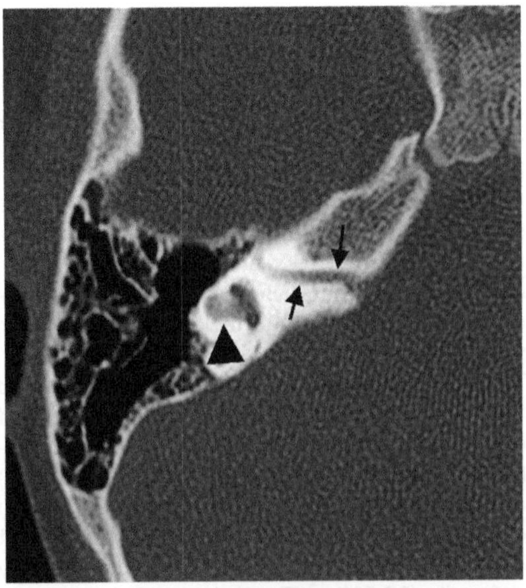

Fig. 21. Narrow IAC. Axial CT image of right temporal bone shows a narrow internal auditory canal (*arrows*). The patient had dysplastic vestibule and SCC which is partially seen (*arrowhead*).

Abnormalities in the course of the facial nerve (**Fig. 24**) are seen in 14% to 16% of children with inner ear malformations.[33] The aberrant nerve characteristically runs below the processus cochleariformis and then across the promontory to reach the round window. In X-linked deafness, the main facial trunk is hypoplastic and the aberrant facial nerve may have several different abnormal courses. Facial nerve anomalies occur commonly with common cavity, hypoplastic cochleae, and children with craniofacial syndromes.[10] The risk of meningitis with certain types of cochlear dysplasia is well known.[4,22,34] A potential space for CSF leak and subsequent meningitis occurs between the subarachnoid space of the IAC and the middle ear cavity because of a defect in the lateral wall of the IAC. Cochlear abnormalities that are associated with increased risk of meningitis include enlarged vestibular aqueduct, common cavity, and IP I malformations. Except for enlarged vestibular aqueduct, both common cavity and IP I

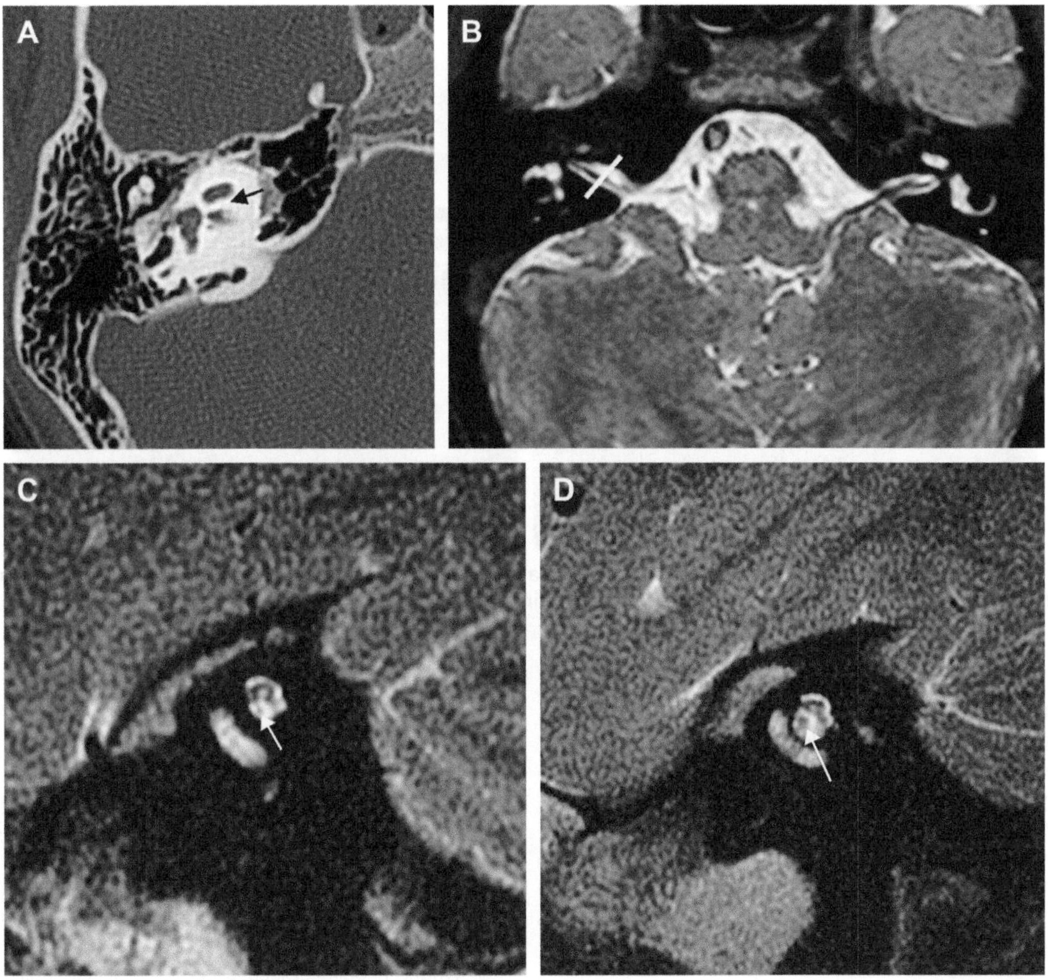

Fig. 22. Cochlear nerve canal hypoplasia. Axial CT image (*A*) of the right temporal bone markedly small cochlear nerve canal in its expected location (*arrow*). Such patients should undergo MR imaging to look for cochlear nerve abnormality. Axial (*B*) T2-weighted MR imaging through the level of the internal auditory canal with oblique sagittal image (*C*) at the level of mid portion (*solid white line*) of the right IAC shows small and hypoplastic dot of cochlear nerve at anterior inferior aspect (*arrow*). (*D*) Compare with normal 4 nerves in IAC, with normal cochlear division at the anterior inferior corner (*arrow*).

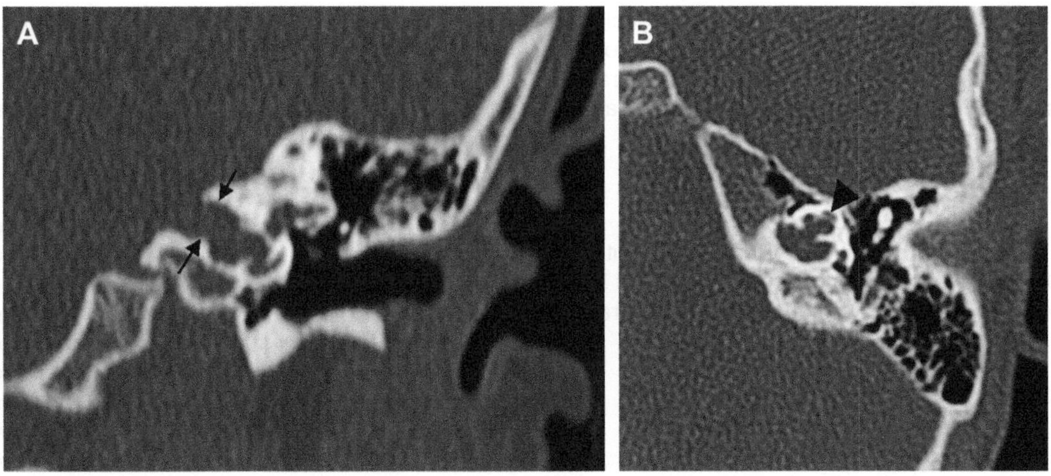

Fig. 23. X-linked anomaly. Coronal (*A*) and axial (*B*) CT images of the left temporal bone show wide patulous IAC (*arrows*) with dysplastic cochlea (*arrowhead*) with absent cochlear modiolus. These patients are at increased risk for perilymphatic hydrops and a gusher if the stapes is disturbed.

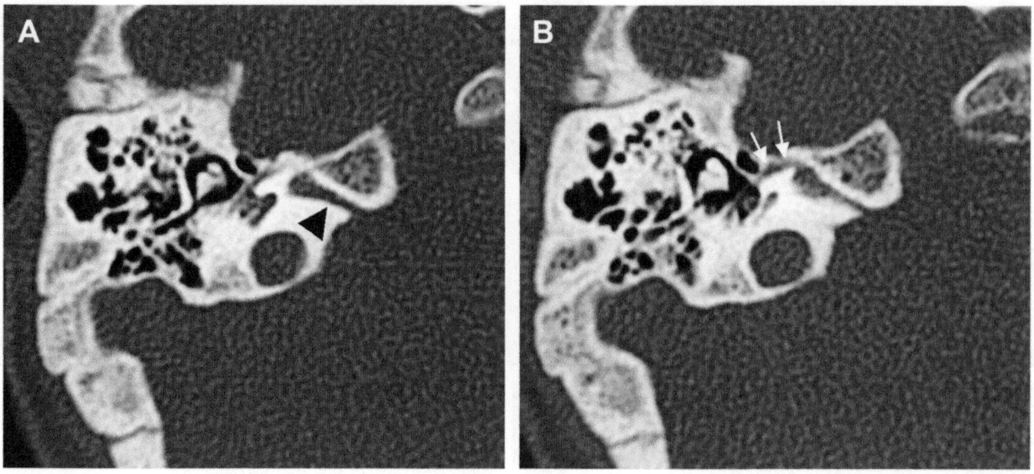

Fig. 24. Facial nerve canal dysplasia. Axial CT image in a patient with common cavity malformation shows anomalous course of the IAC (*A*) (*arrowhead*) and labyrinthine segment (*B*) of right facial nerve (*arrows*).

anomalies have a deficient basal turn of the cochlea as well as deficient modiolus. Phelps and colleagues[23] in 1994, in a paper on cochlear dysplasia and meningitis, strongly asserted that, with normal basal turn of the cochlea, there is no potential for an abnormal communication between the IAC and the middle ear.

SUMMARY

Temporal bone malformations are common and, with newer imaging techniques, even subtle deformities can now be identified. External ear and middle ear malformations occur more commonly together, whereas inner ear malformations are likely to occur independently because of the different embryogenesis of the outer, middle, and inner ears. A multidisciplinary approach including the pediatricians, geneticists, otolaryngologists, radiologists, and audiology and speech therapists is the standard of care for management of patients with temporal bone malformations.

ACKNOWLEDGMENTS

The authors thank Cheryl Langford, Editor III, Department of Otolaryngology, University of Texas Medical Branch, Galveston, TX for the illustrations used in this article.

REFERENCES

1. Graham JM, Phelps PD, Michaels L. Congenital malformations of the ear and cochlear implantation in children: review and temporal bone report of common cavity. J Laryngol Otol Suppl 2000;25:1–14.
2. Weber BP, Dillo W, Dietrich B, et al. Pediatric cochlear implantation in cochlear malformations. Am J Otol 1998;19:747–53.
3. Sennaroglu L, Saatci I. A new classification for cochleovestibular malformations. Laryngoscope 2002; 112:2230–41.
4. Park AH, Kou B, Hotaling A, et al. Clinical course of pediatric congenital inner ear malformations. Laryngoscope 2000;110:1715–9.
5. Wright T, editor. Diseases of the ear. 6th edition. London: Arnold; 1998.
6. Schucknecht H, editor. Pathology of the ear. 2nd edition. Philadelphia: Lea and Febiger; 1993.
7. Hasso A, Casselman J, Broadwell R. Temporal bone congenital anomalies. In: Som P, Curtin H, editors. Head and neck imaging. St Louis (MO): Mosby; 1996. p. 1351–90.
8. Kösling S, Omenzetter M, Bartel-Friedrich S. Congenital malformations of the external and middle ear. Eur J Radiol 2009;69:269–79.
9. Digoy GP, Cueva RA. Congenital aural atresia: review of short- and long-term surgical results. Otol Neurotol 2007;28:54–60.
10. Casselman JW, Offeciers EF, De Foer B, et al. CT and MR imaging of congenital abnormalities of the inner ear and internal auditory canal. Eur J Radiol 2001;40:94–104.
11. Ishimoto S, Ito K, Yamasoba T, et al. Correlation between microtia and temporal bone malformation evaluated using grading systems. Arch Otolaryngol Head Neck Surg 2005;131:326–9.
12. Westerhof JP, Rademaker J, Weber BP, et al. Congenital malformations of the inner ear and the vestibulocochlear nerve in children with sensorineural hearing loss: evaluation with CT and MRI. J Comput Assist Tomogr 2001;25:719–26.

13. Mayer TE, Brueckmann H, Siegert R, et al. High-resolution CT of the temporal bone in dysplasia of the auricle and external auditory canal. AJNR Am J Neuroradiol 1997;18:53–65.
14. Jahrsdoerfer RA, Yeakley JW, Aguilar EA, et al. Grading system for the selection of patients with congenital aural atresia. Am J Otol 1992;13:6–12.
15. Phelps PD, Annis JA, Robinson PJ. Imaging for cochlear implants. Br J Radiol 1990;63:512–6.
16. Benton C, Bellet PS. Imaging of congenital anomalies of the temporal bone. Neuroimaging Clin N Am 2000;10:35–53.
17. Schuknecht HF. Congenital aural atresia. Laryngoscope 1989;99:908–17.
18. Robson CD, Robertson RL, Barnes PD. Imaging of pediatric temporal bone abnormalities. Neuroimaging Clin N Am 1999;9:133–55.
19. Aguilar EA III. Congenital auricular malformations. In: Bailey BJ, editor. Head and neck surgery–otolaryngology. Philadelphia: Lippincott Williams & Wilkins; 2001. p. 2374–87.
20. Smith SD, Harker LA. Single gene influences on radiologically–detectable malformations of the inner ear. J Commun Disord 1998;31:391–408.
21. Giesemann AM, Goetz F, Neuburger J, et al. From labyrinthine aplasia to otocyst deformity. Neuroradiology 2010;52:147–54.
22. Slattery WH 3rd, Luxford WM. Cochlear implantation in the congenital malformed cochlea. Laryngoscope 1995;105:1184–7.
23. Phelps PD, King A, Michaels L. Cochlear dysplasia and meningitis. Am J Otol 1994;15:551–7.
24. Phelps PD, Coffey RA, Trembath RC, et al. Radiological malformations of the ear in Pendred syndrome. Clin Radiol 1998;53:268–73.
25. Okuno T, Takahashi H, Shibahara Y, et al. Temporal bone histopathologic findings in Alagille's syndrome. Arch Otolaryngol Head Neck Surg 1990;116:217–20.
26. Propst EJ, Blaser S, Gordon KA, et al. Temporal bone findings on computed tomography imaging in branchio–oto–renal syndrome. Laryngoscope 2005;115:1855–62.
27. Jackler RK, Hwang PH. Enlargement of the cochlear aqueduct: fact or fiction? Otolaryngol Head Neck Surg 1993;109:14–25.
28. Casselman JW, Offeciers FE, Govaerts PJ, et al. Aplasia and hypoplasia of the vestibulocochlear nerve: diagnosis with MR imaging. Radiology 1997;202:773–81.
29. Phelps PD, Reardon W, Pembrey M, et al. X–linked deafness, stapes gushers and a distinctive defect of the inner ear. Neuroradiology 1991;33(4):326–30.
30. Sennaroglu L, Sarac S, Ergin T. Surgical results of cochlear implantation in malformed cochlea. Otol Neurotol 2006;27:615–23.
31. Papsin BC. Cochlear implantation in children with anomalous cochleovestibular anatomy. Laryngoscope 2005;115:1–26.
32. McElveen JT Jr, Carrasco VN, Miyamoto RT, et al. Cochlear implantation in common cavity malformations using a transmastoid labyrinthotomy approach. Laryngoscope 1997;107:1032–6.
33. Gray RF, Ray J, Baguley DM, et al. Cochlear implant failure due to unexpected absence of the eighth nerve–a cautionary tale. J Laryngol Otol 1998;112:646–9.
34. Phelps PD, Proops D, Sellars S, et al. Congenital cerebrospinal fluid fistula through the inner ear and meningitis. J Laryngol Otol 1993;107:492–5.

Congenital Cystic Lesions of the Head and Neck

Mohannad Ibrahim, MD[a,*], Khaled Hammoud, MS[b], Mohit Maheshwari, MD[c], Amit Pandya, MD[a]

KEYWORDS

- Congenital neck lesions • Cystic neck masses
- Head and neck masses • Thyroglossal duct cysts
- Cystic hygroma • Thymic cysts • Bronchogenic cysts

Congenital cervical cystic masses comprise an uncommon group of lesions that is usually encountered during infancy and childhood. The prevalence of these lesions varies from common (thyroglossal duct cysts, branchial cleft cysts, and cystic hygromas) to very rare (thymic and cervical bronchogenic cysts). The absolute number remains unknown. Thyroglossal duct (TGD) cysts are the most common mass found in the midline of the neck in children.[1] Anomalies of the branchial apparatus include branchial, thymic, and parathyroid anomalies, which may manifest as cysts, sinuses, fistulae, and ectopic glands.[2]

Clinical history and physical examination of the patient are important elements in the evaluation of a suspected congenital neck mass (**Table 1**). Familiarity with the embryology and anatomy of the cervical region frequently allows the differential diagnosis to be narrowed. Congenital cervical cystic lesions are usually slow-growing masses and typically cause symptoms only due to enlargement or infection. A painless soft or fluctuant cervical mass is the first clinical manifestation in most cases.

Following physical examination, ultrasonography (US) is usually performed. US helps to confirm the cystic nature of the lesion and extent of the mass, and to demonstrate its relationship to surrounding normal structures. Computed tomography (CT) also provides this information, and is ideally suited for evaluation of larger masses that cannot be entirely visualized with US. Moreover, CT is superior for detecting calcification and, when contrast material is administered, the vascularity of lesions. Magnetic resonance (MR) imaging demonstrates the full extent of the mass and provides important supplemental information for accurate preoperative planning. This information can be especially relevant in cases of extension into the mediastinum or deep spaces of the neck. Furthermore, MR imaging offers superior resolution for evaluating masses located in anatomically complex areas, such as the floor of the mouth.

THYROGLOSSAL DUCT CYST

Embryology

During the fourth week of gestation, the thyroid gland originates as a diverticulum from the floor of the pharynx (tuberculum impar) at a site that later becomes the foramen cecum of the base of the tongue.[3] The gland then grows caudally into the loose prepharyngeal connective tissues, just anterior to or through the eventual location of the hyoid bone, to rest in the lower midline of the neck. As the gland moves downward, it leaves behind an epithelial trace attached to the foramen cecum, known as the thyroglossal tract. The thyroglossal tract runs ventral to the developing hyoid

[a] Department of Radiology, University of Michigan Health System, 1500 East Medical Center Drive, Ann Arbor, MI 48109-0302, USA
[b] College of Human Medicine, Michigan State University, Lansing, MI 48824, USA
[c] Department of Radiology, Medical College of Wisconsin, Milwaukee, WI 53226, USA
* Corresponding author.
E-mail address: mibrahim@umich.edu

Neuroimag Clin N Am 21 (2011) 621–639
doi:10.1016/j.nic.2011.05.006
1052-5149/11/$ – see front matter

Table 1
Clinical features of congenital cervical lesions

Lesion	Peak Prevalence (Age in Years)	Sex Predilection	Usual Location
Thyroglossal duct cyst	<10	Equal	Hyoid level or below (80%), within 2 cm of midline
Branchial cleft cyst			
First	Middle age	F > M	Parotid, external auditory canal
Second	10–40	Equal	Upper neck, mandibular angle, lateral to carotid vessels
Third	10–30	—	Left posterior cervical triangle
Fourth	Any age	—	Sinus tract arising from left pyriform sinus
Cystic hygroma	<2	Equal	Posterior cervical triangle, oral cavity
Dermoid cyst	10–30	Equal	Floor of mouth
Epidermoid cyst	Infancy	Equal	Floor of mouth
Thymic cyst	2–13	M > F	Low anterolateral neck (L > R)
Bronchogenic cyst	Any age	M > F	Low anterolateral neck

Abbreviations: F, female; L, left; M, male; R, right.

bone, then assumes a curved course behind it, as the hyoid bone rotates and takes its adult position. It then continues downward anterior to the thyrohyoid membrane. The thyroglossal duct generally obliterates between the fifth and tenth week of gestation, leaving behind a proximal remnant at the foramen cecum (at the base of the tongue) and a distal remnant (pyramidal lobe of the thyroid). The duct is intimately associated with developing hyoid bone, either within the periosteum of the hyoid bone or even passing through it.[4,5] Failure of the thyroglossal duct to obliterate before the formation of the mesodermal anlage of the hyoid bone results in its persistence during development and after birth. An embryologically defined line extending from the tongue base to the thyroid gland determines the site of anomalies of the thyroglossal duct (**Fig. 1**). The majority of thyroglossal duct cysts are either juxtahyoid or infrahyoid.[1,5]

Thyroglossal duct anomalies constitute the vast majority of congenital midline cervical masses seen in children, accounting for 70% of congenital neck anomalies,[1] and the second most common benign neck mass in pediatric patients after benign lymphadenopathy.[6] About 50% of patients present before 20 years of age, with a second group of patients presenting in young adulthood.[5,7] No gender predilection has been reported.[1,5] Rare cases of hereditary thyroglossal duct cysts have been reported; typically these cysts have an autosomal dominant pattern of transmission and occur in prepubertal girls.[8]

Clinical Characteristics

TGD cysts are epithelial remnants of the thyroglossal tract located adjacent to the hyoid bone (60%), between the hyoid bone and base of the tongue (24%), between the hyoid bone and pyramidal lobe of the thyroid gland (13%); the remainder

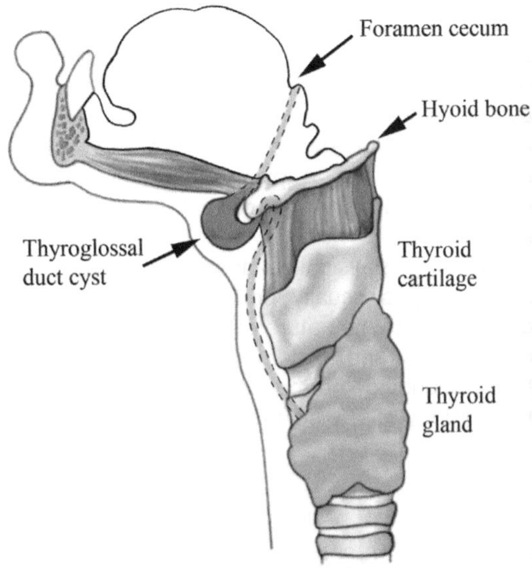

Fig. 1. Thyroglossal duct (TGD) pathway. Embryologic thyroglossal duct from the foramen cecum through the developing hyoid bone to the pyramidal lobe of the thyroid.

are intralingual (3%).[1,5] TGD cysts are located in the midline (75%) or slightly off-midline (25%) in the anterior neck, usually within 2 cm of the midline.[1] Of the lesions in a paramedian location, most will occur on the left for unclear reasons.[1]

The TGD cyst arises as a cystic expansion of a remnant of the thyroglossal duct tract.[1] The stimulus for the expansion is not known; one postulate is that lymphoid tissue is associated with the tract hypertrophies at the time of a regional infection, thereby occluding the tract with resultant cyst formation.[9] The majority of patients have a history of a preceding upper respiratory tract infection.[5] A retention phenomenon with blocked thyroglossal duct and accumulation of secretions has been described as another possibility.[10]

Patients with TGD cysts usually present with a palpable asymptomatic midline neck mass in a pediatric or young adult patient at or below the level of the hyoid bone.[1,5] Midline location and close association with the hyoid bone are the only nearly universal traits of these lesions. The mass moves during swallowing or on protrusion of the tongue, due to its attachment to the tongue via the tract of thyroid descent. Some patients will have neck or throat pain, or dysphagia.[1] Up to half of TGD cysts are not diagnosed until adult life.[5] TGD anomalies occur in approximately 7% of the population, although only a minority of these is ever symptomatic.[11] The tract can lie dormant for years or even decades until a stimulus leads to cystic dilation. Many cystic remnants of the thyroglossal tract are never detected clinically. Infection can sometimes cause the transient appearance of a mass or enlargement of the cyst, at times with periodic recurrences. Spontaneous drainage may also occur.[5]

Approximately 15% to 33.8% of thyroglossal anomalies present as fistulae.[1] The fistulous openings are almost always considered to be a secondary feature, resulting from infection with either a spontaneous or a surgical drainage.[1] Congenital fistulae in the newborn have been described.[5,12] Approximately 1% to 2% of patients presenting with TGD cysts have an ectopic thyroid gland within the wall of the cyst.[13]

Radiologic Features

At sonography, TGD cysts have a variable, complex sonographic pattern ranging from a typical anechoic to pseudosolid appearance.[14] The finding of an anechoic mass with no perceptible or thin outer wall in the midline anterior neck is characteristic of a thyroglossal duct cyst (**Fig. 2**A, B). However, this classic appearance is seen in less than half of the cases.[14] More commonly, these cysts appear as homogeneous or heterogeneous complex hypoechoic masses, often with increased through-transmission.[14] The cysts may have variable degrees of fine to coarse internal echoes and, infrequently, septa.[14,15] Hyperechoic, pseudosolid appearance is occasionally seen in adults; however, their cystic nature is only confirmed with posterior enhancement or shift of the lesion's content after application of transducer pressure (see **Fig. 2**C).[15] There is no correlation between the sonographic appearance and pathologic evidence of hemorrhage, infection, and inflammation.[14] Heterogeneity seen in thyroglossal duct cysts on sonography is more likely due to the proteinaceous content of the fluid secreted from the cyst wall rather than to infection.[14] Preoperative sonographic visualization of normal thyroid tissue is sufficient to exclude a diagnosis of ectopic thyroid tissue and obviates routine thyroid scintigraphy.[14]

A low-density cystic midline mass is usually seen on CT scan along the expected course of the thyroglossal duct with a smooth, thin, well-defined wall (**Fig. 3**). The mass has homogeneous low attenuation, the values of which correspond to those of fluid (10–18 HU). Elevated attenuation values of the fluid cyst reflect increased protein content and generally correlate with a history of prior infection.[16] Although thyroglossal duct cysts are usually unilocular, septations may be seen occasionally. A peripheral rim of enhancement is usually seen on contrast-enhanced scans.[16] The fascial planes adjacent to the cyst can be preserved. Abnormal fascial planes, manifesting as thickening of the platysma or strap muscle with cutaneous thickening and induration of the subcutaneous fat, are usually related to postinflammatory changes (**Fig. 4**).[16]

An uncomplicated thyroglossal duct cyst has low signal intensity on T1-weighted images and is hyperintense on T2-weighted images, findings that reflect its fluid content. The rim will be nonenhancing unless inflammation is present.[17] Unlike the wall of the cyst, the cyst's contents will not enhance. In case of infection or hemorrhage, a thick irregular rim may be visualized, and the signal intensity of the fluid becomes variable, related to the presence of proteinaceous debris.

BRANCHIAL CLEFT CYST

A variety of congenital anomalies of branchial origin are found in the neck region, including sinus, fistula, or cyst.[11] Branchial anomalies comprise approximately 30% of congenital neck masses.[11]

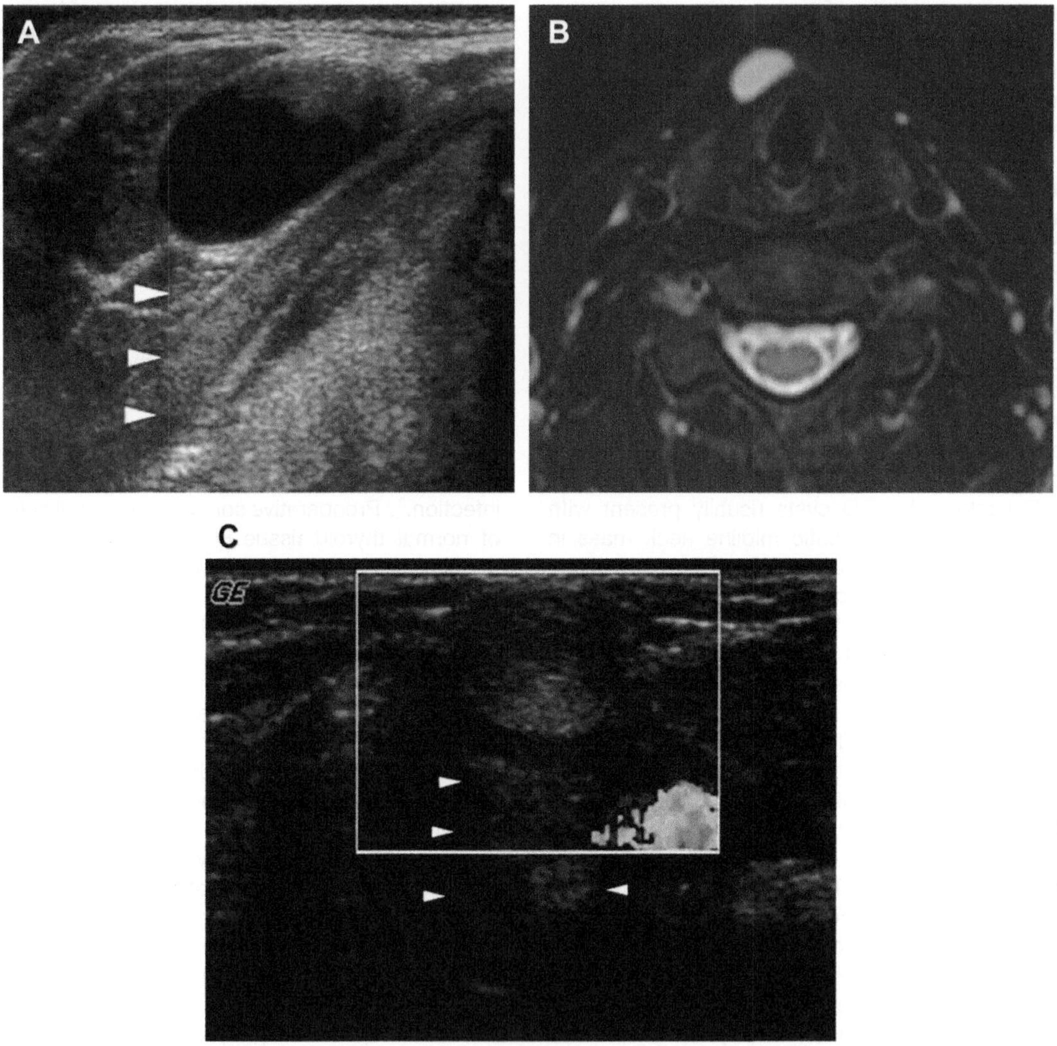

Fig. 2. TGD cyst in a 29-year-old woman with neck mass. (*A*) Ultrasonography demonstrates anechoic, avascular lesion with minimal posterior enhancement (*arrowheads*). (*B*) Axial T2-weighted image in the same patient confirms the cystic nature of the lesion with high T2 signal. (*C*) Ultrasonography in a different patient with TGD cyst. The lesion is hyperechoic with posterior enhancement (*arrowheads*), confirming the cystic nature of the lesion.

A branchial cyst is defined as a cyst with no internal or external openings. A branchial sinus has an external or internal opening, and may or may not have a cyst connected to it. Branchial sinuses with external openings are usually associated with the first and second branchial anomalies. Third and fourth branchial anomalies are usually associated with branchial sinuses with internal openings. A branchial fistula has both an internal and external opening. The majority of the branchial lesions manifest as cyst (75%), fistula (25%), or as skin tags (1%).[7] Patients with branchial cleft cysts are usually older children or young adults, in contrast to patients with fistulae, who are usually infants or young children.

Embryology

During the fourth through the seventh weeks of human embryonic development, 6 paired branchial arches appear and disappear forming the lower face and neck.[18,19] Separating the 6 arches are 5 paired ectodermal-lined branchial clefts (grooves) and 5 endodermal-lined pharyngeal pouches. A closing membrane is present at the interface of the pharyngeal pouches and the branchial clefts.[18,19] The external auditory canal normally forms from the first cleft; and the tympanic cavity, mastoid air cell, and Eustachian tube form from the first pouch. The palatine tonsil and tonsillar fossa develop from the second pouch,

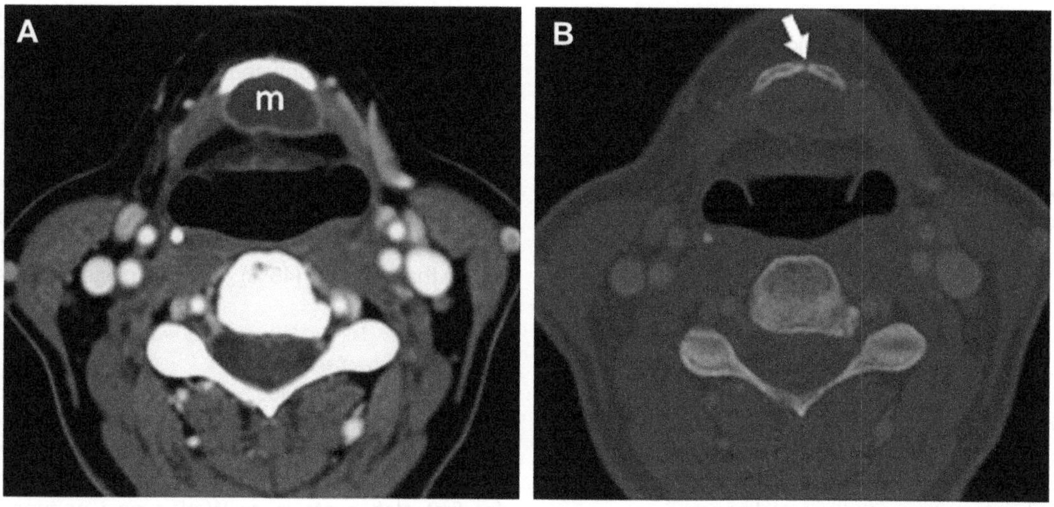

Fig. 3. TGD cyst in a 52-year-old woman. (*A*) Axial contrast-enhanced CT scan shows a hypoattenuated cystic mass (m) in the anterior midline of the neck just posterior to the hyoid bone. (*B*) Axial CT scan with bone windows demonstrating a tiny notch (*arrow*) within the central aspect of the hyoid bone.

with the second cleft normally disappearing completely.

Numerous theories have been offered to explain the pathogenesis of congenital cervical cysts.[20] It is possible that there are in fact several different mechanisms by which the cysts are formed in the lateral aspect of the neck. The most widely accepted hypothesis for their development is incomplete obliteration of the branchial apparatus, primarily the cleft; in the case of sinuses or fistulae, the closing membrane and pouch are implicated as well. Cystic changes in regional lymph nodes caused by epithelial entrapment within the node at the time of development have also been implicated in the development of lateral cervical cysts.[21] Persistence of vestiges of the precervical sinus was also proposed as the source of these anomalies. Some investigators doubt a common etiology between the cysts and sinuses, though many surgeons believe that congenital lateral cervical sinuses and fistulae result from the branchial apparatus.

Despite the different theories on the origin of congenital cervical cysts, the most popularly believed concerns branchial remnants, with anomalies of the second branchial apparatus comprising

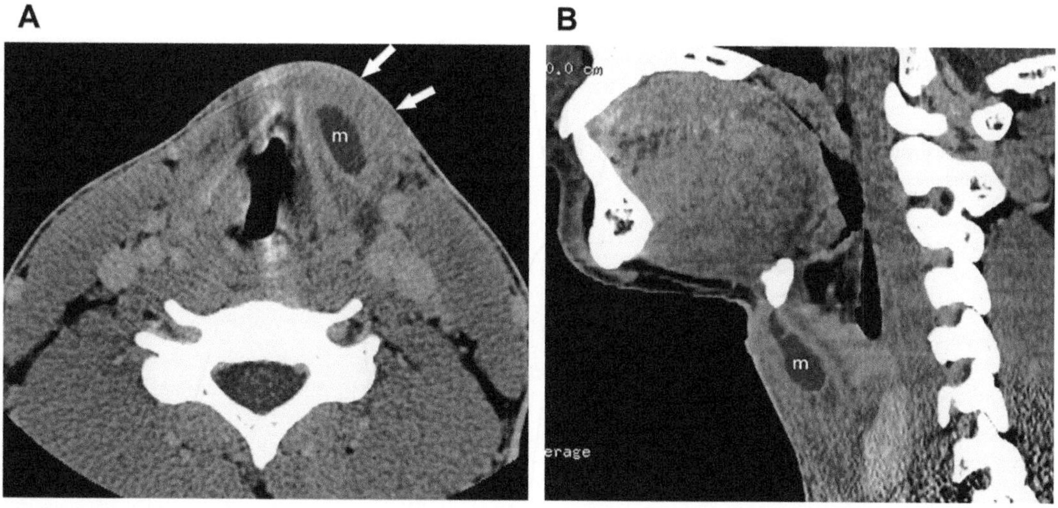

Fig. 4. Infected thyroglossal duct cyst in a 10-year-old boy. Axial (*A*) and reformatted sagittal (*B*) contrast-enhanced CT scans show a hypoattenuated mass (m) in the left strap muscles. There is enhancing rim with thickening of the muscle and subcutaneous induration (*arrows*).

the majority of these lesions.[22] As the head and neck develop, the second branchial arch overgrows the second, third, and fourth branchial clefts, finally fusing with the lateral branchial wall (**Fig. 5**). In the process, an ectoderm-lined cavity called the cervical sinus of His is formed. The incomplete obliteration of the cervical sinus plays an important role in the development of second branchial cleft anomalies. An embryologically defined line extending from the oropharyngeal tonsillar fossa to the supraclavicular region of the neck defines the site of anomalies of the second branchial cleft.[23] Anomalies of the first branchial cleft can occur anywhere along a residual embryologic tract extending from the submandibular triangle and terminating at the cartilaginous/bony junction of the external auditory canal, coursing through the parotid gland and variably interacting with the facial nerve.[23]

First Branchial Cleft Cyst

Closure of the first branchial cleft is concurrent with the emergence of the developing parotid gland and migration of the facial nerve; thus, first branchial cleft anomalies are typically closely related to these structures.[2] These anomalies can be extraparotid or can be related to the parotid gland, particularly the superficial lobe. These lesions may be confused with preauricular pits and sinuses, which result from failure of the auricular hillocks to fuse. Such lesions account for only 5% to 8% of all branchial clef defects[24] and are most commonly seen in middle-aged women.[25] Lesions have been classified as fistula, sinus, or cyst. Fistulae occur slightly more commonly (52%) than sinuses (48%), whereas cysts are least common.[26]

Clinical characteristics

The cystic anomalies classically present as enlarging mass near the lower pole of the parotid gland, or as a mass along the external auditory canal. The most common classification system for first cleft cysts is as Work type I or type II lesions (**Fig. 6**).[27] Type I lesions are described as duplications of the membranous external auditory canal, and contain ectodermal elements only. It is characteristically found medial to the concha of the ear in a parallel course with the external auditory canal, but may extend into the retroauricular area. Type II lesions are composed of ectoderm and mesoderm, and therefore may contain

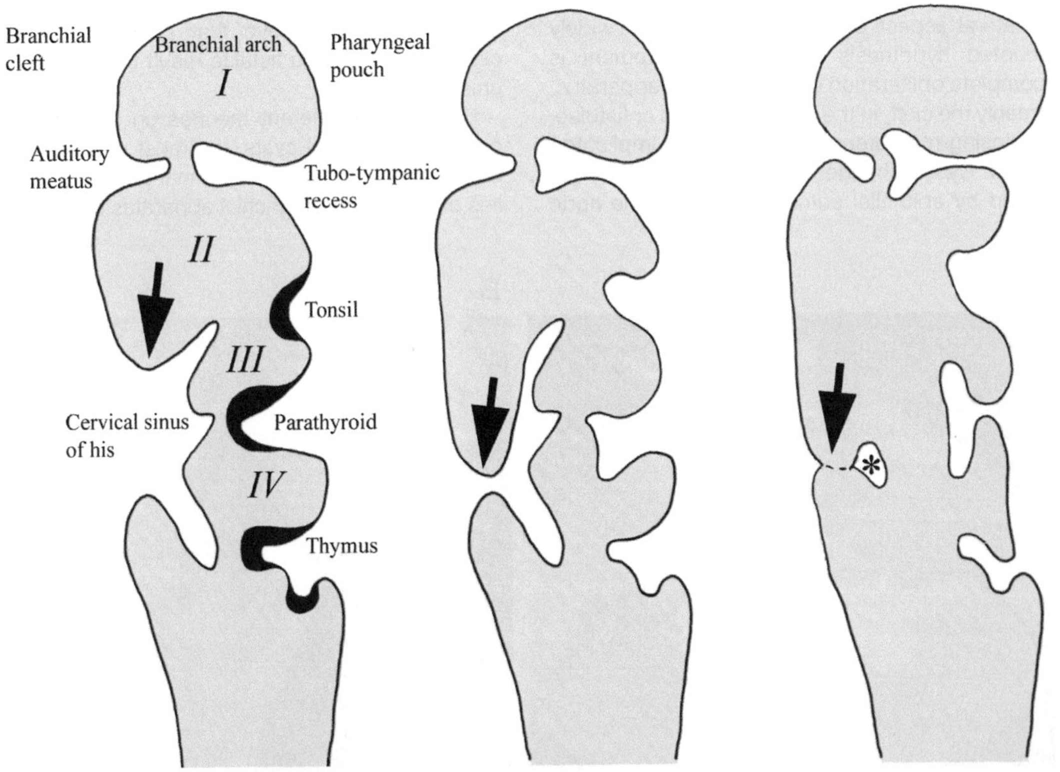

Fig. 5. The developing branchial apparatus. During development, the second arch grows caudally (*arrow*) and predominates forming the sinus of His (*asterisk*). Indentations between each arch form clefts on the external surface of the embryo and pharyngeal pouches internally. Incomplete fusion may lead to fistulae or sinus tracts.

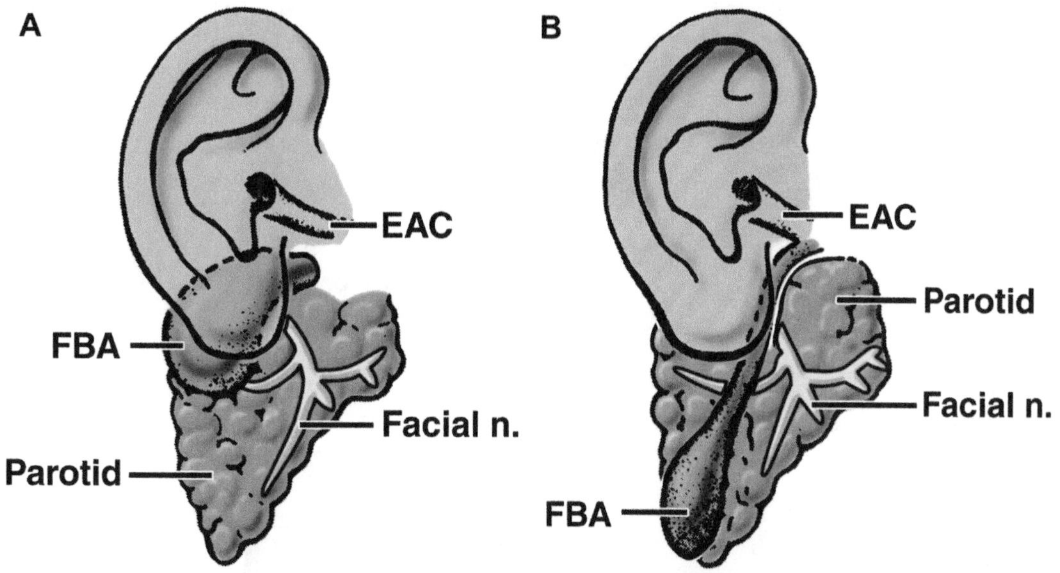

Fig. 6. Work type I (*A*) and type II (*B*) first branchial anomaly (FBA) cysts. (*A*) Type I cyst is principally a duplication anomaly of the membranous external auditory canal (EAC). The EAC and middle ear are normal. (*B*) Type II cyst may have a sinus stoma in the membranous EAC, with the lesion is extending medial or lateral to the facial nerve. The middle ear is normal. (*From* Mukherji SK, Fatterpekar G, Castillo M, et al. Imaging of congenital anomalies of the branchial apparatus. Neuroimaging Clin N Am 2000;10:75–93; with permission.)

cartilage. These lesions involve both the external auditory canal and cartilaginous pinna, or are associated with the parotid gland.

Radiologic features

These lesions are usually related to the parotid gland and/or the lower margin of the pinna. The cyst can be parallel to the membranous external auditory canal (**Fig. 7**), or can be either within, superficial to, or deep to the parotid gland (**Fig. 8**), with occasionally a tract directed toward the external auditory canal. A first branchial cleft cyst appears as an oval or round cystic mass with variable wall thickness and enhancement.[24] The cyst contents are of fluid attenuation (10–25 HU) on CT scan, while on MR imaging there is mainly low to intermediate T1-weighted and high T2-weighted signal intensity (see **Fig. 7**B, C).

In most cases, neither the CT nor MR imaging appearance of these cysts is characteristic enough to allow differentiating a first branchial cleft cyst from any other cystic mass of the parotid gland; particularly if a tract connecting to the external auditory canal cannot be identified. Any tumor of the parotid or periparotid region can mimic a first branchial cleft cyst clinically. If the CT appearance is that of a cystic mass, a branchial cleft cyst should be included in the differential diagnosis along with an inflammatory parotid cyst, benign cystic tumors, and necrotic adenopathy of squamous cell carcinoma.

Second Branchial Cleft Cyst

Anomalies of the second branchial cleft account for 95% of all branchial cleft anomalies, with cysts being more common than sinuses or fistulae combined.[28] Second branchial cleft anomalies pass close to the glossopharyngeal and hypoglossal nerves and then enter the pharynx at the level of the tonsillar fossa. These lesions are subclassified into 4 types.[29] Type I lesions are anterior to the sternocleidomastoid (SCM) muscle and are not in contact with the carotid sheath. Type II lesions are the most common second arch anomalies and are deep to the SCM muscle, either anterior or posterior to the carotid artery. Type III lesions pass between the internal and external carotid arteries and are adjacent to the pharynx. Type IV lesions are medial to the carotid sheath and are in close proximity to the pharynx adjacent to the tonsillar fossa.

Clinical characteristics

Second branchial cleft cysts occur most frequently at the mandibular angle. However, the cysts can occur anywhere along the potential tract from the oropharyngeal tonsillar fossa to the supraclavicular region of the neck (**Fig. 9**).[24] This tract follows a characteristic course determined during embryologic development. If a fistula is present, the ostium is usually seen within the anterior neck just above the clavicle, along the anterior border of the junction of the mid and lower third of the SCM muscle (**Fig. 10**).

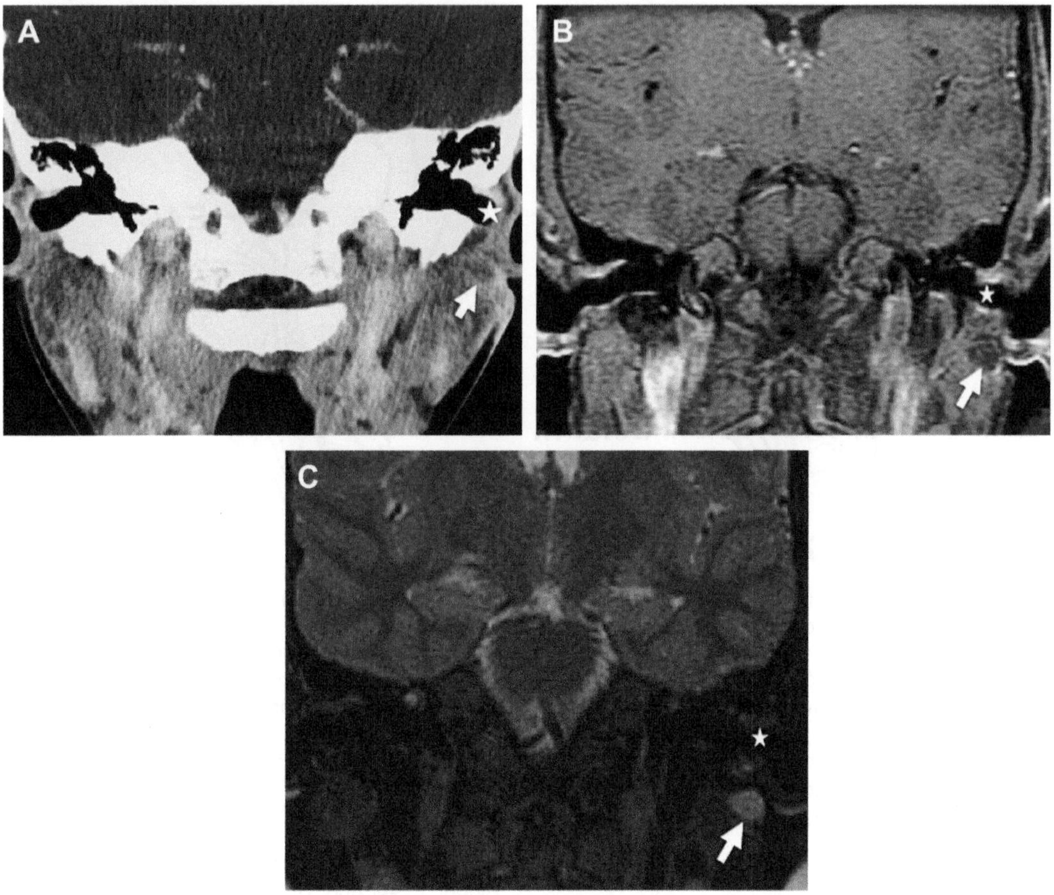

Fig. 7. (*A*) Coronal reformatted CT scan demonstrating Work type I cyst (*arrow*) that is parallel to the membranous EAC (*star*). Coronal contrast-enhanced T1-weighted (*B*) and T2-weighted (*C*) images demonstrating the hypointense T1 signal and hyperintense T2 signal of the lesion, and the lack of enhancement.

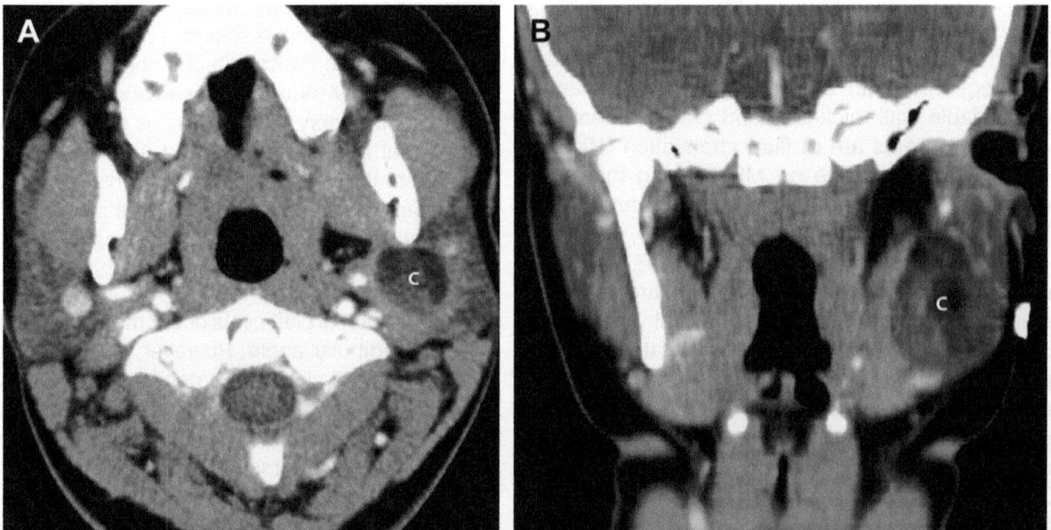

Fig. 8. Axial (*A*) and coronal reformatted (*B*) enhanced CT images demonstrate a left intraparotid Work type II, first branchial cleft cyst (c).

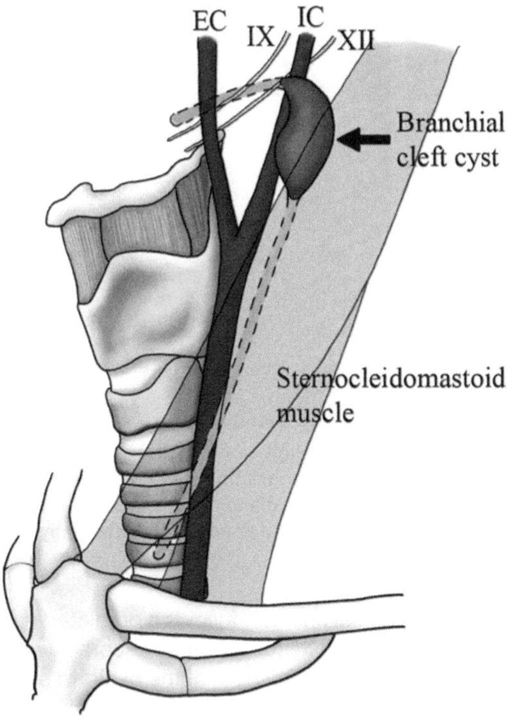

Fig. 9. The path of second branchial cleft anomalies, which can occur anywhere along a line from the supraclavicular region to the oropharyngeal mucosa. The path travels lateral to the common carotid artery, then heads medially between the external carotid and internal carotid arteries under the glosspharyngeal nerve and above the hyopglossal nerve, terminating medially as an opening within the tonsillar fossa.

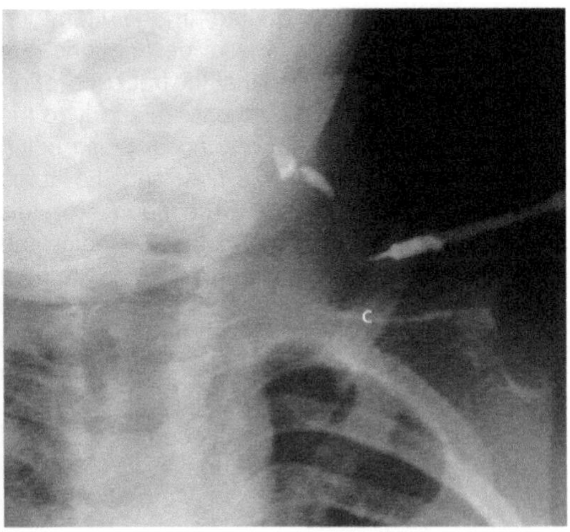

Fig. 10. Second branchial cleft sinus tract in a 1-year-old male with intermittent drainage in the left lower neck. A fistulogram demonstrates the sinus tract starting slightly above the clavicle (c) and extending superiorly and medially. There is no definite communication to the oropharynx or the pyriform sinus.

These cysts usually appear as painless, fluctuant masses in the lateral neck adjacent to the anteromedial border of the SCM muscle, most commonly at the mandibular angle.[29] The mass enlarges slowly over time, and may become painful and tender if secondarily infected.

Radiologic features

At US, the second branchial cleft cyst is seen as a well-marginated, anechoic mass with an imperceptible peripheral wall that displaces the surrounding soft tissues.[30] The majority of the lesions demonstrate posterior acoustic enhancement. Occasionally the cyst can be hyperechoic and show a pseudosolid appearance; or the lesion is hypoechoic with fine, indistinct internal echoes, representing debris.[30] In adult patients, some cysts can infrequently demonstrate thick wall or multiloculation with septations within a single cyst.[30]

At CT, these cysts are typically well-circumscribed masses of homogeneous low attenuation (**Fig. 11**).[24] The classic location of these cysts is at the mandibular angle, along the anteromedial border of the SCM muscle, lateral to the carotid space, and at the posterior margin of the submandibular gland.[24] The cyst typically displaces the SCM muscle posteriorly or posterolaterally, the vessels of the carotid space medially or posteromedially, and the submandibular gland anteriorly. It may also be seen more medially extending from the oropharyngeal region to the base of the skull within the parapharyngeal space. Wall thickness, enhancement, and surrounding deep tissue edema vary depending on the severity of the associated inflammatory process (**Fig. 12**).

MR imaging better depicts the deep tissue extent of a second branchial cleft cyst, which allows accurate preoperative planning. The cyst fluid varies from hypointense to intermediate signal relative to muscle on T1-weighted images, and is usually hyperintense on T2-weighted images (**Fig. 13**).[25] Mural thickness and enhancement vary, depending of the presence and severity of any associated inflammatory process.[24] Occasionally a beak sign may be seen on axial CT or MR images. This sign represents a curved rim of tissue or "beak" pointing medially between the internal and external carotid arteries. It is considered a pathognomonic imaging feature of a second branchial cleft cyst, specifically a type III cyst.[31]

Third and Fourth Branchial Cleft Anomalies

Third and fourth arch anomalies are extremely rare, most commonly seen on the left side of the neck.[32,33] Both of these anomalies typically present with a long history of neck infections and abscesses.[33] Anomalies of the fourth branchial

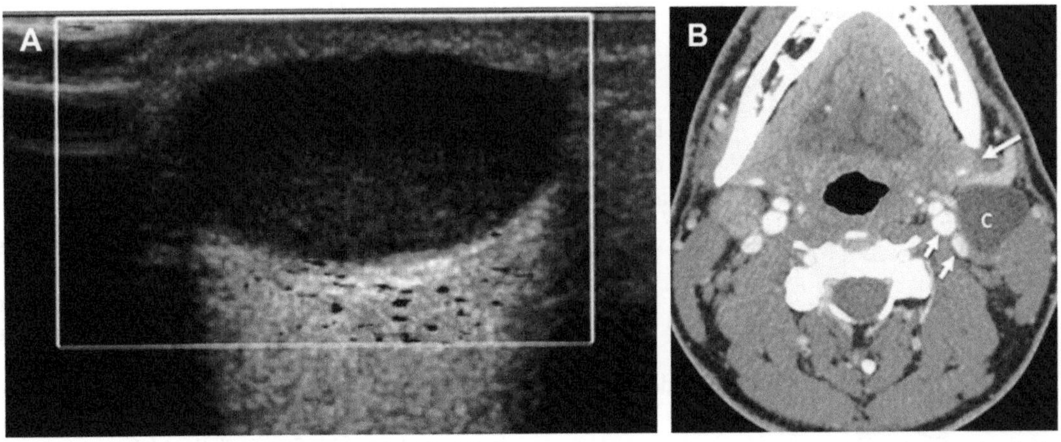

Fig. 11. (*A*) Ultrasonography of a left mandibular angle lump demonstrates elliptical-shaped avascular lesion filled with internal echoes. The cystic nature of the lesion is confirmed by posterior enhancement. (*B*) Axial CT scans show a cystic lesion (c) at the mandibular angle displacing the submandibular gland anteriorly (*long arrow*), the sternocleidomastoid muscle posterolaterally, and the vascular structures (*short arrows*) posteromedially, the classic location for a Bailey type II cyst.

cleft usually manifest as a sinus tract rather than a cyst or fistula. Distinguishing third branchial cleft anomalies from fourth branchial cleft anomalies may be difficult, because both have relationships with the pyriform sinus.[33] The difference between the two lesions lies in their relationships to the superior laryngeal nerve (the nerve of the fourth arch).[23] Those above this structure are of third branchial cleft origin, whereas those below are derived from the fourth branchial cleft.

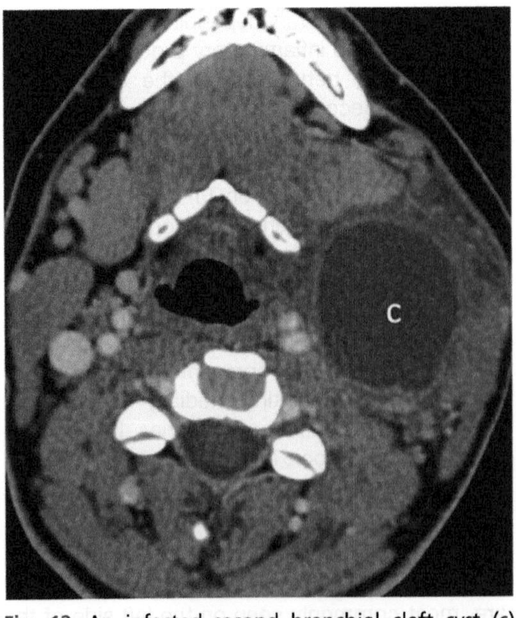

Fig. 12. An infected second branchial cleft cyst (c) seen in its most common location as a thick-walled round cystic mass just posteroinferior to the mandibular angle.

Third branchial anomaly follows a predicted embryologic course extending from the supraclavicular fossa to the lateral aspect of the pyriform sinus (**Fig. 14**).[2] The opening of a third branchial cleft fistula is found along the anterior border of the SCM muscle, usually more caudal than the opening of a second branchial anomaly. The tract passes posterior to the common or internal carotid artery between the hypoglossal nerve below and the glossopharyngeal nerve above.[2,23] The tract enters the thyroid membrane above the internal branch of the superior laryngeal nerve and enters the pharynx at the pyriform sinus.

Although the courses of fourth branchial arch anomalies are widely quoted in the literature, case reports matching these descriptions are rare.[2] It has been proposed that the tract of a fourth pouch sinus or fistula should pass inferiorly to the remnants of the fourth arch arteries, those being the subclavian artery on the right and the aortic arch on the left (**Fig. 15**).[2] The course of this anomaly is from the pyriform fossa medial and inferior to the superior laryngeal nerve. It then descends in the tracheoesophageal groove parallel to the recurrent laryngeal nerve into the mediastinum. It loops under the aortic arch on the left side and subclavian artery on the right, follows the dorsal aspect of the common carotid artery, then exits at the skin surface.

Radiologic features

Third branchial cleft cyst most commonly appears as a unilocular cystic mass centered in the posterior cervical space on CT and MR images (**Fig. 16**). Mural thickness, enhancement, and surrounding edematous changes vary depending on the

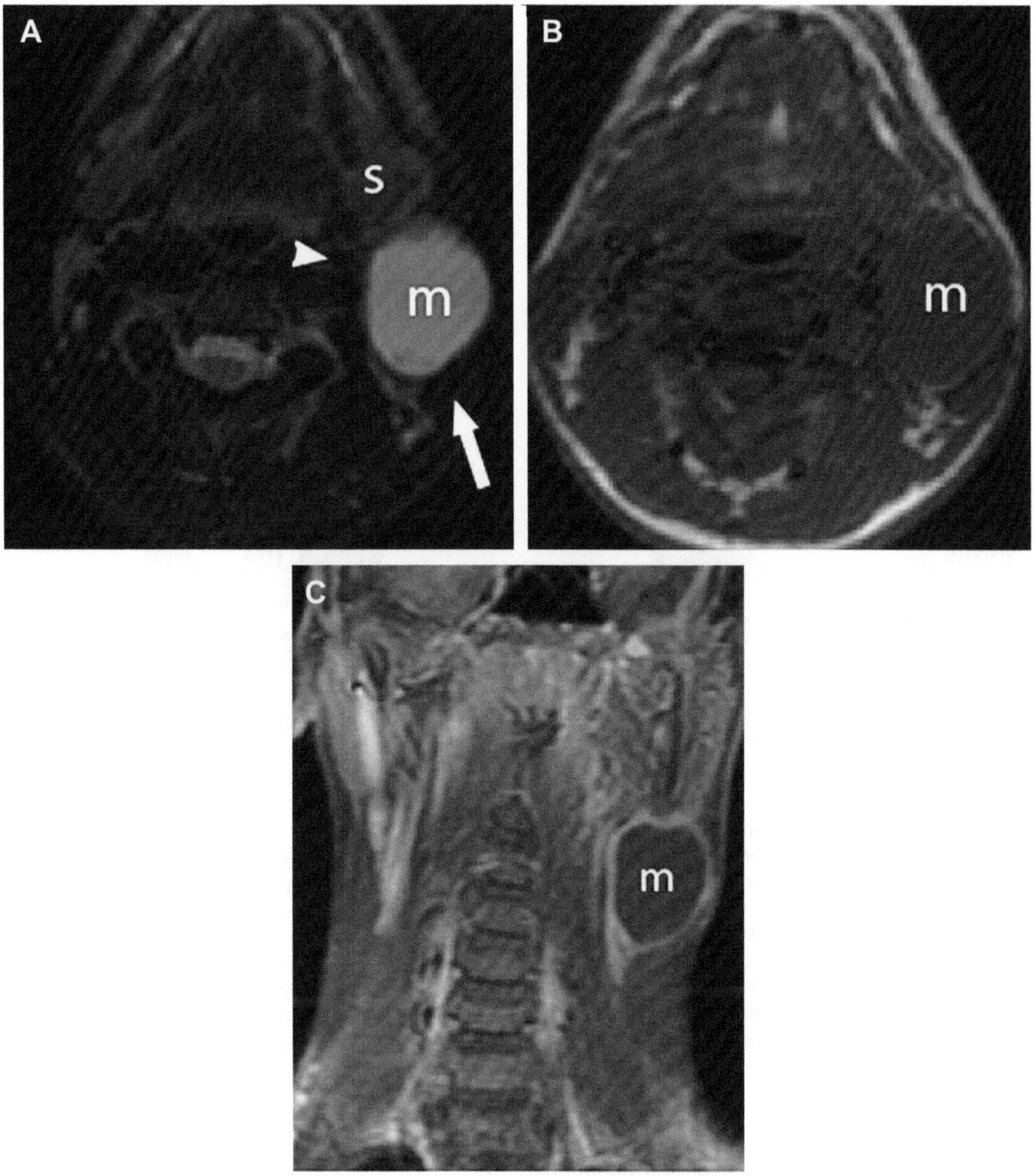

Fig. 13. A second branchial cleft cyst in a 10-year-old girl with a history of a mass in the left neck. (*A*) Axial T2-weighted image with fat suppression shows a well-defined mass (m) along the anterior-medial border of the left sternocleidomastoid muscle (*long arrow*), lateral to the carotid space (*arrowhead*), and posterior to the submandibular gland (s). (*B*) Axial T1-weighted image reveals mild hypointensity of the mass (m). (*C*) Coronal contrast-enhanced T1-weighted image with fat suppression shows mild rim enhancement of the mass (m).

severity of the associated inflammatory process. As with other branchial cleft cysts, the cyst fluid may vary in signal intensity on T1-weighted images depending on the protein concentration, and is typically hyperintense relative to muscle on T2-weighted images.[25]

Although controversial, the literature supports the fact that an internal fistula arising from the apex of the pyriform sinus would be a fourth pouch remnant (**Fig. 17**).[2,34] Benson and colleagues[2] reported a fourth branchial cleft cyst that connected with the pyriform sinus and appeared similar to an external or mixed laryngocele.

CYSTIC HYGROMA

Cystic hygromas are developmental tumors of the lymphatic system that affect any anatomic subsite in the human body. Cystic hygroma usually affects the head and neck (approximately 75%), with a

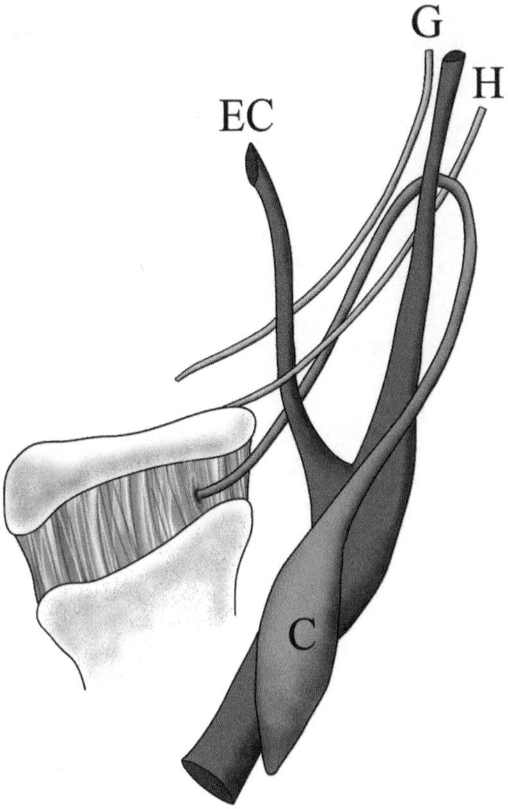

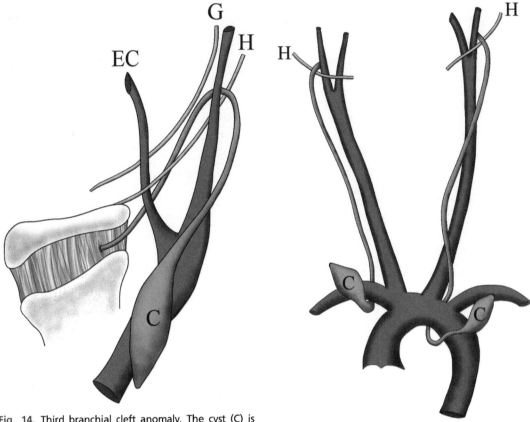

Fig. 14. Third branchial cleft anomaly. The cyst (C) is posterior to the sternocleidomastoid muscle (not shown), and the tract ascends posterior to the internal carotid artery. It then extends medially to pass between the hypoglossal (H) and glossopharyngeal (G) nerves. It pierces the thyroid membrane to enter the mid aspect of the pyriform sinus. EC, external carotid artery. (*From* Mukherji SK, Fatterpekar G, Castillo M, et al. Imaging of congenital anomalies of the branchial apparatus. Neuroimaging Clin N Am 2000;10:75–93; with permission).

Fig. 15. Fourth branchial cleft anomaly. Cysts (C) are located anterior to the aortic arch on either side. The tract loops around either the aortic arch (*left*) or the subclavian artery (*right*), then courses superiorly to loop over the hypoglossal nerve (H) toward the tip of the pyriform sinus (not shown). (*From* Mukherji SK, Fatterpekar G, Castillo M, et al. Imaging of congenital anomalies of the branchial apparatus. Neuroimaging Clin N Am 2000;10:75–93; with permission).

left-sided predilection. Cystic hygroma accounts for about 5% of benign tumors of infancy and childhood.[35] Lymphangiomas are classified into 3 histologic types based on the size of the abnormal lymphatic spaces: (a) simple lymphangiomas, which have capillary size lymphatic channels, (b) cavernous lymphangiomas, which contain dilated lymphatics and fibrous adventitia, and (c) cystic hygromas, which are macroscopic multilocular cystic masses with cysts of varying size.[36] All 3 types of lymphangioma often coexist within a single lesion. The cysts tend to form along tissue planes, often making complete surgical removal difficult.

The lymphatic system develops from 5 primitive sacs derived from the venous system: paired jugular and posterior sacs and one retroperitoneal sac.[37] It is postulated that lymphangiomas arise from early sequestration of the lymphatic tissue that retain their embryonic growth potential. The tumors then enlarge by continued, rapid growth of these lymphatic rests and by accumulation of fluid in the isolated lymphatics.[37] Alternatively, a cystic hygroma may arise from a failure of the juguloaxillary lymphatic sac to connect to the venous system, producing a congenital obstruction of lymphatic drainage.[37]

Clinical Characteristics

Cystic hygromas are usually diagnosed in infancy. About 50% are discovered at birth, and 90% are evident before the end of the second year.[38] There is no predilection for either sex. These lesions most commonly appear as slow-growing,

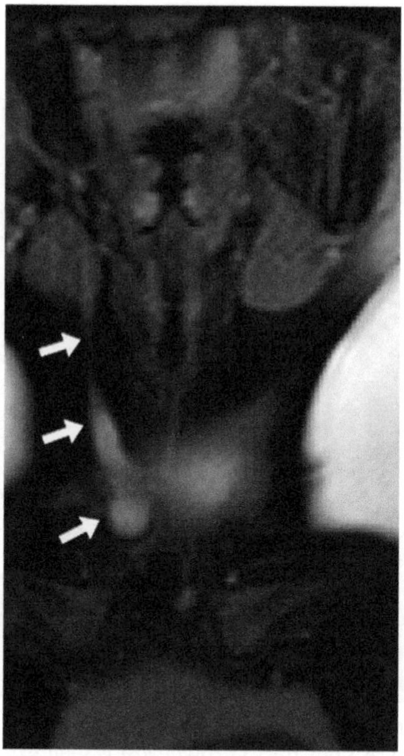

Fig. 16. Third branchial cleft cyst and sinus tract. Coronal T2-weighted image with fat suppression demonstrating a cyst in the right lower neck with a sinus tract extending toward the lateral wall of the pyriform sinus (*arrows*).

asymptomatic soft tissue mass. Sudden enlargement can occur owing to intralesional hemorrhage, inflammation, or even intercurrent respiratory tract infection or trauma. In young infants, however, compression of the airway and esophagus may lead to severe, sometimes life-threatening, dyspnea and difficulty swallowing. Their most common location is in the neck, where 75% occur, classically in the posterior neck; 3% to 10% extend into the mediastinum, and an additional 20% are found in the axilla.[38]

Radiologic Features

On US scans, most cystic hygromas manifest as a complex, multilocular cystic mass with septa of variable thickness (**Fig. 18**).[39] The echogenic portions of the lesion correlate with clusters of small, abnormal lymphatic channels.[39] Fluid-fluid levels can be observed with a characteristic echogenic "hemorrhagic" component layering in the dependent portion of the lesion.[39] Prenatal US may demonstrate a cystic hygroma in the posterior neck soft tissues.

On CT images, cystic hygromas tend to appear as poorly circumscribed, multiloculated, hypoattenuated masses with homogeneous fluid attenuation (**Fig. 19**).[40] Infected or hemorrhagic lesions commonly show higher attenuation than that seen in simple fluid. Usually the mass is centered in the posterior triangle or in the submandibular space. It is not uncommon for some of these lesions to extend from one space in the neck into another as a result of their infiltrative nature.

MR imaging better depicts the extent of cystic hygroma and its relationship to adjacent soft tissues of the neck (see **Fig. 19**). The most common pattern is that of a mass with low or intermediate signal intensity on T1-weighted images and hyperintensity on T2-weighted images. This lesion infrequently may be hyperintense on T1-weighted images, a finding associated with clotted blood or high lipid content. Fluid-fluid level is commonly seen in hemorrhagic lesions.

DERMOID AND EPIDERMOID CYST

Dermoid cysts account for up to 25% of midline cervical anomalies, with thyroglossal duct cyst the most common midline anomaly.[41] The literature is somewhat confusing concerning the relationship between dermoid and teratoma as to origin, definition, and classification. Dermoid cysts are lined by epithelium and differ from epidermoid cysts in that they contain some evidence of epithelial appendages, such as hair, hair follicles, or sebaceous glands within the cyst wall.[42] Complex dermoid cyst contains mesodermal elements (cartilage, bone, and fat); in contrast to the simple dermoid which contains only skin components, that is, epidermis, derma, and dermal glands.[42] That these lesions typically occur along embryonic lines of fusion suggests that they exist as the result of entrapment of epithelial elements during development. Teratomas are characterized by their pluripotential ability to produce virtually any adult tissue (mature teratoma) and fetal tissue (immature teratoma).

Clinical Characteristics

Only 7% of dermoid inclusion cysts occur in the head and neck, with the lateral eyebrow being the most common location.[43] The most common clinical appearance of a dermoid cyst in the neck is a midline, suprahyoid, slowly growing mass in the floor of the mouth.[43,44] Typically the mass is soft, mobile, and unattached to overlying skin. Unlike thyroglossal duct cysts, these lesions have no intimate association with the hyoid bone and therefore do not move with tongue protrusion. Epidermoid cysts of the neck are rare congenital lesions, much less common than dermoid cysts

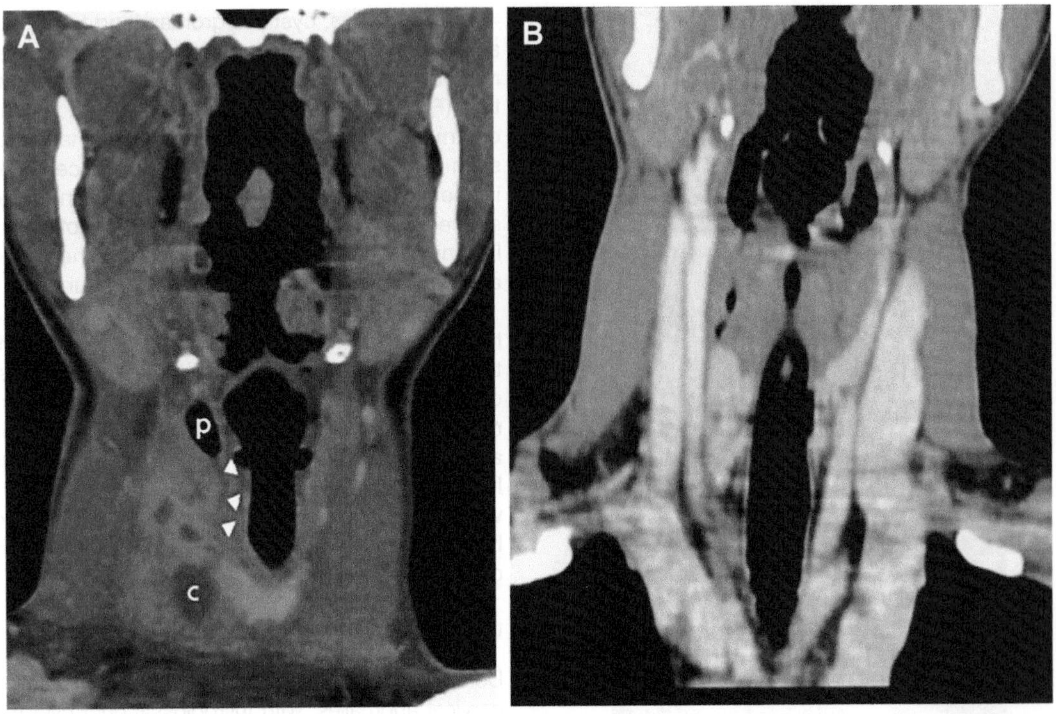

Fig. 17. Infected fourth branchial cleft cyst. (*A*) Reformatted coronal contrast enhanced CT scan demonstrating infected cyst (c) adjacent to the right lobe of the thyroid gland. A sinus tract (*arrowheads*) is seen extending toward the tip of the pyriform sinus (p). (*B*) Following treatment, there is residual sinus tract filled with air extending toward the pyriform sinus.

in the head and neck. These lesions appear earlier than dermoid cysts, with most being evident during infancy. About 5% of dermoid cysts undergo malignant degeneration into squamous cell carcinoma.[44]

Radiologic Features

Dermoid cysts appear as thin-walled, unilocular masses, located in the submandibular or sublingual space. On CT scan, the lesion's content appears as homogeneous, hypoattenuating fluid material (**Fig. 20**) (0–18 HU). Coalescence of fat into small nodules within the fluid matrix gives the cyst a "sack-of-marbles" appearance; which is virtually pathognomonic for a dermoid cyst in this location.[45] The cyst uncommonly may be heterogeneous on CT scans because of the various germinal components. Fluid-fluid levels with supernatant lipid are possible. The rim of these cysts often is enhanced following administration of contrast material.

MR imaging depicts the location and extent of cystic lesions in the floor of the mouth, and is useful for determining their relationship to the surrounding muscles. Most dermoid cysts are located superior to the mylohyoid muscle and will be removed with an intraoral approach.[46] Less commonly, the lesion is inferior to this muscle and will be removed with an external submandibular approach.[46] Dermoid cysts have variable signal intensity on T1-weighted images. The cysts may be hyperintense (because of the presence of sebaceous lipid) or isointense relative to muscle on T1-weighted images, and are usually hyperintense on T2-weighted images. The mass has a clearly demarcated rim but frequently has a heterogeneous internal appearance.[17]

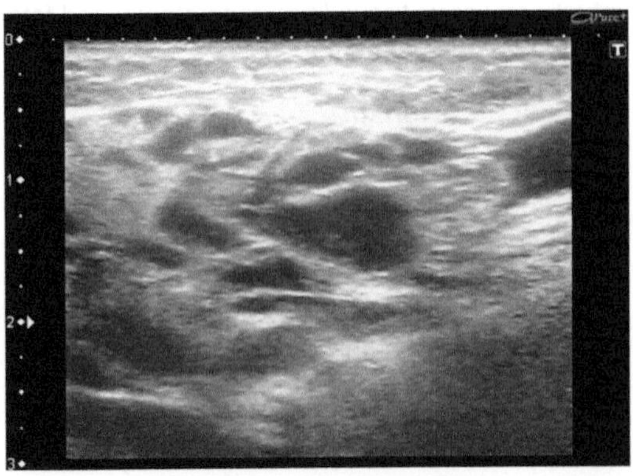

Fig. 18. Cystic hygroma in 6-month-old male with right upper neck mass. Ultrasonography shows a large, multiseptated, anechoic mass of the anterior neck.

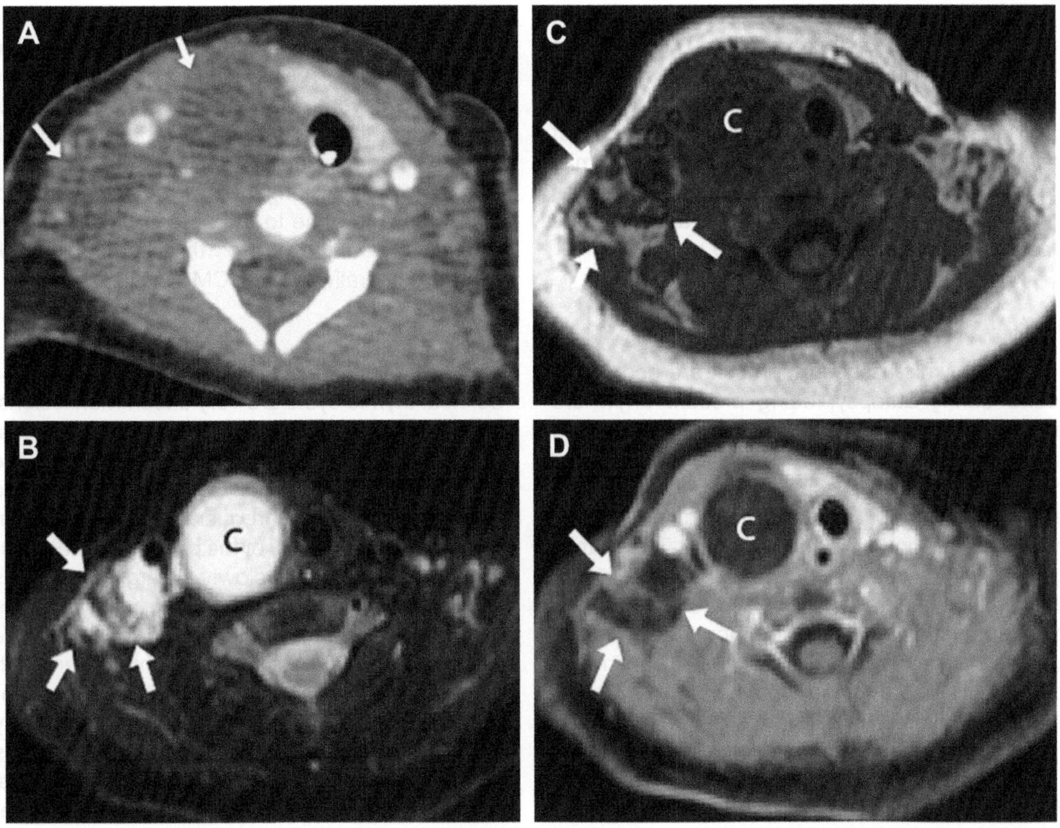

Fig. 19. Cystic hygroma in 5-day-old female with right neck mass. (*A*) Axial contrast-enhanced CT scan demonstrates bilobed cystic lesion (*arrows*) in the right anterior and posterior neck, with tracheal displacement. (*B*) Axial T2-weighted images with fat suppression demonstrate the lesion (c) is predominantly T2 hyperintense. (*C, D*) Axial T1 and fat-saturated enhanced T1-weighted images; the lesion is T1 hypointense with a rim of enhancement. There is heterogeneous T2 hypointense with T1 hyperintense signal in the posterior component (*arrows*), suggestive of intralesional hemorrhage.

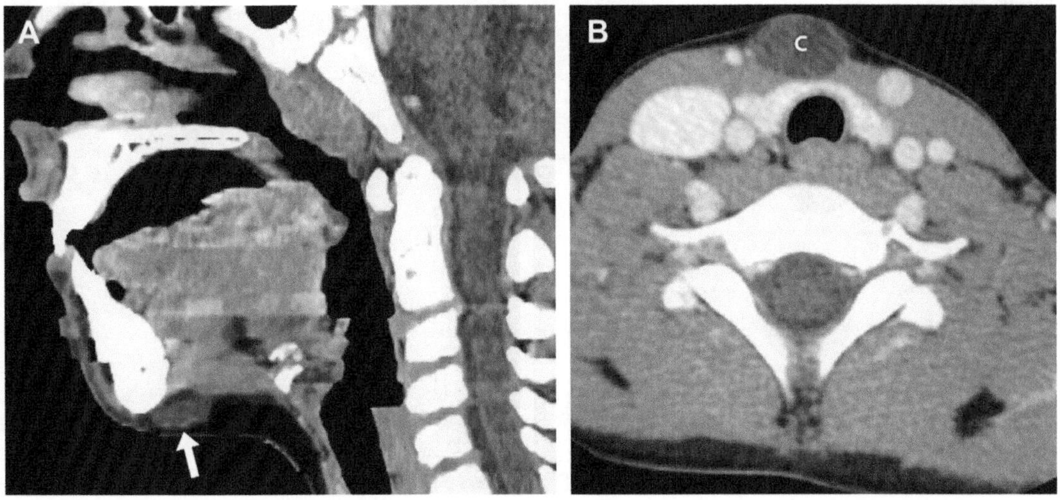

Fig. 20. Two different patients with dermoid cysts. (*A*) Sagittal CT scan demonstrates a hypoattenuated lesion in a typical submental region (*arrow*). (*B*) Axial CT scan demonstrates a midline dermoid cyst (c) in an atypical infrahyoid location at the level of the thyroid gland.

Epidermoid cysts are unilocular and have fluid attenuation on CT scans (**Fig. 21**). These lesions are hypointense on T1-weighted images and hyperintense on T2-weighted images, following the signal intensity of fluid.[17] An epidermoid cyst located entirely within the sublingual space may be difficult to distinguish from other cystic lesions in the floor of mouth (eg, a simple ranula) on the basis of imaging criteria alone.

THYMIC CYST

Nests of thymic tissue in the neck are commonly found during autopsy, being present anywhere along a path from the angle of the mandible to the mediastinum (**Fig. 22**).[47] However, the majority of the cervical thymic tissues remain dormant; with a scarcity of clinical cases of thymic cysts in the neck being reported in the literature. The pathogenesis of thymic cyst remains controversial, with several separate possibilities to explain their development.[48] The most common theory postulates that thymic cysts probably arise from embryonic remnants of the thymopharyngeal duct.[49] Alternatively, other investigators believe that they result from acquired, progressive cystic degeneration of thymic (Hassall) corpuscles and the epithelium reticulum of the thymus.

Embryologically, the thymus is formed from ventral sacculation of the third pharyngeal pouch during the sixth week of development.[50] The thymopharyngeal tract elongates and descends into the mediastinum, with obliteration of the lumen during the seventh and eighth weeks. Fusion of the tracts in the mediastinum occurs by the ninth week. Anatomic location of the thymic cysts occurs anywhere along the thymopharyngeal tract from the hyoid bone to the anterior mediastinum, immediately adjacent to the carotid sheath bordered laterally by the SCM muscles.

Clinical Characteristics

Cervical thymic cysts are very uncommon lesions, with two-thirds of the lesions detected in the first decade of life and the remaining one-third in the second and third decades. Overall, cervical thymic cysts are found more frequently in males than in females.[51] The majority of the patients characteristically present with a slowly enlarging, painless mass in the lateral portion of the neck near the thoracic inlet, either anterior or deep to the SCM muscle.[51] Few patients might present with dysphagia, hoarseness, and dyspnea. Occasionally a cervical thymic cyst can become suddenly evident or abruptly painful after an initially painless course.[47,51] Approximately 50% of all cervical thymic cysts extend into the mediastinum, either by direct extension or by connection to a vestigial remnant or a solid cord.[51] There is preferential

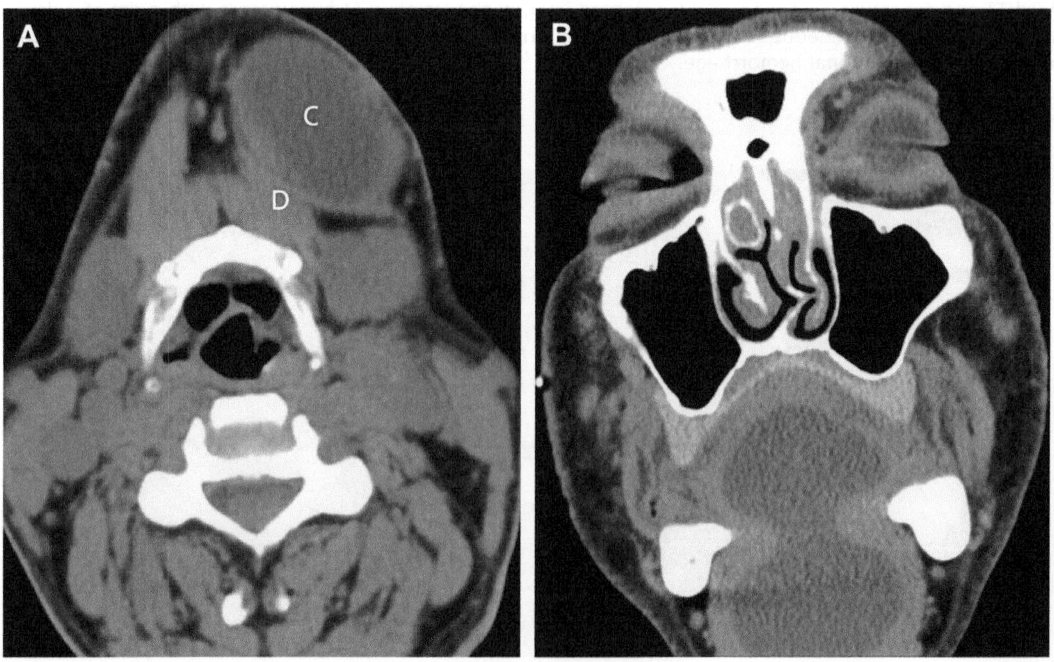

Fig. 21. Epidermoid cysts. (*A*) Axial CT scan demonstrating a submandibular hypoattenuating cyst (C) displacing the anterior belly of the digastric muscle (D). (*B*) Coronal reformatted CT scan in a different patient demonstrating a bilobed sublingual epidermoid cyst.

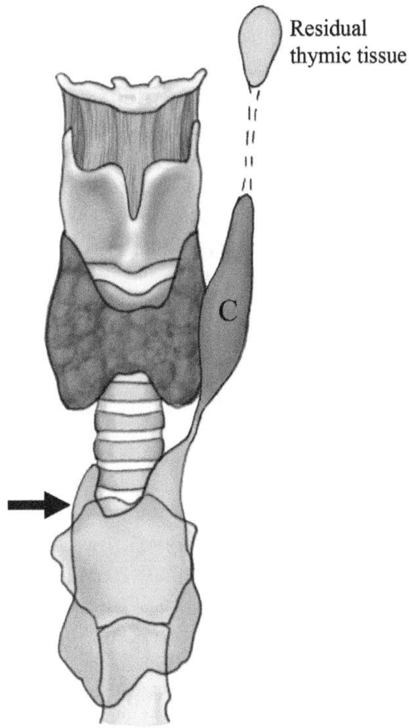

Fig. 22. Thymic cyst anomaly (C). The thymopharyngeal tract courses inferiorly in the tracheoesophageal groove and then to the superior mediastinum.

involvement of the left side of the neck by these lesions.[49] The diagnosis is seldom suspected preoperatively, most likely because of the rarity of the lesions.

The differential diagnosis of cervical thymic cysts includes the more common branchial cleft cyst, thyroglossal duct cyst, cystic hygroma, dermoid cyst, cystic teratoma, and cystic thymoma.[47] A branchial cleft cyst tends to occur in the upper half of the neck, in contrast to the more inferior location of a cervical thymic cyst. Cystic hygromas frequently present as painless soft masses in the posterior triangle and, not uncommonly, the floor of the mouth. Approximately 3% to 10% of cervical cystic hygromas have a mediastinal extension,[38] compared with up to 50% of cervical thymic cysts. Mediastinal extension does not occur in branchial cleft cysts. Up to 90% of cystic hygromas are detected in children younger than 2 years.[38] Branchial cysts are more common in the second and third decades, whereas cervical thymic cyst has a peak incidence between the ages of 2 and 13 years, and are uncommon before the age of 1 year.[47]

Radiologic Features

At US a thymic cyst appears as anechoic, unilocular or multilocular, cystic mass extending just parallel to the SCM muscle within the lower neck, usually on the left. The CT appearance is that of a large, unilocular or multilocular, hypoattenuated cystic mass adjacent to the carotid space with extension into the mediastinum.[52,53] The CT attenuation values of the contents of the cyst range from 10 to 25 HU (**Fig. 23**). After contrast administration, there is usually a peripheral thin rim of enhancement.[53] The signal intensity of thymic cysts on MR images is hypointensity on T1-weighted images and hyperintensity on T2-weighted images.

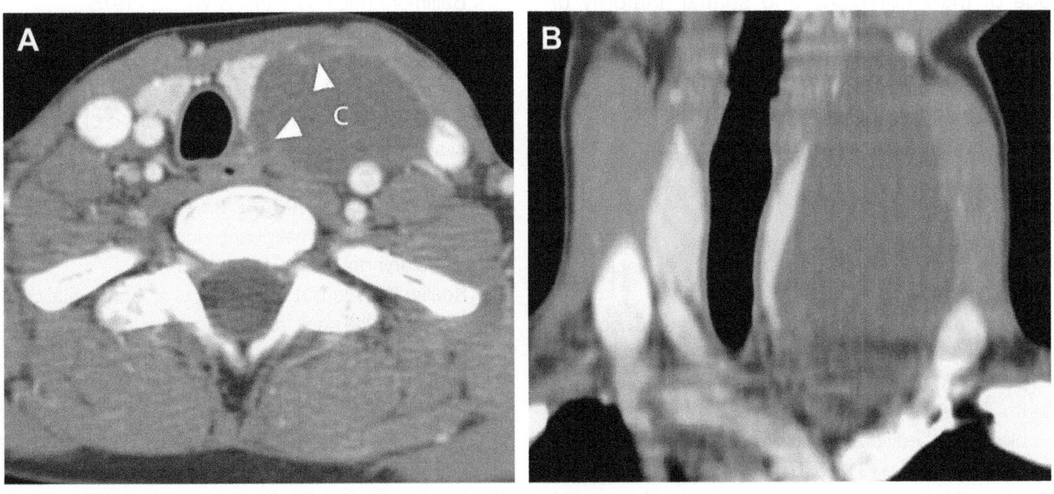

Fig. 23. Axial (*A*) and coronal reformatted (*B*) enhanced CT images demonstrate large thymic cyst (C) in the left anterior neck with multiple loculations (*arrowheads*). The lesion extends from the level of the oropharynx to the superior mediastinum.

CERVICAL BRONCHOGENIC CYST

Cervical bronchogenic cysts are extremely rare. These lesions result from an anomalous foregut development, but it is unclear why these cysts reach an aberrant position in the neck. Cervical bronchogenic cysts have been reported in infants as well as in adults, and occur more commonly in males.[44]

Clinical Characteristics

Cervical bronchogenic cysts are seldom recognized clinically, and may manifest as a swelling or draining sinus, usually located in the suprasternal notch or supraclavicular area.[44]

Radiologic Features

Three of the 4 cases of cervical bronchogenic cyst reported in the literature occurred before the advent of CT. In the solitary case seen at CT, the cyst had a tubular configuration anterior to the trachea.[54] This cyst was infected at the time of imaging, which accounted for the presence of air within the lesion.

SUMMARY

A variety of congenital cystic lesions are encountered in the neck. These lesions are uncommon and are usually seen during infancy or childhood, but detection may be delayed until adulthood. Such lesions often manifest as slow-growing masses, and cause symptoms only after enlarging sufficiently or after infection. Sinuses and fistulae are usually diagnosed at an earlier age than cysts. The clinical manifestations combined with knowledge of the embryology and spatial anatomy of the head and neck often provide clues for a correct diagnosis. Different imaging modalities are important in confirming the cystic nature of the lesion and determining the extent of the lesions in the neck for optimal preoperative planning.

REFERENCES

1. Allard R. The thyroglossal cyst. Head Neck Surg 1982;5:134–46.
2. Benson MT, Dalen K, Mancuso AA, et al. Congenital anomalies of the branchial apparatus: embryology and pathologic anatomy. Radiographics 1992;12(5):943–60.
3. In: Sadler TW, editor. Langman's medical embryology. 6th edition. Baltimore (MD): Williams and Wilkins; 1990. p. 312–3. Chapter 16.
4. Filston H. Common lumps and bumps of the head and neck in infants and children. Pediatr Ann 1989;18:180–6.
5. El-Silimy OE, Bradley PJ. Thyroglossal tract anoma lies. Clin Otolaryngol 1985;10:329–34.
6. Park Y. Evaluation of neck masses in children. An Fam Physician 1995;51:1904–12.
7. Telander R, Deane S. Thyroglossal and branchia cleft cysts and sinuses. Surg Clin North Am 1977 57:779–91.
8. Greinwald JJ, Leichtman L, Simko E. Hereditary thyroglossal duct cysts. Arch Otolaryngol Head Neck Surg 1996;122:1094–6.
9. Noyek AM, Friedberg J. Thyroglossal duct and ectopic thyroid disorders. Otolaryngol Clin North Am 1981;14(1):187–201.
10. Bailey H. Thyroglossal cysts and fistulae. Br J Surg 1925;12:579–89.
11. Enepekides DJ. Management of congenital anoma lies of the neck. Facial Plast Surg Clin North Am 2001;9:131–45.
12. Marshall SF, Becker WF. Thyroglossal cysts and sinuses. Ann Surg 1949;129:642–51.
13. Ostlie DJ, Burjonrappa SC, Snyder CL, et al. Thyroglossal duct infections and surgical outcomes J Pediatr Surg 2004;39:396–9.
14. Wadsworth D, Siegel M. Thyroglossal duct cysts variability of sonographic findings. AJR Am J Roentgenol 1994;163:1475–7.
15. Ahuja AT, King AD, King W, et al. Thyroglossal duct cysts sonographic appearances in adults. AJNR Am J Neuroradiol 1999;20(4):579–82.
16. Reede DL, Bergeron RT, Som PM. CT of thyroglossa duct cysts. Radiology 1985;157(1):121–5.
17. Vogl T, Steger W, Ihrier S, et al. Cystic masses in the floor of the mouth: value of MR imaging in planning surgery. AJR Am J Roentgenol 1993;161:183–6
18. Moore K. The developing human. 3rd edition. Philadelphia: Saunders; 1988.
19. Langmann J. Medical embryology. 3rd edition. Baltimore (MD): Williams & Wilkins; 1975.
20. Golledge J, Ellis H. The aetiology of lateral cervical (branchial) cysts: past and present theories. J Laryngol Otol 1994;108:653–9.
21. Bhaskar SN, Bernier JL. Histogenesis of branchial cysts: a report of 468 cases. Am J Pathol 1959;35 407–14.
22. Burton DM, Pransky SM. Practical aspects of managing non-malignant lumps of the neck. J Otolaryngol 1992;21:398–403.
23. Koeller KK, Alamo L, Adair CF, et al. Congenital cystic masses of the neck: radiologic-pathologic correlation. Radiographics 1999;19(1):121–46 [quiz: 152–3].
24. Harnsberger H, Mancuso A, Muraki A, et al. Branchial cleft anomalies and their mimics: computed tomographic evaluation. Radiology 1984; 152:739–48.
25. Faerber E, Swartz J. Imaging of neck masses in infants and children. Crit Rev Diagn Imaging 1991; 31:283–314.

26. Whetstone J, Branstetter BF 4th, Hirsch BE. Fluoroscopic and CT fistulography of the first branchial cleft. AJNR Am J Neuroradiol 2006;27(9):1817–9.
27. Work WP. Newer concept of first branchial cleft defects. Laryngoscope 1972;9:1581–93.
28. Acierno SP, Waldhausen JH. Congenital cervical cysts, sinuses and fistulae. Otolaryngol Clin North Am 2007;40(1):161–76.
29. Bailey H. Branchial cysts and other essays on surgical subjects in the facio-cervical region. London: Lewis; 1929.
30. Ahuja AT, King AD, Metreweli C. Second branchial cleft cysts- variability of sonographic appearances in adult cases. AJNR Am J Neuroradiol 2000;21(2): 315–9.
31. Harnsberger H. Handbook of head and neck imaging. 2nd edition. St Louis (MO): Mosby-Yearbook; 1995.
32. James A, Stewart C, Warrick P, et al. Branchial sinus of the piriform fossa: reappraisal of third and fourth branchial anomalies. Laryngoscope 2007;117(11):1920–4.
33. Waldhausen JH. Branchial cleft and arch anomalies in children. Semin Pediatr Surg 2006;15(2):64–9.
34. Mukerji SS, Parmar H, Ibrahim M, et al. An unusual cause of recurrent pediatric neck abscess: pyriform sinus fistula. Clin Imaging 2007;31(5):349–51.
35. Donnelly LF, Adams DM, Bisset GS 3rd. Vascular malformations and hemangiomas: a practical approach in a multidisciplinary clinic. AJR Am J Roentgenol 2000;174(3):597–608.
36. Bill AH, Sumner DS. A unified concept of lymphangioma and cystic hygroma. Surg Gynecol Obstet 1975;120:79–86.
37. Sahin FR. The lymphatic system in human embryos with consideration of the morphology of the system as a whole. Am J Anat 1909;9:43–9.
38. Emery PJ, Bailey CM, Evans JN. Cystic hygroma of the head and neck. J Laryngol Otol 1984;98:613–9.
39. Sheth S, Nussbaum AR, Hutchins GM, et al. Cystic hygromas in children: sonographic-pathologic correlation. Radiology 1987;162(3):821–4.
40. Silverman P, Korobkin M, Moore A. CT diagnosis of cystic hygroma of the neck. J Comput Assist Tomogr 1983;7:519–20.
41. Foley DS, Fallat ME. Thyroglossal duct and other congenital midline cervical anomalies. Semin Pediatr Surg 2006;15(2):70–5.
42. Erich JB, Johnsen DS. Congenital dermoid cyst. Am J Surg 1953;85(1):104–7.
43. Erich JB. Dermoid cysts of head and neck. Surg Gynecol Obstet 1937;65:48.
44. Som P. Cystic lesions of the neck. Postgrad Radiol 1987;7:211–36.
45. Hunter TB, Paplanus SH, Chernin MM, et al. Dermoid cyst of the floor of the mouth: CT appearance. AJR Am J Roentgenol 1983;141(6):1239–40.
46. Howell C. The sublingual dermoid cyst. Oral Surg Oral Med Oral Pathol 1985;59:578–80.
47. Nguyen Q, deTar M, Wells W, et al. Cervical thymic cyst: case reports and review of the literature. Laryngoscope 1996;106(3 Pt 1):247–52.
48. Speer FD. Thymic cysts. NY Med Coll Flower Hosp Bull 1938;1:142–50.
49. Mikal S. Cervical thymic cyst: case report and review of the literature. Arch Surg 1974;109:558–62.
50. Barrick B, O'Kell RT. Thymic cysts and remnant cervical thymus. J Pediatr Surg 1969;4:355–8.
51. Guba AM Jr, Adam AE, Jaques DA, et al. Cervical presentation of thymic cysts. Am J Surg 1978; 136(4):430–6.
52. Burton EM, Mercado-Deane MG, Howell CG, et al. Cervical thymic cysts: CT appearance of two cases including a persistent thymopharyngeal duct cyst. Pediatr Radiol 1995;25(5):363–5.
53. Daga BV, Chaudhary VA, Dhamangaokar VB. Case Report: CT diagnosis of thymic remnant cyst/thymopharyngeal duct cyst. Indian J Radiol Imaging 2009; 19(4):293–5.
54. McManus K, Holt G, Aufdemorte T, et al. Bronchogenic cyst presenting as deep neck abscess. Otolaryngol Head Neck Surg 1984;92:109–14.

Hemangiomas and Vascular Malformations of the Head and Neck: A Simplified Approach

Aaron H. Baer, MD[a,*], Hemant A. Parmar, MD[a], Michael A. DiPietro, MD[a], Steven J. Kasten, MD[b], Suresh K. Mukherji, MD[a]

KEYWORDS

- Vascular anomalies • Birthmarks • Hemangioma
- Congenital • Vascular malformations
- Cavernous hemangioma • Cystic hygroma

Vascular anomalies of childhood, sometimes called birthmarks, are among the most common of all congenital and neonatal abnormalities.[1,2] Many descriptive or histopathologic terms have previously been used to describe these anomalies (eg, strawberry hemangioma, port-wine stain, cavernous hemangioma). Although colorful, these terms were used inconsistently and often erroneously, potentially leading to inappropriate clinical management.

In a landmark publication in 1982, Mulliken and Glowacki[3] proposed a system that now represents the international standard for classification of vascular anomalies in children. By examining the clinical and histopathologic features of vascular anomalies, these investigators sought to simplify categorization, thereby clarifying proper clinical management. After further refinement by multiple contributors, the modern classification scheme for vascular anomalies was accepted by the International Society for the Study of Vascular Anomalies (ISSVA) in 1992.[4–6] **Table 1** contains terms commonly used in the literature to describe vascular anomalies categorized based on that classification system.

Vascular anomalies are now divided into 2 categories: vascular tumors, hemangiomas being by far the most common; and vascular malformations (**Table 2**). The term hemangioma describes a lesion that undergoes a phase of proliferation involving high mitotic activity followed by a period of involution. In contrast, a vascular malformation shows normal endothelial turnover and growth commensurate with the child without spontaneous resolution.[3] This category comprises malformations of arterial, venous, capillary, lymphatic, and mixed vascular endothelium. There are other vascular tumors (eg, Kaposiform hemangioendothelioma, tufted angioma, hemangiopericytoma) that are distinct from hemangiomas. These tumors are significantly less common and are not discussed in detail in this article.

In most instances, accurate diagnosis of a hemangioma or vascular malformation requires consideration of both clinical findings and diagnostic imaging. Ultrasonography, magnetic resonance

[a] Department of Radiology, University of Michigan Health System, 1500 East Medical Center Drive, Ann Arbor, MI 48109, USA
[b] Department of Plastic Surgery, University of Michigan Health System, 1500 East Medical Center Drive, Ann Arbor, MI 48109, USA
* Corresponding author. Department of Radiology, Room UH B1-D502, University of Michigan Health System, 1500 East Medical Center Drive, Ann Arbor, MI 48109-5030.
E-mail address: abaer@umich.edu

Neuroimag Clin N Am 21 (2011) 641–658
doi:10.1016/j.nic.2011.05.007
1052-5149/11/$ – see front matter

Table 1
Common colloquial terms for vascular anomalies

Category[a]	Colloquial Term
Hemangioma	Strawberry hemangioma Strawberry mark Mixed hemangioma Capillary hemangioma Capillary-cavernous hemangioma Juvenile hemangioma Cellular hemangioma
Vascular malformation	Port-wine stain (capillary) Port-wine hemangioma (capillary) Cavernous malformation (venous) Cavernous hemangioma (venous)

[a] Based on the ISSVA-accepted classification approved in 1992. Note that the colloquial terms are inconsistently used in the literature. Consequently, the categorization in Table 1 is not applicable in all cases. For example, although the term port-wine stain has most frequently been used to describe capillary malformations, it has also been used to describe venous malformations in the past.

(MR) imaging, computed tomography (CT), and conventional angiography each have a role in assisting diagnosis, but ultrasound and MR imaging are optimal first-line diagnostic tools. These imaging modalities also play a central role in identifying appropriate treatment and assessing treatment efficacy.

HEMANGIOMAS

Mulliken and Glowacki[3] suggested that the term hemangioma be reserved for true neoplasms that arise during infancy, experience a proliferative phase, and eventually involute to some degree.[3] Identifying this characteristic clinical course is vital to accurate diagnosis. The term hemangioma continues to be erroneously used to describe many birthmarks, vascular malformations or otherwise. Hemangiomas can be further divided into hemangiomas of infancy and congenital hemangiomas, which are less common and have generally completed their proliferative phase at the time of birth.

Although many hemangiomas can be diagnosed clinically, diagnostic imaging can assist in clarifying questionable diagnoses, excluding malignancies of similar appearance, identifying lesion depth and organ involvement for surgical planning, and in assessing treatment response. Histologically, the proliferative phase is characterized by high mitotic activity and the involutional phase by fibrosis and decreased cellularity. These cellular changes account for imaging findings that are specific to each evolutionary phase, particularly with MR imaging.

Hemangioma of Infancy

Also referred to as the infantile hemangioma or common infantile hemangioma, the hemangioma of infancy is the most common head and neck tumor of childhood.[1,3,7,8] It is present in approximately 1% to 2% of all neonates and is approximately 5 times more common in girls than in

Table 2
Categorization and flow characteristics of common vascular anomalies

Category	Subcategory	Flow Characteristic
Tumor	Hemangioma of infancy	
	Proliferative phase	High[a]
	Involutional phase	Low[a]
	RICH	High
	NICH	High
Malformation	Arterial malformation	
	Arteriovenous malformation	High
	Arteriovenous fistula	High
	Venous malformation	Low
	Capillary malformation	Low
	Lymphatic malformation	Low
	Mixed vascular malformations	Variable

Abbreviations: NICH, noninvoluting congenital hemangioma; RICH, rapidly involuting congenital hemangioma.
[a] Just as the proliferative, quiescent, and involutional phases of hemangioma development exist as a continuum, so too do the respective flow velocities.

boys.[9–11] The incidence is reportedly even higher in white infants, 10% to 12% in full-term deliveries, and higher still in those born prematurely.[6,11] Although most lesions (80%) are solitary, approximately 20% of affected infants present with more than 5 lesions.[8,9,12]

The most commonly involved locations are the head and neck (60%), followed by the trunk (25%), and extremities (15%).[12,13] Within the head and neck, lesions have been identified in the forehead (**Fig. 1**), temple, cheek, orbital/periorbital region, lips, nasal cavity, larynx, within glands, and in the deep spaces of the neck.

Most hemangiomas of infancy are not visible at birth, but present within the first several weeks of infancy. The proliferative phase, which begins in early infancy, involves rapid growth and can continue for 4 to 10 months.[9] This is followed by a quiescent period and, later, an involutional phase of gradual regression in the next 6 to 10 years. Lesion appearance depends largely on depth, and 2 classic presentations have been described, although myriad forms have been reported. Superficial hemangioma (previously called strawberry hemangioma) describes a hemangioma of infancy that is superficial in location and generally bright red in color. In contrast, deep hemangioma (previously called mixed or cavernous hemangioma) describes a deeper lesion that may be colorless or have a bluish hue.[14]

Complications can result from hemorrhage, ulceration, infection, or from a compromising lesion location. For example, orbital and periorbital hemangiomas can result in vision impairment or amblyopia.[9] Airway involvement is common, particularly in those patients with hemangiomas of the chin and jaw line.[9] Although most lesions ultimately leave no visible cosmetic defect,

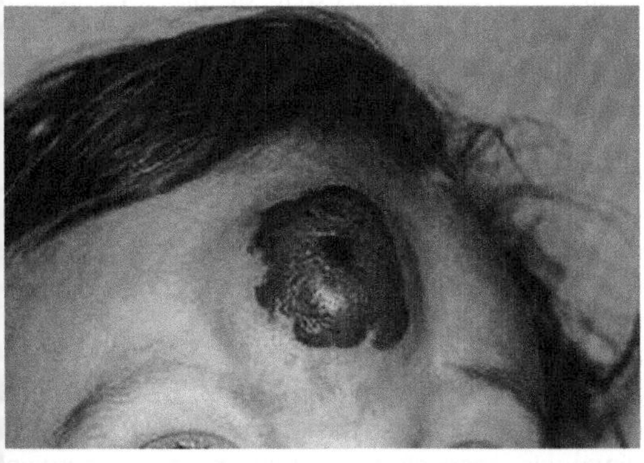

Fig. 1. Hemangioma of infancy, proliferative phase. Eight-month-old girl with a painless, protuberant, pigmented lesion of the forehead. At birth, the structure was pink and minimally raised. Soon thereafter it began enlarging.

a minority can result in permanent pigmentation, scarring, or fibrofatty tissue.[3,9]

Several syndromes have been associated with hemangiomas, such as PHACES syndrome (posterior fossa malformations, hemangiomas, arterial anomalies, coarctation of the aorta and other cardiac defects, and eye abnormalities), and, traditionally, Kasabach-Merritt phenomenon. Characteristics of PHACES also include sternal clefts or supraumbilical raphes (**Fig. 2**). Despite contradictions in the literature, Kasabach-Merritt (K-M) phenomenon (consumptive coagulopathy and thrombocytopenia) does not have an association with true hemangiomas. Current evidence suggests that the discolored, raised cutaneous lesions believed to be hemangiomas in K-M are kaposiform hemangioendotheliomas or tufted angiomas.[15] The literature also contains associations with many other syndromes including Dandy-Walker, Klippel-Trenaunay, Sturge-Weber, Beckwith-Wiedemann, von Hippel-Lindau, and Osler-Weber-Rendu syndrome.[14]

Some of these lesions involute spontaneously without cosmetic defect, and, in these cases, conservative watchful management is preferred. However, consideration must always be given to the anatomic area involved and the rate of growth of the lesion. The need for late surgical reconstruction can often be avoided by early intervention for hemangiomas located in critical areas such as the ear or nasal tip. Long-term functional sequelae from the temporary lesions must also be considered. For example, periocular hemangiomas frequently mandate treatment to prevent permanent vision impairment.

Treatment options include surgical excision, pharmacotherapy, chemotherapy, and laser therapy. Intralesional injection of corticosteroids is a common and effective means of promoting involution, particularly with small lesions. Oral corticosteroids have been shown to be effective in treating hemangiomas, with a 70% to 90% response rate.[9] Systemic treatment is typically reserved for problematic lesions because potential side effects are numerous, including hypertension, fat deposition, mood alteration, and relative immunosuppression. However, these side effects can be easily minimized with the appropriate administration regimen. β-Blockers have recently been examined as a possible safe and effective alternative to corticosteroids.[16,17] The risk/benefit ratio of this method, in comparison with corticosteroid therapy, remains to be established. In cases of life-threatening hemangiomas with failed prior therapy, vincristine and interferon-α have been used with high success rates.[9] Laser therapy has also been used with variable success, particularly

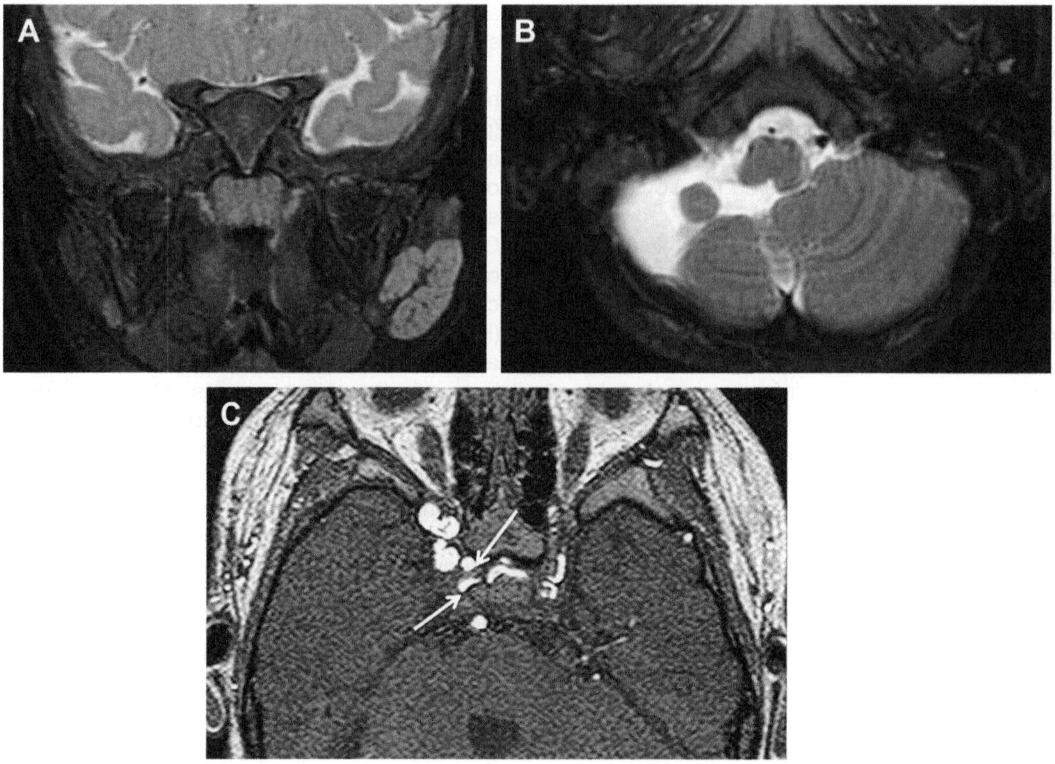

Fig. 2. PHACES syndrome. Ten-month-old infant with PHACES syndrome. Coronal T2-weighted image (*A*) shows a homogeneous and mildly T2-hyperintense mass in the left masticator space, typical for a hemangioma of infancy. Axial T2-weighted image (*B*) shows dysplasia of the right cerebellar hemisphere. Further, a time-of-flight MR angiogram source image shows an anomalous vessel connecting the right internal carotid artery to the basilar artery (*C, arrows*), suggesting a persistent trigeminal artery.

for thin hemangiomas causing skin irregularity and in treating areas of ulceration in larger hemangiomas. Intravenous steroids and surgical excision are the treatments of choice for life-threatening hemangiomas, those causing a loss of function, lesions unresponsive to less-invasive treatments, and for cases in which excessive redundant tissue is expected to persist after involution.[9]

Congenital Hemangioma

The term congenital hemangioma refers to a hyperproliferative vascular lesion that completes its proliferative phase before birth. It has yet to be elucidated whether the congenital hemangioma is histopathologically distinct from, or simply a variant of, the hemangioma of infancy, but the natural history is distinct. Imaging characteristics of congenital and infantile hemangiomas are similar, but immunohistochemical analysis confirms that they are distinct entities. A specific glucose transporter protein, GLUT-1, has been identified that is specific to hemangiomas of infancy but expressed by neither congenital hemangiomas nor vascular malformations.[3,8,10]

Two forms exist, the rapidly involuting congenital hemangioma (RICH) and the noninvoluting congenital hemangioma (NICH).[10] Differentiating between congenital and infantile hemangiomas is done primarily with clinical information. RICHs complete involution more rapidly than hemangiomas of infancy, usually within the first 14 months of life.[14] In contrast, NICHs do not involute but grow commensurately with the child. Because of the rapidity of regression, involuted RICHs can leave redundant skin, which can be cosmetically problematic. Differential diagnosis for the congenital hemangioma includes tufted angioma, embryonic rhabdomyosarcoma, fibrosarcoma, hemangiopericytoma, infantile myofibromatosis, and neuroblastoma.[14]

Imaging characteristics

Although most hemangiomas can be diagnosed clinically, imaging can assist in confirming a clinical diagnosis, assessing tumor extent, and in surgical planning. Ultrasound and MR imaging are both reasonable first-line diagnostic tools for a suspected hemangioma. As a noninvasive, inexpensive, and increasingly available imaging modality,

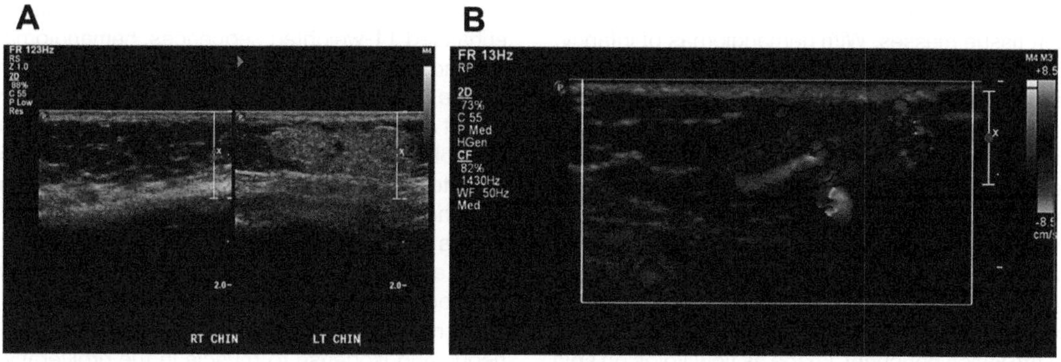

Fig. 3. Hemangioma of infancy, quiescent phase. Two-year-old girl with fullness of the left submental region. Grayscale ultrasound shows a well-circumscribed, echogenic mass in the region of interest (*A*). Color flow Doppler identifies multiple vessels within the mass and a sizeable intervening soft tissue component (*B*).

ultrasonography is ideal for evaluating a suspected hemangioma that is small in size and superficial in location.[18] Particularly deep or large lesions may require MR imaging for complete characterization.

Congenital hemangiomas have the same imaging features as hemangiomas of infancy with a few exceptions. For example, congenital hemangiomas can have intravascular thrombi, which are not seen in the infantile form, larger venous components than infantile hemangiomas, and vascular aneurysms.[16]

Grayscale ultrasonography depicts a well-demarcated structure of variable echogenicity (Fig. 3A). Color flow Doppler shows a highly vascular structure, which, in contrast with a vascular malformation, contains a sizeable parenchymal component (see Fig. 3B). Hemangiomas are characterized by a high flow velocity during the proliferative phase and a lower flow velocity during the involutional phase. Unlike arteriovenous malformations, hemangiomas should not have an increased mean venous velocity.

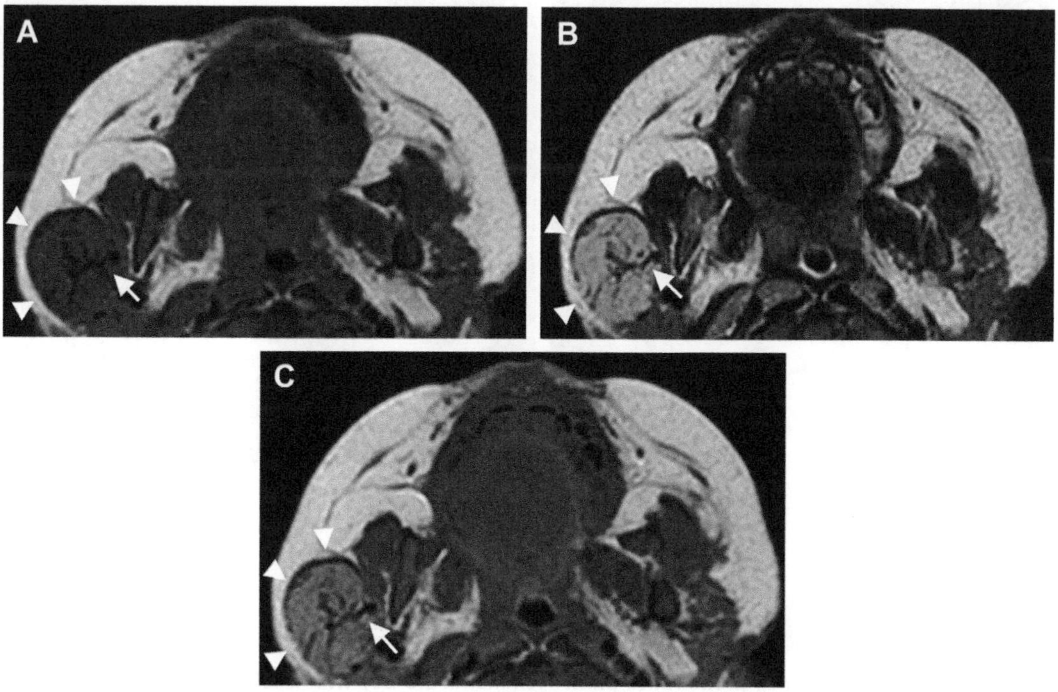

Fig. 4. Hemangioma of infancy, quiescent phase. Three-year-old boy with a firm mass of the left periauricular region. T1-weighted imaging reveals a well-demarcated, homogeneous structure that is isointense to muscle (*A, arrowheads*). T2-weighted imaging shows high signal intensity throughout the lesion (*B, arrowheads*). High-flow internal vasculature is shown by flow voids on both T1-weighted and T2-weighted sequences (*arrows*). Postcontrast T1-weighted imaging shows intense, uniform enhancement (*C, arrowheads*).

MR imaging is helpful in evaluating deep or large soft tissue masses. With hemangiomas of infancy, MR imaging shows a well-marginated soft tissue mass. T1-weighted sequences show a homogeneous lesion with intermediate signal intensity during the proliferative phase, and a heterogeneous lesion with small focal areas of fat replacement during the involutional phase (**Fig. 4**A).[12,16] On T2-weighted images, lesions appear homogeneous and moderately hyperintense during the proliferative phase (see **Fig. 4**B) and more heterogeneous while involuting. High-flow vessels, which are often at the lesion periphery, image as flow voids on spin echo sequences and as high signal intensity on gradient echo sequences.[8,16] On contrast-enhanced T1-weighted sequences, hemangiomas enhance homogeneously (see **Fig. 4**C). In the proliferative phase, MR angiography or venography may depict a large feeding artery or large draining veins (**Fig. 5**D). Phleboliths produce intralesional foci of low intensity, are uncharacteristic of hemangiomas, and should suggest an alternative diagnosis. Phleboliths are commonly seen in venous malformations and in mixed vascular malformations with a venous component.

On nonenhanced CT, lesions appear homogeneous and isodense to muscle in the proliferative phase and heterogeneous with areas of low

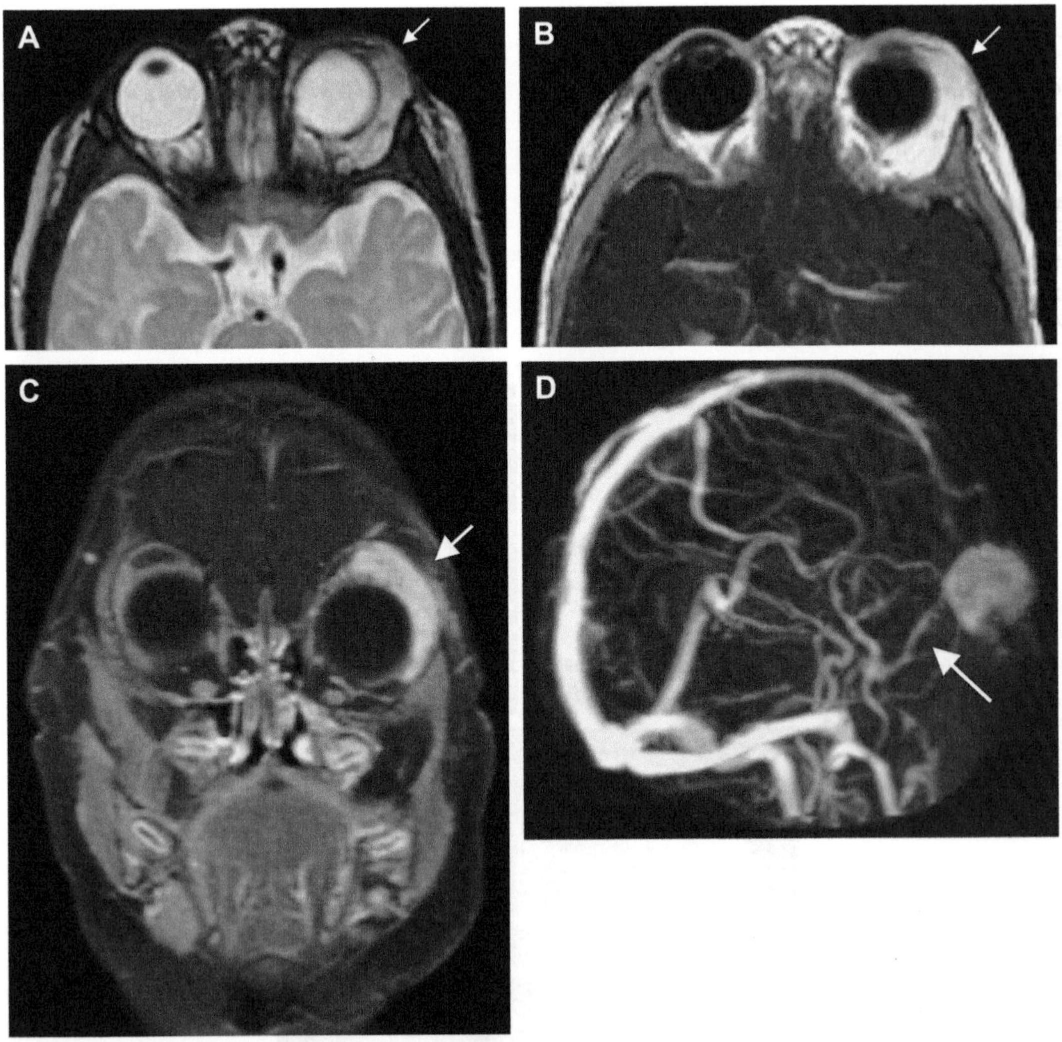

Fig. 5. Hemangioma of infancy, proliferative phase. Ten-month-old boy with a left orbital mass identified at birth. MR imaging shows a T2-hyperintense lesion involving the superior and lateral aspects of the left orbit (*A, arrow*). The tumor shows intense enhancement on postcontrast T1-weighted imaging (*B* and *C, arrows*). MR venography, presented here as a maximum-intensity projection image, shows a prominent draining vein extending posteriorly into the left cavernous sinus (*D, arrow*). This patient was treated successfully with systemic corticosteroids for impairment of eyelid excursion.

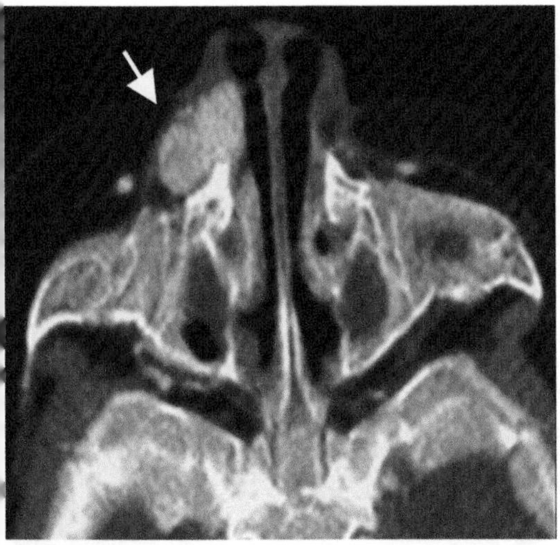

Fig. 6. Hemangioma of infancy, involutional phase. Five-year-old boy with fullness of the right lateral nose. Contrast-enhanced CT depicts a homogeneously and avidly enhancing mass (*arrow*).

attenuation (fat) in the involutional phase.[12] Contrast-enhanced CT images depict a lesion that uniformly enhances (**Fig. 6**). Again, phleboliths are uncommon in true hemangiomas, and, if present, should suggest a vascular malformation with a venous component.

Conventional angiography shows a hypervascular mass with parenchymal enhancement. Enlarged feeding and draining vessels are commonly identified. Arteriovenous shunting has been documented but is uncommon.

VASCULAR MALFORMATIONS

Mulliken and Glowacki[3] suggested that the term vascular malformation be used to describe anomalies of vasculature that are present at birth, grow proportionally with the child, have normal endothelial turnover, and do not spontaneously regress.[3] Rather than a product of cellular hyperproliferation or neoplasia, these lesions result from abnormal vascular morphogenesis. This category includes arterial, venous, capillary, and lymphatic malformations, and any combination thereof.

Vascular malformations are categorized by primary constituent channel type (eg, arterial, venous, capillary) and subcategorized by relative flow velocity. These categories vary widely in potential complications and treatment challenges.

As with hemangiomas, the clinical presentation of vascular malformations depend on location and depth. By definition, these lesions are present at birth. However, they may not be visible or recognized until much later. Although the natural history of these lesions does not include a proliferative phase, they can grow in size. Hormonal changes, infection, trauma, and surgical injury can all result in enlargement. Unlike hemangiomas, vascular malformations can produce significant distortion of underlying bone.[7,19]

Histologically, the vascular channels have normal cellularity and are lined with mature endothelium. Mitotic activity is not accelerated in these dysplastic structures, and they do not express biologic markers characteristic of vascular tumors, such as GLUT-1, FcγRII, merosin, and Lewis Y antigen.[2]

Optimal treatment is dependent on subtype. Surgical resection, intralesional sclerotherapy, laser photocoagulation, chemotherapy, and pharmacotherapy have all been performed with varying degrees of success.

Venous Malformations

Venous malformations (VMs) are the most common of all vascular malformations.[8] They are second only to hemangiomas as the most common vascular abnormality of the head and neck in childhood.[3,20] The VM is frequently referred to as a cavernous hemangioma, although the entity is not a hemangioma.

These lesions, like all vascular malformations, are said to be present at birth, although they are frequently not identified until later in life. Composed of venous sinusoids of varying size, VMs have been described in intradermal, subcutaneous, intramuscular, and intraosseous locations.[2] Common head and neck locations include the subcutaneous tissues of the face, muscles of

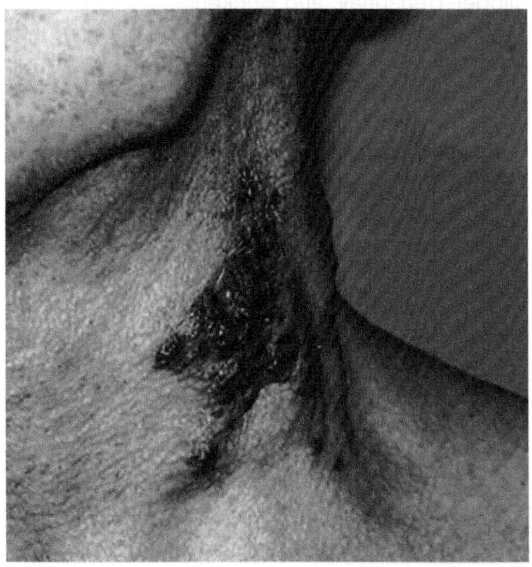

Fig. 7. Venous malformation. An irregular, slightly raised, purple-colored lesion of the left neck. On physical examination, the venous malformation was easily compressible and expanded slightly with Valsalva.

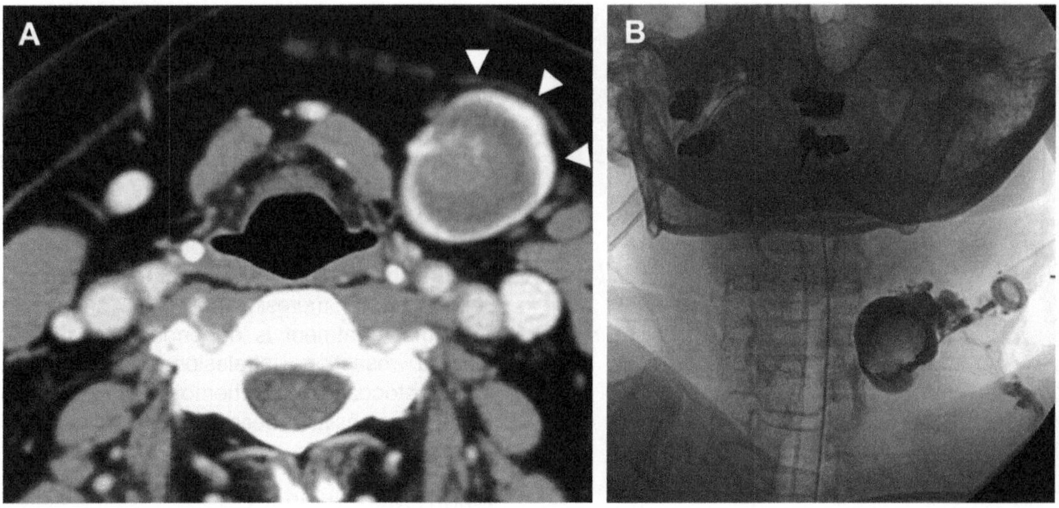

Fig. 8. Venous malformation. Three-year-old girl with left neck mass that increases in size when she is crying. Contrast-enhanced CT shows late enhancement (*A, arrowheads*). Localization with direct injection of contrast under fluoroscopy identified this as a low-flow venous malformation. Multistage sclerotherapy was performed with pure ethanol, resulting in eventual regression of the lesion (*B*).

mastication, periorbital region, and deep neck spaces. Lesion depth and location dictate clinical presentation. Superficial VMs are bluish in color, soft, and compressible (**Fig. 7**). Some superficial lesions enlarge with Valsalva maneuver or with high-volume states. In contrast with arterial or arteriovenous malformations, these venous anomalies should not produce an auscultatory bruit or palpable thrill. Several syndromes are associated with VMs, including blue rubber bleb nevus, familial cutaneomucosal venous malformation, Klippel-Trenaunay, and Bockenheimer syndrome.

Conservative management, such as a compression device, is frequently preferred for uncomplicated lesions. Complications that indicate treatment include disfigurement, hemorrhage (including gastrointestinal bleeding), pain, and venous thrombosis.[16] Traditionally, small focal lesions undergo complete surgical resection. Laser photocoagulation has also been used with reported success. At present, sclerotherapy is a commonly used first-line treatment of many low-flow anomalies including VMs.[4] Sclerosants used in the treatment of VMs include ethanol, sodium tetradecyl sulfate, polidocanol, and ethanolamine oleate (**Fig. 8**B).[4]

Imaging characteristics

When any vascular malformation is suspected, ultrasound is an ideal first-line diagnostic study, because the modality can characterize the lesion as low or high flow.[18] MR imaging and CT are useful in defining lesion extent, involvement of vital organs, and identifying bone destruction. The low-flow characteristic of VMs accounts for many of their imaging features.

Grayscale ultrasound depicts the VM as a poorly marginated structure with vascular channels that are often compressible (**Fig. 9**). The lesion is usually hypoechoic and heterogeneous and can appear infiltrative.[16] Doppler spectral analysis shows monophasic low-velocity internal flow with no identifiable arterial waveform. Phleboliths, highly suggestive of a VM, image as echogenic foci with distal acoustic shadowing.

The use of intravenous gadolinium-based contrast is strongly recommended when low-flow lesions such as venous and lymphatic

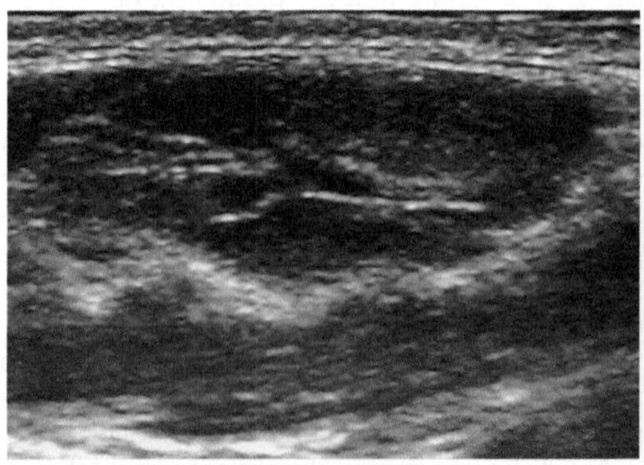

Fig. 9. Venous malformation. Seven-year-old boy with blue-colored posterior neck swelling. Grayscale ultrasonography shows an ill-defined, superficial structure with large compressible hypoechoic components. Doppler examination (not shown) shows low flow velocity with no identifiable arterial waveform.

malformations are suspected. On T1-weighted imaging, these lobulated lesions appear hypointense to isointense compared with muscle (**Fig. 10**A). Heterogeneous signal may be perceived in the setting of intralesional hemorrhage or thrombosis.[16] T2-weighted appearance varies with vascular channel size. Large channels produce a cystic and hyperintense appearance, secondary to the blood within, whereas smaller channels appear more solid with intermediate signal intensity (see **Fig. 10**B).[12] Venous thrombi produce low signal intensity on T2-weighted sequences. Unlike high-flow lesions, VMs generally do not produce flow voids on MR imaging. However, gradient echo sequences may show an absence of signal within lesion vessels, suggesting a low flow velocity. Phleboliths, highly suggestive of venous malformations, image as focal signal voids on T2-weighted studies. Contrast-enhanced MR imaging produces heterogeneous delayed enhancement (see **Fig. 10**C).

On CT, VMs appear as lobulated or multilobulated lesions, isodense to muscle, that can infiltrate multiple spaces of the head and neck.[12] In contrast with hemangiomas, hyperdense rounded phleboliths may be present and are considered by some to be pathognomonic for the VM (**Fig. 11**). In this respect, CT can prove a valuable modality in the diagnosis of VMs, because it readily identifies small calcified phleboliths. CT can also reveal bone remodeling adjacent to the lesion, a finding characteristic of VMs but uncommon to hemangiomas. Although they are benign lesions, the poor margination of VMs can give them an incongruously aggressive appearance. These low-flow lesions have small feeding arteries but may have enlarged draining veins. Contrast-enhanced CT usually shows enhancement, although to a variable extent because of the low-flow characteristic (see **Fig. 8**A).

If prior imaging shows a low-flow lesion, conventional angiography provides little benefit from

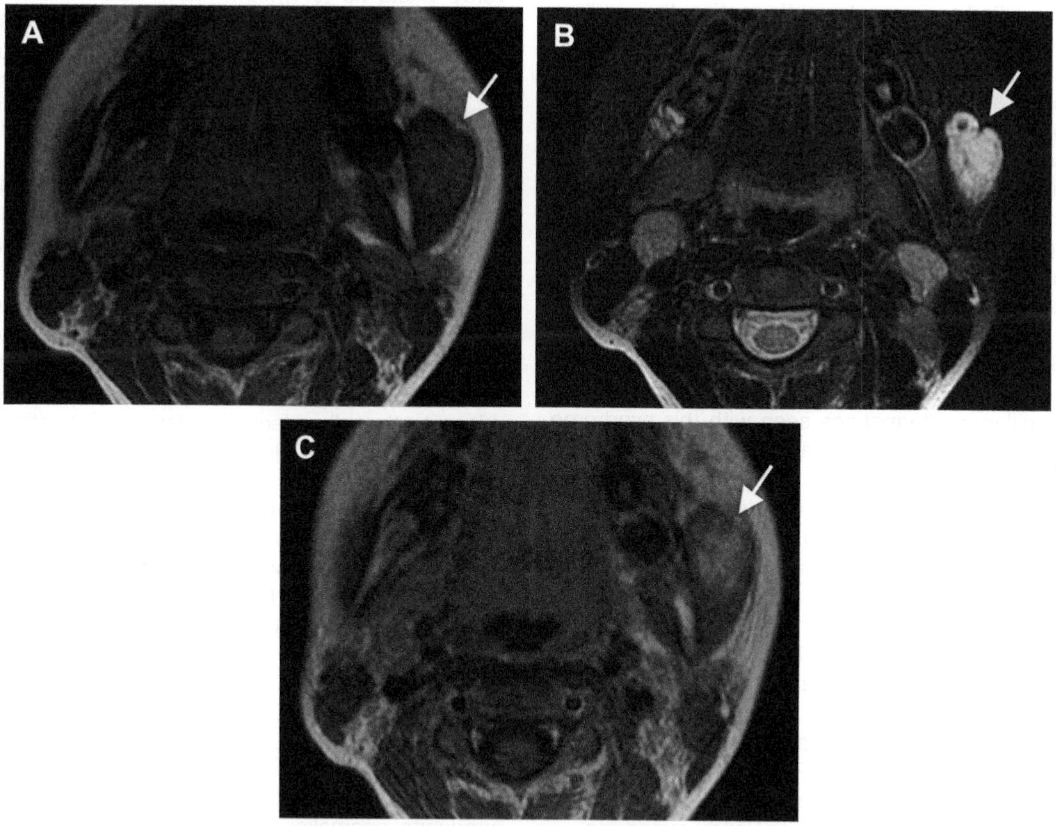

Fig. 10. Venous malformation. Eight-year-old boy with subtle swelling of the left cheek (*arrows*). On T1-weighted imaging, the lesion is isointense to muscle (*A*). T2-weighted MR imaging with fat saturation shows a well-demarcated, heterogeneous structure with high signal intensity (*B*). After intravenous gadolinium-based contrast administration, fat-saturated T1-weighted images show heterogeneous, delayed enhancement (*C*). Findings are consistent with a venous malformation consisting of large vascular channels and no identifiable soft tissue component. Incidental enlarged level II lymph nodes are seen bilaterally.

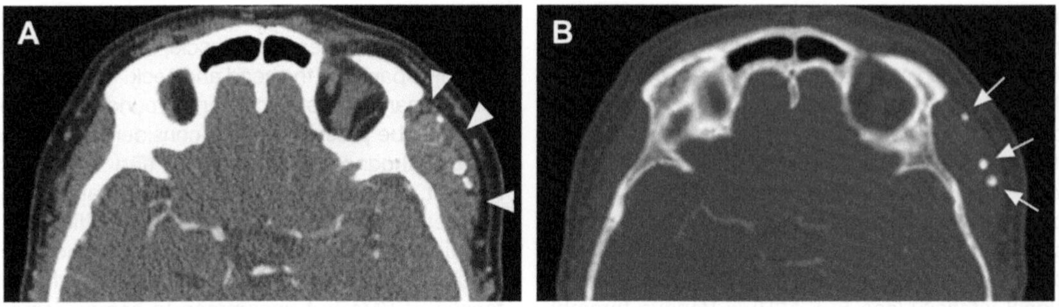

Fig. 11. Venous malformation. Eleven-year-old boy with a soft, compressible swelling of the left temple. With soft tissue windows, contrast-enhanced CT shows a lesion within the left temporalis muscle without significant arterial-phase enhancement (*A, arrowheads*). In bone windows, multiple round foci of high attenuation are seen, reflecting phleboliths within the intramuscular lesion (*B, arrows*).

a diagnostic perspective. The modality is insensitive for the detection of these low-flow lesions, although a known VM can be well visualized with direct injection of contrast (see **Fig. 8**B). Normal arterial and capillary phases are expected.

Capillary Malformations

Classified as a vascular malformation, the capillary malformation was previously termed port-wine stain, capillary hemangioma, nevus flammeus, angel's kiss, and stork's bite.[2,7] Like other vascular malformations, CM are present at birth and grow commensurately with the child. The superficial dermal location of these lesions accounts for their characteristic appearance. Color can range from light pink to dark purple, and the lesions frequently appear as macules or patches of the forehead, eyelids, nose, and neck.[2]

Port-wine stains have long been associated with Sturge-Weber syndrome, a rare disorder also known as encephalotrigeminal angiomatosis. Capillary malformations seen with this syndrome are characteristically located in the distribution of the ophthalmic division of the trigeminal nerve (V1). The syndrome involves leptomeningeal angiomatosis ipsilateral to the facial lesion, and patients can experience seizures, transient neurologic deficits, glaucoma, and a multitude of other neurologic complications.[1] To ensure early diagnosis, all children born with a cutaneous lesion in the characteristic V1 distribution should undergo contrast-enhanced MR imaging to assess for underlying leptomeningeal angiomatosis. CT should be considered if MR imaging is contraindicated. Other associated syndromes include Louis-Barr and Osler-Weber-Rendu syndrome.

In a review of 415 patients with facial CM, Geronemus and Ashinoff[21] found that 65% of all subjects had significant lesion hypertrophy and/or nodularity by the fifth decade of life. Photocoagulation with pulsed dye laser (PDL) has been shown to be effective in improving appearance, with varying reported degrees of improvement. In one study, patients experienced greater than 75% clearance of lesional color after multiple treatment sessions.[22] Another study reported an average of approximately 40% reduction in lesional color by colorimetry following similar treatment.[23] Controversy exists as to whether early PDL treatment provides long-term benefit, because perceived pigment lightening during infancy (with or without treatment) may in part be caused by normal physiologic changes.[23,24]

Imaging characteristics

The CM diagnosis is primarily clinical, with little role for imaging except to exclude more serious disorders, such as in the setting of possible Sturge-Weber syndrome, as described earlier.

Like venous malformations, CM are low-flow structures. Because of small channel size, the ultrasonographic features of CM are nonspecific, and the primary usefulness of ultrasound is to rule out other disorders. Capillary malformations are frequently not identifiable on MR imaging. When visible, they may appear simply as skin thickening or abnormality of the subcutaneous tissue signal (**Fig. 12**A). Lesions may enhance with intravenous contrast administration (see **Fig. 12**B). CT imaging findings are often negligible, even with extensive disease. The diagnostic value of CT in diagnosing CM is in ruling out more serious disorders.

Arterial Malformations

The term arterial malformation describes high-flow congenital anomalies including arteriovenous malformations (AVM) and arteriovenous fistulae (AVF). All AVM operate as a shunt to some degree. AVM are characterized by an aberrant connection between feeding arteries and draining veins without a normal intervening capillary network.

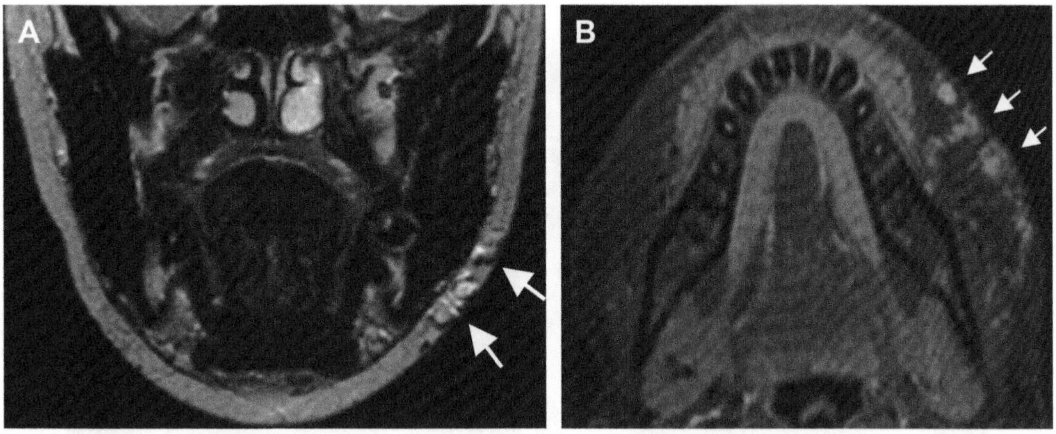

Fig. 12. Capillary malformation. One-year-old girl with dark red patch over her left jaw. T2-weighted imaging shows an ill-defined structure of mixed signal intensity within the subcutaneous soft tissues of the jaw (*A, arrows*). After contrast administration, T1-weighted imaging with fat saturation shows subtle enhancement within the lesion (*B, arrows*).

On physical examination, AVM may be warm to the touch or produce a palpable thrill or auscultatory bruit. The neck and craniofacial region are common sites of occurrence. Like venous and capillary malformations, AVM have mature endothelium with normal mitotic activity. Rapid growth is not a characteristic of the lesion's natural history. However, hormonal change, trauma, and partial surgical resection can result in enlargement. Complications include pain, hemorrhage, and cerebrovascular accident. Large AVM or AVF have also resulted in high-output heart failure. Associated syndromes include Wyburn-Mason, Osler-Weber-Rendu, capillary malformation-arteriovenous malformation, Cobb, and Parkes-Weber syndrome. For complicated lesions, a combination of endovascular embolization and surgical resection has been used with good outcomes.[25]

Imaging characteristics

Arterial malformations are high-flow lesions without a normal capillary network between lesion arteries and veins, features that contribute to their characteristic imaging findings.

The AVM has no parenchymal component and, as such, images on grayscale ultrasonography as a poorly defined heterogeneous structure. Fat is often seen around the AVM. Doppler ultrasound shows a network of multiple arteries with increased diastolic flow and arterialized draining veins with a biphasic waveform.[16]

MR angiography can be valuable in visualizing the characteristic appearance of AVM: dilated feeding arteries and draining veins without normal intervening capillaries or parenchyma. Venous enhancement is early and intense and venous lakes are generally not present.[16] Like proliferating hemangiomas, these high-flow lesions produce flow-voids on spin echo sequences and high signal intensity on gradient echo imaging (**Fig. 13**)[16]

AVMs appear as multiple intertwined enhancing vessels on CT. In contrast with the hemangioma, the AVM is not associated with a soft tissue/parenchymal component. CT may show hypertrophy of adjacent bone. As with MR imaging, contrast-enhanced CT shows large feeding arteries, an absence of a capillary network, and intense early venous enhancement (**Fig. 14**).[16]

Conventional angiography shows a high-flow structure with large feeding arteries, an absent capillary network, and large draining veins with early venous filling (see **Fig. 13**C).

Lymphatic Malformations

The term lymphatic malformation (LM) refers to vascular anomalies resulting from abnormal lymphangiogenesis. LMs account for approximately 6% of all benign lesions of childhood.[7] Most of these lesions are present at birth and nearly all are identified by 2 years of age.

Previously used terms such as lymphangioma, cavernous lymphangioma, and cystic hygroma are no longer preferred, because the histologically based classification has no prognostic significance. The current preferred terms include macrocystic, microcystic, and mixed macrocystic and microcystic LMs. These subcategories correlate with treatment response and prognosis.[26,27]

Like arterial, venous, and capillary malformations, LM are characterized by a structural abnormality rather than abnormal endothelial proliferation or neoplasia. The exact pathophysiology of LM

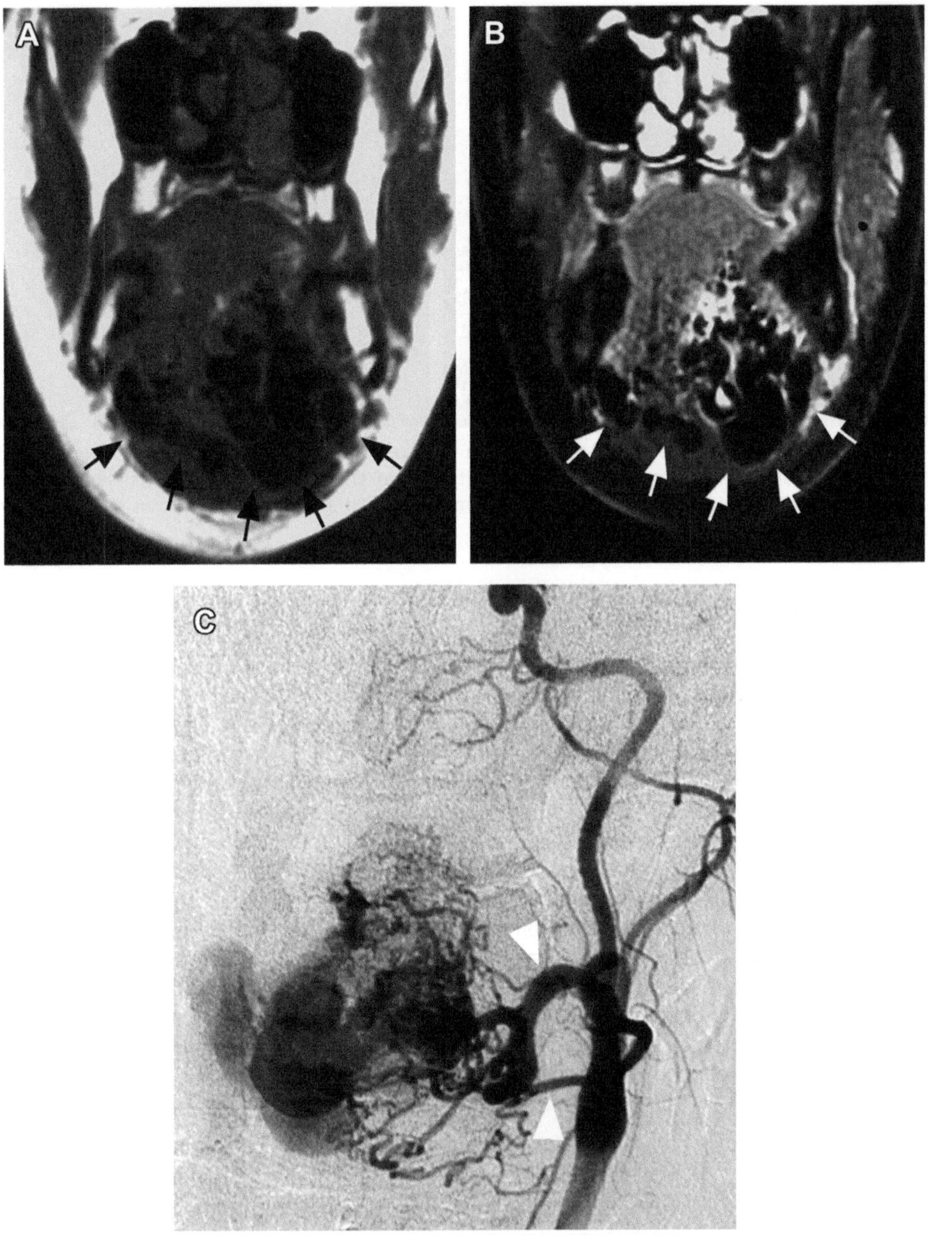

Fig. 13. Arteriovenous malformation. Eight-year-old boy with known AVM of the sublingual and submandibular region. T1-weighted and T2-weighted images with fat saturation show an extensive, ill-defined structure in the submandibular region with large internal flow voids (*A* and *B*, *arrows*). Conventional angiography shows an entangled vascular structure with vessels of varying size supplied by branches of the external carotid artery (*C*, *arrowheads*).

formation has yet to be established. Proposed mechanisms of formation include abnormal budding of lymphatic tissue, lymphatic sequestration, and failed development of normal lymphatic-venous drainage channels.[7] It has also been proposed that the expression of specific vascular endothelial growth factors unique to LM, and not found in normal lymph tissue or other vascular malformations, plays a central role in LM formation.[27,28]

LMs can be found anywhere in the body where lymphatic tissue exists, but approximately 75% of lesions are located in the head and neck. Another 20% are found in the axilla.[8,29] Within the neck, the posterior triangle is commonly

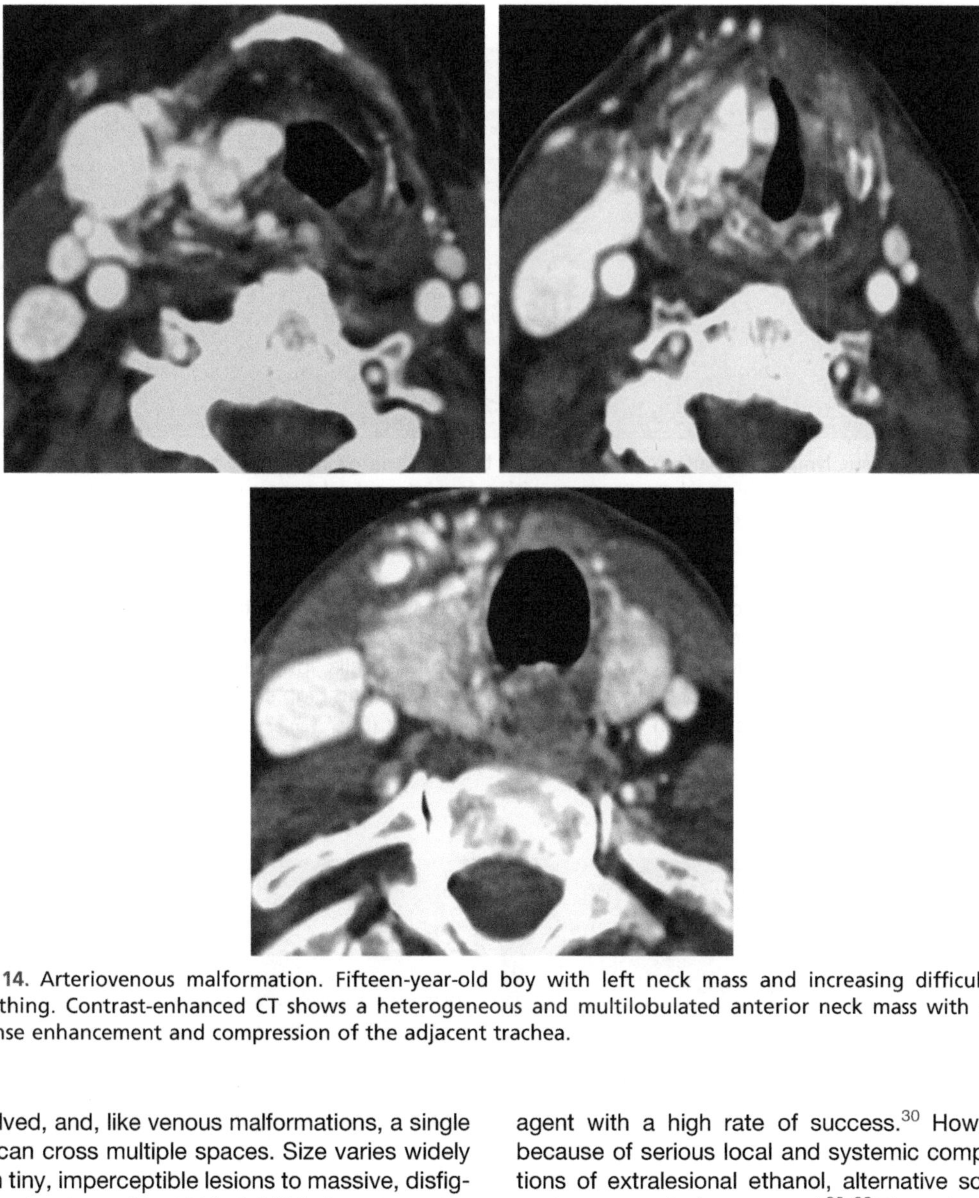

Fig. 14. Arteriovenous malformation. Fifteen-year-old boy with left neck mass and increasing difficulty in breathing. Contrast-enhanced CT shows a heterogeneous and multilobulated anterior neck mass with early, intense enhancement and compression of the adjacent trachea.

involved, and, like venous malformations, a single LM can cross multiple spaces. Size varies widely from tiny, imperceptible lesions to massive, disfiguring structures. Most LMs (>95%) do not spontaneously regress.[26] Associated syndromes include Klippel-Trenaunay, Maffucci, and Proteus syndrome. The most serious potential complication of LM is respiratory compromise. Skeletal distortion is another common complication of craniofacial LM, including mandibular overgrowth, bite abnormalities, and osteolysis.[27]

Optimal treatment is case dependent and can include surgical excision, which is frequently staged, pharmacotherapy, and sclerotherapy. At this time, percutaneous sclerotherapy is the preferred first-line treatment of LM, although surgical excision remains the treatment of choice for microcystic LM refractory to sclerotherapy. Pure ethanol has also been used as a sclerosing agent with a high rate of success.[30] However, because of serious local and systemic complications of extralesional ethanol, alternative sclerosants are now being pursued.[30–33] The sclerosant OK-432 (picibanil) is an effective treatment option for macrocystic LM, although it seems to have little or no effect on the microcystic variety.[32]

The differential diagnosis for LM includes other cystic lesions of the neck, such as the second branchial cleft cyst, thyroglossal duct cyst, thymic cyst, suppurative lymph node, and neck abscess.[12]

Imaging characteristics

As with most venous and capillary malformations, the LM is a low-flow structure, an attribute reflected in imaging. The microcystic or macrocystic morphology also influences imaging characteristics.

Ultrasonography is the first-line diagnostic imaging study for suspected LM.[18] Macrocystic

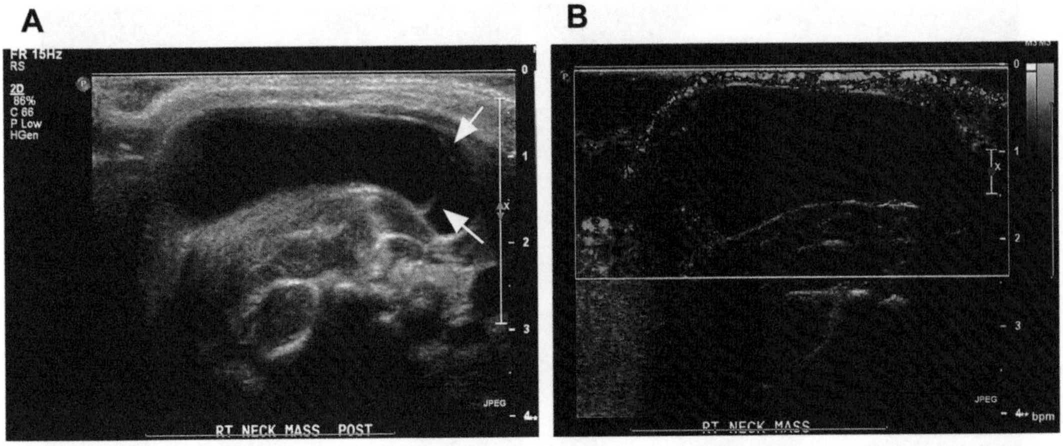

Fig. 15. Macrocystic lymphatic malformation. Neonate born with large right neck mass. Grayscale ultrasonography shows a large, primarily anechoic structure with a few internal echogenic septae (*A, arrows*). Color flow Doppler shows an absence of appreciable flow within the lesion (*B*).

lesions appear as hypoechoic, multiloculated cystic structures on grayscale ultrasound (**Fig. 15**).[16] Microcystic LMs are hyperechoic because of their numerous closely packed septae, which are vascularized, as shown on Doppler analysis.[16]

LMs appear as septated cystic structures on MR imaging. The cystic components of LM have imperceptible walls, low signal intensity on T1-weighted imaging, and high signal intensity on T2-weighted imaging (**Fig. 16**). Hemorrhage within an LM can produce visible fluid-fluid levels with high signal

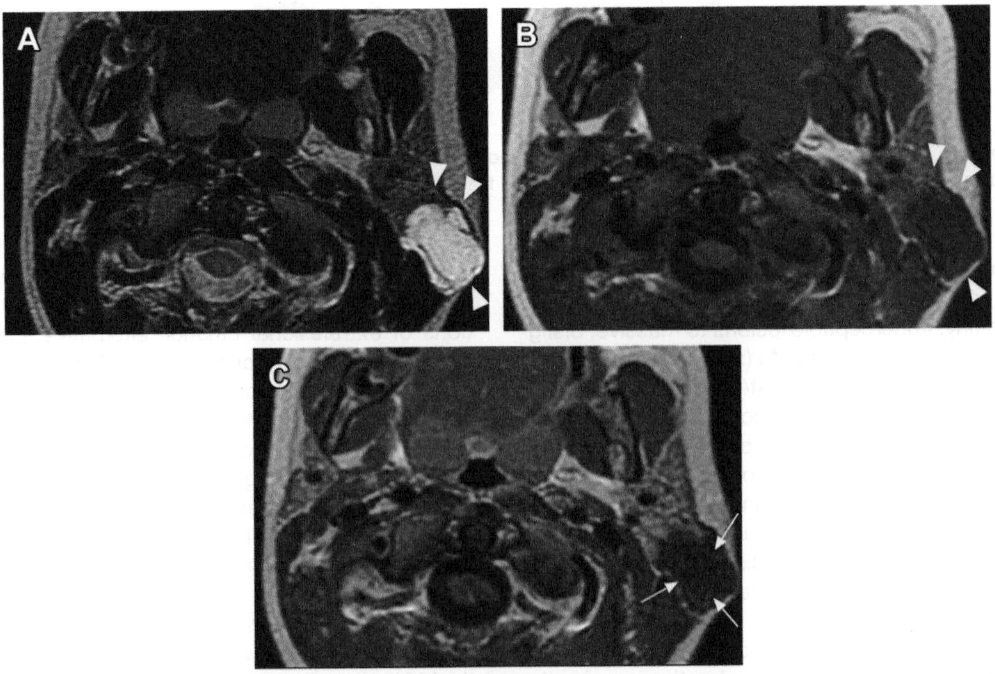

Fig. 16. Macrocystic lymphatic malformation. Fifteen-year-old with asymptomatic mass of the left postauricular scalp. T2-weighted MR imaging shows a well-demarcated cystic structure of the scalp soft tissues (*A, arrowheads*) with internal septae of low signal intensity. T1-weighted imaging depicts the lesion as isointense to muscle (*B, arrowheads*). After intravenous gadolinium administration, there is minimal enhancement of the internal septae (*C, arrows*) without enhancement of the cystic spaces.

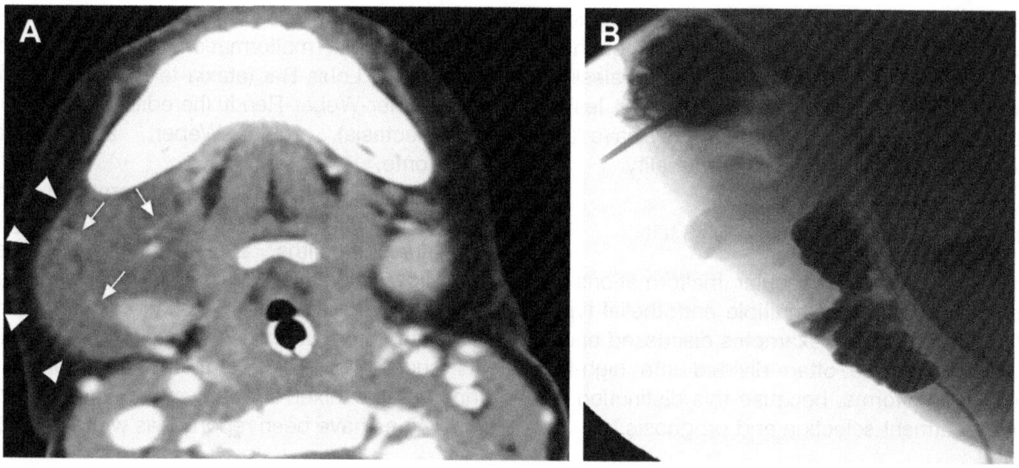

Fig. 17. Macrocystic lymphatic malformation. Six-month-old girl with painless right submandibular swelling. On contrast-enhanced CT, the lymphatic malformation appears as a low-attenuation cystic structure (*A*, *arrowheads*) with subtly enhancing septae (*A*, *arrows*). This low-flow lesion was visualized by direct injection of contrast under fluoroscopy and resolved after several rounds of sclerotherapy (*B*).

on T1-weighted sequences. The cystic components of these lesions do not enhance with contrast administration but the vascularized internal septae often do.[8] In macrocystic LMs, the enhancing septae are subtle in appearance (see **Fig. 16**C). However, microcystic LMs with crowded septae can show an apparent slight enhancement of the entire lesion, potentially leading to misdiagnosis.[8]

On CT, LM appear as low-attenuation masses (10–25 HU) with imperceptible walls and a lack of contrast enhancement except within the septae (**Fig. 17**A).[7] The exception is an LM complicated by infection whose walls can become visibly thickened and show contrast enhancement.[7] Similar findings can be seen with an incompletely resected LM.

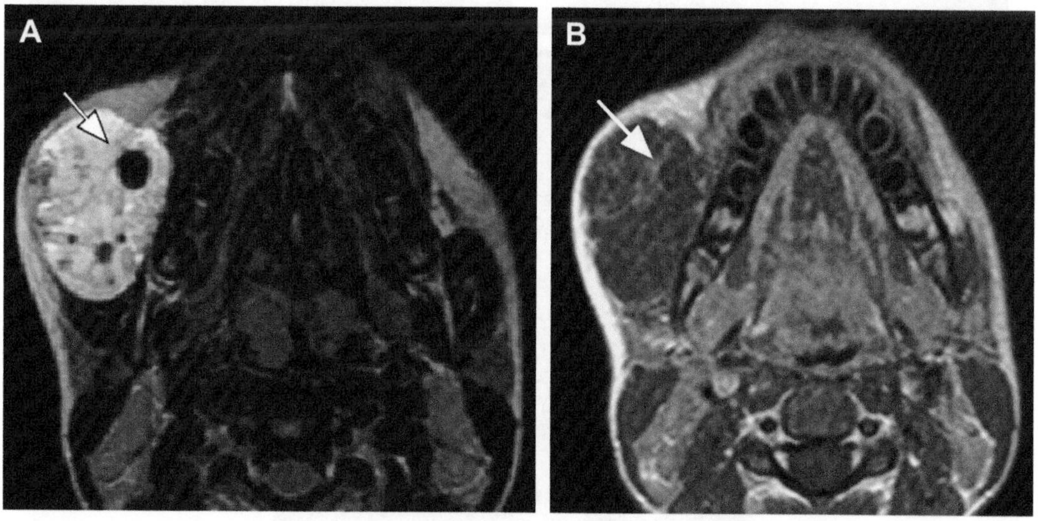

Fig. 18. Venolymphatic malformation. Thirteen-year-old boy with mass of the right jaw. T2-weighted (*A*) and contrast-enhanced T1-weighted (*B*) images show a large, heterogeneous, but predominantly T2-hyperintense lesion in the right masticator/buccal space. There is a T1-hypointense and T2-hypointense focus (*arrows*) suggestive of a phlebolith. On the postcontrast image (*B*), only some areas (venous components) show contrast enhancement, whereas the more posterior regions (lymphatic components) do not enhance. This low-flow malformation was amenable to sclerotherapy.

As low-flow lesions, the diagnostic value of conventional angiography is limited, although LM can be well visualized with direct intralesional contrast injection (see **Fig. 17**B). Mixed lesions with an angiomatous component may have large feeding vessels visible with this modality.

MIXED VASCULAR MALFORMATIONS

Mixed or combined vascular malformations are vascular anomalies of multiple endothelial types. AVMs and AVF are 2 examples discussed earlier. Mixed lesions are often divided into high-flow and low-flow forms, because this distinction can guide treatment selection and prognosis.

There are numerous syndromes associated with mixed vascular malformations, including Klippel-Trenaunay, Louis-Bar (ataxia-telangiectasia), Maffucci, Osler-Weber-Rendu (hereditary hemorrhagic telangiectasia), Parkes-Weber, and Proteus syndrome.[4,14]

Imaging characteristics are determined by the constituent tissues: venous components often contain phleboliths, arterial components have high flow velocities, and so forth. Venolymphatic (**Fig. 18**) and capillary-lymphatic malformations are both common entities with low flow velocities. As such, first-line treatment is sclerotherapy. Innumerable mixed arterial-venous-lymphatic malformations have been reported as well (**Fig. 19**).

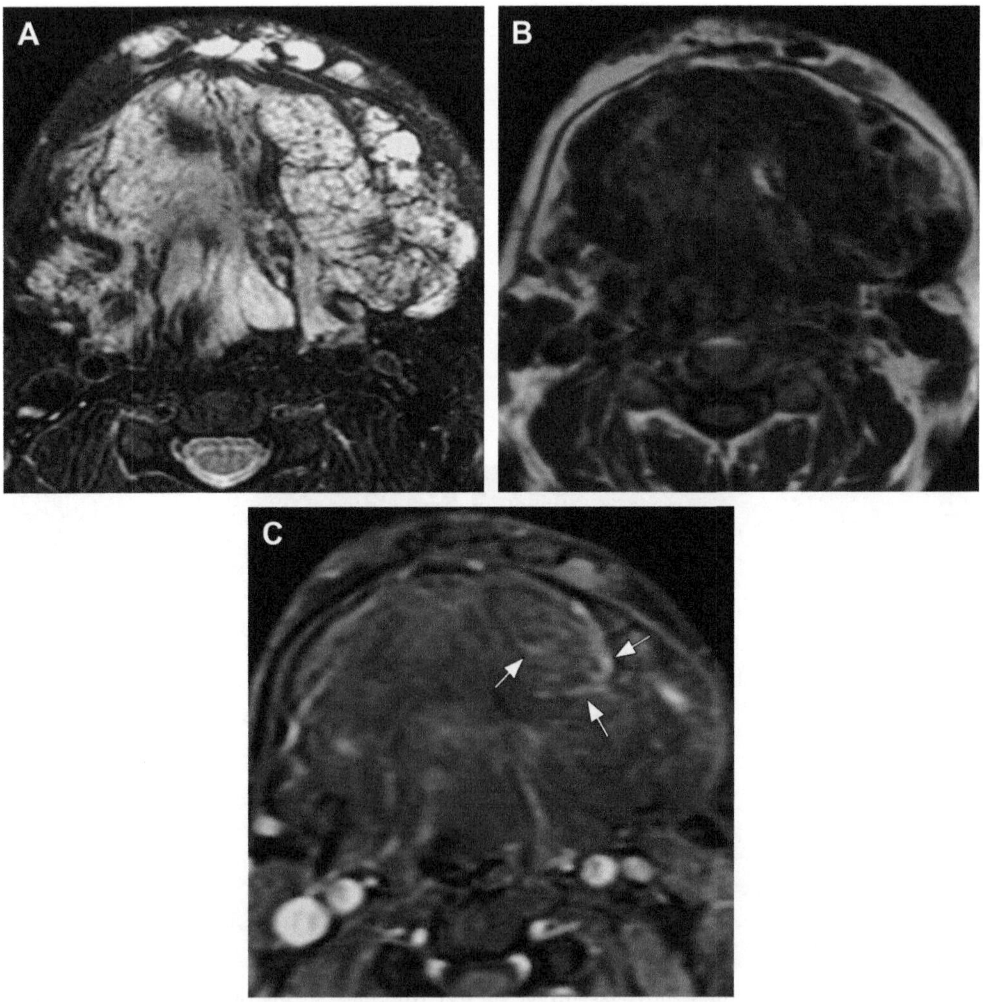

Fig. 19. Mixed vascular malformation. Ten-year-old girl with large jaw mass. Axial T2-weighted image (*A*) shows an ill-defined, multicompartmental lesion in the left sublingual and submandibular space. The structure is heterogeneous but predominantly T2-hyperintense. The lesion was isointense on T1-weighted imaging (*B*). Postcontrast-enhanced T1-weighted images show a linear pattern of enhancement in some areas (*C, arrows*). This lesion was a mixed vascular malformation with venous, capillary, and lymphatic components at histology.

SUMMARY

Vascular anomalies, including vascular tumors and vascular malformations, are common in childhood and vary widely in their presentation, natural course, complications, and treatment. Outcomes tend to be favorable, but accurate diagnosis, with clinical and radiographic contributions, is vital to ensure proper management and to reduce morbidity. **Box 1** summarizes imaging characteristics that are central to the accurate diagnosis of vascular anomalies.

Box 1
Key imaging features of common vascular anomalies

- Hemangioma
  - Ultrasound is an ideal first-line diagnostic study for suspected vascular anomalies.[18]
  - If a suspected hemangioma images as a soft tissue mass with few vessels or surrounding edema, other tumors should be considered.[16]
  - Hemangiomas are highly vascular but also have an associated soft tissue mass, whereas no parenchymal component is associated with an arteriovenous malformation.
  - All hemangiomas, infantile or congenital, can produce high signal intensity on T2-weighted imaging and show enhancement on contrast-enhanced T1-weighted imaging.
- Venous malformation
  - Phleboliths are considered by many to be pathognomonic for a venous malformation (or a venous component of a mixed lesion).
  - Remodeling of adjacent bone is common with venous malformations and uncharacteristic of hemangiomas.
  - Often poorly circumscribed, the benign venous malformation can have an aggressive appearance.
  - Venous malformations are frequently compressible and should contain no arterial waveform on ultrasound.
- Lymphatic malformation
  - In distinguishing between venous and lymphatic components, contrast-enhanced T1-weighted MR imaging with fat saturation is frequently valuable.
  - Macrocystic LMs appear as predominantly cystic, transspatial lesions.
  - The cystic components of lymphatic malformations do not enhance, but the vascularized internal septae often do.
- Arteriovenous malformation
  - Contrast-enhanced CT or MR imaging shows large feeding arteries, an absence of capillary network, and intense early venous enhancement.
  - Identification of a high-flow lesion with arteriovenous shunting is a contraindication to percutaneous sclerotherapy.

REFERENCES

1. Thomas-Sohl K, Vaslow D, Maria B. Sturge-Weber syndrome: a review. Pediatr Neurol 2004;30(5):303–10.
2. Elluru R, Azizkhan R. Cervicofacial vascular anomalies. II. Vascular malformations. Semin Pediatr Surg 2006;15(2):133–9.
3. Mulliken JB, Glowacki J. Hemangiomas and vascular malformations in infants and children: a classification based on endothelial characteristics. Plast Reconstr Surg 1982;69(3):412–22.
4. Legiehn G, Heran MK. Venous malformations: classification, development, diagnosis, and interventional radiologic management. Radiol Clin North Am 2008;46(3):545–97, vi.
5. Burrows PE, Mulliken JB, Fellows KE, et al. Childhood hemangiomas and vascular malformations: angiographic differentiation. AJR Am J Roentgenol 1983;141(3):483–8.
6. Tucci F, De Vincentiis G, Sitzia E, et al. Head and neck vascular anomalies in children. Int J Pediatr Otorhinolaryngol 2009;73(Suppl 1):S71–6.
7. Som PM, Curtin HD. Head and neck imaging. St Louis (MO): Mosby; 2003.
8. Navarro O, Laffan E, Ngan B. Pediatric soft-tissue tumors and pseudo-tumors: MR imaging features with pathologic correlation: Part 1. Imaging approach, pseudotumors, vascular lesions, and adipocytic tumors. Radiographics 2009;29(3):887–906.
9. Adams D, Lucky A. Cervicofacial vascular anomalies. I. Hemangiomas and other benign vascular tumors. Semin Pediatr Surg 2006;15(2):124–32.
10. Berenguer B, Mulliken J, Enjolras O, et al. Rapidly involuting congenital hemangioma: clinical and histopathologic features. Pediatr Dev Pathol 2003;6(6):495–510.
11. Buckmiller LM, Richter GT, Suen JY. Diagnosis and management of hemangiomas and vascular malformations of the head and neck. Oral Dis 2010;16(5):405–18.
12. Harnsberger HR. Diagnostic imaging. Head and neck. Salt Lake City (UT): Amirsys; 2004.
13. Fishman SJ, Mulliken JB. Hemangiomas and vascular malformations of infancy and childhood. Pediatr Clin North Am 1993;40(6):1177–200.
14. Enjolras O, Mulliken JB. Vascular tumors and vascular malformations (new issues). Adv Dermatol 1997;13:375–423.

15. Enjolras O, Wassef M, Mazoyer E, et al. Infants with Kasabach-Merritt syndrome do not have "true" hemangiomas. J Pediatr 1997;130(4):631–40.
16. Dubois J, Alison M. Vascular anomalies: what a radiologist needs to know. Pediatr Radiol 2010;40(6): 895–905.
17. Haider K, Plager D, Neely D, et al. Outpatient treatment of periocular infantile hemangiomas with oral propranolol. J AAPOS 2010;14(3):251–6.
18. Paltiel HJ, Burrows PE, Kozakewich HP, et al. Soft-tissue vascular anomalies: utility of US for diagnosis. Radiology 2000;214(3):747–54.
19. Boyd JB, Mulliken JB, Kaban LB, et al. Skeletal changes associated with vascular malformations. Plast Reconstr Surg 1984;74(6):789–97.
20. Flis C, Connor S. Imaging of head and neck venous malformations. Eur Radiol 2005;15(10):2185–93.
21. Geronemus RG, Ashinoff R. The medical necessity of evaluation and treatment of port-wine stains. J Dermatol Surg Oncol 1991;17(1):76–9.
22. Geronemus RG, Quintana AT, Lou WW, et al. High-fluence modified pulsed dye laser photocoagulation with dynamic cooling of port-wine stains in infancy. Arch Dermatol 2000;136(7):942–3.
23. van der Horst CM, Koster PH, de Borgie CA, et al. Effect of the timing of treatment of port-wine stains with the flash-lamp-pumped pulsed-dye laser. N Engl J Med 1998;338(15):1028–33.
24. Cordoro K, Speetzen L, Koerper M, et al. Physiologic changes in vascular birthmarks during early infancy: mechanisms and clinical implications. J Am Acad Dermatol 2009;60(4):669–75.
25. Sekhar L, Biswas A, Hallam D, et al. Neuroendovascular management of tumors and vascular malformations of the head and neck. Neurosurg Clin N Am 2009;20(4):453–85.
26. Smith RJ. Lymphatic malformations. Lymphat Res Biol 2004;2(1):25–31.
27. Bloom D, Perkins J, Manning S. Management of lymphatic malformations. Curr Opin Otolaryngol Head Neck Surg 2004;12(6):500–4.
28. Huang HY, Ho CC, Huang PH, et al. Co-expression of VEGF-C and its receptors, VEGFR-2 and VEGFR-3, in endothelial cells of lymphangioma. Implication in autocrine or paracrine regulation of lymphangioma. Lab Invest 2001;81(12):1729–34.
29. Siegel M. Magnetic resonance imaging of musculoskeletal soft tissue masses. Radiol Clin North Am 2001;39(4):701–20.
30. Puig S, Aref H, Brunelle F. Double-needle sclerotherapy of lymphangiomas and venous angiomas in children: a simple technique to prevent complications. AJR Am J Roentgenol 2003;180(5):1399–401.
31. Ernemann U, Kramer U, Miller S, et al. Current concepts in the classification, diagnosis and treatment of vascular anomalies. Eur J Radiol 2010; 75(1):2–11.
32. Poldervaart M, Breugem C, Speleman L, et al. Treatment of lymphatic malformations with OK-432 (picibanil): review of the literature. J Craniofac Surg 2009;20(4):1159–62.
33. Hall N, Ade-Ajayi N, Brewis C, et al. Is intralesional injection of OK-432 effective in the treatment of lymphangioma in children? Surgery 2003;133(3):238–42.

Imaging of Congenital Spine and Spinal Cord Malformations

Stephanie Rufener, MD[a,b], Mohannad Ibrahim, MD[a], Hemant A. Parmar, MD[a,*]

KEYWORDS

- Spine • Congenital • Spinal cord • Spine embryology
- Spine imaging

SPINAL CORD DEVELOPMENT

There are 3 basic embryologic stages to spinal development.[1,2] The first stage occurs during the second or third week of embryonic development and is referred to as gastrulation. During gastrulation, the embryonic disk converts from a bilaminar disk to a trilaminar disk composed of ectoderm, mesoderm, and endoderm. Primary neurulation is the second stage in spinal development and occurs during weeks 3 to 4. During primary neurulation, the notochord and overlying ectoderm interact to form the neural plate, which then bends and folds to form the neural tube. The neural tube then closes bidirectionally in a zipperlike manner (**Fig. 1**). Secondary neurulation is the final stage of spinal development and occurs during weeks 5 and 6. During secondary neurulation, the secondary neural tube is formed by the caudal cell mass. The secondary neural tube is initially solid, subsequently cavitates, and eventually forms the tip of conus medullaris and filum terminale via a process called retrogressive differentiation. Abnormalities in any of these developmental stages can lead to spine or spinal cord malformations.

CATEGORIZATION OF SPINAL DYSRAPHISMS

Spinal dysraphisms can be broadly divided into open and closed types.[1–3] Open spinal dysraphisms describe entities that have an overlying skin defect with neural tissue exposed to the environment. Closed spinal dysraphisms describe entities in which the overlying skin remains intact. Closed spinal dysraphisms can be further subcategorized based on whether a subcutaneous mass is present or absent.[4] The key features of open and closed spinal dysraphisms are summarized in **Table 1**.

OPEN SPINAL DYSRAPHISMS

Myelomeningocele and Myelocele

Myelomeningocele and myelocele result from defective closure of the primary neural tube and are characterized clinically by neural placode exposure through a midline skin defect on the back. Myelomeningoceles account for greater than 98% of open spinal dysraphisms.[1] Myeloceles are rare. Because open spinal dysraphisms are often diagnosed clinically (often antenatally), imaging of these entities is not

[a] Department of Radiology, University of Michigan Health System, 1500 East Medical Center Drive, Ann Arbor, MI 48109, USA
[b] Mount Scott Diagnostic Imaging Center, 9200 SE 91st Avenue, Suite 330, Portland, OR 97086, USA
* Corresponding author. Department of Radiology, University of Michigan Health System, Taubman Center/B1/132 F, 1500 East Medical Center, Ann Arbor, MI 48109-0302.
E-mail address: hparmar@umich.edu

Neuroimag Clin N Am 21 (2011) 659–676
doi:10.1016/j.nic.2011.05.011
1052-5149/11/$ – see front matter

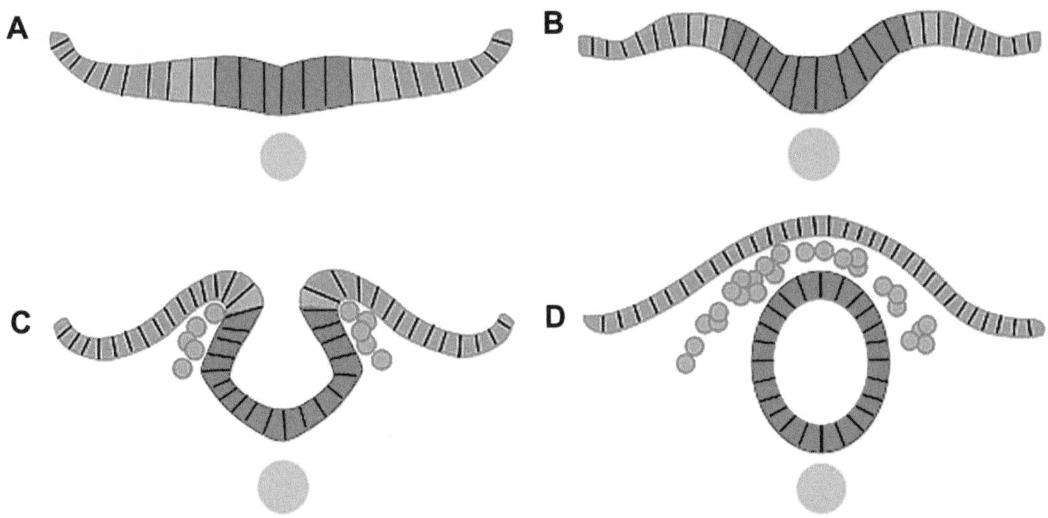

Fig. 1. Primary neurulation. (*A–D*) Stages of primary neurulation. Interaction of the notochord (*circle*) and overlying ectoderm results in formation of the neural plate (*dark green*), which then bends to form the neural tube and ultimately closes in a zipperlike fashion. (*Reprinted from* Rufener SL, Ibrahim M, Raybaud CA, et al. Congenital spine and spinal cord malformations–pictorial review. Am J Roentgenol 2010;194:S26–37; with permission.)

always performed. When imaging is performed, the main differentiating feature between a myelomeningocele and myelocele is neural placode position relative to the skin surface.[2] With a myelomeningocele, the neural placode protrudes above the skin surface (**Fig. 2**). With a myelocele, the neural placode is flush with the skin surface (**Fig. 3**).

Hemimyelomeningocele and Hemimyelocele

Hemimyelomeningocele and hemimyelocele have been described but are rare.[5] These entities occur when a myelomeningocele or myelocele is associated with diastematomyelia (cord splitting) and one hemicord fails to neurulate.

CLOSED SPINAL DYSRAPHISMS WITH A SUBCUTANEOUS MASS

Lipomas with a Dural Defect

Lipomas with a dural defect can be characterized as lipomyelocele or lipomyelomeningocele and occur as a result of defective primary neurulation whereby mesenchymal tissue enters the neural tube and forms lipomatous tissue.[6] Clinically, lipomyeloceles and lipomyelomeningoceles are characterized by the presence of a subcutaneous fatty mass above the intergluteal crease. The position of the placode-lipoma interface is the main differentiating feature between a lipomyelocele and lipomyelomeningocele.[4] If the placode-lipoma interface lies within the spinal canal, it is characterized as a lipomyelocele (**Fig. 4**). If the placode-lipoma interface lies outside of the spinal canal because of expansion of the subarachnoid space, it is characterized as a lipomyelomeningocele, (**Fig. 5**).

Meningocele

A meningocele is characterized by herniation of a cerebrospinal fluid-filled sac lined by dura and arachnoid mater. The spinal cord may be tethered to the neck of the cerebrospinal fluid-filled sac but is not located within the meningocele itself. Posterior meningoceles refer to herniation of the cerebrospinal fluid-filled sac through a posterior spina bifida (osseous defect of posterior spinal elements) and are most commonly lumbar or sacral in location but can also occur in the occipital and cervical regions (**Fig. 6**). Anterior

Table 1
Summary of spinal dysraphisms

Open Spinal Dysraphisms-Not covered by intact skin	
Myelocele	Neural placode flush with skin surface
Myelomeningocele	Neural placode protrudes above skin surface
Hemimyelocelee	Myelocele associated with diastematomyelia
Hemimyelomeningocele	Myelomeningocele associated with diastematomyelia
Closed Spinal Dysraphisms-Covered by intact skin *With a Subcutaneous Mass:*	
Lipomyelocele	Placode-lipoma interface within the spinal canal
Lipomyelomeningocele	Placode-lipoma interface outside of the spinal canal
Meningocele	Herniation of CSF filled sac lined by dura
Terminal myelocystocele	Terminal syrinx herniating into posterior meningocele
Myelocystocele	Dilated central canal herniating through posterior spina bifida
Without a Subcutaneous Mass: Simple Dysraphic States	
Intradural lipoma	Lipoma within the dural sac
Filar lipoma	Fibrolipomatous thickening of filum
Tight filum terminale	Hypertrophy and shortening of filum
Persistent terminal ventricle	Persistent cavity within conus medullaris
Dermal sinus	Epithelial lined fistula between neural tissue and skin surface
Complex Dysraphic States	
Dorsal enteric fistula	Connection between bowel and skin surface
Neurenteric cyst	More localized form of dorsal enteric fistula
Diastematomyelia	Separation of cord into two hemicords
Caudal agenesis	Total or partial agenesis of spinal column
Segmental spinal dysgenesis	Various segmentation anomalies

meningoceles are most commonly presacral in location but can also occur elsewhere (**Fig. 7**).[7]

Terminal Myelocystocele

A terminal myelocystocele is herniation of a large terminal syrinx (syringocele) into a posterior meningocele through a posterior spinal defect (**Fig. 8**).[2] The meningocele component communicates with the subarachnoid space and the terminal syrinx component communicates with the central canal. The meningocele and terminal syrinx components do not usually communicate with each other.[8]

Myelocystocele

A nonterminal myelocystocele refers to herniation of a dilated central canal through a posterior spina bifida defect (**Fig. 9**). Myelocystoceles are covered with skin and are most commonly seen in the cervical or cervicothoracic regions but can occur at any level.[9]

CLOSED SPINAL DYSRAPHISMS WITHOUT A SUBCUTANEOUS MASS

Closed spinal dysraphisms without a subcutaneous mass can be subcategorized into simple and complex dysraphic states.

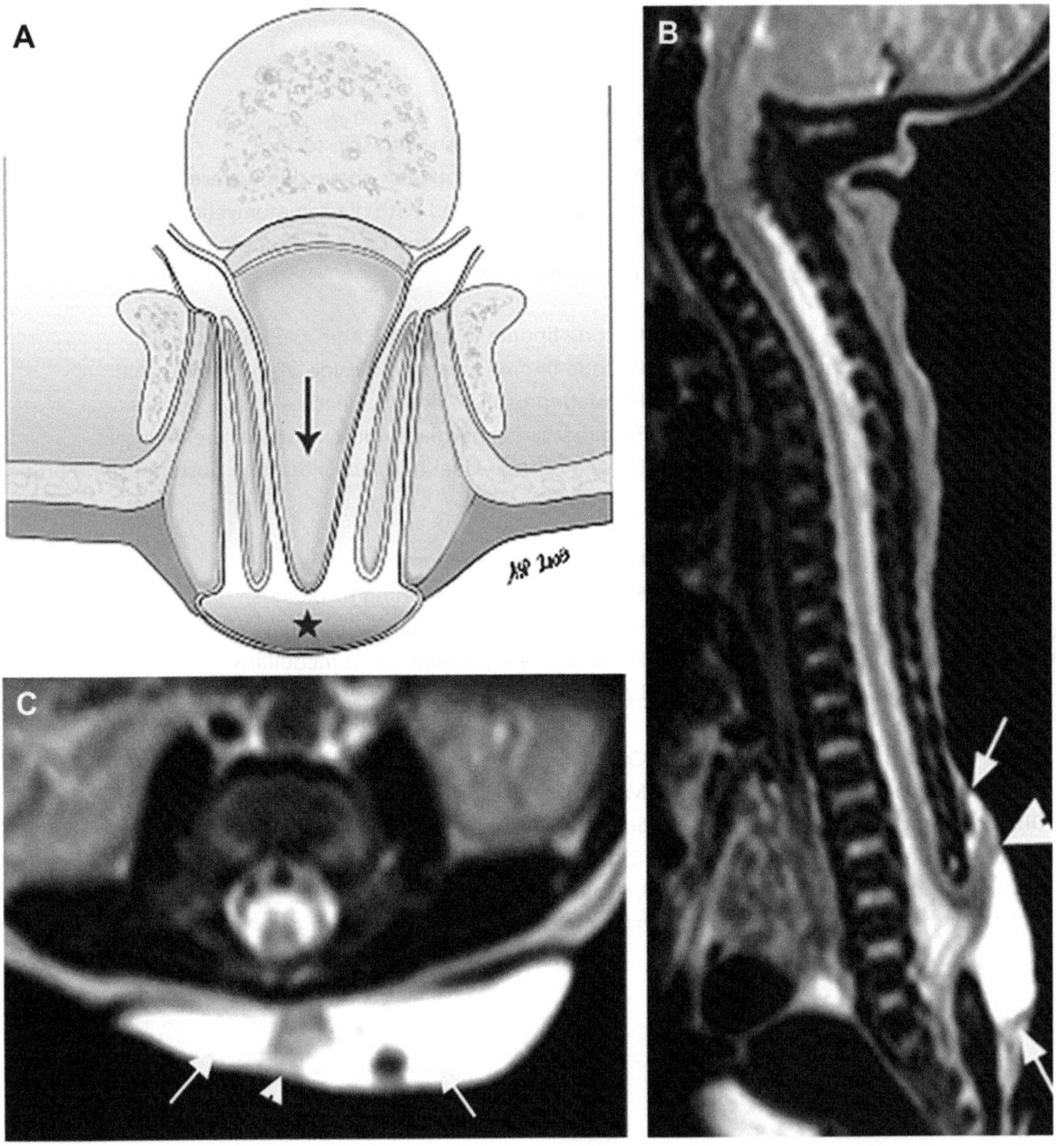

Fig. 2. Myelomeningocele. (*A*) Axial diagram. Expansion of underlying subarachnoid space (*arrow*) results in protrusion of the neural placode (*star*) above the skin surface. (*B*) Sagittal and (*C*) axial T2-weighted magnetic resonance (MR) images in a newborn with Chiari II malformation show large open defect in the lower lumbar spine (*small arrows*). There is extension of the neural placode (*arrowhead*) to the skin surface caused by expansion of the underlying subarachnoid space, which is characteristic of a myelomeningocele. (Part [*A*] *Reprinted from* Rufener SL, Ibrahim M, Raybaud CA, et al. Congenital spine and spinal cord malformations–pictorial review. Am J Roentgenol 2010;194:S26–37; with permission.)

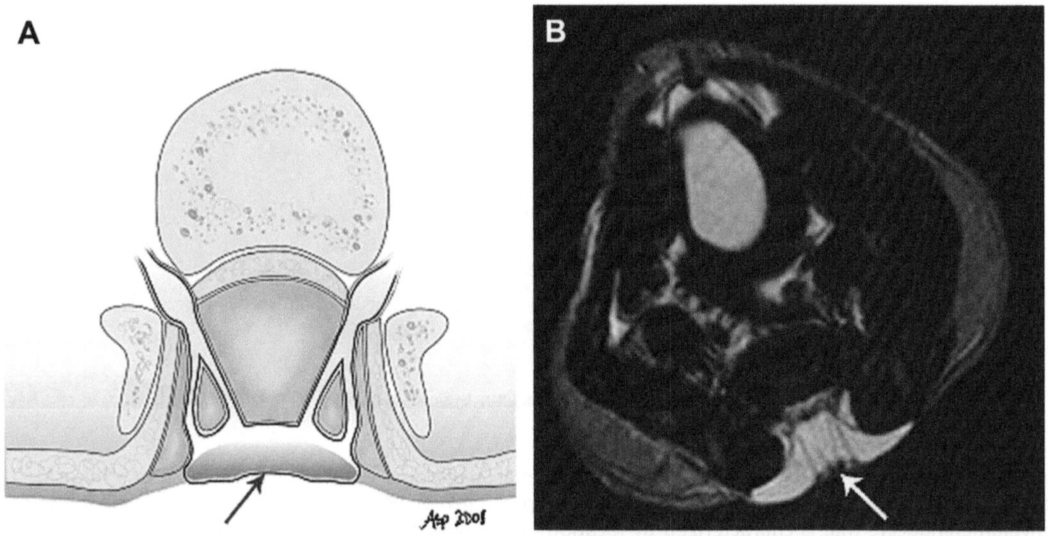

Fig. 3. Myelocele. (*A*) Axial diagram. The exposed neural placode (*arrow*) is flush with the skin surface. (*B*) Axial T2-weighted MR image shows an exposed neural placode (*arrow*) that does not protrude above the skin surface, consistent with a myelocele. There is no expansion of the underlying subarachnoid space. (*Reprinted from* Rufener SL, Ibrahim M, Raybaud CA, et al. Congenital spine and spinal cord malformations–pictorial review. Am J Roentgenol 2010;194:S26–37; with permission.)

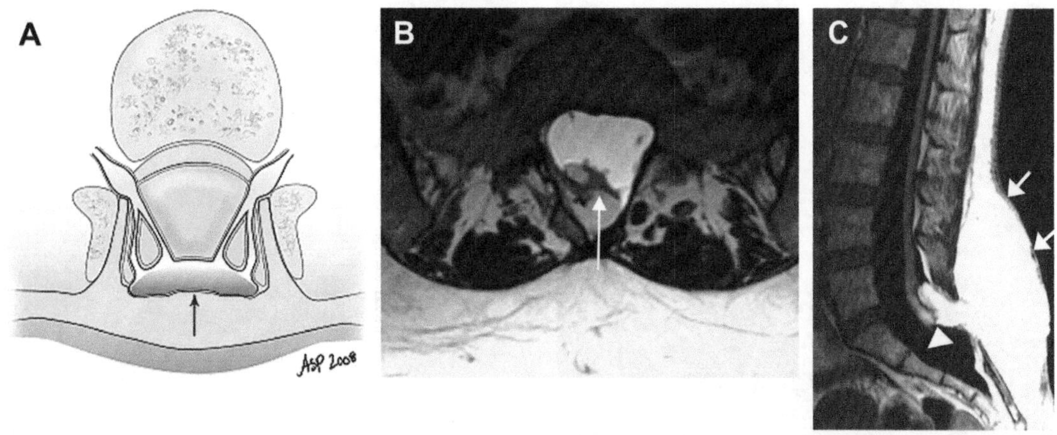

Fig. 4. Lipomyelocele. (*A*) Axial diagram. Placode-lipoma interface (*arrow*) is located within the spinal canal. (*B*) Axial T2-weighted MR image shows the placode-lipoma interface (*arrow*) within the spinal canal, characteristic for a lipomyelocele. (*C*) Sagittal T1-weighted MR image shows a subcutaneous fatty mass (*arrow*) and placode-lipoma interface (*arrowhead*) that is located within the spinal canal. (Part [*A*] *Reprinted from* Rufener SL, Ibrahim M, Raybaud CA, et al. Congenital spine and spinal cord malformations–pictorial review. Am J Roentgenol 2010;194:S26–37; with permission.)

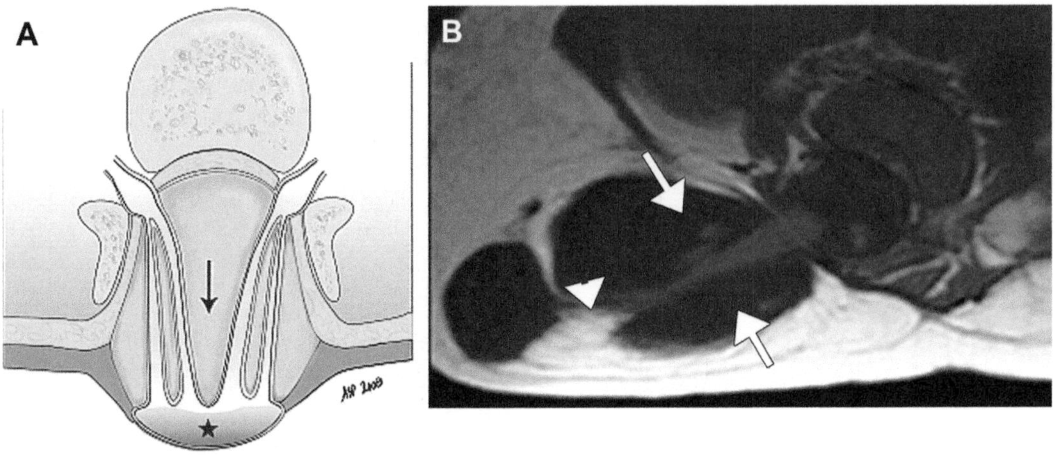

Fig. 5. Lipomyelomeningocele (*A*) Axial diagram. The placode-lipoma interface (*star*) is positioned outside the spinal canal because of expansion of the subarachnoid space (*arrow*). (*B*) Axial T1-weighted MR image shows a lipomyelomeningocele that is characterized by location of the placode-lipoma interface (*arrowhead*) outside the spinal canal because of expansion of the subarachnoid space (*arrows*). (Part [A] *Reprinted from* Rufener SL, Ibrahim M, Raybaud CA, et al. Congenital spine and spinal cord malformations–pictorial review. Am J Roentgenol 2010;194:S26–37; with permission.)

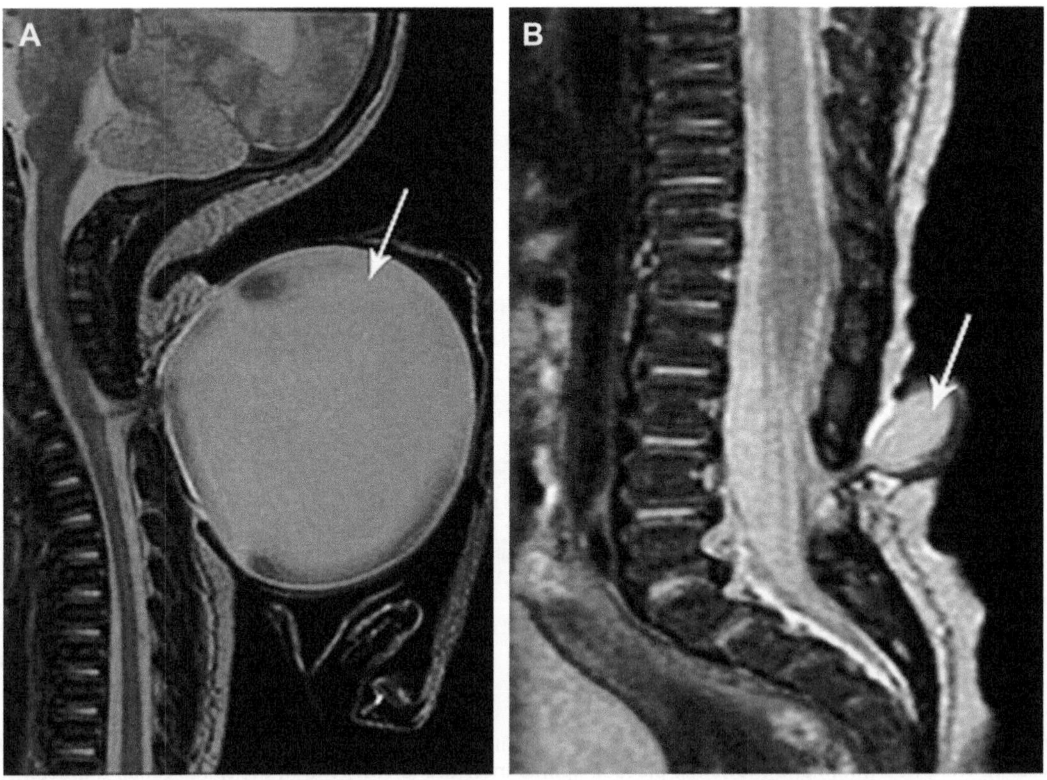

Fig. 6. Posterior meningocele (*A*) Sagittal T2-weighted MR image shows a large posterior cervical meningocele (*arrow*). (*B*) Sagittal T2-weighted MR image shows a small posterior lumbar meningocele (*arrow*). Both of these were skin covered (closed) defects. (*Reprinted from* Rufener SL, Ibrahim M, Raybaud CA, et al. Congenital spine and spinal cord malformations–pictorial review. Am J Roentgenol 2010;194:S26–37; with permission.)

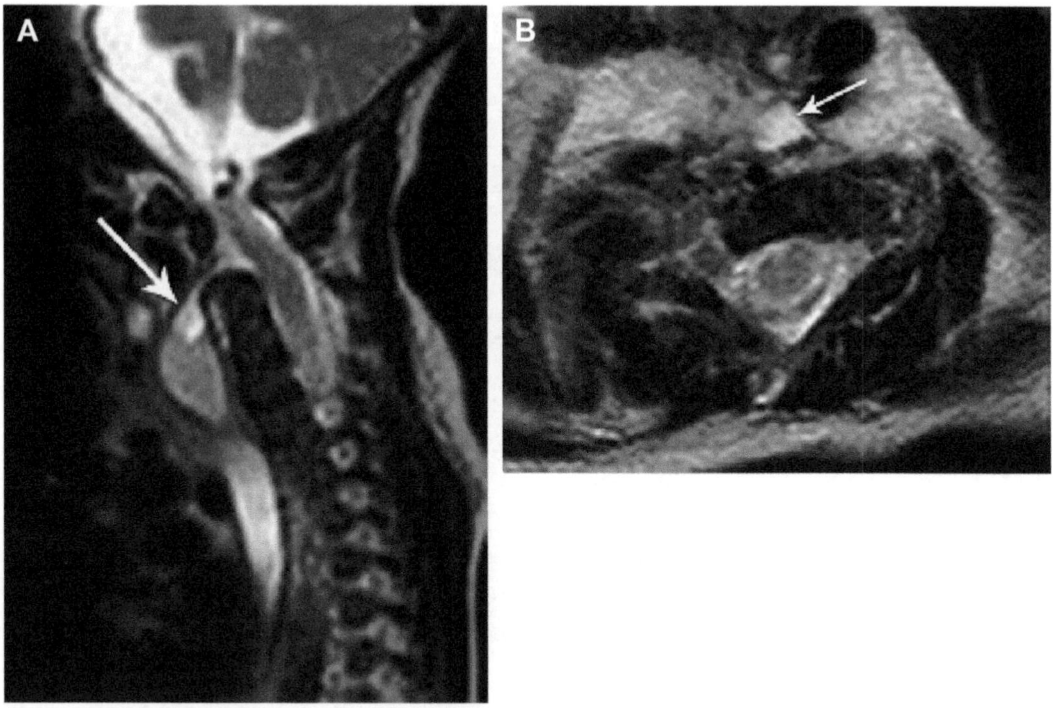

Fig. 7. Anterior meningocele. Sagittal (*A*) and axial (*B*) T2-weighted MR images in a patient with a small anterior meningocele in the cervical region (*arrows*). (*Reprinted from* Rufener SL, Ibrahim M, Raybaud CA, et al. Congenital spine and spinal cord malformations–pictorial review. Am J Roentgenol 2010;194:S26–37; with permission.)

Simple Dysraphic States

Simple dysraphic states consist of intradural lipoma, filar lipoma, tight filum terminale, persistent terminal ventricle, and dermal sinus.

Intradural Lipoma

An intradural lipoma is characterized by a dorsal midline lipoma that is contained within the dural sac without an associated open spinal dysraphism (**Fig. 10**). Intradural lipomas are usually lumbosacral in location and most often present with tethered cord syndrome, a clinical syndrome of progressive neurologic abnormalities in the setting of traction on a low-lying conus medullaris.[2]

Filar Lipoma

A filar lipoma refers to fibrolipomatous thickening of the filum. On magnetic resonance imaging, a filar lipoma appears as a strip of T1 signal hyperintensity within a thickened filum terminale (**Fig. 11**). In the absence of clinical evidence of tethered cord syndrome, filar lipomas can be considered a normal variant.[10,11]

Tight Filum Terminale

Hypertrophy and shortening of the filum terminale is seen with a tight filum terminale (**Fig. 12**). This condition causes impaired ascent of the conus medullaris and tethering of the spinal cord. The conus medullaris is low lying relative to its normal position, which is usually superior to the L2-L3 disc level.[2]

Persistent Terminal Ventricle

A persistent terminal ventricle refers to persistence of a small ependyma-lined cavity within the conus medullaris (**Fig. 13**). Location immediately superior

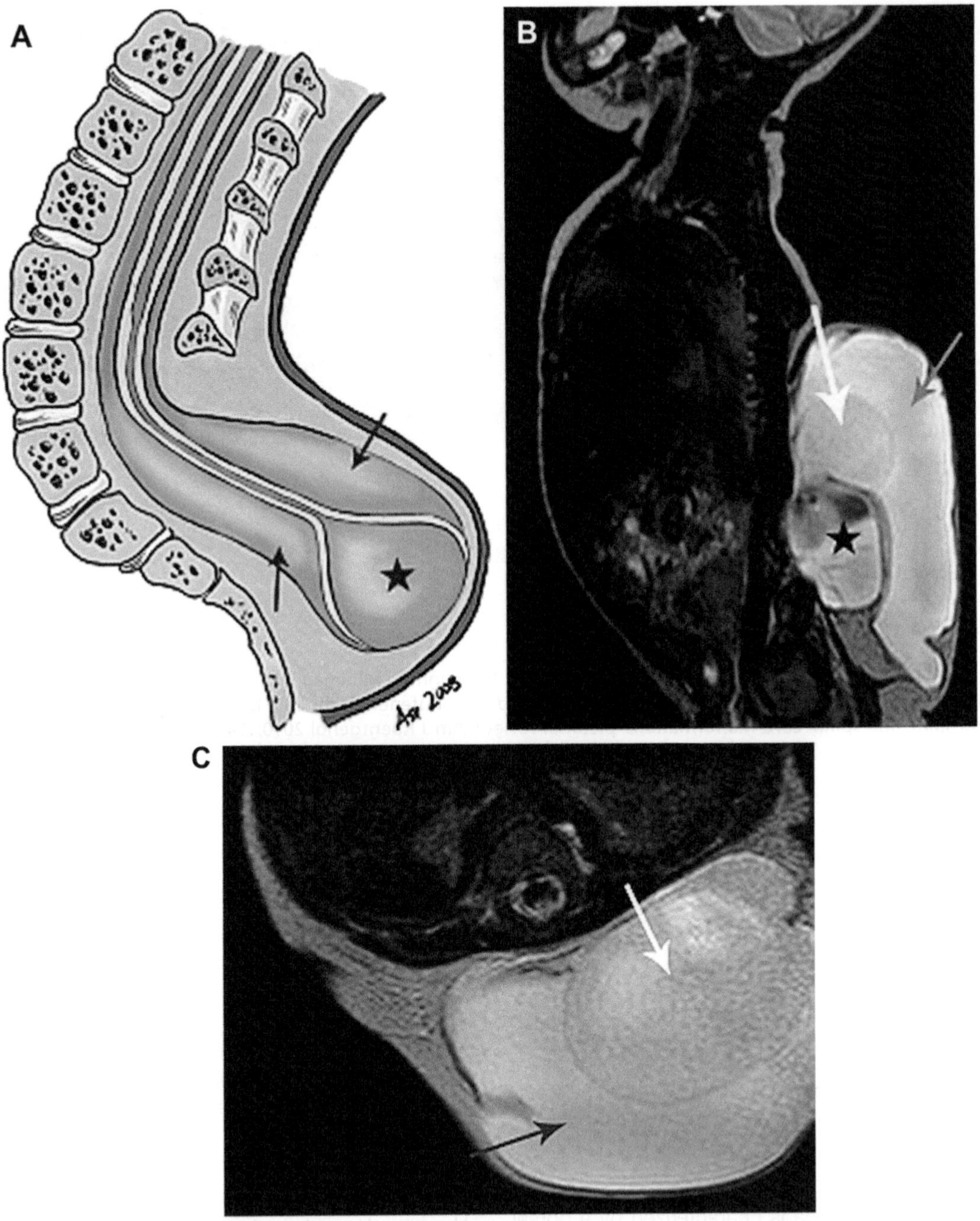

Fig. 8. Terminal myelocystocele. (*A*) Sagittal diagram of a terminal syrinx (*star*) herniating into a large posterior meningocele (*arrows*). Sagittal (*B*) and axial (*C*) T2-weighted MR images of a patient with a terminal syrinx (*white arrows*) herniating into a large posterior meningocele component (*gray arrows*). The sagittal image shows turbulent flow within the more anterior meningocele component (*star*). (*Reprinted from* Rufener SL, Ibrahim M, Raybaud CA, et al. Congenital spine and spinal cord malformations–pictorial review. Am J Roentgenol 2010;194:S26–37; with permission.)

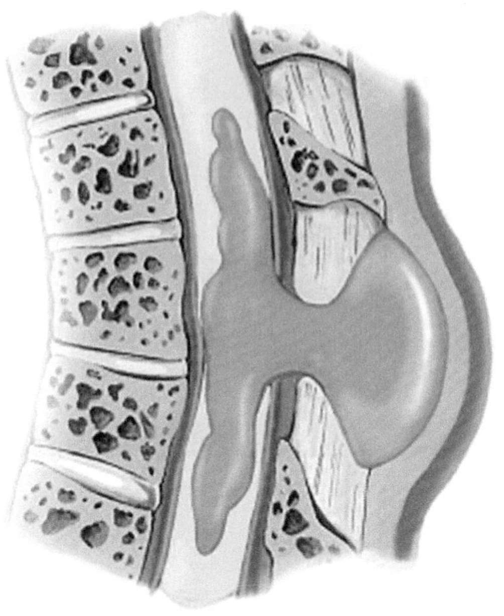

Fig. 9. A nonterminal myelocystocele showing a dilated central canal herniating through a posterior spinal defect. (*Reprinted from* Rufener SL, Ibrahim M, Raybaud CA, et al. Congenital spine and spinal cord malformations–pictorial review. Am J Roentgenol 2010;194:S26–37; with permission.)

to the filum terminale and lack of associated contrast enhancement help to differentiate this entity from other cystic lesions of the conus medullaris.[12]

Dermal Sinus

A dermal sinus refers to an epithelium-lined fistula connecting neural tissue and/or meninges to the skin surface. Dermal sinuses occur most commonly in the lumbosacral region and are often associated with a spinal dermoid/epidermoid cyst at the level of the conus medullaris or cauda equina (**Figs. 14** and **15**). Patients present clinically with a midline dimple and may also have an associated hairy nevus, hyperpigmented patch, or capillary hemangioma.[13] Because the fistulous connection between neural tissue and the skin surface can result in infectious complications like meningitis and abscess, surgical repair is of great importance.

Complex Dysraphic States

Complex dysraphic states can be subcategorized into 2 groups: disorders of midline notochordal integration, which includes dorsal enteric fistula, neurenteric cyst, and diastematomyelia, and disorders of notochordal formation, which includes caudal agenesis and segmental spinal dysgenesis.

Disorders of Midline Notochordal Integration

Dorsal enteric fistula and neurenteric cyst

A dorsal enteric fistula is an abnormal connection with the skin surface; a more localized form of a dorsal enteric fistula is called a neurenteric cyst (**Fig. 16**). These entities are lined with mucin-secreting epithelium similar to the gastrointestinal tract and are most commonly located in the cervicothoracic spine anterior to the spinal cord.[14]

Diastematomyelia

Diastematomyelia occurs when there is separation of the spinal cord into 2 hemicords. The 2 hemicords are usually symmetric in caliber, although the length of separation varies. Two types of diastematomyelia have been described. In type 1, there are 2 individual dural tubes separated by an osseous or cartilaginous septum (**Fig. 17**). In type 2, there is a single dural tube containing both hemicords, and an intervening fibrous septum may be seen (**Fig. 18**).[15] Diastematomyelia can clinically present with scoliosis and tethered cord syndrome. A distinctive finding that may be present on physical examination is a hairy tuft on the patient's back.[16]

Disorders of Notochordal Formation

Caudal agenesis

Total or partial agenesis of the spinal column is referred to as caudal agenesis (**Fig. 19**) and can be associated with other findings, including anal imperforation, genital anomalies, renal dysplasia or aplasia, pulmonary hypoplasia, and/or limb abnormalities. Caudal agenesis can be categorized into 2 types. In type I, the conus medullaris is high in position and abruptly terminates. In type 2, the conus medullaris is low lying and may be tethered.[17]

Segmental Spinal Dysgenesis

The clinical-radiological spectrum of segmental spinal dysgenesis includes multiple entities, including segmental agenesis/dysgenesis of the thoracic and/or lumbar spine, segmental abnormality of the spinal cord or nerve roots, congenital paraparesis or paraplegia, and congenital lower limb deformities. Three-dimensional computed tomography reconstructions can be useful for demonstration of various vertebral segmentation anomalies (**Fig. 20**).[18]

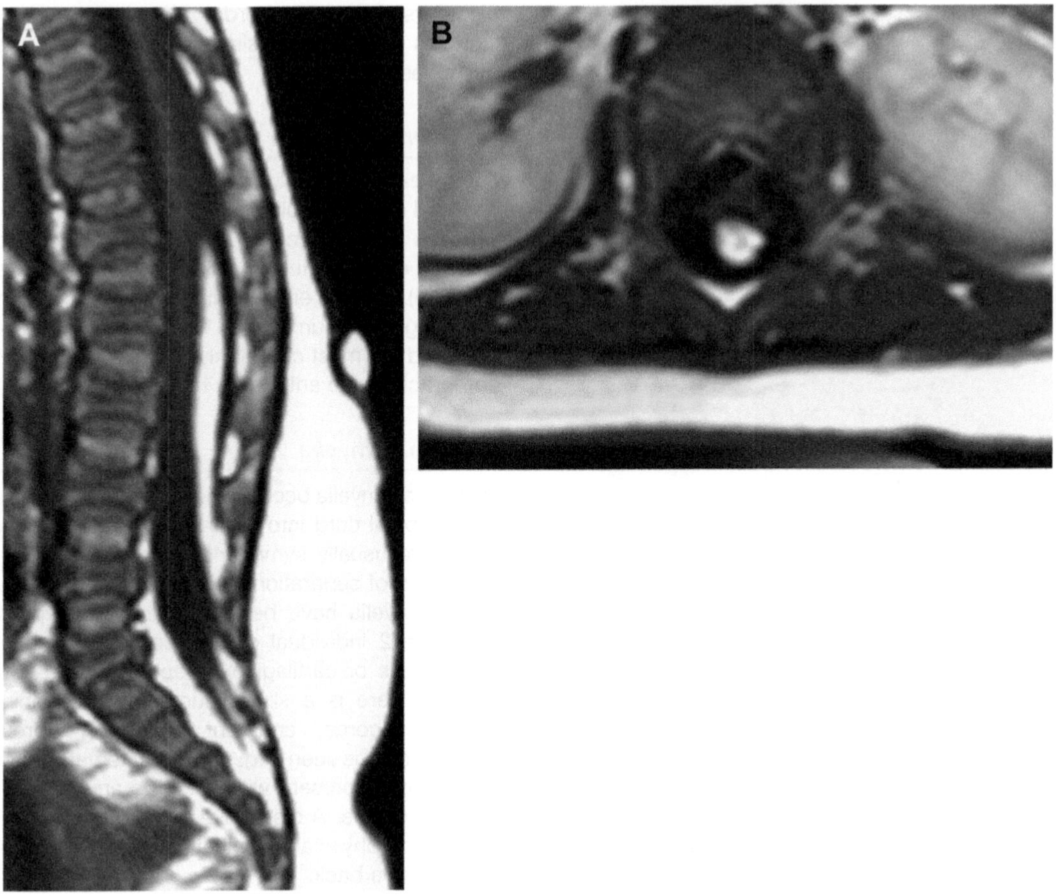

Fig. 10. Intradural lipoma. Sagittal T1-weighted MR image (*A*) and axial T1-weighted MR image (*B*) show a large intradural lipoma that shows hyperintense signal on the T1 image. The lipoma is attached to the dorsal aspect of the conus medullaris.

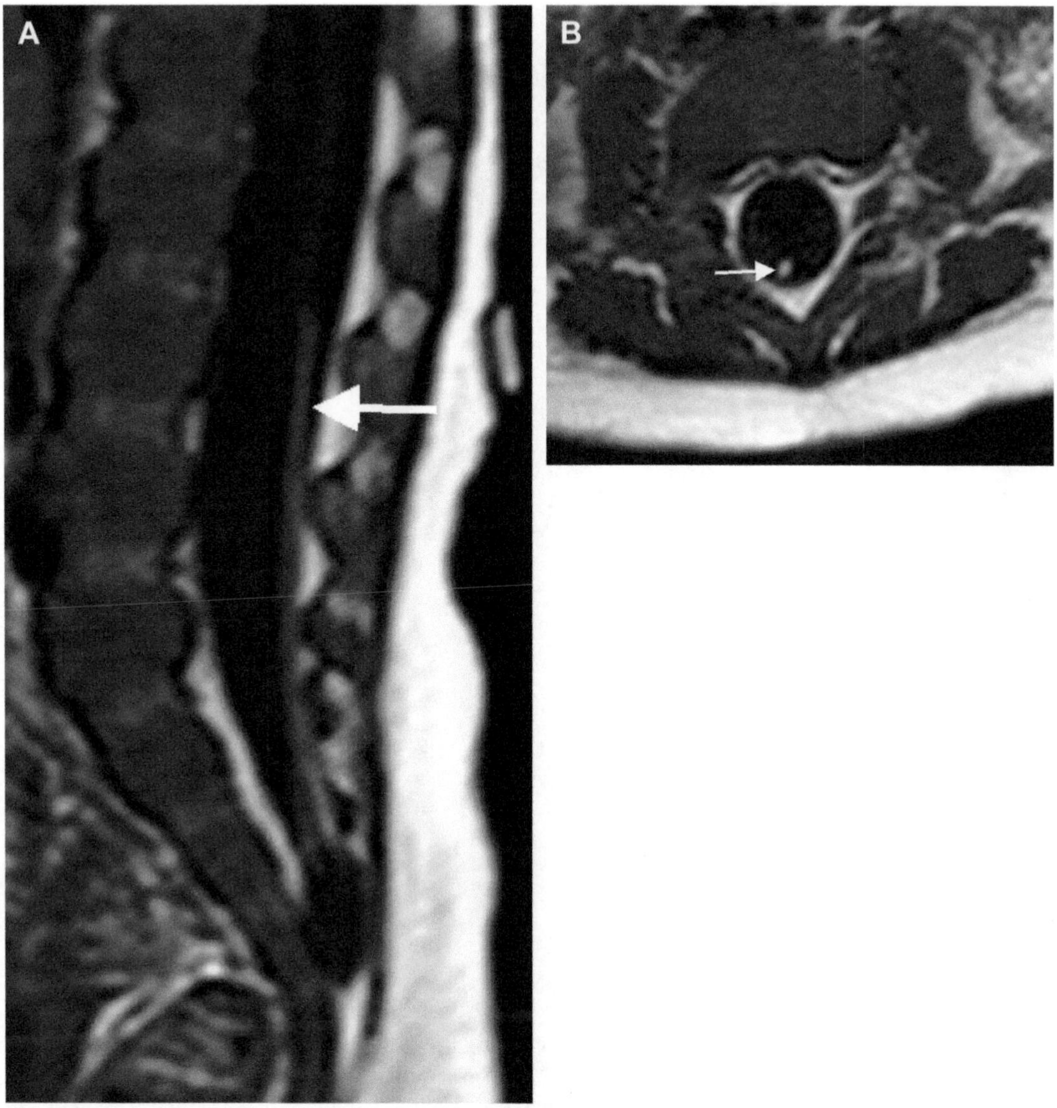

Fig. 11. Filum terminale lipoma. Sagittal (*A*) and axial (*B*) T1-weighted MR images show a filar lipoma (*arrows*) with characteristic T1 hyperintensity and marked thickening of the filum terminale.

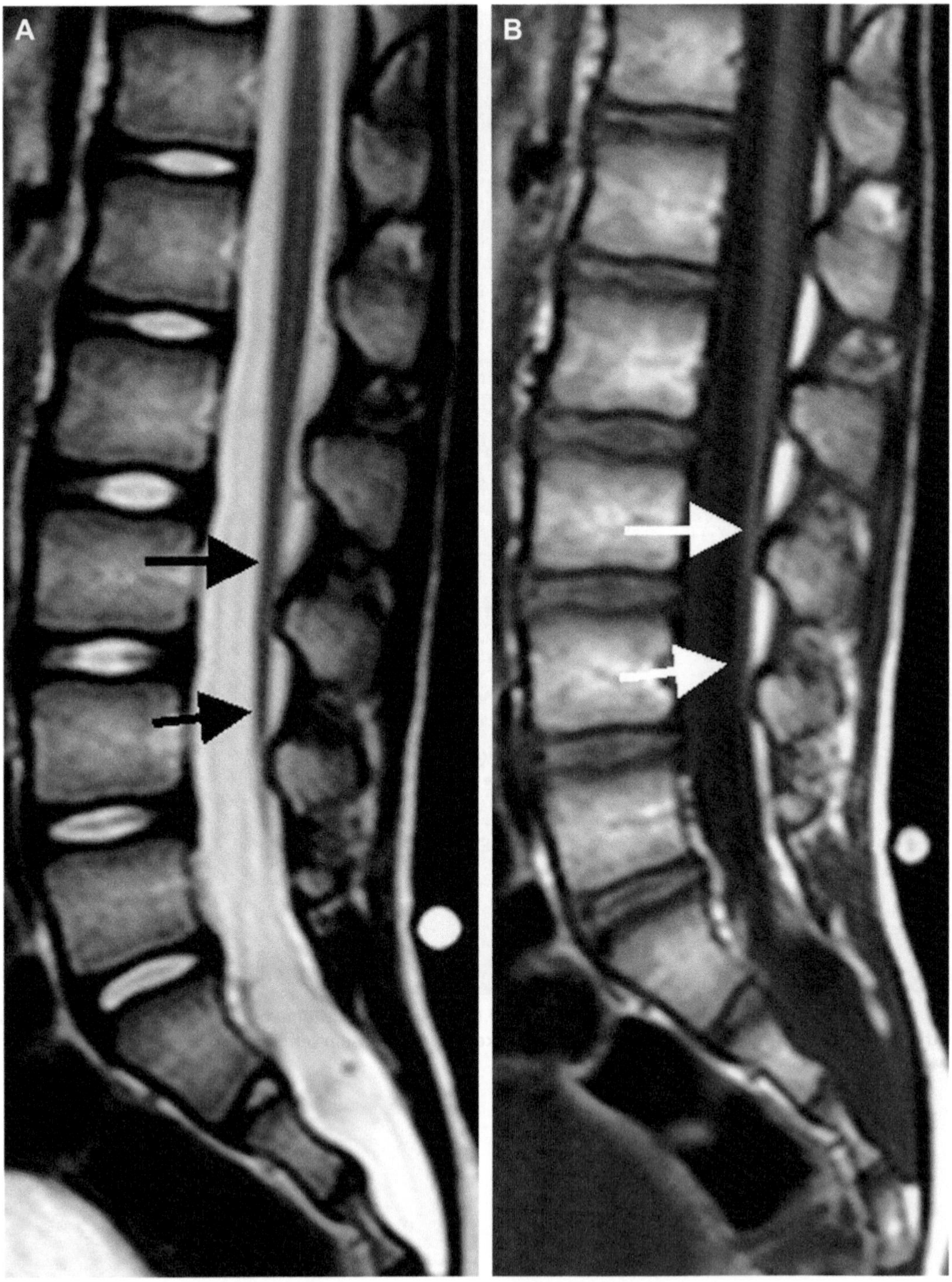

Fig. 12. Tight filum terminale. (*A*) Sagittal T2-weighted and (*B*) T1-weighted MR images show thickening of the filum terminale (*arrows*) with a low-lying conus medullaris, which is characteristic for a tight filum terminale.

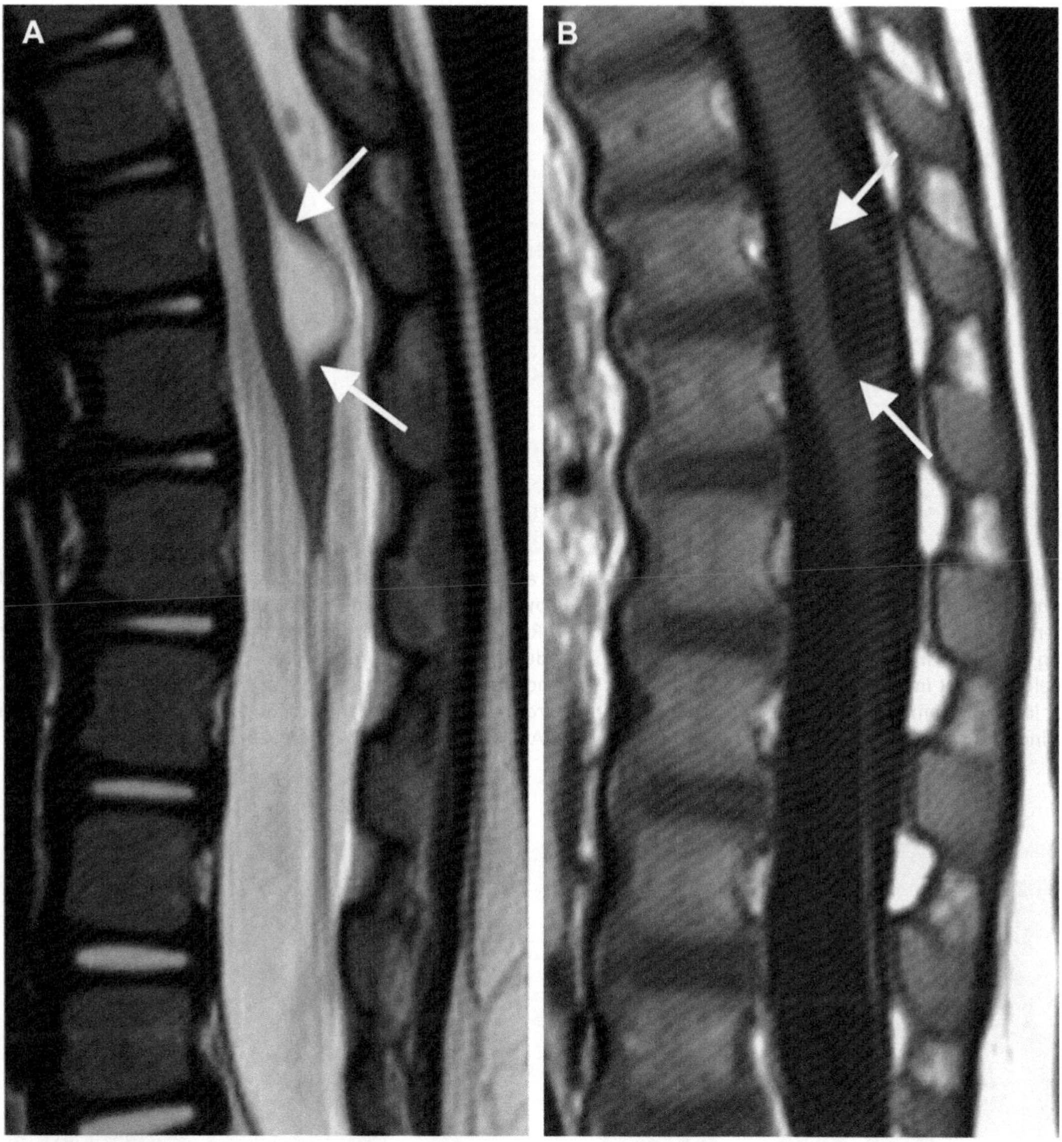

Fig. 13. Terminal ventricle. Sagittal T2-weighted (*A*) and T1-weighted (*B*) MR images show a persistent terminal ventricle that manifests as a cystic structure (*arrows*) at the inferior aspect of the conus medullaris. There was no enhancement noted on the postcontrast enhanced images (not shown). Also note a small fatty lipoma of the filum terminale.

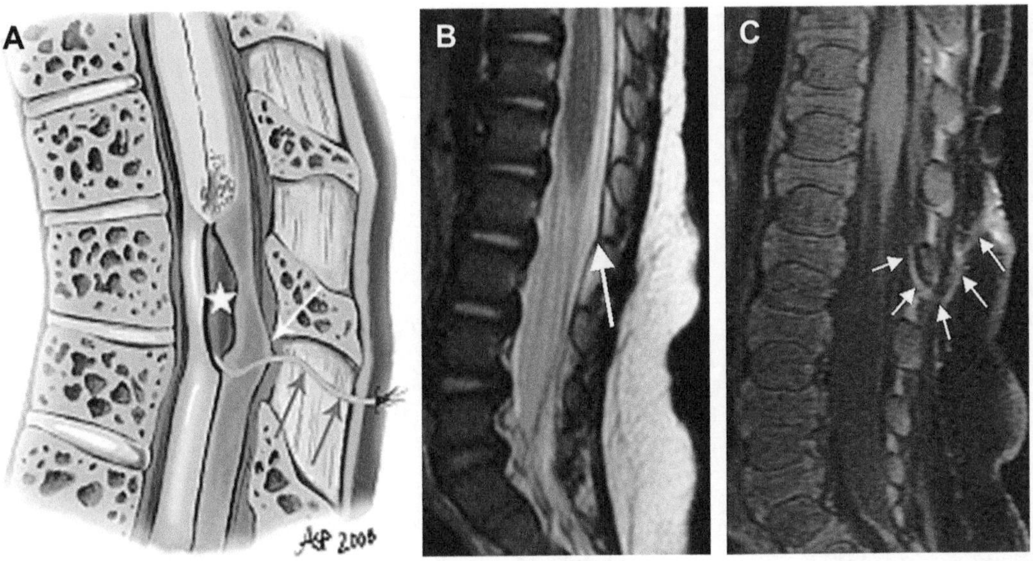

Fig. 14. Dorsal dermal sinus. Sagittal diagram (*A*) shows an intradural dermoid (*stars*) and associated tract extending from the central canal to the skin surface (*gray arrows*). There is tenting of the dural sac at the origin of the dermal sinus (*white arrow*). (*B*) Sagittal T2-weighted MR image in a patient with dorsal dermal sinus shows tenting of the posterior dura (*arrow*) at the site of intradural connection. (*C*) Sagittal postcontrast enhanced T1-weighted MR image with fat suppression shows enhancement of the dorsal dermal sinus tract (*arrows*), caused by local inflammation of the tract. (Part [*A*] *Reprinted from* Rufener SL, Ibrahim M, Raybaud CA, et al. Congenital spine and spinal cord malformations–pictorial review. Am J Roentgenol 2010;194:S26–37; with permission.)

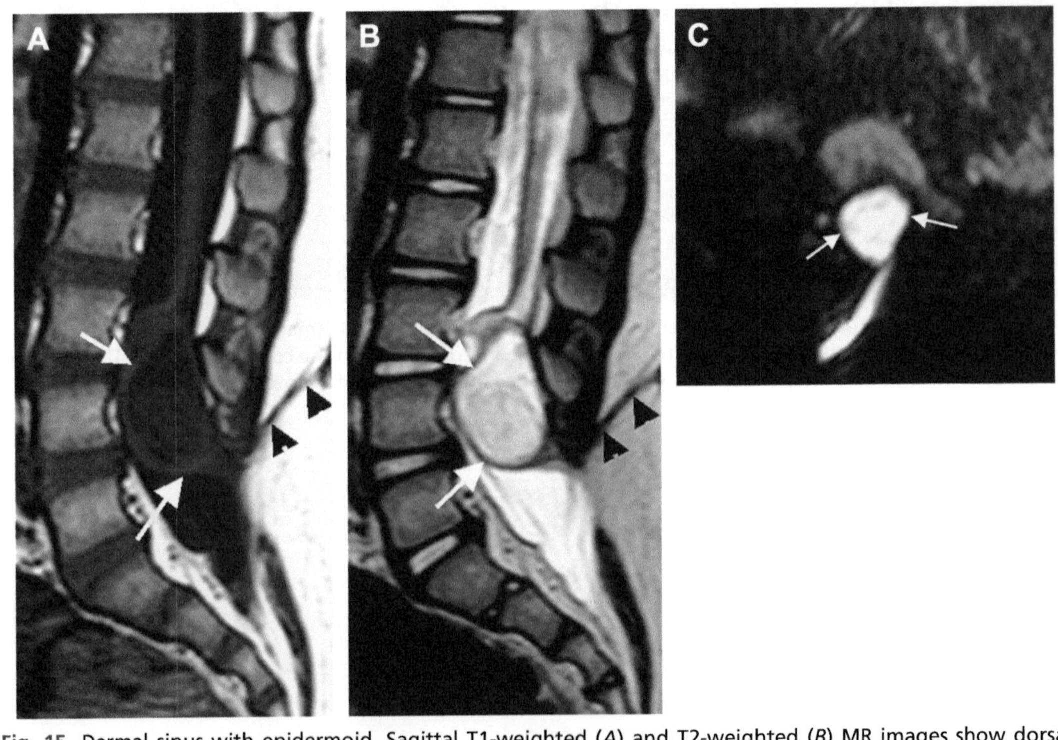

Fig. 15. Dermal sinus with epidermoid. Sagittal T1-weighted (*A*) and T2-weighted (*B*) MR images show dorsal dermal sinus tract in the lower lumbar spine (*arrowheads*). There is a large epidermoid (*arrows*) seen intraspinally associated with the dermal sinus. (*C*) Axial diffusion-weighted image at the level of the lower lumbar spine show hyperintensity within the intradural epidermoid (*arrows*).

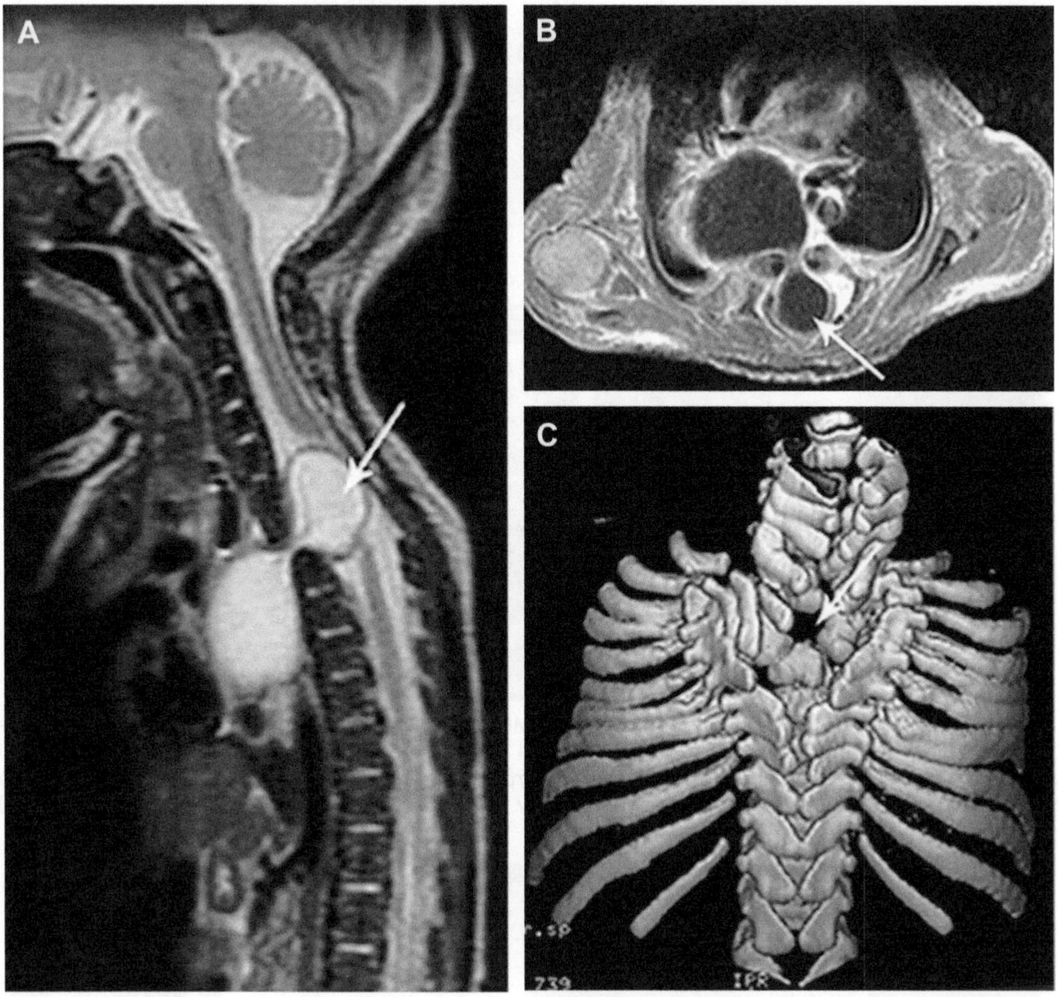

Fig. 16. Neurenteric cyst. Sagittal T2-weighted MR image (*A*) and axial T1-weighted MR image (*B*) show a neurenteric cyst with bilobed configuration (*arrows*) extending from the central canal into the posterior mediastinum. (*C*) Three-dimensional (3-D) computed tomography (CT) reconstruction image from the same patient shows the osseous opening (*arrow*) through which the neurenteric cyst passes; this opening is called the Kovalesky canal. (*Reprinted from* Rufener SL, Ibrahim M, Raybaud CA, et al. Congenital spine and spinal cord malformations–pictorial review. Am J Roentgenol 2010;194:S26–37; with permission.)

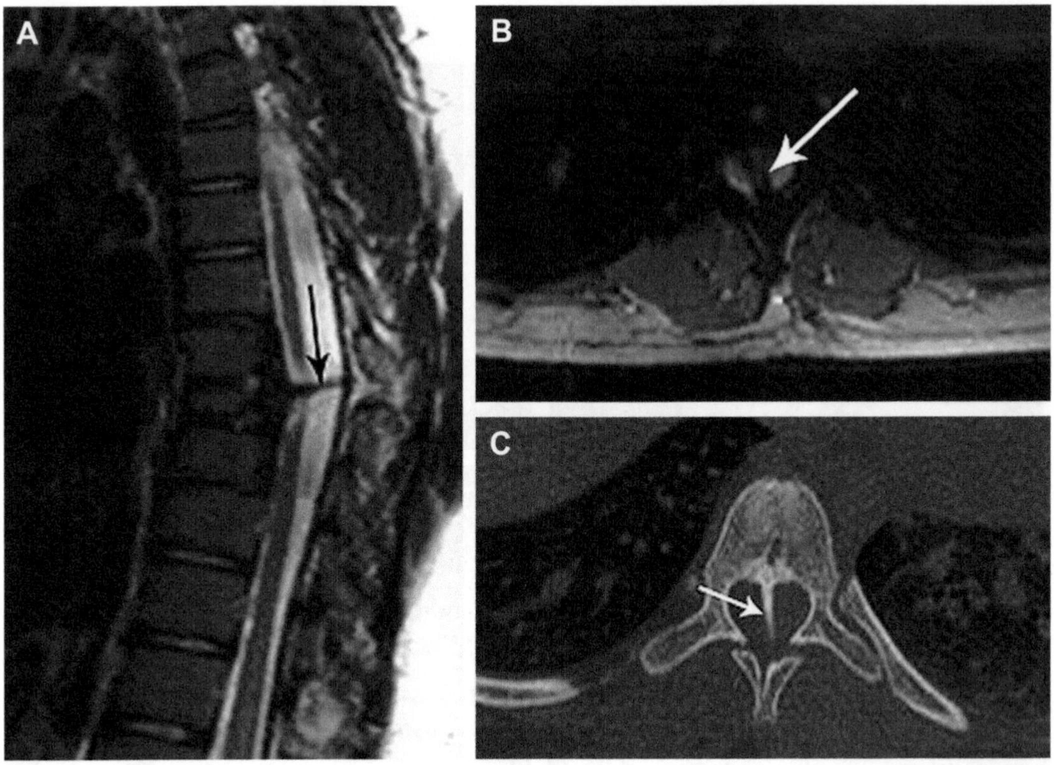

Fig. 17. Diastematomyelia (type I). Sagittal T2-weighted MR image (*A*), axial T2-weighted MR image (*B*), and axial CT image using bone algorithm (*C*) show 2 separate dural tubes separated by an osseous septum (*arrows*), which is characteristic for type 1 diastematomyelia. (*Reprinted from* Rufener SL, Ibrahim M, Raybaud CA, et al. Congenital spine and spinal cord malformations–pictorial review. Am J Roentgenol 2010;194:S26–37; with permission.)

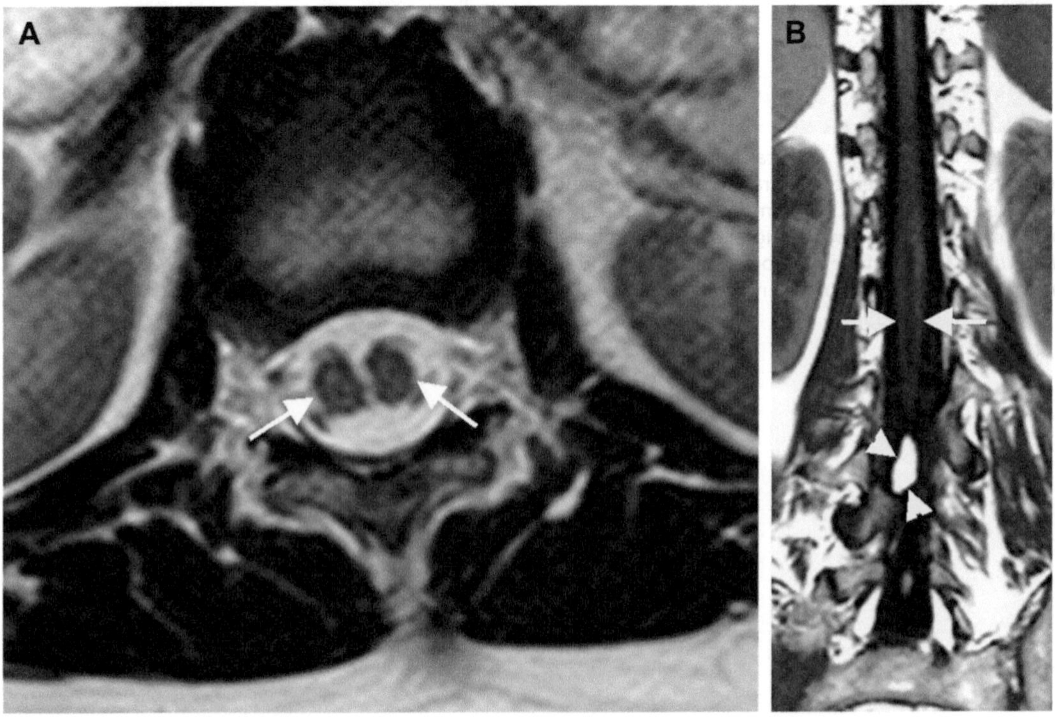

Fig. 18. Diastematomyelia (type II). Axial T2-weighted MR image (*A*) and coronal T1-weighted MR image (*B*) show a single dural tube containing 2 hemicords (*white arrows*), which is characteristic for type 2 diastematomyelia. Also note a small lipoma associated with the right hemicord (*arrowheads*).

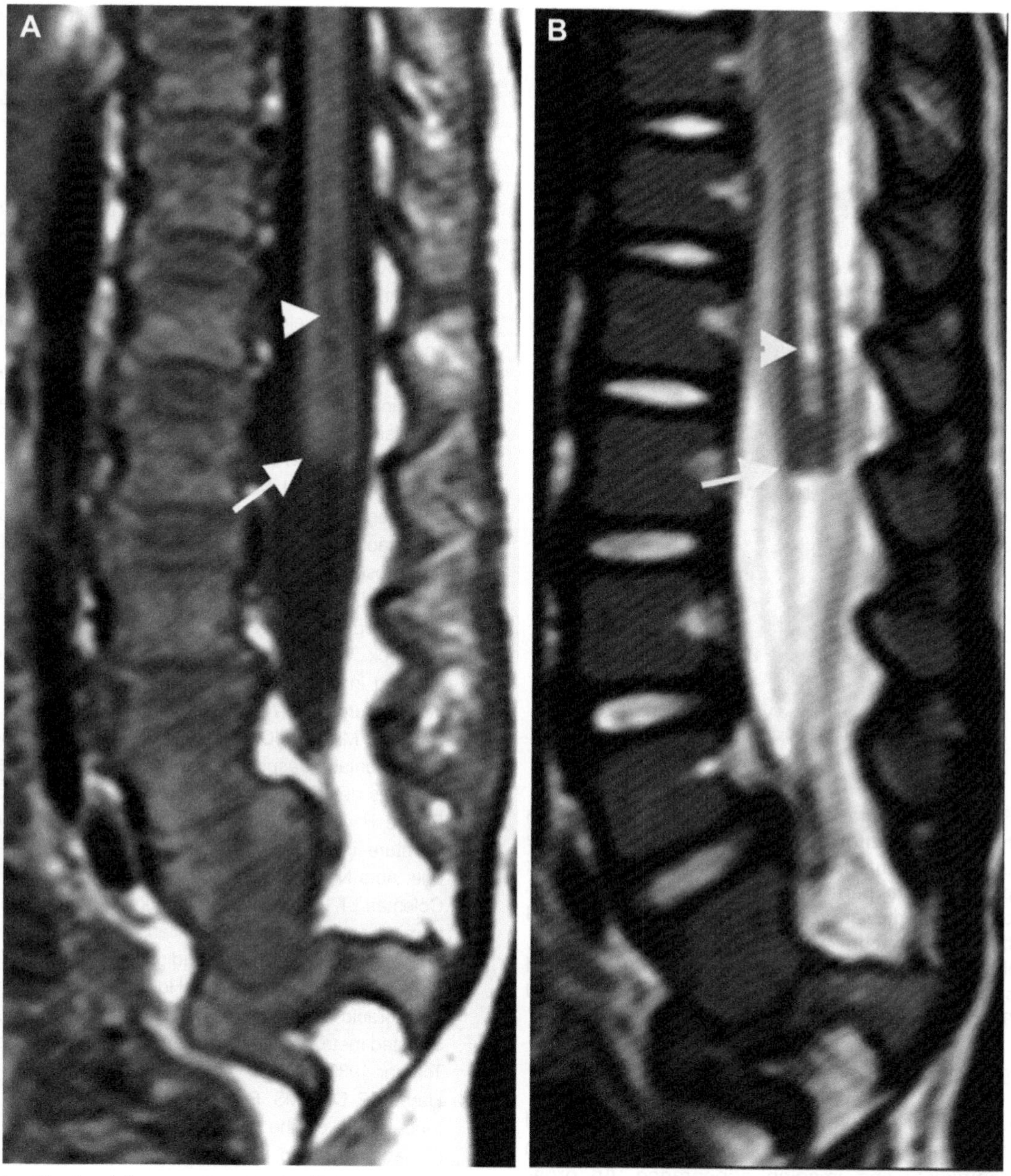

Fig. 19. Caudal regression. Sagittal T1-weighted MR image (*A*) and sagittal T2-weighted MR image (*B*) show sacral agenesis. The conus medullaris is wedge shaped (*arrow*) because of abrupt termination. Appearance is characteristic of type I caudal agenesis. A distal cord syrinx (*arrowhead*) is also noted.

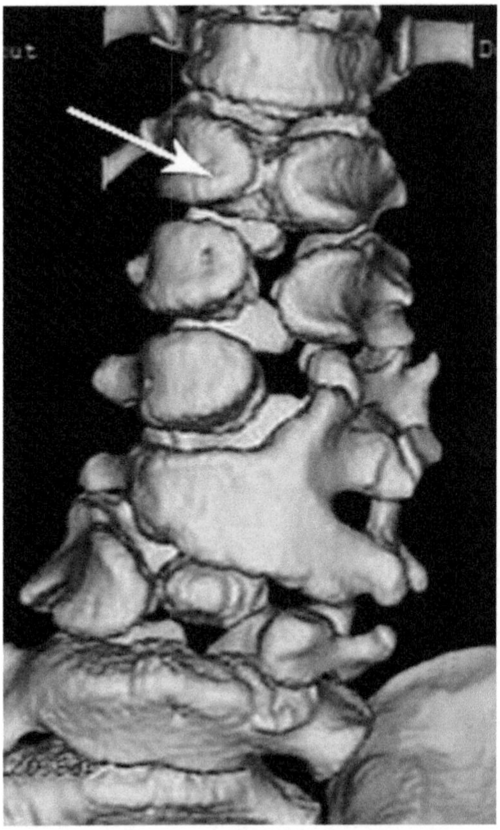

Fig. 20. Segmentation fusion anomaly. (*A, B*) Various types of segmentation anomalies in the lumbar spine (superior to inferior, beginning at level of *arrow*): partial sagittal partition, butterfly vertebra, hemivertebra, tripedicular vertebra, and widely separated butterfly vertebra. (*Reprinted from* Rufener SL, Ibrahim M, Raybaud CA, et al. Congenital spine and spinal cord malformations–pictorial review. Am J Roentgenol 2010;194:S26–37; with permission.)

SUMMARY

Congenital malformations of the spine and spinal cord include numerous entities that vary in complexity and imaging appearance. An organized approach to evaluation of imaging findings with consideration of clinical and developmental factors allows for greater ease in diagnosis.

ACKNOWLEDGMENTS

The authors would like to thank Anne Philips, medical illustrator from the Department of Radiology at the University of Michigan, for providing various illustrations used in this article.

REFERENCES

1. Tortori-Donati P, Rossi A, Cama A. Spinal dysraphism: a review of neuroradiological features with embryological correlations and proposal for a new classification. Neuroradiology 2000;42:471–91.
2. Barkovich AJ. Pediatric neuroradiology. 4th edition. Philadelphia: Lippincott Williams & Wilkins; 2005. p. 801–68.
3. Anderson FM. Occult spinal dysraphisms: diagnosis and management. J Pediatr 1968;73:163–78.
4. Rossi A, Biancheri R, Cama A, et al. Imaging in spine and spinal cord malformations. Eur J Radiol 2004;50:177–200.
5. Parmar H, Shah J, Patkar D, et al. Diastematomyelia and terminal myelocystocele arising from one hemicord: case report. Clin Imaging 2003;27:41–3.
6. Naidich TP, McLone DG, Mutleur S. A new understanding of dorsal dysraphism with lipoma (lipomyeloschisis): radiological evaluation and surgical correction. AJNR Am J Neuroradiol 1983;4:103–16.
7. Lee KS, Gower DJ, McWhorter JM, et al. The role of MR imaging in the diagnosis and treatment of anterior sacral meningocele. Report of 2 cases. J Neurosurg 1988;69:628–31.
8. McLone DG, Niadich TP. Terminal myelocystocele. Neurosurgery 1985;16:36–43.
9. Peacock WJ, Murovic JA. Magnetic resonance imaging in myelocystoceles. Report of two cases. J Neurosurg 1989;70:804–7.
10. Brown E, Matthes JC, Bazan C III, et al. Prevalence of incidental intraspinal lipoma of the lumbosacral spine as determined by MRI. Spine 1994;19:833–6.
11. Guiffre R. Intradural spinal lipomas: review of the literature (99 cases) and report of an additional one. Acta Neurochir (Wien) 1966;14:69–95.
12. Coleman LT, Zimmerman RA, Rorke LB. Ventriculus terminalis of the conus medullaris: MR findings in children. AJNR Am J Neuroradiol 1995;16:1421–6.
13. Scotti G, Harwood-Nash DC, Hoffman HJ. Congenital thoracic dermal sinuses: diagnosis by computer assisted metrizamide myelography. J Comput Assist Tomogr 1980;4:675–7.
14. Harris CP, Dias MS, Brockmeyer DL, et al. Neurenteric cysts of the posterior fossa: recognition, management and embryogenesis. Neurosurgery 1991;29:893–7.
15. Pang D, Dias MS, Ahab-Barmada M. Split cord malformation, part I: a unified theory of embryogenesis for double spinal cord malformations. Neurosurgery 1992;31:451–80.
16. Schijman E. Split spinal cord malformations: report of 22 cases and review of the literature. Childs Nerv Syst 2003;19:96–103.
17. Nievelstein RA, Valk J, Smit LM, et al. MR of the caudal regression syndrome: embryologic implications. AJNR Am J Neuroradiol 1994;15:1021–9.
18. Tortori-Donati P, Fondelli M, Rossi A, et al. Segmental spinal dysgenesis: neuroradiologic findings with clinical and embryologic correlation. AJNR Am J Neuroradiol 1999;20:445–56.

Fetal Neuroimaging

Karuna Shekdar, MD*, Tamara Feygin, MD

KEYWORDS

• Fetal MR • Neuroimaging • Anomalies

FETAL NEUROIMAGING

The primary imaging method for routine examination of the fetal nervous system is ultrasonography (US).[1–4] Magnetic resonance (MR) imaging with its multiplanar imaging ability and high signal-to-noise ratio is highly accurate in illustrating the morphologic changes of the developing brain and fetal brain abnormalities.[4,5] With the development of fast imaging and excellent anatomic detail provided by MR imaging, fetal MR imaging has become a valuable tool in prenatal evaluation.[6] Furthermore, MR imaging can provide excellent anatomic resolution images even when US is limited by patient habitus, fetal presentation, or oligohydramnios.[7] Evaluation of the fetal brain by MR imaging is not limited by the calvarium. MR imaging allows superior delineation of the cortex, ventricles, the subarachnoid spaces, and posterior fossa structures. This article of fetal neuroimaging is primarily focused on evaluation of fetal brain, spine, face, and neck using MR imaging.

Safety of Fetal MR Imaging

Since the initial use of fetal MR imaging in the mid-1980s, there has been no consistent or convincing evidence to suggest harmful effects from short-term exposure of the fetus to changing electromagnetic fields that occur during MR imaging.[8,9] Experimental studies have not shown any deleterious side effects of MR imaging on the developing embryo or in the long-term outcome of children who had undergone fetal MR imaging between 21 weeks of gestation and term.[10] MR imaging is now accepted as a safe and valuable imaging tool in prenatal evaluation of the fetus.[11,12]

Even though it is considered safe, MR imaging is not performed in the first trimester of organogenesis. Fetal MR imaging is generally performed in the second trimester of gestation, usually from 18 weeks onwards. It is difficult to obtain good-quality images in very young fetuses by MR imaging.[11] There is Food and Drug Administration approval for fetal MR imaging using magnets up to field strength of 1.5 Tesla.

Fetal Neuroimaging MR Techniques

Different types of coils can be used. A body coil alone or a body phased-array coil in combination with a surface coil positioned on the mother's abdomen is generally used. Considering the developing brain, the imaging parameters have to be optimized. T2-weighted (T2W) images, in particular, are used to assess the changes in brain tissue water content in the developing brain. Images are routinely obtained in orthogonal planes (ie, sagittal, coronal, and axial planes) relative to the fetal head. Fast T2W images provide the majority of the diagnostic information.[12,13] The half-Fourier single-shot turbo spin-echo (HASTE) sequence provides heavily T2W images with low susceptibility weighting in a very short time. Sequential slice capability and interleaving allow for good quality images even with physiologic fetal movement. The utility of T1-weighted (T1W) images is limited in the high water content of the developing nonmyelinated brain. T1W imaging is performed in addition to routine T2W imaging in fetuses older than 28 weeks of gestation, when satisfactory T1W signal-to-noise and contrast resolution can be achieved. Gradient-echo images especially the fast low-angle shot (FLASH) sequences allow for excellent differentiation between the cortical ribbon and white matter and the ventricular walls. Extremely rapid gradient-echo, echo planar imaging (EPI), with its high

Disclosure statement: the authors have nothing to disclose.
Neuro-radiology Division, Department of Radiology, The Children's Hospital of Philadelphia, University of Pennsylvania, 34th & Civic Center Boulevard, Philadelphia, PA 19104, USA
* Corresponding author.
E-mail address: shekdar@email.chop.edu

Neuroimag Clin N Am 21 (2011) 677–703
doi:10.1016/j.nic.2011.05.010

sensitivity to paramagnetic susceptibility, is used in identification of hemorrhage and mineralization as well as osseous and vascular structures. Diffusion-weighted imaging and apparent diffusion coefficient maps can also be obtained and are valuable in assessment of ischemic damage.[14]

At the authors' institution, fetal cine imaging is routinely included along with fetal morphologic imaging. Fetal cine imaging is useful in assessing dynamic movements, such as swallowing and fetal extremity movements. The entire duration of a typical fetal neuroimaging examination is approximately 30 to 40 minutes. No maternal or fetal sedation is used at the authors' institution. Contrast agents are not used in evaluation of pregnant patients for fetal MR imaging, because gadolinium crosses the placenta. The toxicity of gadolinium to the fetus is not known.

Indications for Fetal Neuroimaging

MR imaging is not used as a screening tool in evaluation of the fetus. MR imaging is usually performed because of abnormal findings on US evaluation. The most common indications for fetal neuroimaging are listed in **Box 1**[11] in order of frequency with the most common indication, ventriculomegaly, listed first.

A special note should be made of the indications when a fetal MR evaluation is obtained even when brain US study is normal. These include possibility of potentially destructive brain lesions related to maternal coagulation disorders, maternal hypoxia, maternal trauma, and fetal demise in multiple gestation. In all these indications, the role of MR imaging is to assess for brain damage, which is difficult to be evaluated by US.[11] Other indications include maternal infection or a fetus presenting with extracerebral multiple malformations, because of the high incidence of extracerebral lesions associated with brain lesions. Known central nervous system (CNS) malformations or chromosomal aberrations in siblings and family history of genetic disorders involving the CNS also warrant MR evaluation, even with a preceding normal US examination.

Box 1
Common indications for fetal neuroimaging

Ventriculomegaly
Suspected malformation
Potential destructive lesion
Multiple malformations in the fetus
Malformation in siblings/known family history of genetic disease
Maternal infection

MR imaging is usually not indicated in cases of intrauterine growth restriction.[11] However, MR imaging can provide useful information when intrauterine growth restriction is associated with progressive microcephaly or other abnormalities, such as fetal hydrops or arthrogryposis.

Development of the Fetal Brain on MR Imaging

MR imaging appearance of the developing fetal brain reflects changes of histogenesis and myelination. Subsequent changes are seen in the brain volume, surface configuration (ie, sulcation), and internal configuration (**Figs. 1–3**).

Table 1 describes cortical landmarks demonstrated in almost 75% of developing fetal brains with respect to gestational ages.[5,11,15]

There is ongoing research to develop MR-based findings for assessing brain maturation and development. One study has developed a semiquantitative scale and scoring system for assessing brain maturation. Defined visual imaging indices, including specific areas of myelination, presence, and location of germinal matrix, cortical infolding, and sulcal depth, have been used.[16]

ANOMALIES OF THE FETAL BRAIN

Ventriculomegaly

Ventriculomegaly is one of the most common indications for performing fetal brain MR imaging.

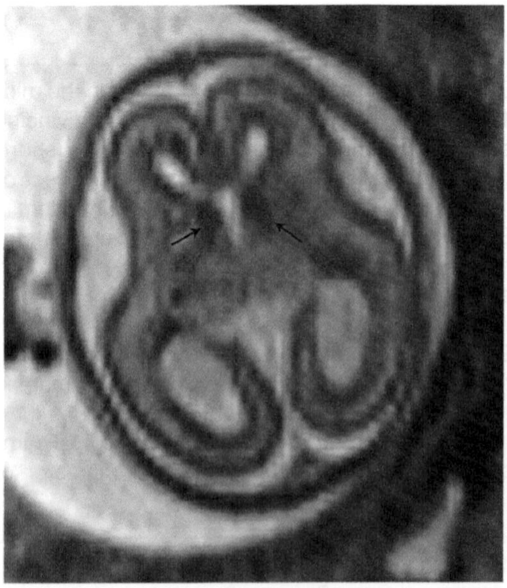

Fig. 1. Axial HASTE image in a 20-week gestational age fetus. Note the smooth appearance of the brain surface with shallow concavity at the location of the future sylvian fissure. Small black arrows point to the developing germinal matrix.

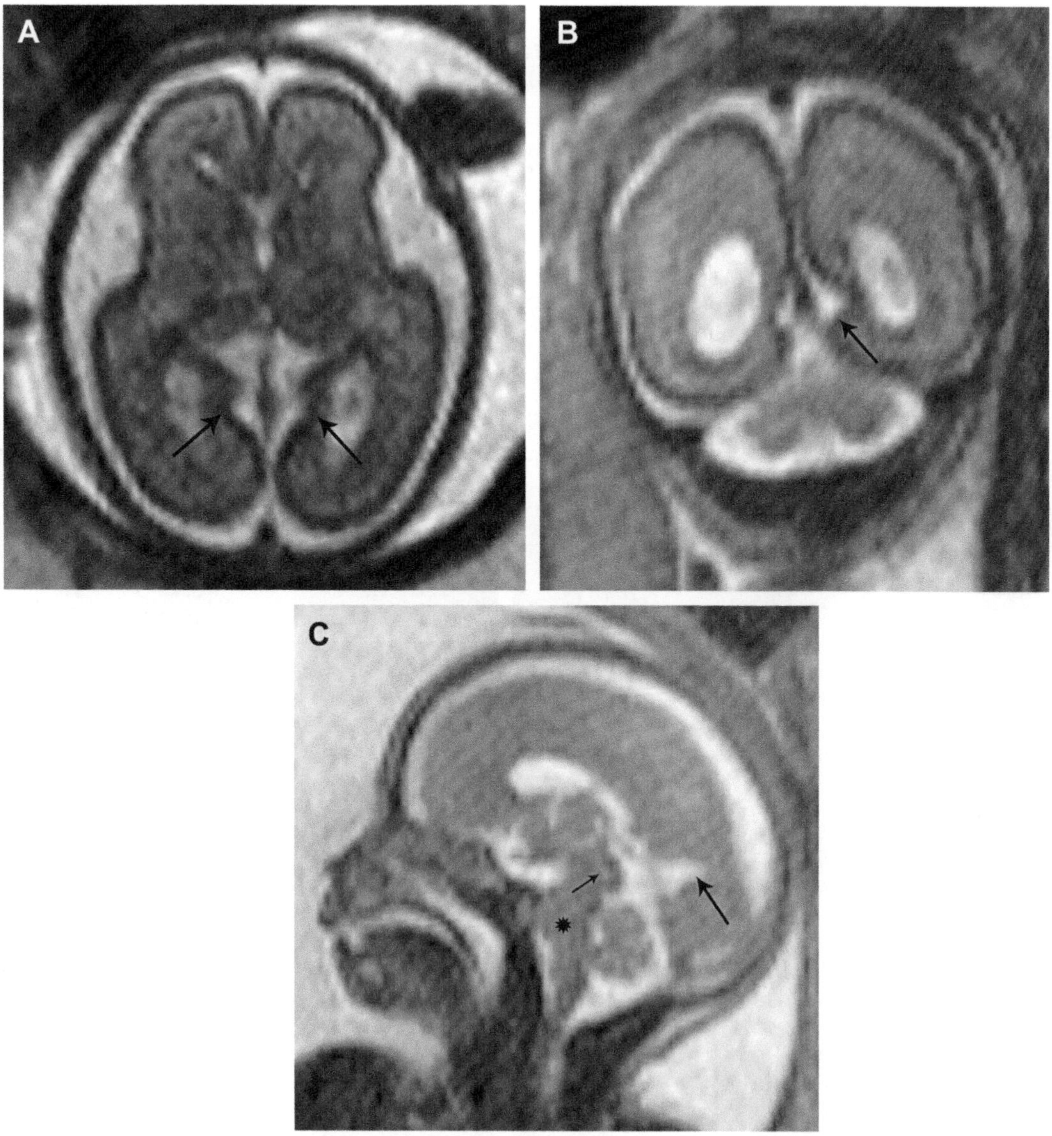

Fig. 2. HASTE images of 23-week gestational age fetal brain in the axial (*A*), coronal (*B*), and sagittal (*C*) planes. Long black arrows point to the calcarine fissure. Small black arrow points toward the normal cerebral aqueduct and black asterisk shows normal-sized brainstem.

Ventriculomegaly may be due to an apparent cause, which can be detected by imaging in approximately 60% of cases.[17] In approximately 40% of cases no apparent cause can be detected on imaging.[11]

Ventriculomegaly is defined as ventricular size, measured at the atrial level, greater than 10 mm.[18] Ventriculomegaly can be divided into mild (10 to 15 mm) (**Fig. 4**), moderate (>15 mm with >3 mm of adjacent cortical thickness), and severe ventriculomegaly (with <2 mm of adjacent cortical thickness) (**Fig. 5**). The causes of ventriculomegaly may be several. If it is mild, it could be transient and possibly a normal finding. Ventriculomegaly may be related to cerebral dysgenesis example corpus callosal anomalies. It could be the result of an ex vacuo phenomenon secondary to atrophy, infections, or infarction. It may also be related to hydrocephalus

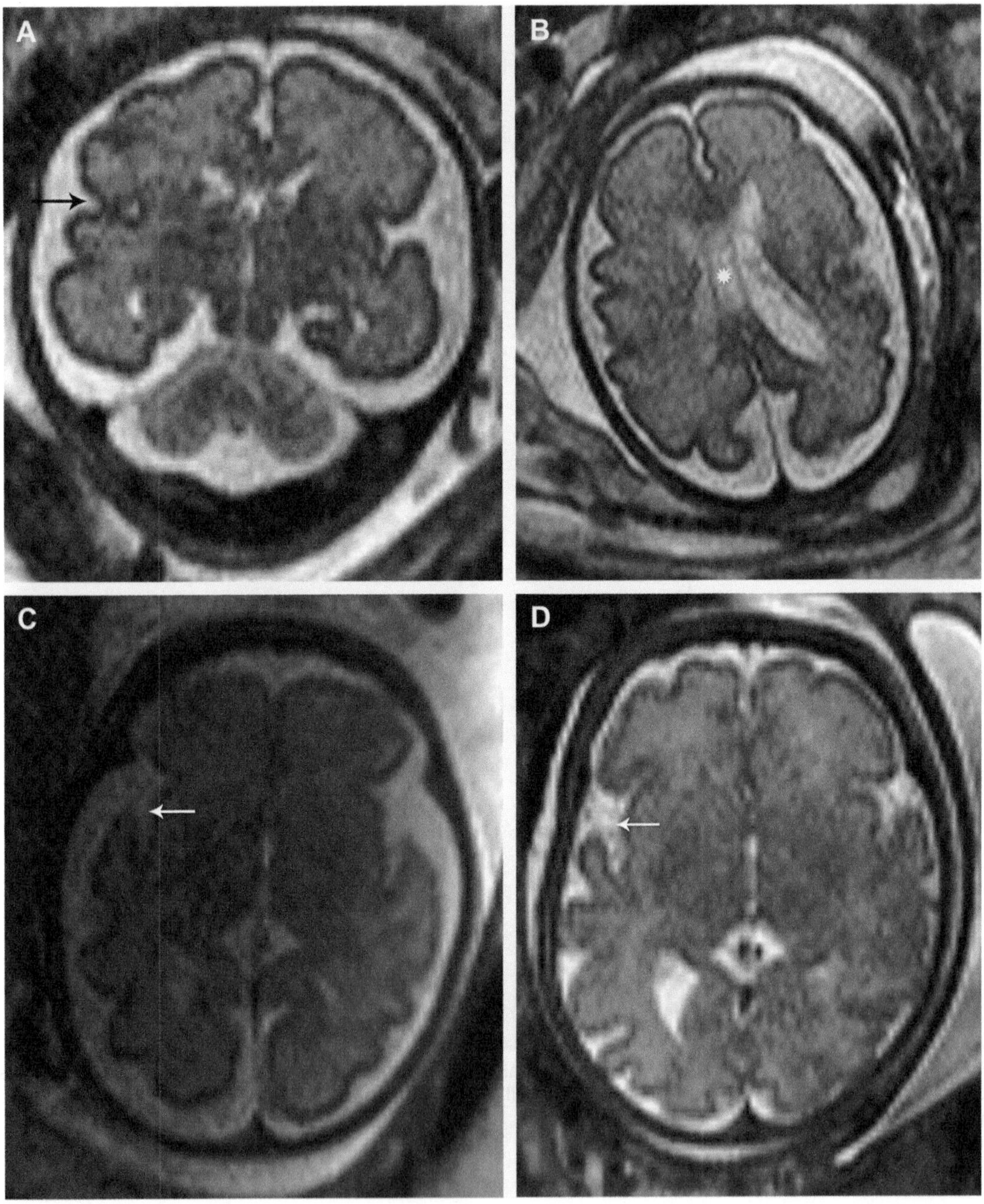

Fig. 3. HASTE images of 28-week gestational age fetal brain in the coronal (*A*) and axial (*B*) planes demonstrating further elaborated cortex (*black arrow*) and normal cavum septum pellucidum (*white asterisk*). HASTE images of a 32-week (*C*) and 36-week (*D*) gestational age fetal brain, demonstrating progressive development of the sylvian fissure (*white arrows*).

associated with disorder of cerebrospinal fluid (CSF) dynamics.[19]

The prognosis of ventriculomegaly depends on the cause of the ventricular dilatation, the gestational age at which occurs, and its progression. Mild isolated ventriculomegaly (10 to 12 mm) is not associated with adverse postnatal outcomes in majority of the cases.[20] Developmental delay is associated with mild isolated ventriculomegaly, however, in the range of 19% to 36%.[20] Ventriculomegaly with

Table 1
Developing sulcation in fetal brains

Sulci/ Fissures	Appears	Deepens	Developed
Parieto-occipital	16 to 17 wk	18 to 20 wk	20 to 22 wk
Calcerine	16 to 17 wk	18 to 20 wk	24 wk
Central sulcus	24 to 25 wk	31 wk	35 wk
Precentral sulcus	26 to 27 wk	31 wk	35 wk
Postcentral sulcus	28 to 29 wk	31 wk	35 wk

Data from Refs.[5,11,15]

dysmorphic appearance is usually a feature of neural tube defects. A box-shaped configuration of the frontal horns is often associated with absence of septum pellucidum. Colpocephaly, which is disproportionate dilatation of the atria and occipital horns with small frontal horns, is often present with hypogenesis of the corpus callosum. Enlarged ventricles, with effacement of the extracerebral CSF spaces along with large head size, usually denote an obstructive component to the ventriculomegaly. When there is preservation of extracerebral CSF spaces or prominence with ventriculomegaly, however, hypogenesis is usually the cause. In some cases, hypogenesis and hydrocephalus can coexist.

Corpus Callosum Abnormalities

Agenesis of the corpus callosum could be complete or partial (hypogenesis). This could result either from a vascular or inflammatory insult occurring in the early (before 12 weeks) gestation. In agenesis of the corpus callosum, the interhemispheric axonal fibers do not cross the midline. As a result the fibers are distributed longitudinally as Probst bundles and located along the superomedial margin of the lateral ventricles. Colpocephaly is present with a high-riding third ventricle. Associated findings include ventriculomegaly, parallel orientation of the frontal horns, absence of the septum pellucidum, and small head size. The cingulate sulcus is absent in complete agenesis of corpus callosum (**Fig. 6**).

Corpus callosum agenesis is often associated with other malformations, chromosomal abnormalities, and genetic syndromes. Corpus callosal agenesis may be present along with Dandy-Walker malformation as well as other neural tube defects, such as Chiari II malformation. Interhemispheric clefts and cysts with hypogenesis of the corpus callosum have also been documented (**Fig. 7**).

Partial hypogenesis of corpus callosum could result from from incomplete formation or from a postformational destructive process. When there is massive ventriculomegaly, it may be difficult to visualize the corpus callosum. Fetal MR imaging in corpus callosal agenesis can delineate other

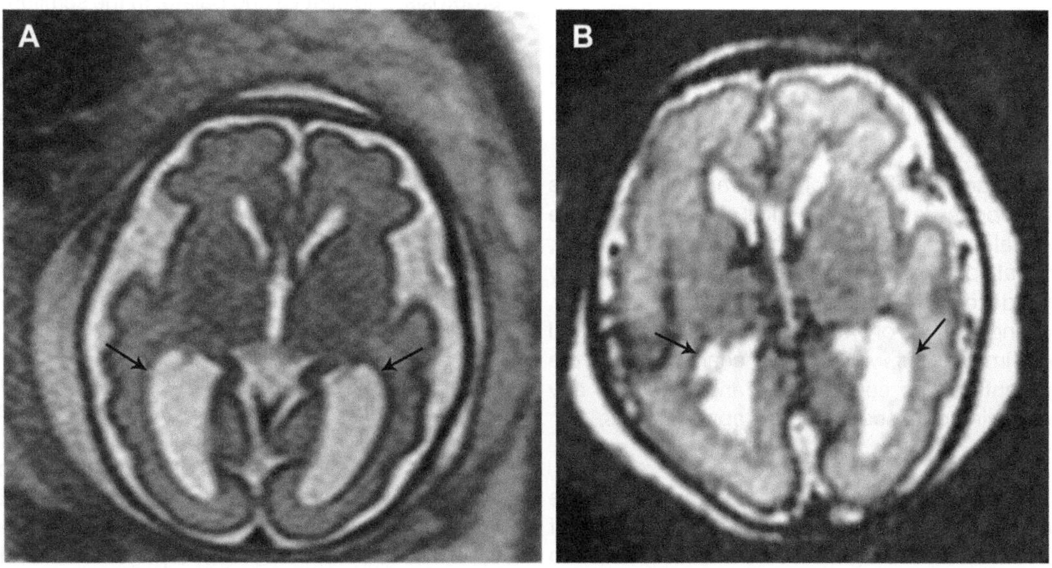

Fig. 4. Axial HASTE image (*A*) and axial EPI image (*B*) demonstrating mild ventriculomegaly (*black arrows*).

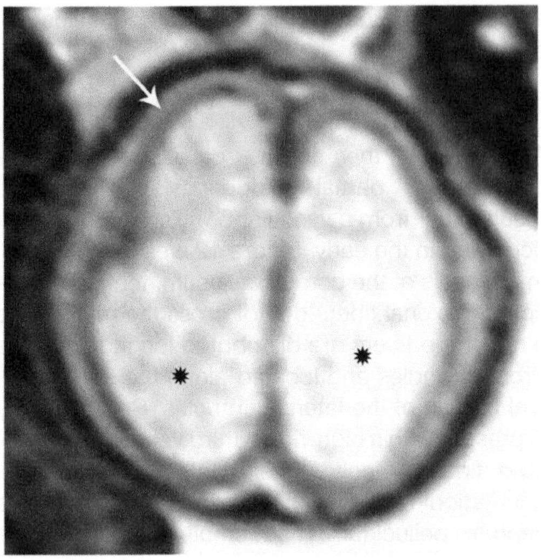

Fig. 5. Severe ventriculomegaly (*black asterisks*) with only thin mantle of overlying cerebral cortex (*white arrow*).

findings, such as pericallosal lipoma, interhemispheric cysts (see **Fig. 7**), and gyral abnormalities as well as heterotopias.[17,21,22] Retrospective studies have demonstrated that 43% of cases of confirmed corpus callosal agenesis were detected by fetal MR but not by US.[7]

Disorders of Dorsal Neural Tube Development

Disorders of dorsal neural tube development associated with defects of primary neurulation include anencephaly, cephalocele, myelomeningocele, and the Chiari II malformation.

Cephaloceles

Cephalocele is protrusion of intracranial contents via a bony defect of the skull. Locations of the cephaloceles, in order of occurrence, are occipital, frontal, parietal, and basal. The protrusion may include only meninges and CSF or, in addition, varying portions of brain parenchyma (**Fig. 8**). Fetal MR imaging is valuable in characterizing the contents of the cephaloceles and detecting any underlying or associated brain abnormalities.[11,17]

Chiari II malformation

Typical stigmata of Chiari II malformation include small posterior fossa and downward herniation of the hindbrain through the foramen magnum into the upper cervical spinal canal. This is best depicted on midline sagittal MR images (**Fig. 9**). Additional findings include varying degrees of ventriculomegaly and dysmorphic appearance of ventricles. There may be concurrent corpus callosal abnormalities. Associated findings of gray matter heterotopias (**Fig. 10**) may be present and can be detected on MR imaging.

Myelomeningocele (MMC) is associated with Chiari II malformation. Fetal MR imaging is important in selecting and triaging patients with MMC and Chiari II malformation, who may be potential candidates for in utero surgical repair.[17,23]

Spinal findings of neural tube defects on fetal MR imaging are discussed separately in the spine section of the article.

Disorders of Ventral Neural Tube Development

Disorders of ventral neural tube development occur due to insults to the rostral end of the embryo (which contribute in formation of the face and the brain during 5 to 10 weeks of gestational age). Abnormalities of frontal induction include the holoprosencephalies, septo-optic dysplasia, cerebral and cerebellar hypoplasia, and the Dandy-Walker spectrum.

Holoprosencephaly

In the alobar form, the interhemispheric fissure and the falx are absent. There is a large monoventricle and the thalami are fused (**Fig. 11**). There is microcephaly and abnormal frontal sloping with protuberant orbits. Facial anomalies are usually associated with the alobar holoprosencephaly, such as cyclopia, hypotelorism, anophthalmia, proptosis, and cleft lip and palate. In the semilobar form, there is partial separation of the cerebral hemispheres posteriorly, but there remains a single ventricular cavity and varying degrees of fusion of the basal ganglia and thalami. Lobar holoprosencephaly is the least severe form in which there is near complete separation of the hemispheres but there is fusion at the level of the cingulate gyrus and frontal horns of the lateral ventricles (**Fig. 12**). The septum pellucidum is usually absent. It may be difficult to distinguish between lobar holoprosencephaly and septo-optic dysplasia. Fetal MR imaging can distinguish holoprosencephaly with large monoventricle from agenesis of the corpus callosum with associated large midline clefts or cysts.[11,17,24] MR imaging is particularly useful in demonstrating subtle findings of lobar holoprosencephaly, which are likely to be missed by US. Fusion of the frontal lobes and continuity of the cortex across the midline are depicted on the MR imaging in lobar holoprosencephaly.

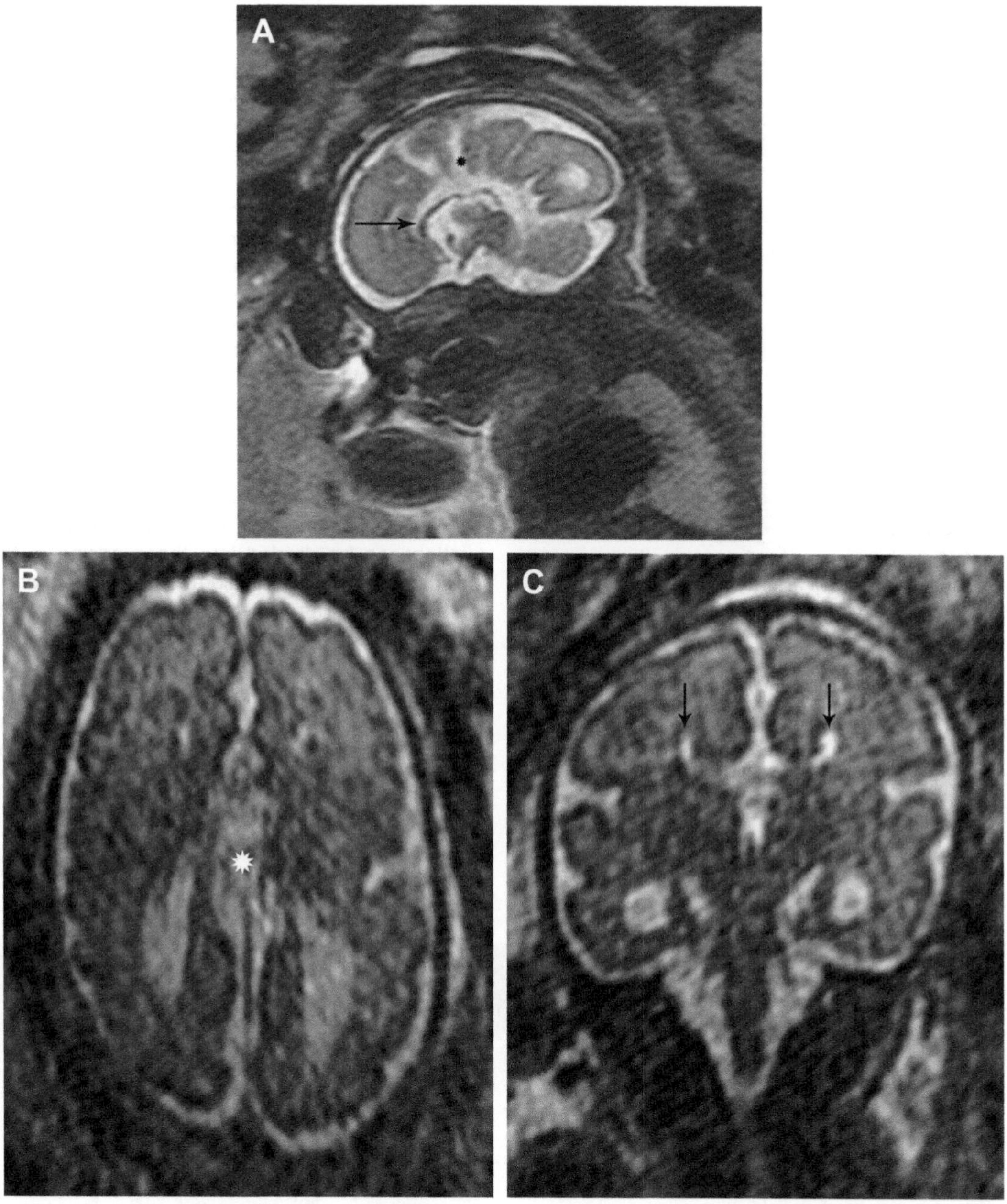

Fig. 6. Corpus callosum agenesis. Sagittal HASTE (*A*) shows complete absence of the corpus callosum, converging medial hemispheric sulci (*black asterisk*). Prominent anterior commissure (*black arrow*) should not be mistaken for corpus callosum. Axial HASTE (*B*) shows parallel orientation of lateral ventricles and high-riding third ventricle (*white asterisk*). Coronal HASTE (*C*) shows steer-horn–shaped frontal horns (*arrows*), resulting from impression of Probst bundles.

Dandy-Walker Spectrum

Although US is adequate in demonstrating severe forms of the Dandy-Walker malformation, MR imaging is superior in delineation of dural structures, position of the tentorium, and other associated abnormalities.[24] The Dandy-Walker malformation is characterized by large posterior fossa cyst in continuity with the fourth ventricle along with vermian agenesis or hypogenesis and elevation of the torcula (**Fig. 13**). Hydrocephalus is usually present. The cerebellar hemispheres

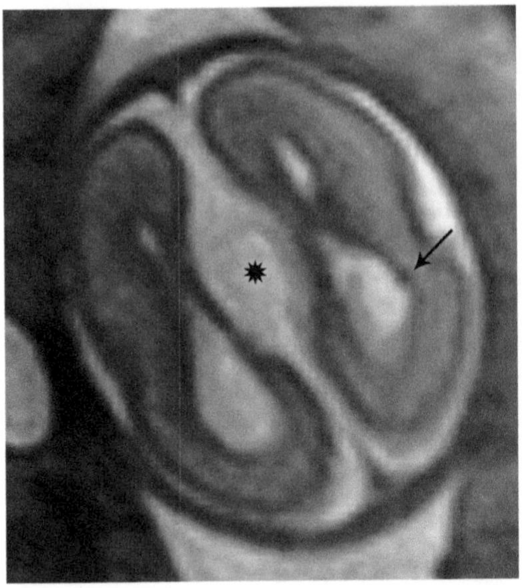

Fig. 7. Complete agenesis of corpus callosum, interhemispheric cyst (*black asterisk*), and gray matter subependymal heterotopia (*black arrow*) in a patient with Aicardi syndrome.

are usually hypoplastic and compressed laterally by the large posterior fossa cyst.

Posterior fossa cystic malformations also includes the Dandy-Walker variant, mega cisterna magna, Blake pouch cyst, and retrocerebellar arachnoid cyst. The midline sagittal view is helpful in characterizing these abnormalities and also in characterizing the cerebellar vermis (**Figs. 14** and **15**). It may sometimes be difficult to distinguish Dandy-Walker variant from Blake pouch cyst or retrocerebellar arachnoid cyst.

Dandy-Walker malformations are usually associated with other CNS or systemic abnormalities, including chromosomal abnormalities, corpus callosal agenesis, holoprosencephaly, and disorders of cortical migration organization, such as the Walker-Warburg syndrome, which can be seen on MR imaging.

Disorders of Proliferation, Differentiation and Histogenesis

Disorders of neural, glial, and mesenchymal proliferation can be divided into those arising in the premigration stage, the migration, and the postmigration stage. These disorders are not commonly evident on US; hence, MR imaging is most appropriate technique for detection of such malformations. This information from MR imaging is useful for genetic counseling for future pregnancies because the majority of these malformations have a genetic basis of origin.[11]

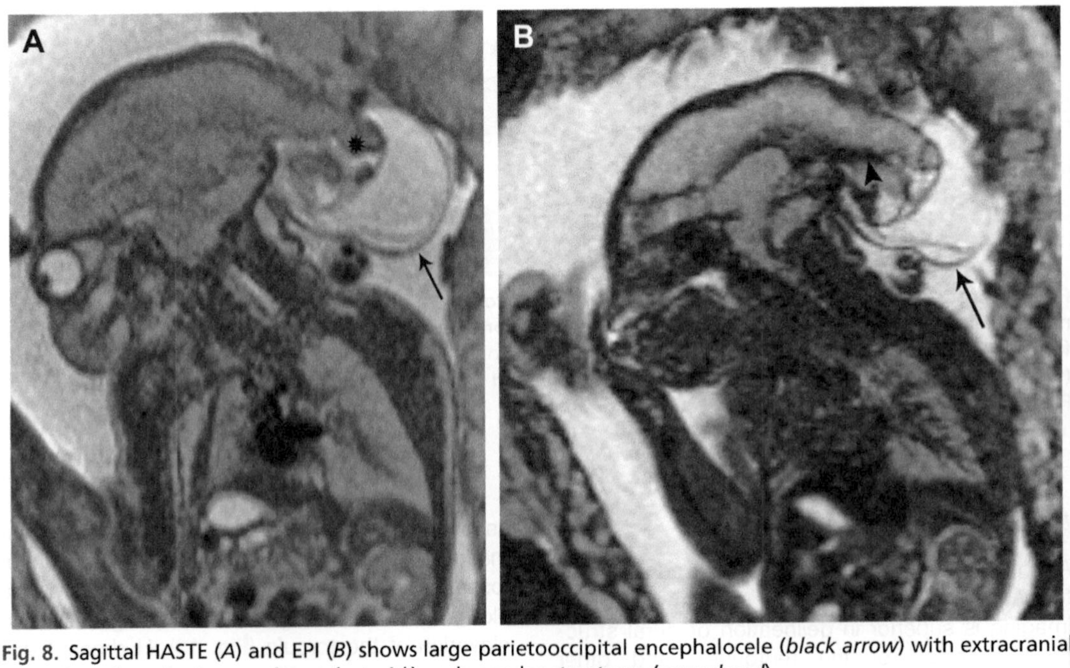

Fig. 8. Sagittal HASTE (*A*) and EPI (*B*) shows large parietooccipital encephalocele (*black arrow*) with extracranial extension of cerebral parenchyma (*asterisk*) and vascular structures (*arrowhead*).

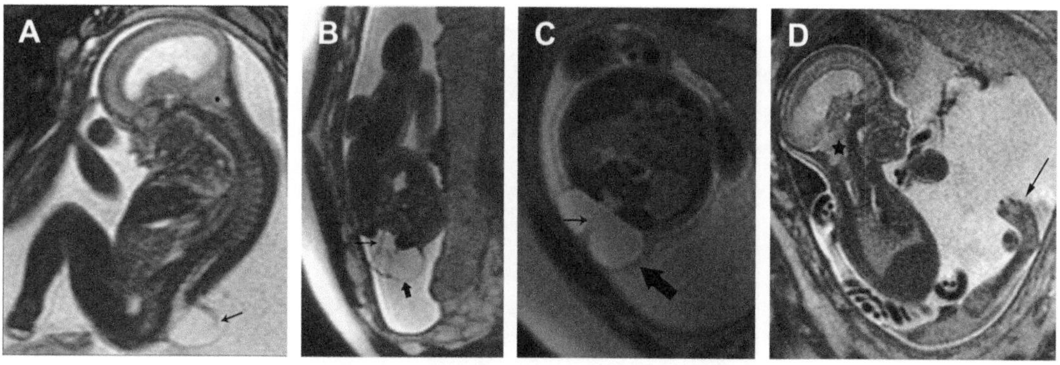

Fig. 9. Chiari II and myelomeningocele—sagittal (*A*) and axial (*B, C*) HASTE images demonstrating findings of small posterior fossa with hindbrain herniation (*black star*), lumbosacral MMC sac (*thick black arrow*) and neural placode elements within the sac (*thin black arrow*). Note clubfoot deformity (*D*) (*long black arrow*).

Neuronal migrational disorders

Neuronal migrational disorders occur during neuronal migration characterized by the disturbance of normal neuronal arrangement. This group of abnormalities consists of lissencephaly, including type I (agyria and pachygyria) and type II (Walker-Warburg syndrome) (**Fig. 16**); polymicrogyria; gray matter heterotopias (nodular and laminar heterotopia); and microcephaly.

Lissencephaly type I is characterized by thickening of the cortical ribbon with broad flat gyri and primitive shallow sulcation (**Fig. 17**). This may be associated with corpus callosal hypogenesis. The type II lissencephaly (for example, cobblestone lissencephaly) has thickened and severely disorganized cortex. Meninges are thickened and densely adherent to the cortex and obliterate the subarachnoid space. There may be associated subcortical heterotopias. Other associated abnormalities include callosal hypogenesis, micropthalamia, and cerebellar vermian hypoplasia. Muscular dystrophy, congenital eye malformations, and posterior cephaloceles are some other known associations. Fetal MR imaging can characterize and detect all these findings in these cases.[25]

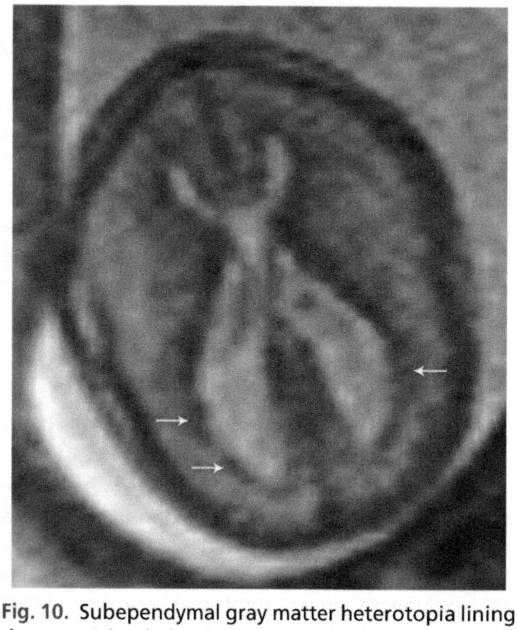

Fig. 10. Subependymal gray matter heterotopia lining the ventricles (*white arrows*) in this fetus, who also had Chiari II malformation.

Posterior fossa histogenetic disorders include cerebellar hypogenesis, cerebellar cortical dysplasias, and heterotopias. These abnormalities result from nonformation of one or both cerebellar hemispheres. In hypoplasia the cerebellar hemispheres may be formed but are small. In some cases there is vermian hypogenesis with or without cerebellar hypogenesis. Many cases of fetal ventriculomegaly are usually associated with cerebellar hypogenesis.

Postmigratory Organization Disorders

Polymicrogyria

The most common entity in this category is the polymicrogyria, which is characterized by multiple small and irregular sulci associated with enlarged overlying subarachnoid spaces (**Fig. 18**). Ventricular dilatation may be present. Polymicrogyria due to an infectious cause, such as cytomegalovirus (CMV) infection, can be suspected when calcifications may be evident.

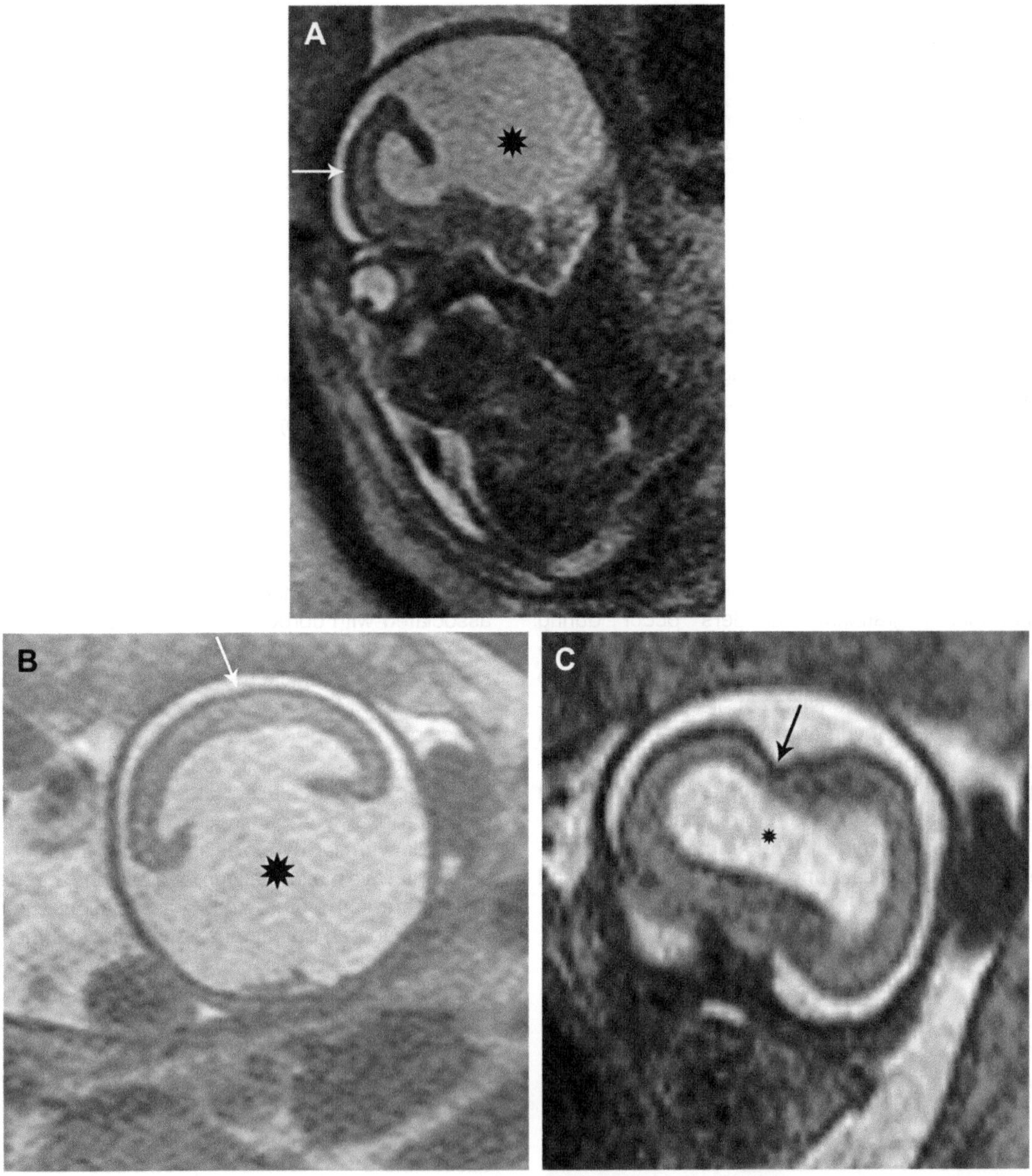

Fig. 11. Alobar holoprosencephaly—sagittal HASTE (*A*) shows only minimal frontal cerebral mantle (*white arrows in A and B*) and replacement of majority of the brain with CSF (*asterisk*). Axial (*B*) and coronal (*C*) HASTE showing complete absence of falx, interhemispheric fissure and corpus callosum. Horseshoe-shaped monoventricle communicating with a dorsal cyst (*asterisk*). Pancake-like residual brain tissue anteriorly (*black arrow*).

Schizencephaly

Schizencephaly, although included in the postmigratory group of abnormalities, is mostly considered to be of destructive origin resulting from insult developing before 16 weeks of gestation. Schizencephaly is characterized by a CSF-filled, gray matter–lined cleft that extends from the cortex to the wall of the lateral ventricle (**Fig. 19**). Associated malformations include ventriculomegaly, polymicrogyria, heterotopias, corpus callosal agenesis, and absence of the cavum septum pellucidum.[12,26,27]

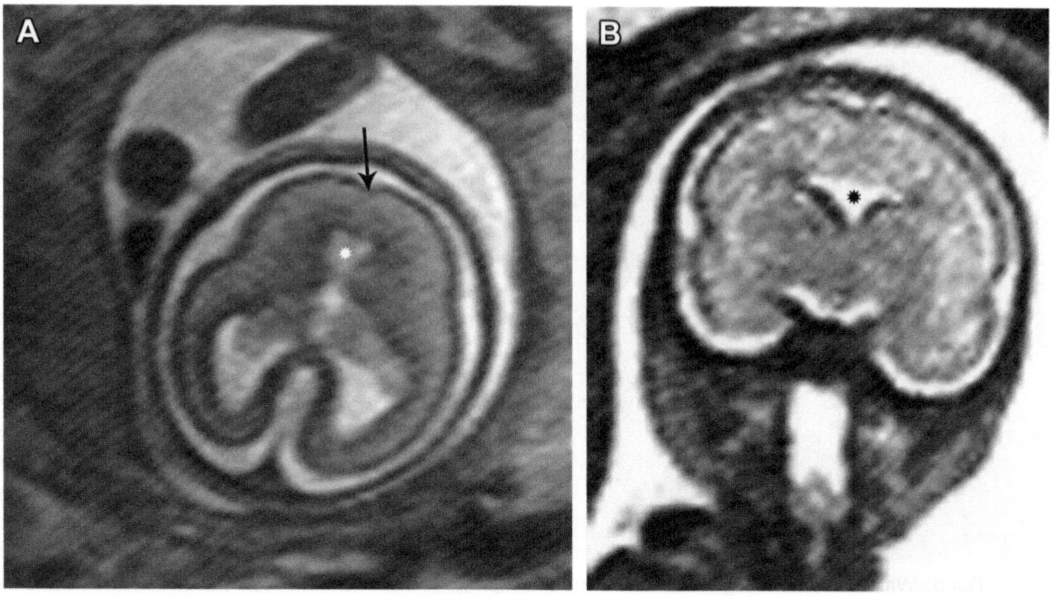

Fig. 12. Lobar holoprosencephaly—axial (*A*) and coronal (*B*) HASTE images showing relatively better separation of the midline structures posteriorly but fused frontal horns (*white asterisk in A and black asterisk in B*) and anterior frontal lobe (*black arrow*).

Neuronal heterotopias

Heterotopias represent gray matter in abnormal locations as result of abnormality in the stage of migration. Several causes are postulated, including vascular and environmental causes, such as trisomy 13, fetal alcohol syndrome, and maternal infections. Most patients with subependymal heterotopias have seizures (see **Fig. 10**). Those

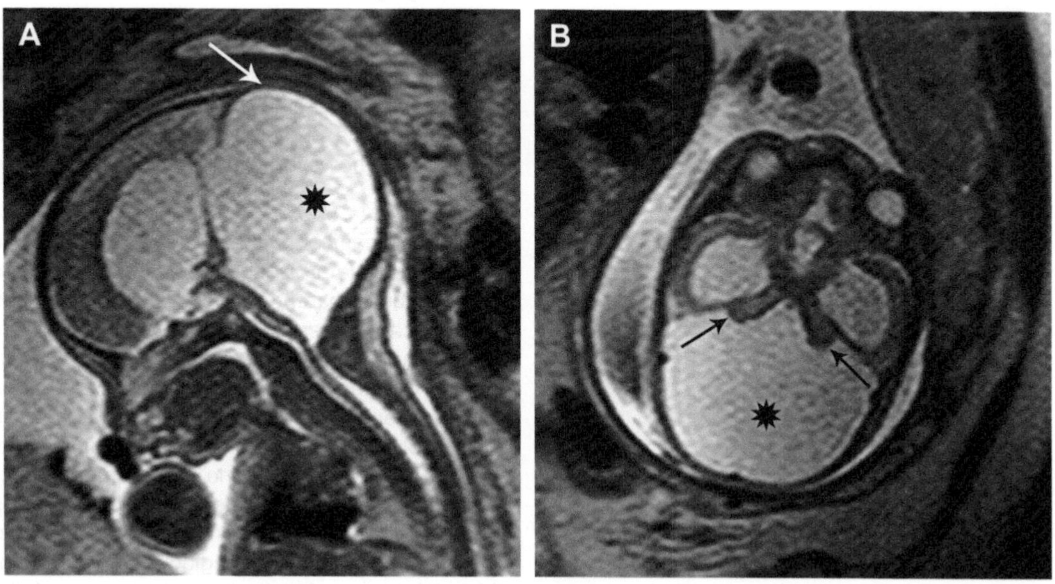

Fig. 13. Dandy-Walker malformation—sagittal (*A*) and axial (*B*) HASTE showing enlarged posterior fossa (*asterisk*) with absence of the vermis and large posterior fossa cyst (*asterisk in A and B*) and winged-outward appearance of hypoplastic cerebellar hemispheres (*small black arrows*). Note the elevated torcula (*white arrow*). (*From* Shekdar K. Posterior fossa malformations. Semin Ultrasound CT MR 2011;32:228–41; with permission.)

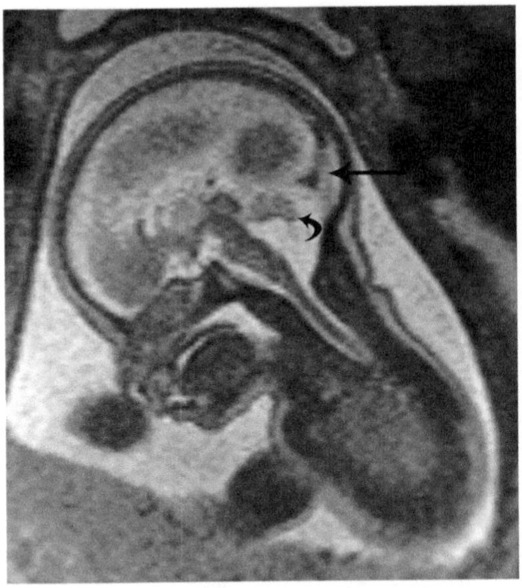

Fig. 14. Dandy-Walker variant—sagittal HASTE shows small rotated vermis (*curved arrow*) and direct communication of fourth ventricle with retrocerebellar CSF space. Torcular herophili is normally positioned (*arrow*).

patients with laminar or band heterotopias may have developmental delay and earlier onset of seizures. It may be necessary in young fetuses to repeat the MR imaging examination in few weeks

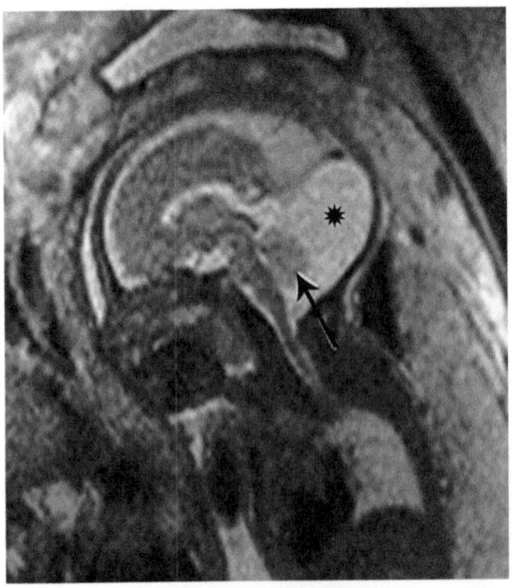

Fig. 15. Posterior fossa arachnoid cyst—sagittal HASTE shows expanded posterior fossa, retrocerebellar CSF collection (*asterisk*) and normal cerebellum (*arrow*).

after the initial examination to better appreciate the findings of polymicrogyria.[17,24,28]

Clastic Abnormalities of the Developing Fetal Brain

Clastic lesions include hemorrhage, infarction, porencephaly, encephalomalacia, leukomalacia, atrophy, and hydranencephaly.

Hemorrhage

Hemorrhage intracranially could occur in the extra-axial space, intraventricular or within the brain parenchyma. Although the timetable of evolution of fetal hemorrhage is not precisely established, the blood products can be seen as high signal intensity on T1W images and low signal intensity on T2W images. If the hemorrhage is remote, then presence of blood products could be identified by secondary findings of focal ventriculomegaly, porencephalic cyst, cavities, or atrophy. The EPI gradient sequences can identify remote blood products as focal increased susceptibility from hemosiderin staining (**Fig. 20**). There are many reports that show MR imaging identifying hemorrhage, which is not seen on US. Intraventricular hemorrhage could be identified as irregular T2 hypointensity of the choroid plexus itself or in ventricles besides the choroid plexus. The cause of hemorrhage may not be evident by imaging alone; however, information about underlying causes, such as vascular malformations or mass lesions, can be demonstrated on MR imaging. MR imaging is also more sensitive in identifying sequelae of hemorrhage, such as porencephaly and encephalomalacia.[24] Isolated small germinal matrix hemorrhage may be visualized on MR imaging, which may not be seen by US. The clinical significance of isolated fetal germinal matrix hemorrhage, however, is not known.[29]

Ischemia/infarction

Fetal MR imaging is the preferred modality to demonstrate fetal ischemia or infarction. This may not be apparent by US. Diffusion-weighted imaging can further aid in demonstration of acute to subacute ischemic lesions.[14] The classic ischemia of arterial distribution is not the common pattern seen in utero. Ischemia in the fetal brain may involve the cortical ribbon and white matter or just the white matter alone. Hemorrhagic infarction is more common. Ischemic cerebral changes in utero may result in white matter necrosis or leukomalacia. On fetal MR imaging, particular attention should be paid to the morphology of the germinal matrix to identify presence of any focal areas of T2 hypointensity or increased susceptibility on gradient images. Sometimes this may be

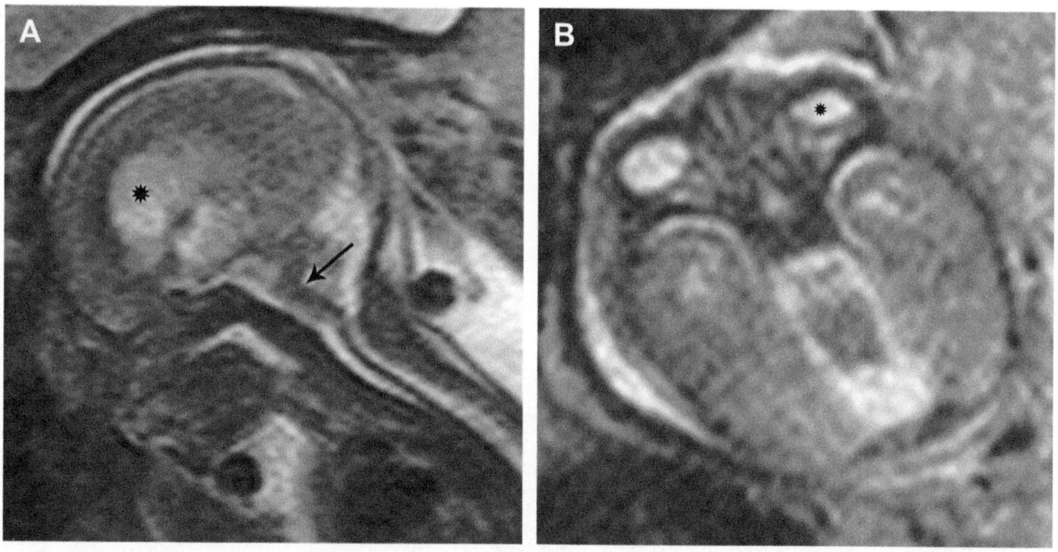

Fig. 16. Walker-Warburg syndrome—sagittal HASTE (*A*) shows supatentorial hydrocephalus (*asterisk*) and kinked, Z-shaped brainstem (*arrow*). Axial HASTE (*B*) through the orbits shows left microphthalmia (*asterisk*).

evident only as a focal irregular dilatation of the ventricle. In contrast, larger areas of ischemia and the sequelae with diffuse necrosis are easy to identify on MR imaging (**Fig. 21**).

Hydranencephaly

Hydranencephaly is considered to be a sequel of ischemic event in the distribution of internal carotid arteries, which has occurred after the basic brain

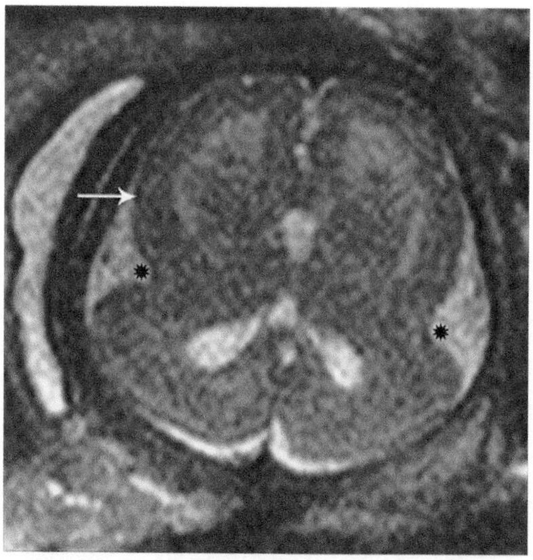

Fig. 17. Lissencephaly—32-week gestational age axial HASTE shows smooth cortex with shallow sylvian fissures (*asterisks*), imparting characteristic figure-of-8 appearance, thin outer cortical layer (*white arrow*), and thick band of inner cortex, indicative of arrest.

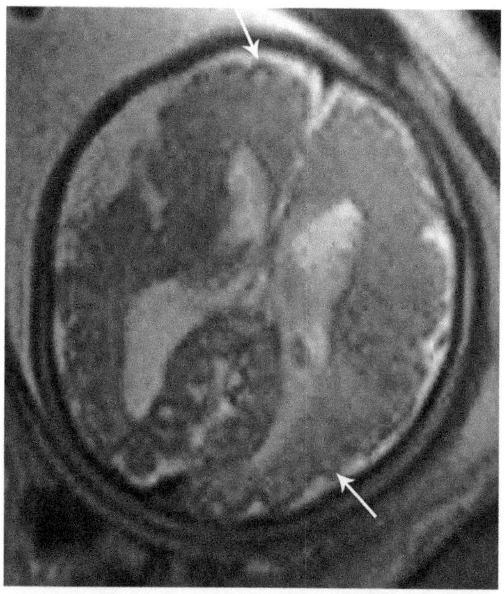

Fig. 18. Polymicrogyria—32-week gestational age fetus with increased number of irregular gyri in frontal and posterior temporal regions (*white arrows*).

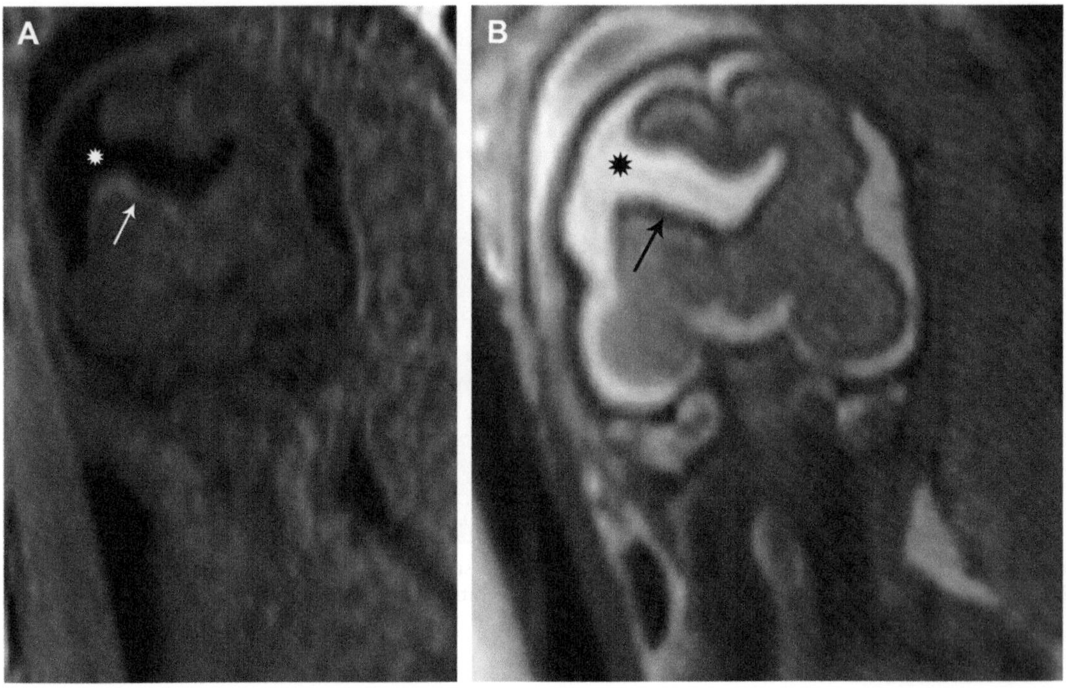

Fig. 19. Open lip schizencephaly—coronal T1 (*A*) and coronal HASTE (*B*). Large CSF-filled cleft (*asterisk*), lined by gray matter (*arrow*), extending from lateral ventricle to extra-axial space.

structure was formed. Large portions of the involved cerebral hemispheres are replaced with fluid-filled cavities (**Fig. 22**). When these areas of involvement are large, it can be confusing to differentiate hydranencephaly from alobar holoprosencephaly. The differentiating feature, however, is presence of an intact falx, which is noted in hydranencephaly that distinguishes it from alobar holoprosencephaly

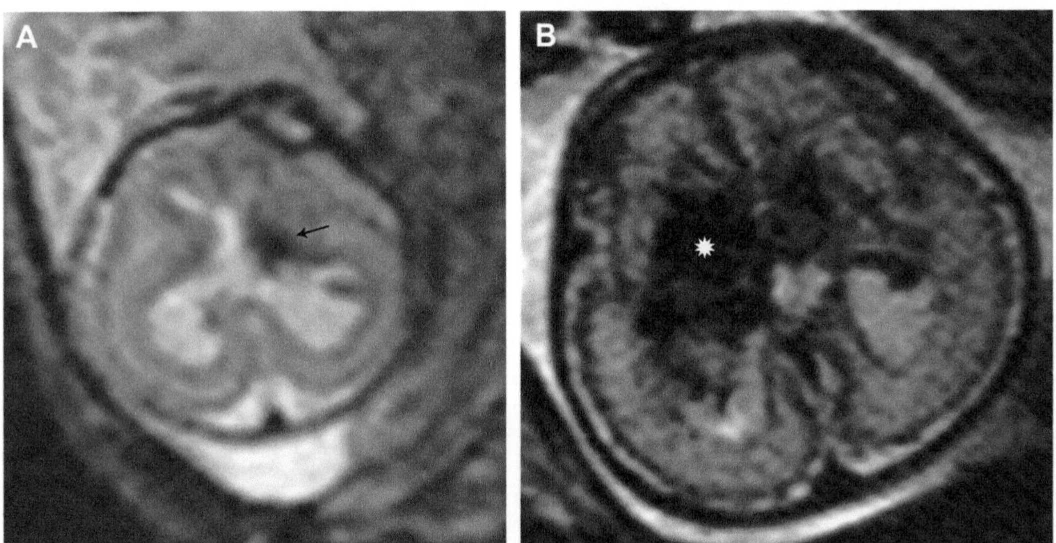

Fig. 20. Germinal matrix hemorrhage. HASTE axial (*A*) showing unilateral grade I germinal matrix bleed (*arrow*). EPI axial (*B*) shows grade IV germinal matrix bleed (*asterisk*).

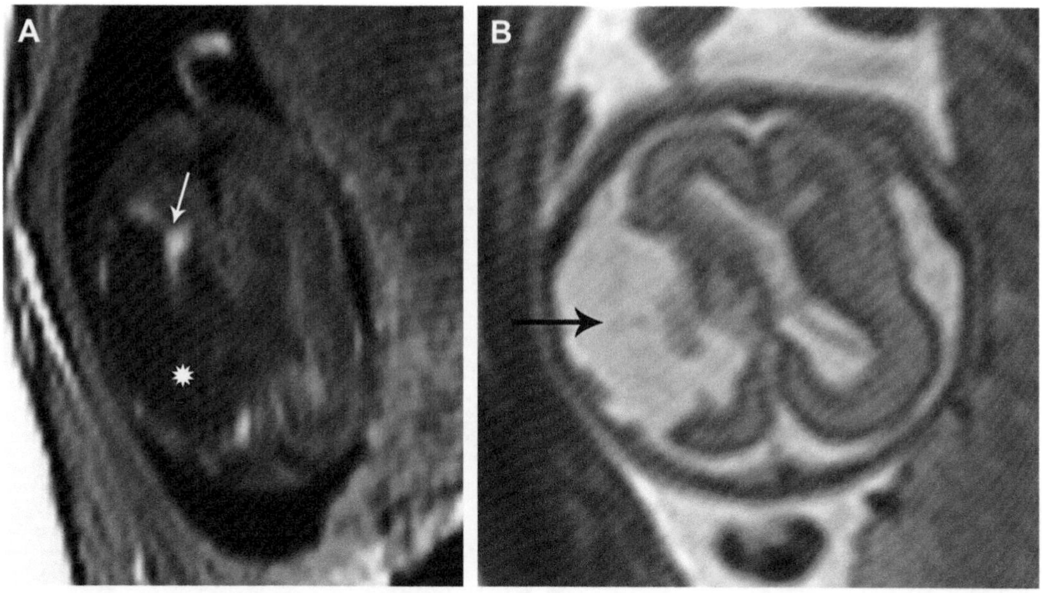

Fig. 21. Porencephaly-axial T1 (*A*) large CSF-filled area (*white asterisk*) with peripheral blood products (*white arrow*). Axial EPI (*B*)—large cyst (*black arrow*) replacing brain tissue in the distribution of the MCA territory directly communicating with lateral ventricle.

(see **Figs. 11** and **22**). Another helpful feature to identify hydranencephaly is foci of susceptibility from hemorrhage or blood products, which may be seen in most of the cases.[11,24]

Porencephaly and encephalomalacia

These are sequelae that may result from hemorrhage, ischemia, infection, or trauma. Fetal MR imaging is helpful in identifying these lesions and in several cases may provide clues regarding their origin. Information obtained from fetal MR imaging is important in estimating the extent of brain injury and predicting outcome.

Infections

CMV infection is the most common congenital CNS infection. Fetal MR imaging reflects the neuropathologic changes of microcephaly, parenchymal destruction, periventricular necrosis, ventricular dilation, cysts, and disorganized cortex and heterotopias (**Fig. 23**).[11] Periventricular calcifications are not readily detected on MR but may be evident on gradient-echo EPI sequences.

Aqueductal Stenosis

Aqueductal stenosis may be sporadic or hereditary, as seen with X-linked hydrocephalus. There is characteristic enlargement of the lateral ventricles and the third ventricle with a normal-sized fourth ventricle (**Fig. 24**). Aqueductal stenosis may be associated with other abnormalities, such as corpus callosal agenesis, and Dandy-Walker malformation. It may result as a sequela of prior hemorrhage or infection.

Neurocutaneous Disorders

The most common neurocutaneous disorder identified in utero is tuberous sclerosis. Tuberous sclerosis is an autosomal dominant multisystem disorder characterized by the triad of epilepsy, mental retardation, and characteristic adenoma sebaceum. This disorder comprises multiple angiomyolipomas, cardiac rhabdomyomas, and intracranial stigmata as well. The intracranial lesions consist of cortical tubers, subependymal nodules, and mixed cell astrocytomas at the foramen of Monro. Cortical tubers as well as subependymal nodules appear as focal T2 hypointensities (**Fig. 25**). When calcified, they may demonstrate focal increased susceptibility. The intracranial stigmata are better identified with MR imaging, especially in the younger fetus.

In Utero Fetal CNS Mass Lesions

Congenital brain tumors are rare. The most common tumors in this category are teratomas

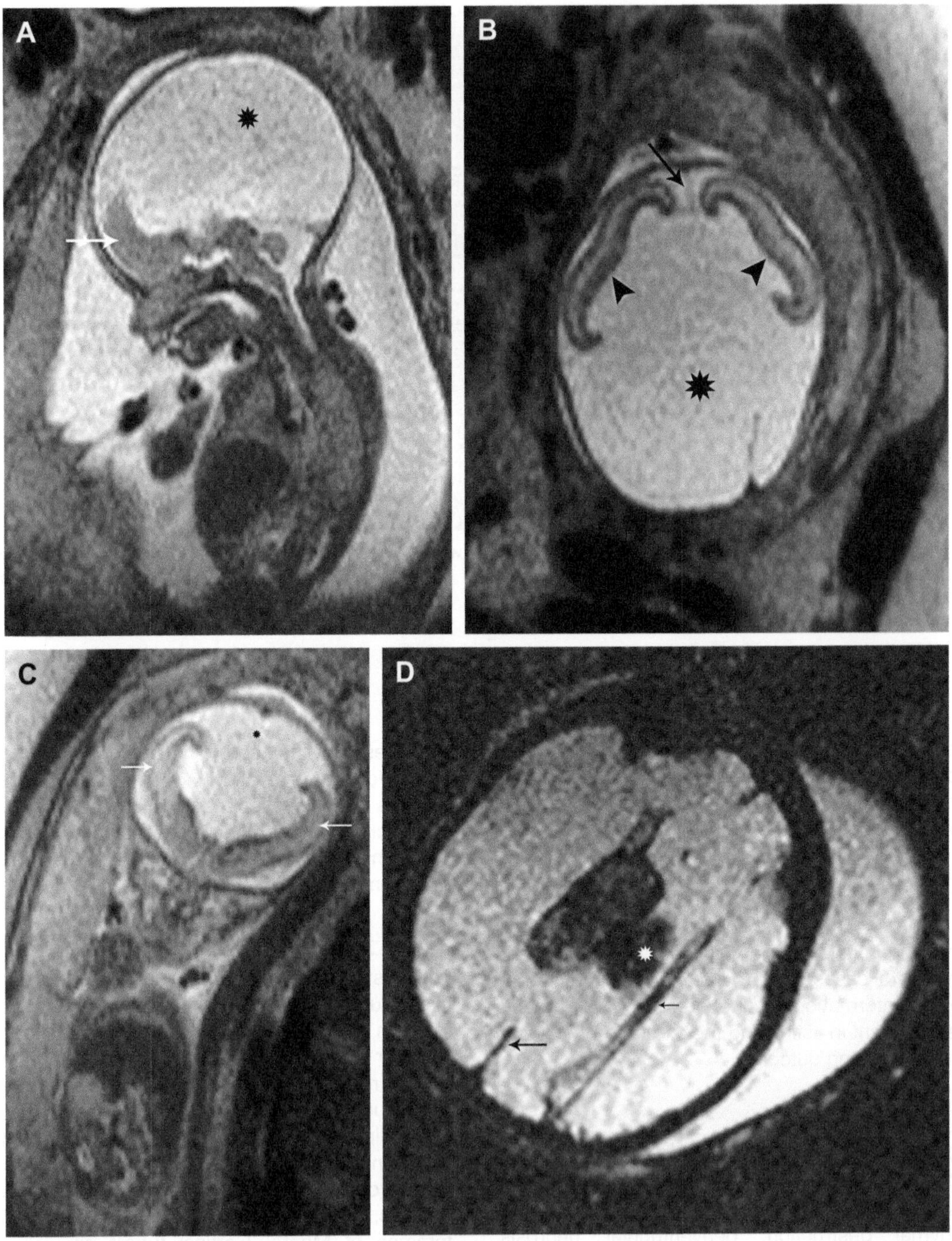

Fig. 22. Hydranencephaly-sagittal (*A*), axial (*B*) and coronal (*C*) show massively enlarged ventricles (*black asterisks in A–C*), destruction of the brain parenchyma with residual cortical tissue (*white arrows in A & C and black arrowheads in B*). Note the formation of the falx, anteriorly (*black arrow*). (*D*) Axial EPI image in another patient with hydranencephaly again demonstrating presence of falx posteriorly (*thick black arrow*). Note hemorrhagic staining of the residual brain tissue (*white asterisk*).

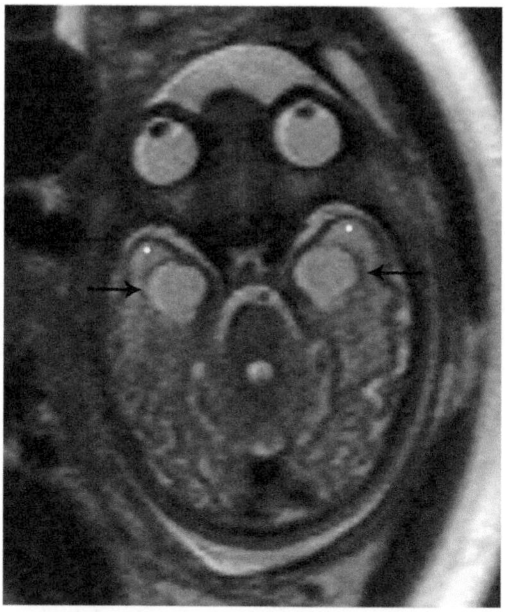

Fig. 23. CMV infection—axial HASTE shows bilateral temporal cysts (*arrows*) and anterior parenchymal signal abnormality (*white asterisk*).

followed by glioblastomas (Fig. 26). Fetal MR imaging is helpful in characterizing the location, extent, morphology, and its effect on surrounding structures.

Intracranial Vascular Malformations of the Fetus

Vein of Galen malformation

The most common cerebrovascular malformation diagnosed in prenatal life is the Galen vein malformation. The pathophysiology of this lesion is abnormal communication of arterial feeders from the circle of Willis as well as the vertebrobasilar arterial system, which anastomose with the galenic venous system, which then becomes aneurysmally dilated (Fig. 27). There is usually accompanying cardiomegaly and high-output congestive heart failure. Cerebral ischemic lesions may occur due to steal phenomenon. When there is obstruction of the venous outflow, hydrocephalus may be present. Prenatal MR evaluation can delineate the abnormally enlarged vessels and the dilated Galen vein. In addition, MR imaging can also identify the cerebral ischemic lesions and hemorrhage as well as hydrocephalus that may also be present.

Arachnoid Cysts and Other Neuroepithelial Cysts

Arachnoid cysts are benign collections of CSF, which develop between the layers of the arachnoid. These could be formed anywhere in brain. It is important to identify posterior fossa arachnoid cysts from other posterior fossa cystic malformations of the Dandy-Walker spectrum. The vermis is usually well formed in an arachnoid cyst (see Fig. 15)

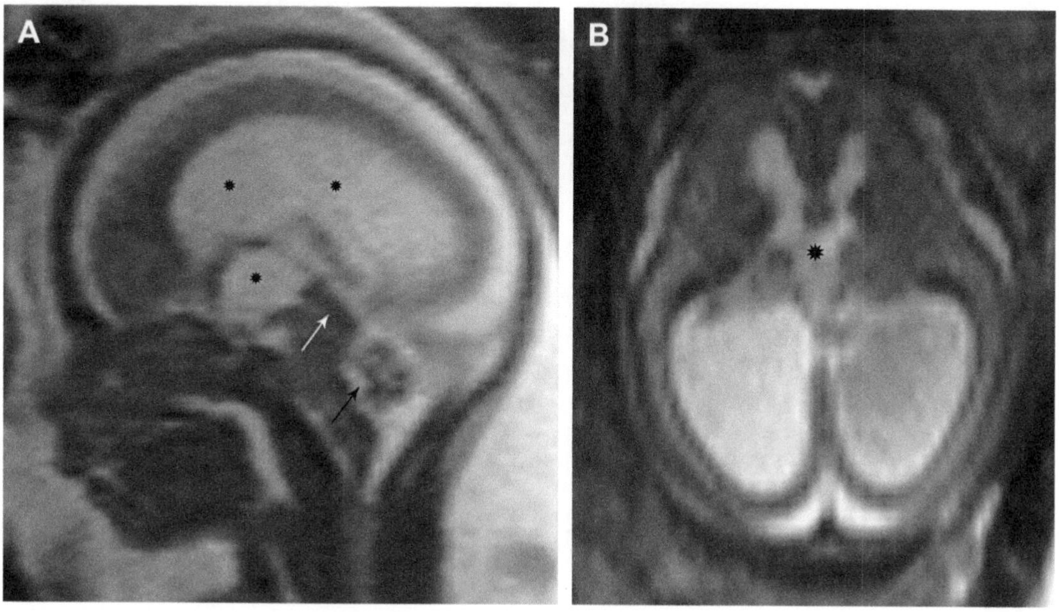

Fig. 24. Aqueduct stenosis—sagittal HASTE (*A*) shows focal narrowing of aqueduct (*white arrow*), dilated lateral (*double asterisk*), and third (*asterisk*) ventricles and normal size fourth ventricle (*black arrow*). Axial HASTE (*B*) shows hydrocephalus with dilated third ventricle (*asterisk*).

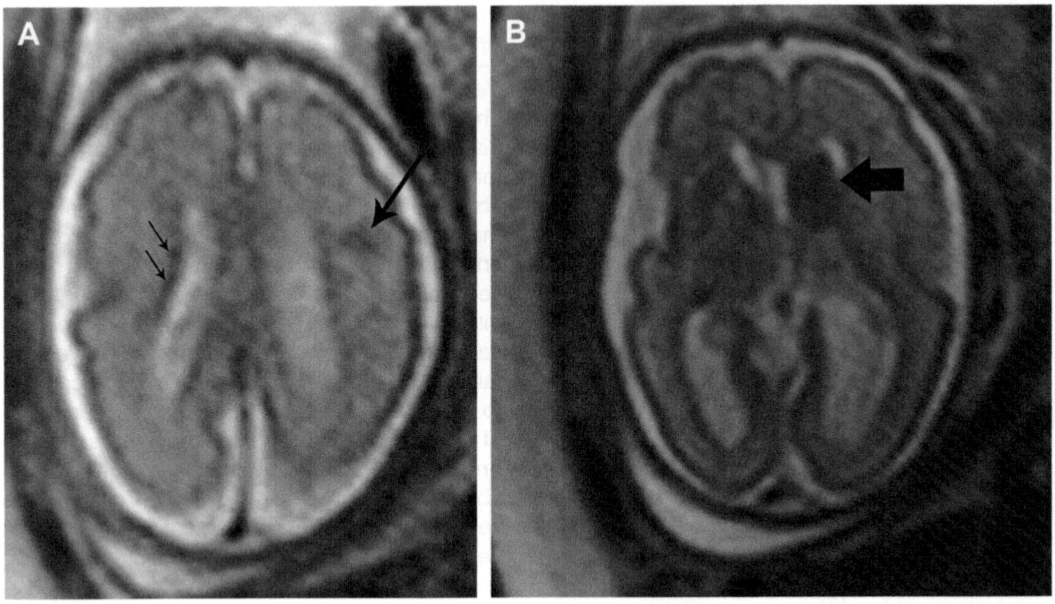

Fig. 25. Tuberous sclerosis—axial HASTE (*A*) shows cortical tuber (*large arrow*) and subependymal nodules (*small arrows*). Axial HASTE (*B*) shows bilateral lesions at foramen of Monro, larger on the left (*thick arrow*), consistent with mixed giant cell tumor.

whereas it is hypoplastic or absent in the Dandy-Walker spectrum (see **Figs. 13** and **14**).

Choroid plexus cyst is the most common neuroepithelial cyst seen in the fetus. It is seen in approximately 1% of normal pregnancies. There is an association of large choroid plexus cysts with trisomy 18.

Anomalies of the Fetal Face and Skull

Anomalies of the fetal face, skull, and neck may be observed as isolated abnormalities. When these abnormalities are detected on US, the role of MR imaging is to detect any associated abnormalities of the brain.[30] More commonly, fetal face, skull,

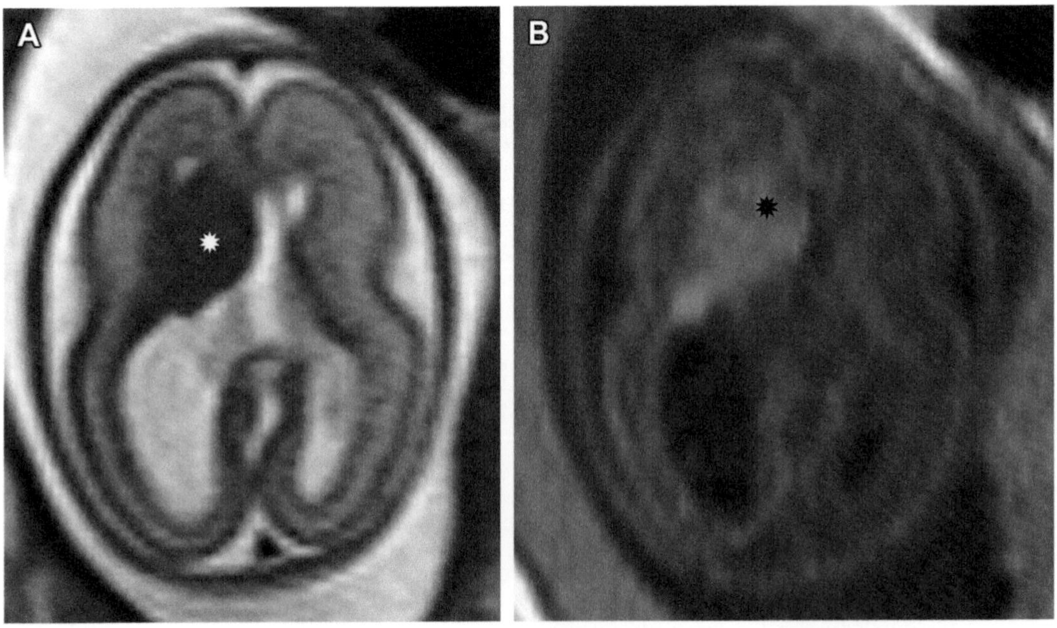

Fig. 26. Congenital tumor (postnatally proved to be a PNET-primitive neuroectodermal tumor). (*A*) T2 Hypointense and (*B*) T1 hyperintense mass lesion (*asterisk*) in the right ventricle, extending into the periventricular parenchyma.

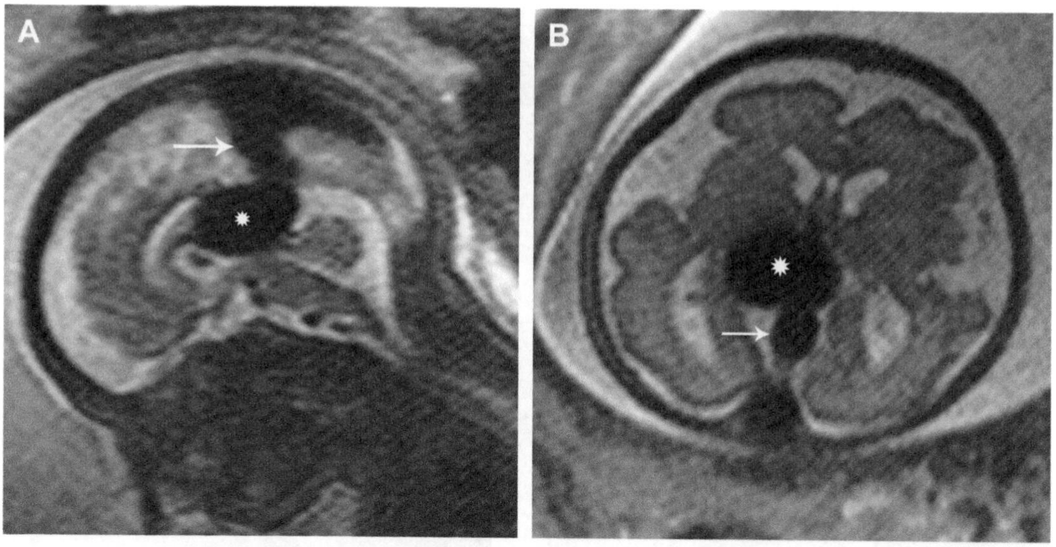

Fig. 27. Galen vein malformation—sagittal (*A*) and axial (*B*) HASTE show large varix (*asterisk*) replacing the Galen vein and prominent promesencephalic vein (*arrow*).

and neck anomalies are visualized in association with CNS abnormalities, chromosomal abnormalities, and syndromes.

Orbit abnormalities

Hypotelorism is defined as decrease in the normal intraocular distance below the fifth percentile for gestational age. Typically, hypotelorism is commonly associated with midline malformations of the brain, such as holoprosencephaly. It can also occur with other chromosomal abnormalities, syndromes, and abnormal calvarial development.

Hypertelorism is defined as increased interocular distance or abnormally wide-set eyes (**Fig. 28**). Hypertelorism may be an isolated abnormality. Hypertelorism is known to occur with anterior cephalocele due to mechanical disruption of migration of the orbits from a lateral to a more anterior position.[31]

When the orbital measurements are less than fifth percentile for gestational age, it is consistent with microphthalmia. Micropthalamia is associated with karyotype abnormalities and sporadic inheritable genetic syndromes (see **Fig. 16**B). Anophthalmia is absence of the optic globe, either unilateral or bilateral. In association, the bony orbit could also be small or absent.

Cleft lip and palate

Cleft lip may occur in isolation or with cleft palate and could be unilateral or bilateral defect. The defect is usually well identified on MR as amniotic fluid filling the cleft (**Fig. 29**).[32] When the cleft is complete, it extends from the upper lip to the nose and the hard palate. Closely apposed clefts, however, may be difficult to be visualized on MR.[33] When the cleft is complete and bilateral, it is usually associated with elevation of the median nasal prominence and characteristic premaxillary protrusion. 3-D reconstructions can be reformatted from the obtained MR images to demonstrate the clefts (see **Fig. 29**).

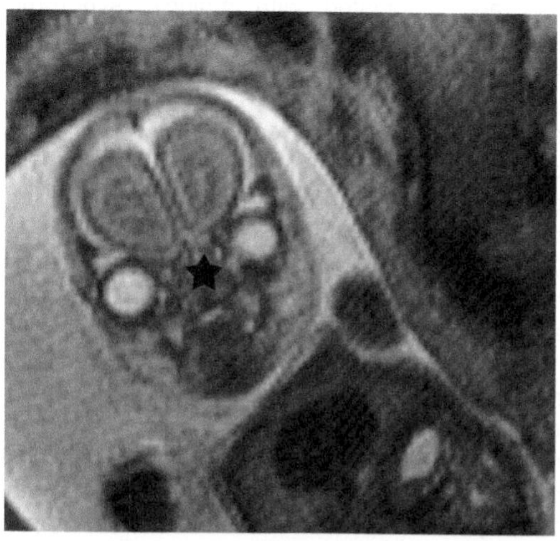
Fig. 28. Hypertelorism-coronal HASTE demonstrating increased interorbital distance (*star*).

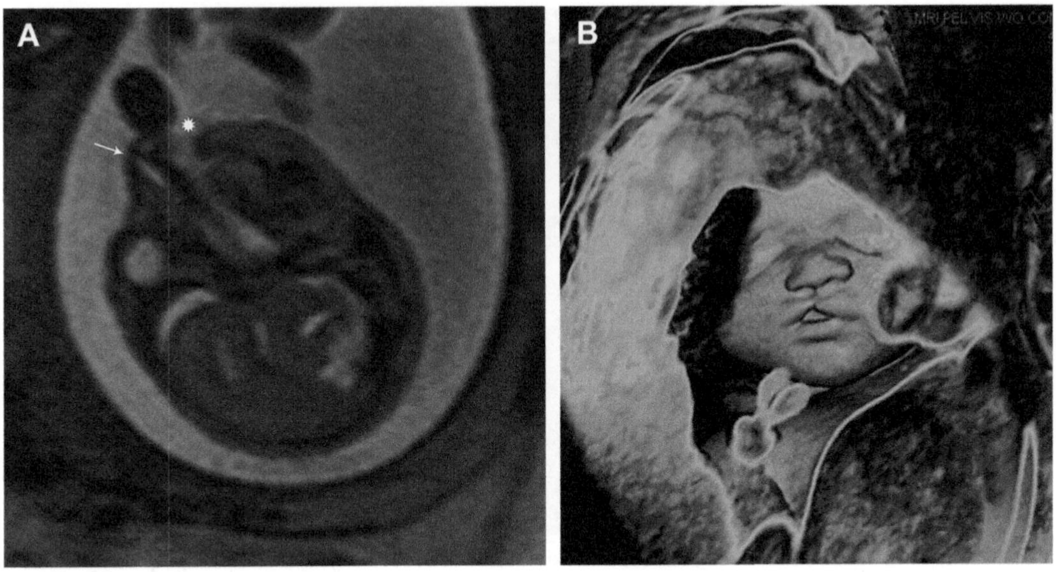

Fig. 29. Bilateral cleft lip—axial HASTE (*A*) shows a small (*arrow*) right-sided and large (*asterisk*) left-sided maxillary defects. MR 3-D reformation in another fetus (*B*) obtained from source images demonstrating fetal face with unilateral cleft lip.

Cleft palate in isolation is much less common. Cleft lip and cleft palate often occur as part of syndromes or chromosomal abnormalities. Information obtained from fetal MR imaging of the brain and face is valuable in diagnosing these complex syndromes and heritable abnormalities, which aids in prenatal genetic counseling.

Mandibular abnormalities

A small or receding mandible (retrognathia) may result in micrognathia. Micrognathia and retrognathia are associated with multiple syndromes and chromosomal abnormalities.[34] Pierre Robin syndrome is one such complex abnormality that is characterized by severe mandibular hypoplasia. Consequent to a small mandible, the size of the oral cavity is significantly reduced with a normal-sized tongue falling back and resulting in airway obstruction. This abnormality can result in the fetus unable to swallow adequately and has significant hazard for airway obstruction.[33] There is associated polyhydramnios (**Fig. 30**).

Similar to fetuses with large facial and cervical masses, which have potential for the fetal airway to be obstructed, fetuses with severe mandibular hypoplasia have risk for airway obstruction. These cases have to be identified prenatally so a safe delivery can be planned via an ex utero intrapartum treatment (EXIT) procedure. An EXIT procedure involves securing of the fetal airway by performing a tracheostomy even before the placenta is clamped off, ensuring patency of the fetal airway.

Abnormalities of the fetal skull shape can occur due to several causes, such as hydrocephalus,

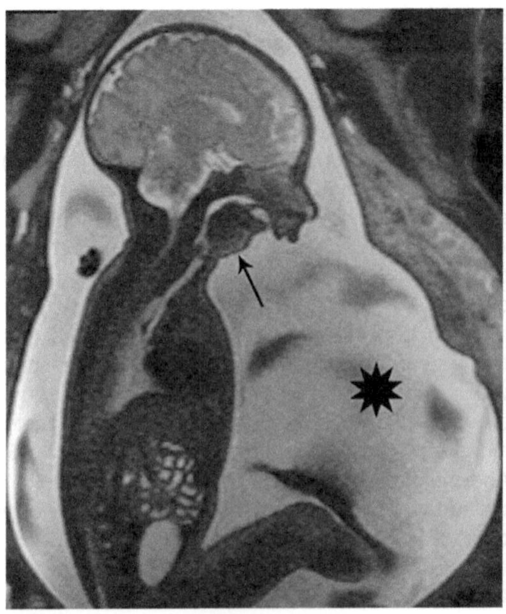

Fig. 30. Pierre Robin syndrome—severe micrognatia (*arrow*), which impairs normal swallowing, resulting in polyhydramnios (*asterisk*).

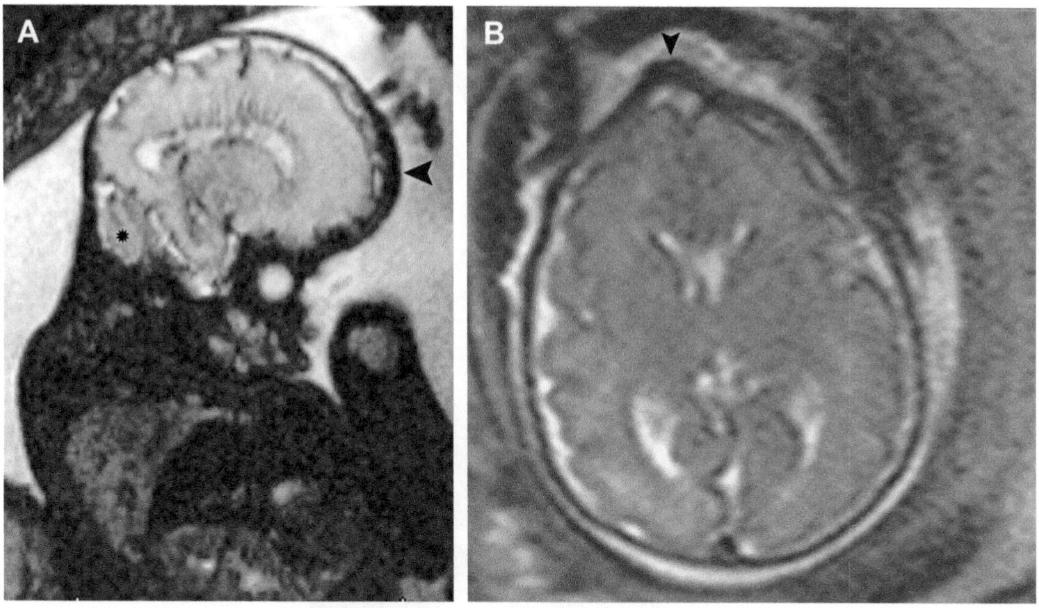

Fig. 31. Apert syndrome—sagittal EPI (*A*) shows dysmorphic skull with frontal bossing (*arrowhead*) and small posterior fossa (*asterisk*). Axial HASTE (*B*) shows trigonocephaly (*arrowhead*) related to premature fusion of metopic suture.

intracranial mass lesions, craniosynostosis, and skeletal dysplasias.[24] Apert syndrome, an inherited form of craniosynostosis, can be identified on fetal MR imaging (**Fig. 31**).

Anomalies of the Fetal Neck

The most common neck mass is cystic hygroma or lymphatic malformation. Cystic hygroma results from an abnormality of the canalization of the lymphatic system. Cystic hygromas are large typically multiloculated cystic masses with transpatial extension.[12] Septations between the locules and sometimes presence of complex fluid or blood products causing fluid-fluid levels can be identified on MR (**Fig. 32**). Cystic hygromas can be large enough and extend into the mediastinum, axilla, and chest wall.

Cystic hygromas may be located in the posterior nuchal region and are frequently associated with fetal hydrops and chromosomal abnormalities, such as trisomy 18, Turner syndrome, and Down syndrome (**Fig. 33**).

The next most common masses seen in the face and neck are teratomas. Teratomas in the fetal neck are typically heterogeneous with solid components and cystic areas, frequently with calcifications and hemorrhage.[12] Presence of hemorrhage and calcification could be identified as areas of susceptibility on EPI (**Fig. 34**).

The large fetal neck masses are associated with the risk of life-threatening airway obstruction at birth. There is also high incidence of polyhydramnios due to impaired fetal swallowing. This can lead to premature labor. US can adequately detect these fetal neck masses. MR imaging, however, is superior in better characterization of these lesions.

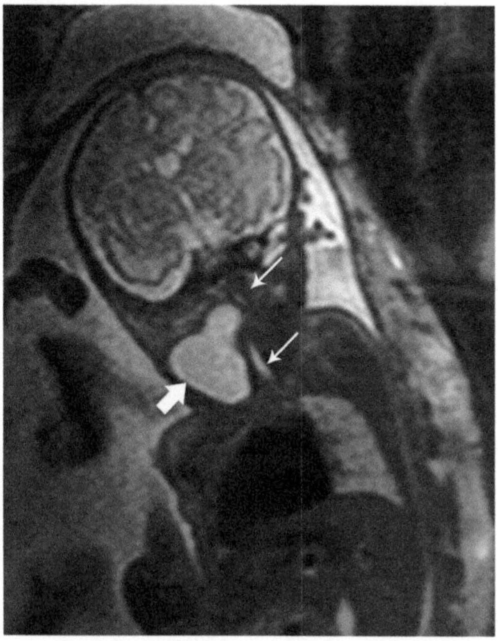

Fig. 32. Cervical lymphatic malformation—coronal HASTE shows unilateral cystic lesion (*thick white arrow*) with deep extension into the neck but with patent airway (*small white arrows*).

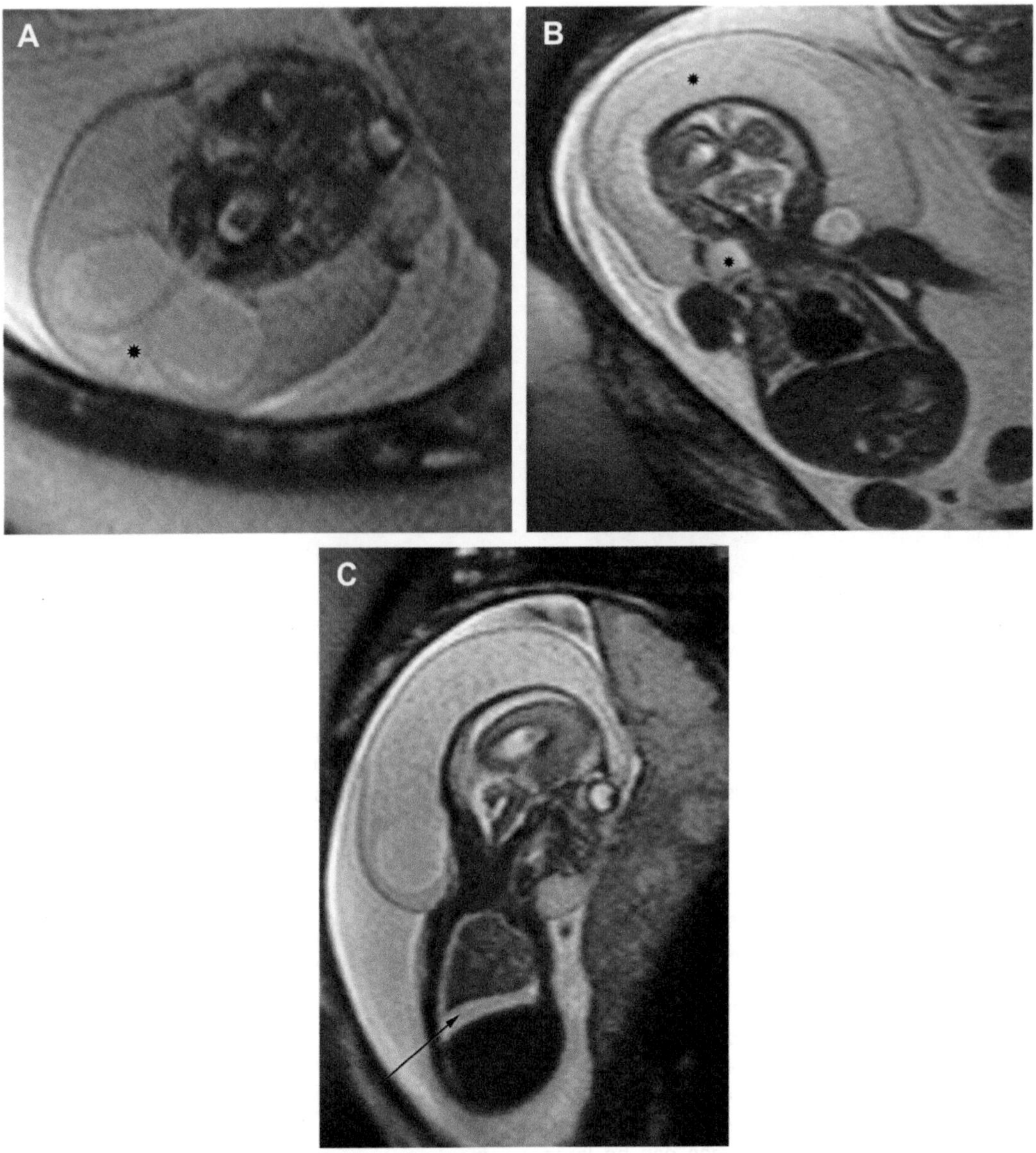

Fig. 33. Large lymphatic malformation, enveloping the fetal head and neck, with multiple locules (*asterisks*) as seen on axial (*A*) and coronal (*B*) HASTE images. Notice pleural effusion (*black arrow*) in same fetus on (*C*).

Important information derived from the fetal MR study is the relationship of the mass with respect to the airway and mass effect exerted. If the fluid-filled trachea cannot be visualized in the region of a neck mass, it is presumed that there is tracheal compression and the airway is compromised. These cases have to be delivered with an EXIT procedure.[35] The fetus is partially delivered and the airway is secured before clamping the umbilical cord. Fetal cine imaging is very helpful in assessing the airway in the presence of large neck masses.

Anomalies of the Fetal Spine

MR imaging of the fetal spine is complementary, often superior, to US for assessment of suspected spinal malformations and also provides better detection of associated CNS and non-CNS anomalies, which have a significant impact on postnatal neurologic outcome and quality of life.[7,12]

Abnormalities in the neurulation can result from defects in disjunction, which is the process by which the neural tube separates from the overlying ectoderm. When the failure of disjunction is small,

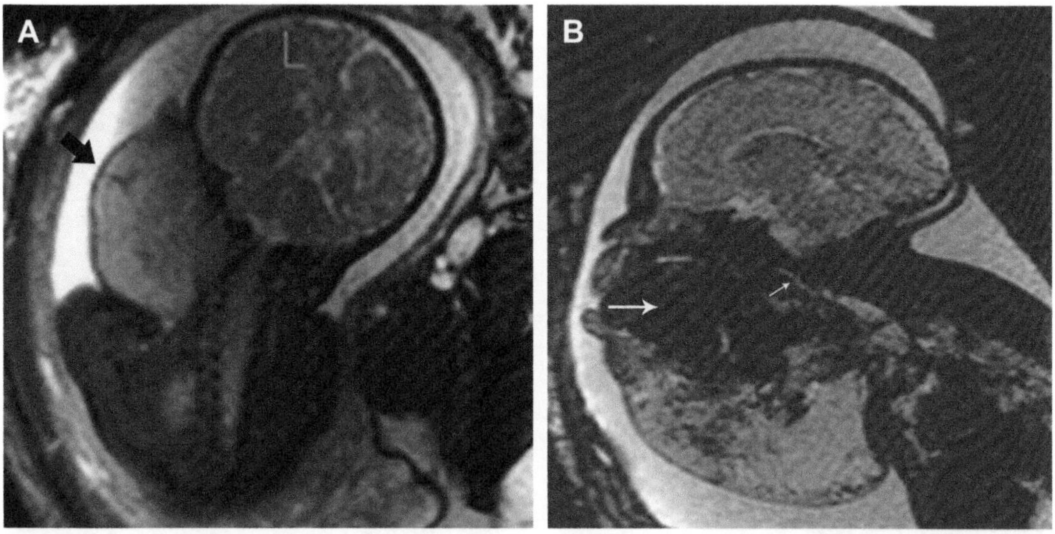

Fig. 34. Teratoma—solid mass lesion in lateral aspect of fetal neck (*A*) with few scattered hypointense foci (*black arrow*), likely vessels. Large teratoma of lower face and neck, in another fetus (*B*). Notice significant heterogeneity and susceptibility (*long white arrow*) from either hemorrhage or mineralization. Mass is narrowing the fetal airway (*short white arrow*).

it may result in myeloschisis and if large results in an MMC. In MMC, the neural placode, along with the expanded subarachnoid space (MMC sac) protruding through the osseous and the cutaneous defect, is elevated with respect to the level of the skin surface, whereas in a myeloschisis or myelocele, the placode does not protrude beyond the plane of the skin surface. MMC is associated with Chiari II malformation (see **Fig. 9**). The size of the MMC sac is variable and could be large or small. Although US may be more accurate in determining the level of the defect and termination of the neural placode, MR imaging provides superior detail and soft tissue resolution, therefore making the two modalities complementary.[23,36]

This valuable information provided by MR imaging is an essential part of prenatal assessment and triaging of patients involved in an ongoing multicenter trial in the United States, comparing the outcome of fetal MMC repair with standard postnatal MMC repair.[36,37] Recently published results from this study indicate that prenatal fetal MMC repair leads to reversal of hindbrain herniation, improvement in lower-extremity function, and decreased need for CSF diversion compared with postnatal repair controls (**Fig. 35**).[38,39]

Premature disjunction of the cutaneous ectoderm from the neuroectoderm allows mesenchyme to contact the inner portion of the developing neural tube. As the neural tube closes, the inducted mesenchyme can interfere with neurulation, resulting in formation of terminal lipoma or a lipomyelomeningocele. These lesions are skin covered and not associated with Chiari II malformation. These abnormalities can be detected with MR imaging, especially in the older fetuses but may be hard to detect on US.[23] Small sites of failure of disjunction can result in dermal sinus and spina bifida. Prenatal diagnosis of a small dermal sinus may be difficult with fetal MR imaging.[23]

Caudal regression syndrome includes a wide spectrum, ranging from the most severe, which is sirenomyelia, to mild sacral dysplasia. MR imaging can identify the more severe forms but the milder forms may be difficult to detect prenatally.[40]

Diastematomyelia or the split cord malformation involves the cord focally divided into two hemicords, often separated by a bony bar or a fibrous septum. Diastematomyelia most commonly occurs in the lumbar region and is associated frequently with vertebral body anomalies. It has been reported that diastematomyelia is present in the upper 40% of MMC cases (**Fig. 36**). All cases of MMC should be checked for presence of diastematomyelia.

The fetal MMC must be distinguished from another entity—the terminal myelocystocele. Terminal myelocystocele is characterized by marked dilatation of

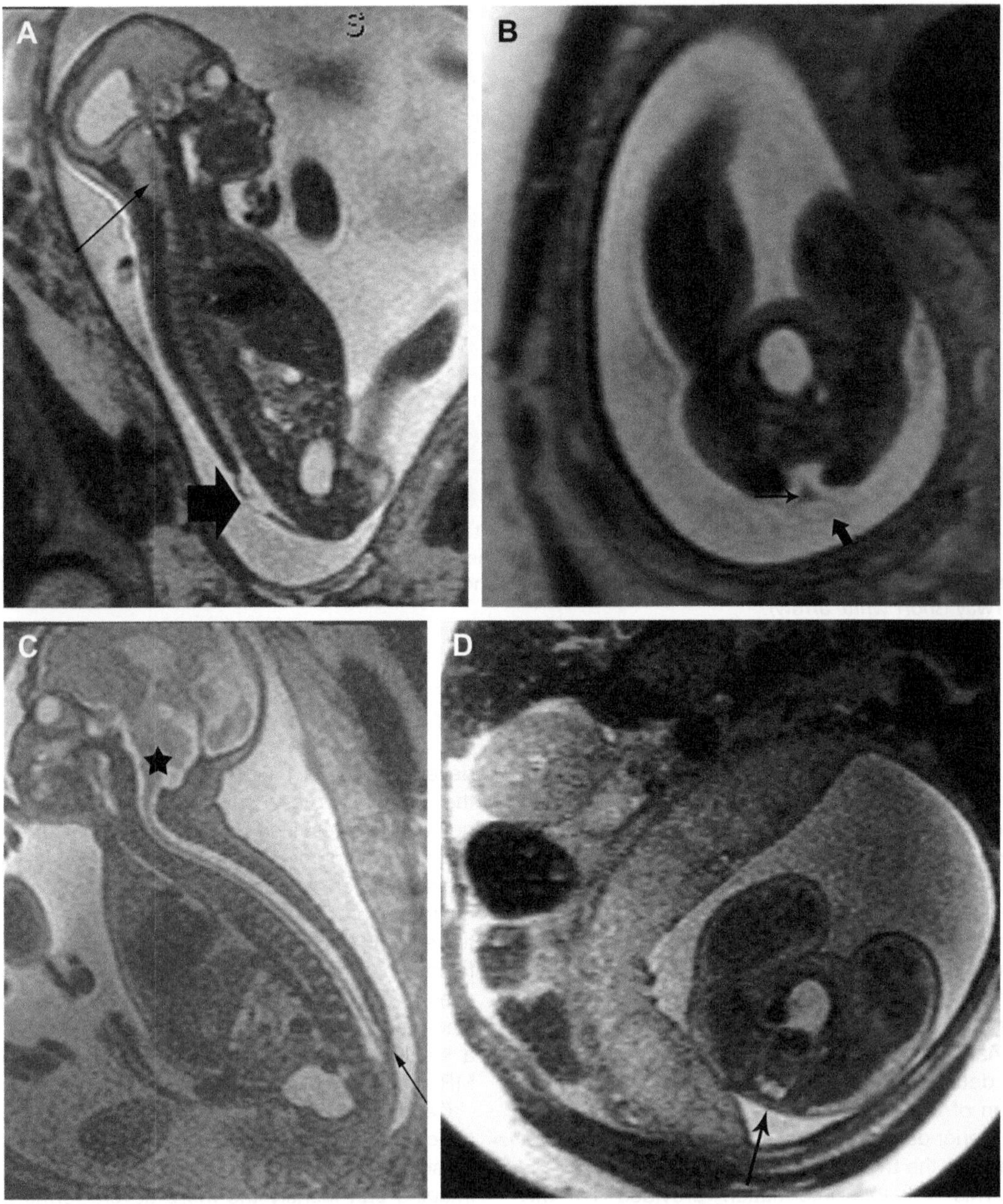

Fig. 35. MMC comparison of appearances preuterine and postintrauterine closure (*A*, *B*) Sagittal and axial images before MMC closure. (*C*, *D*) Corresponding images after intrauterine MMC repair. Notice the surgical closure of the sac (*black arrow*) and remarkable improvement of the hindbrain herniation (*star*) after repair.

the terminal central canal of the spinal cord, which herniates through a lumbosacral spina bifida. This entity can be distinguished prenatally from the MMC by the characteristic thick wall of the protruding sac and absence of Chiari II malformation (**Fig. 37**).

Sacrococcygeal teratoma is a congenital neoplasm arising from the totipotent cells of the caudal cell mass. They are usually heterogeneous with mixed cystic and solid components, although rarely can be purely cystic or solid. Sacrococcygeal teratomas classified into 4 types. Type I is

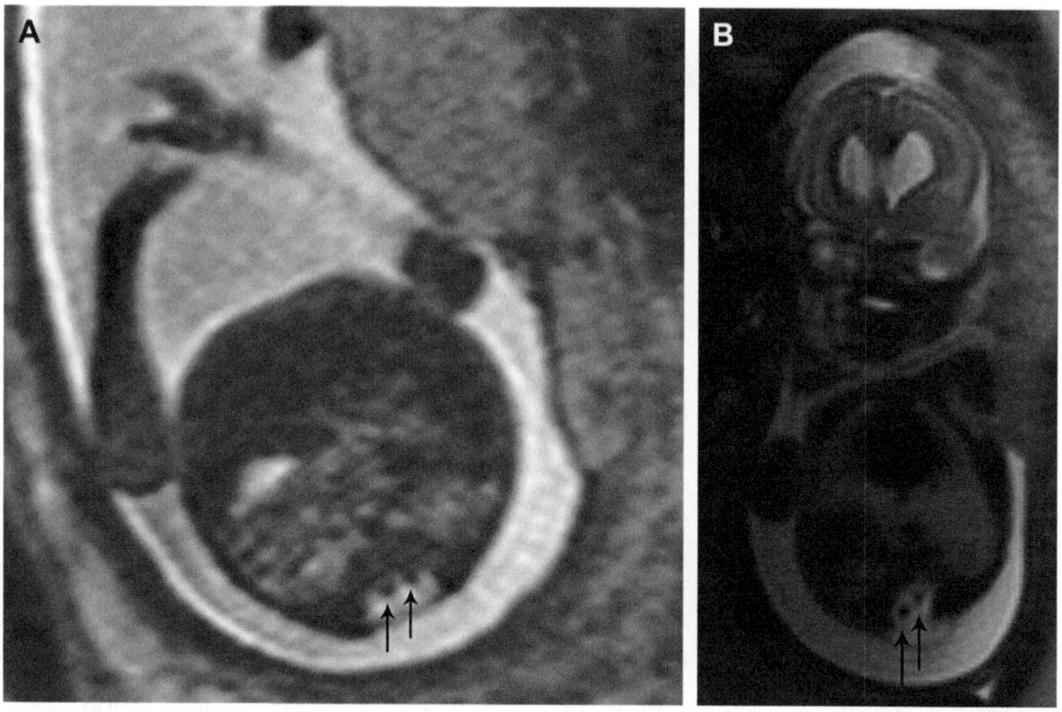

Fig. 36. Diastematomyelia—axial HASTE (*A*), arrows point to the split cord; coronal HASTE (*B*), demonstrates diastematomyelia in patient with Chiari II and MMC.

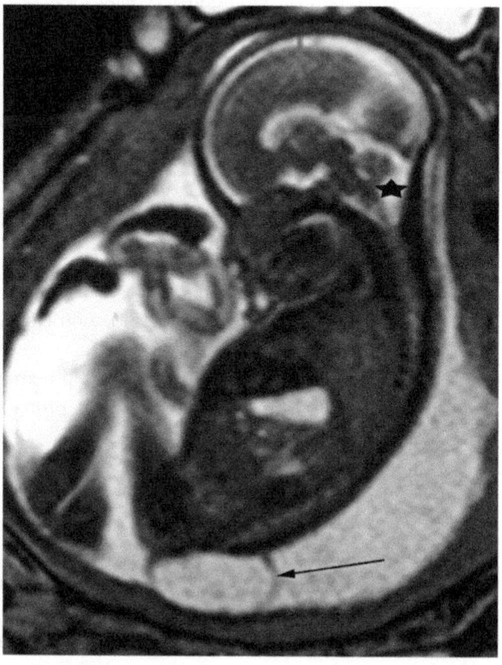

Fig. 37. Myelocystocele-sagittal HASTE image demonstrating thick-walled sac of the myelocystocele (*black arrow*). Note absence of hindbrain herniation (*black star*).

external with a small presacral component (most common). Type II is predominantly external with a small intrapelvic component. Type III has a small extrapelvic component but is predominantly intrapelvic with intra-abdominal extension. Type IV is entirely within the pelvis and abdomen and is known to be frequently malignant.

MR imaging is valuable in determining the full extent of the lesion and its relationship to the surrounding pelvic, abdominal, and spinal structures (Fig. 38). Large sacrococcygeal teratomas with a big solid component can be associated with increased vascularity leading to associated findings of cardiomegaly, congestive cardiac failure, and hydrops fetalis. In fetuses with hydrops, sacrococcygeal tumor has been successfully removed in utero with resolution of hydrops.

Congenital vertebral anomalies are frequently associated with systemic anomalies involving the genitourinary and lower gastrointestinal systems (cloacal abnormalities), and a diligent search should be made for their detection. Some of the more common in this group of constellation of anomalies are VACTERL (vertebral, renal, cardiac, tracheoesophageal, anorectal, and limb anomalies)

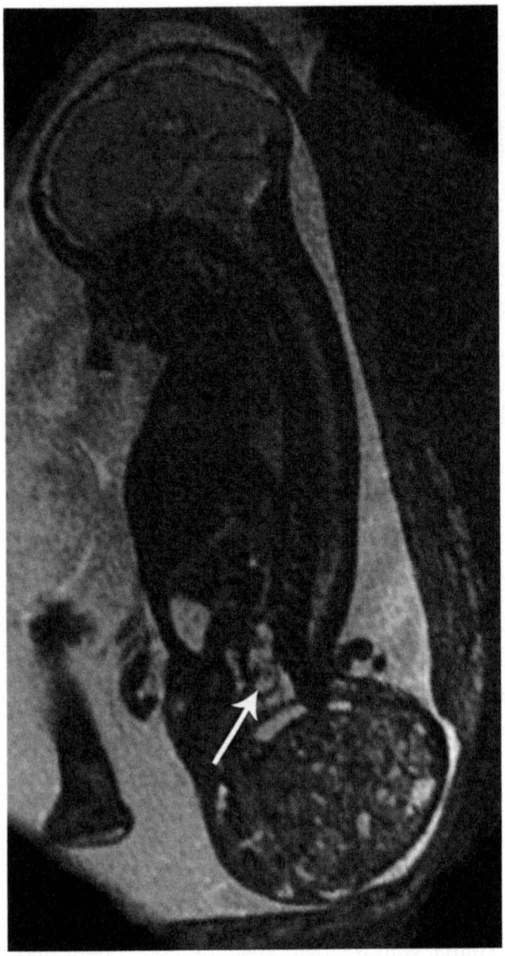

Fig. 38. Sacrococcygeal teratoma—sagittal EPI demonstrating type I sacrococcygeal teratoma with large exophytic component and small pelvic component (*white arrow*).

and OEIS (omphalocele, exstrophy, imperforate anus, and spine abnormalities).

SUMMARY

US remains the screening modality of choice in evaluation of the fetal nervous system. Fetal MR imaging is an established powerful tool for obtaining additional information in evaluation of anomalies of the fetal brain, face, neck, and spine. It is helpful to patients and their health care professionals to make vital management decisions and aids in genetic counseling for future pregnancies.

REFERENCES

1. Economides DL, Braithwaite JM. First trimester ultrasonographic diagnosis of fetal structural abnormalities in a low risk population. Br J Obstet Gynaecol 1998;105(1):53–7.
2. Economides DL, Whitlow BJ, Kadir R, et al. First trimester sonographic detection of chromosomal abnormalities in an unselected population. Br J Obstet Gynaecol 1998;105(1):58–62.
3. Isaksen CV, Eik-Nes SH, Blaas HG, et al. Comparison of prenatal ultrasound and postmortem findings in fetuses and infants with central nervous system anomalies. Ultrasound Obstet Gynecol 1998;11(4):246–53.
4. Girard N, Raybaud C, Dercole C, et al. In vivo MRI of the fetal brain. Neuroradiology 1993;35(6):431–6.
5. Girard N, Raybaud C, Poncet M. In vivo MR study of brain maturation in normal fetuses. AJNR Am J Neuroradiol 1995;16(2):407–13.
6. Dinh DH, Wright RM, Hanigan WC. The use of magnetic resonance imaging for the diagnosis of fetal intracranial anomalies. Childs Nerv Syst 1990;6(4):212–5.
7. Levine D, Barnes PD, Madsen JR, et al. Fetal central nervous system anomalies: MR imaging augments sonographic diagnosis. Radiology 1997;204(3):635–42.
8. Schwartz JL, Crooks LE. NMR imaging produces no observable mutations or cytotoxicity in mammalian cells. AJR Am J Roentgenol 1982;139(3):583–5.
9. Thomas A, Morris PG. The effects of NMR exposure on living organisms. I. A microbial assay. Br J Radiol 1981;54(643):615–21.
10. Baker PN, Johnson IR, Harvey PR, et al. A three-year follow-up of children imaged in utero with echo-planar magnetic resonance. Am J Obstet Gynecol 1994;170(1 Pt 1):32–3.
11. Girard N, Raybaud C, Gambarelli D, et al. Fetal brain MR imaging. Magn Reson Imaging Clin N Am 2001;9(1):19–56, vii.
12. Simon EM, Goldstein RB, Coakley FV, et al. Fast MR imaging of fetal CNS anomalies in utero. AJNR Am J Neuroradiol 2000;21(9):1688–98.
13. Chen Q, Levine D. Fast fetal magnetic resonance imaging techniques. Top Magn Reson Imaging 2001;12(1):67–79.
14. Baldoli C, Righini A, Parazzini C, et al. Demonstration of acute ischemic lesions in the fetal brain by diffusion magnetic resonance imaging. Ann Neurol 2002;52(2):243–6.
15. Levine D, Barnes PD. Cortical maturation in normal and abnormal fetuses as assessed with prenatal MR imaging. Radiology 1999;210(3):751–8.
16. Vossough A, et al. Development and validation of a semiquantitative brain maturation score on clinical fetal MRI. Paper presented at: ASNR annual meeting. Boston (MA), May 15–20, 2010.
17. Hubbard AM, Simon EM. Fetal imaging. Magn Reson Imaging Clin N Am 2002;10(2):389–408.
18. Hilpert PL, Hall BE, Kurtz AB. The atria of the fetal lateral ventricles: a sonographic study of normal atrial size and choroid plexus volume. AJR Am J Roentgenol 1995;164(3):731–4.

19. Girard NJ, Raybaud CA. Ventriculomegaly and pericerebral CSF collection in the fetus: early stage of benign external hydrocephalus? Childs Nerv Syst 2001;17(4-5):239–45.
20. Bloom SL, Bloom DD, DellaNebbia C, et al. The developmental outcome of children with antenatal mild isolated ventriculomegaly. Obstet Gynecol 1997;90(1):93–7.
21. d'Ercole C, Girard N, Cravello L, et al. Prenatal diagnosis of fetal corpus callosum agenesis by ultrasonography and magnetic resonance imaging. Prenat Diagn 1998;18(3):247–53.
22. Levine D, Barnes PD, Madsen JR, et al. Fetal CNS anomalies revealed on ultrafast MR imaging. AJR Am J Roentgenol 1999;172(3):813–8.
23. Simon EM. MRI of the fetal spine. Pediatr Radiol 2004;34(9):712–9.
24. Levine D. MR imaging of fetal central nervous system abnormalities. Brain Cogn 2002;50(3):432–48.
25. Greco P, Resta M, Vimercati A, et al. Antenatal diagnosis of isolated lissencephaly by ultrasound and magnetic resonance imaging. Ultrasound Obstet Gynecol 1998;12(4):276–9.
26. Raybaud C, Girard N, Levrier O, et al. Schizencephaly: correlation between the lobar topography of the cleft(s) and absence of the septum pellucidum. Childs Nerv Syst 2001;17(4–5):217–22.
27. Denis D, Maugey-Laulom B, Carles D, et al. Prenatal diagnosis of schizencephaly by fetal magnetic resonance imaging. Fetal Diagn Ther 2001;16(6): 354–9.
28. Mitchell LA, Simon EM, Filly RA, et al. Antenatal diagnosis of subependymal heterotopia. AJNR Am J Neuroradiol 2000;21(2):296–300.
29. Trop I, Levine D. Hemorrhage during pregnancy: sonography and MR imaging. AJR Am J Roentgenol 2001;176(3):607–15.
30. Babcook C, editor. The fetal face and neck. Philadelphia: W. B. Saunders; 2000. p. 307–30.
31. Cohen MM Jr, Richieri-Costa A, Guion-Almeida ML, et al. Hypertelorism: interorbital growth, measurements, and pathogenetic considerations. Int J Oral Maxillofac Surg 1995;24(6):387–95.
32. Stroustrup Smith A, Estroff JA, Barnewolt CE, et al. Prenatal diagnosis of cleft lip and cleft palate using MRI. AJR Am J Roentgenol 2004;183(1):229–35.
33. Levine D, editor. Atlas of fetal MRI. Boca Raton: Taylor & Francis Group, LLC; 2005.
34. Bromley B, Benacerraf BR. Fetal micrognathia: associated anomalies and outcome. J Ultrasound Med 1994;13(7):529–33.
35. Hubbard AM, Crombleholme TM, Adzick NS. Prenatal MRI evaluation of giant neck masses in preparation for the fetal exit procedure. Am J Perinatol 1998;15(4):253–7.
36. Mangels KJ, Tulipan N, Tsao LY, et al. Fetal MRI in the evaluation of intrauterine myelomeningocele. Pediatr Neurosurg 2000;32(3):124–31.
37. Bruner JP, Tulipan N, Paschall RL, et al. Fetal surgery for myelomeningocele and the incidence of shunt-dependent hydrocephalus. JAMA 1999; 282(19):1819–25.
38. Sutton LN, Adzick NS, Bilaniuk LT, et al. Improvement in hindbrain herniation demonstrated by serial fetal magnetic resonance imaging following fetal surgery for myelomeningocele. JAMA 1999;282(19):1826–31.
39. Tulipan N, Sutton LN, Bruner JP, et al. The effect of intrauterine myelomeningocele repair on the incidence of shunt-dependent hydrocephalus. Pediatr Neurosurg 2003;38(1):27–33.
40. Allen LM, Silverman RK. Prenatal ultrasound evaluation of fetal diastematomyelia: two cases of type I split cord malformation. Ultrasound Obstet Gynecol 2000;15(1):78–82.

Neurosurgical Management of Congenital Malformations of the Brain

Shawn L. Hervey-Jumper, MD[a], Aaron A. Cohen-Gadol, MD, MSc[b], Cormac O. Maher, MD[c,*]

KEYWORDS

- Arachnoid cyst • Arteriovenous malformation • Children
- Chiari malformation • Encephalocele • Pineal cyst

Congenital malformations encompass a diverse group of disorders that often present at birth, either as the result of genetic abnormalities, infection, errors of morphogenesis, or abnormalities in the intrauterine environment. Congenital disorders affecting the brain are now often diagnosed before delivery with the use of prenatal ultrasonography. Over the past several decades, there have been major advances in the understanding and management of these conditions. This article focuses on the most common cranial congenital malformations, limiting the discussion to the neurosurgically relevant aspects of arachnoid cysts, pineal cysts, Chiari malformations, and encephaloceles. In addition, cerebral arteriovenous malformations (AVMs) are included in this discussion, despite increasing evidence that they are not always the congenital and static lesions they were once thought to be.

ARACHNOID CYSTS

Arachnoid cysts are cerebrospinal fluid (CSF)-filled cavities surrounded by a wall of simple arachnoid cells. They develop within the arachnoid membrane as a result of membrane duplications or splitting. Although most arachnoid cysts are congenital, secondary arachnoid cysts result from CSF accumulations in patients after head injury, stroke, or central nervous system (CNS) infection.[1,2] They should be differentiated from dermoid cysts; epidermoid cysts; neuroepithelial cysts; or leptomeningeal cysts occurring secondary to intracranial hemorrhage, infection, or trauma. They are typically asymptomatic and are discovered incidentally in children during evaluation for seizures, headaches, developmental delay, head trauma, or in infants with macrocrania (**Table 1**).[3] They occur in children at a prevalence rate of 0.5% to 2.6% with a male predominance (**Fig. 1**).[3,4] The location of arachnoid cysts has been well described. The most common location is the middle cranial fossa. Other common locations include retrocerebellar, supracerebellar, within the cerebellopontine angle, along the convexities, or in the quadrigeminal cistern (**Table 2**). Middle fossa arachnoid cysts show a strong

Disclosure statement: The authors have nothing to disclose.

[a] Department of Neurosurgery, University of Michigan, 1500 East Medical Center Drive, Ann Arbor, MI 48109-0338, USA
[b] Department of Neurological Surgery, Indiana University, 1801 North Senate Boulevard, Suite 610, Indianapolis, IN 46062, USA
[c] Department of Neurosurgery, University of Michigan, 1500 East Medical Center Drive, Room 3552 Taubman Center, Ann Arbor, MI 48109-5338, USA
* Corresponding author.
E-mail address: cmaher@med.umich.edu

Neuroimag Clin N Am 21 (2011) 705–717
doi:10.1016/j.nic.2011.05.008
1052-5149/11/$ – see front matter

Table 1
Indications for MR imaging in 309 pediatric patients with arachnoid cysts

Indication	Cases (%)
Concern for seizure	16
Headache	14
Cognitive dysfunction or developmental delay	15
Acute neurologic or mental status change	13
History of intracranial tumor	11
Trauma	7
History of hydrocephalus	5
Pituitary/endocrine issues	3
Intracranial hemorrhage	2
Other	15

Data from Al-Holou WN, Yew AY, Boomsaad ZE, et al. Prevalence and natural history of arachnoid cysts in children. J Neurosurg Pediatr 2010;5:578–85.

left-sided predominance for reasons that are not clear.[3]

The etiology and embryology of arachnoid cysts are incompletely understood. Some think their association with other developmental abnormalities, such as autosomal dominant polycystic kidneys, heterotopias, neurofibromatosis type 1, and Marfan disease, suggests an underlying genetic cause.[2] Given the common incidence of arachnoid cysts, however, it is probable that these associations are coincidental and may not carry any pathogenetic implications. Four histologic and ultrastructural differences have been noted between arachnoid cysts and the normal arachnoid membrane: hyperplastic arachnoid cells within the cyst wall, splitting of the arachnoid membrane at the margin of cyst wall, absence of traversing trabecular processes within the cyst, and a thick layer of collagen in the cyst wall.[2,5] Arachnoid cysts are thought to represent developmental variants in the meninx primitiva, which surrounds the neural tube during differentiation of the mesenchyma.[6] These CSF spaces, therefore, develop within the layers of the arachnoid membrane.

The indications for neurosurgical intervention in children with arachnoid cysts vary by institution and treating physician. Most cysts do not require surgical treatment. Indications for intervention in one single-institution review included progressive macrocephaly, headache, hydrocephalus, increased intracranial pressure, developmental delay, traumatic cyst rupture, behavioral concerns, and refractory epilepsy.[3] Arachnoid cysts are common and great care must be taken when attempting to attribute nonfocal neurologic symptoms to an arachnoid cyst. Larger cysts and cysts within the anterior fossa and quadrigeminal plate

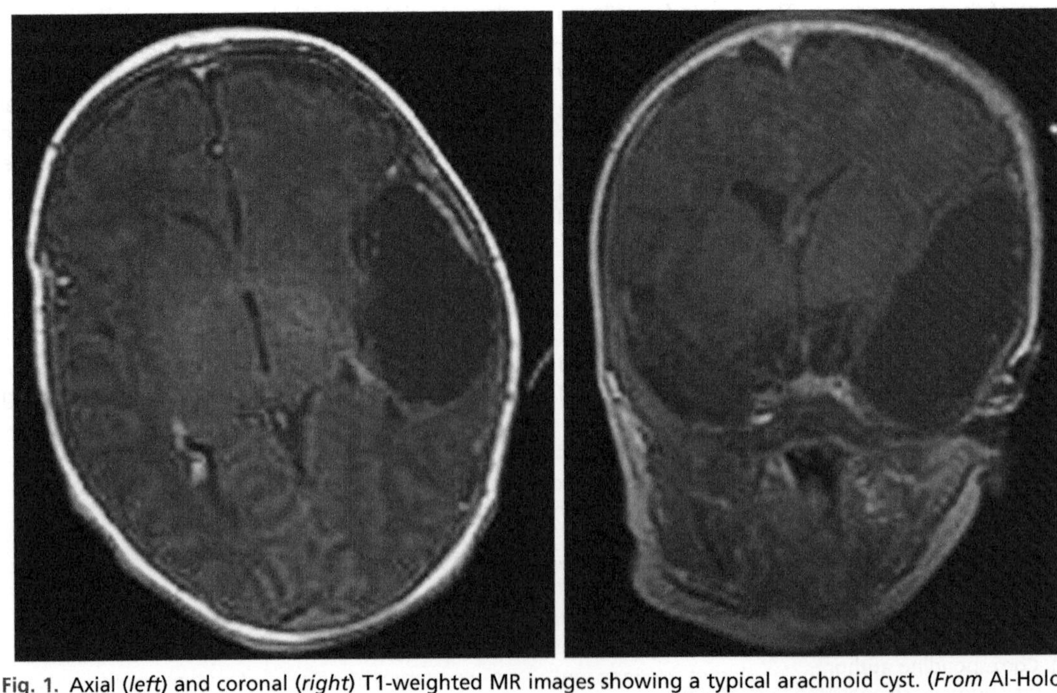

Fig. 1. Axial (*left*) and coronal (*right*) T1-weighted MR images showing a typical arachnoid cyst. (*From* Al-Holou WN, Yew AY, Boomsaad ZE, et al. Prevalence and natural history of arachnoid cysts in children. J Neurosurg Pediatr 2010;5:578–85; with permission.)

Table 2
Location of arachnoid cysts

Lesion Location	Total Number	Left	Right	Midline
Total	309	139	84	86
Anterior fossa	6	1	5	0
Middle fossa	145	96	49	0
Galassi type I	99	64	35	—
Galassi type II	22	17	5	—
Galassi type III	24	15	9	—
Posterior fossa	118	35	25	58
Posterior	89	25	13	52
Superior	8	1	1	6
Cerebellopontine angle	20	9	11	0
Convexity	12	7	5	0
Ventricular	1	0	0	1
Quadrigeminal plate	18	0	0	14
Sellar/suprasellar	5	0	0	5
Interhemispheric	4	0	0	4

Data from Al-Holou WN, Yew AY, Boomsaad ZE, et al. Prevalence and natural history of arachnoid cysts in children. J Neurosurg Pediatr 2010;5:578–85.

were more likely to correlate with patient symptoms and receive recommendation for surgical treatment.[3] Surgical treatments include craniotomy for cyst fenestration, endoscopic cyst fenestration, or CSF diversion with a cyst-to-peritoneum shunt.

The long-term behavior of arachnoid cysts is not well understood. Several case reports and small series have reported changes in cyst size, ranging from enlargement to spontaneous resolution.[7–11] The natural history of arachnoid cysts was reviewed by Al-Holou and colleagues[3] in a large single-institution review. Of 111 patients followed over a mean of 3.5 years, 11 arachnoid cysts increased in size, 13 decreased in size, and 87 remained stable. Younger age at presentation was associated with cyst enlargement and the need for neurosurgical intervention. In that series, no patient older than 4 years of age had cyst enlargement or developed new symptoms. The mechanism by which cysts enlarge is poorly understood; however, a number of theories have been proposed. The most widely accepted theory is that the arachnoid lining may function as a unidirectional ball valve, making CSF entry easier than CSF egress.[2,4,12–15]

PINEAL CYSTS

Pineal cysts are common incidental findings on brain imaging. They have been identified with increasing frequency since the advent of magnetic resonance (MR) imaging (**Fig. 2**).[16–18] Prior studies describing the prevalence of pineal cysts have estimated a population prevalence between 1.1% and 4.3%.[16,17,19–22] A recent large single-institution series identified a 1.9% prevalence of pineal cysts on routine brain imaging in children and young adults, with a slightly increased prevalence in girls and older children.[23]

On MR imaging, pineal cysts must be differentiated from cystic pineal region tumors, including teratomas, pineal parenchymal tumors, germ cell tumors, and low-grade astrocytomas, as well as arachnoid cysts in the adjacent quadrigeminal cistern.[24,25] Although generally considered benign incidental findings, they have rarely been associated with neurologic sequelae, including hydrocephalus from aqueductal compression, Parinaud syndrome, and gaze paresis from tectal plate compression.[18,26–35]

The etiology of pineal cysts is not known. The pineal gland is usually solid and less than 7 mm in diameter. When the pineal gland is greater than 1 cm in size, concern for the possibility of an underlying pineal mass increases.[36] Pastel and colleagues[37] reviewed the ultrastructure of benign pineal-region cysts to determine whether benign cysts have smooth walls or internal structure on MR imaging. The investigators found that the presence of thin walls supports the diagnosis of benign pineal cysts, and that internal septations or small internal cysts are common findings in benign cysts on MR imaging.[37]

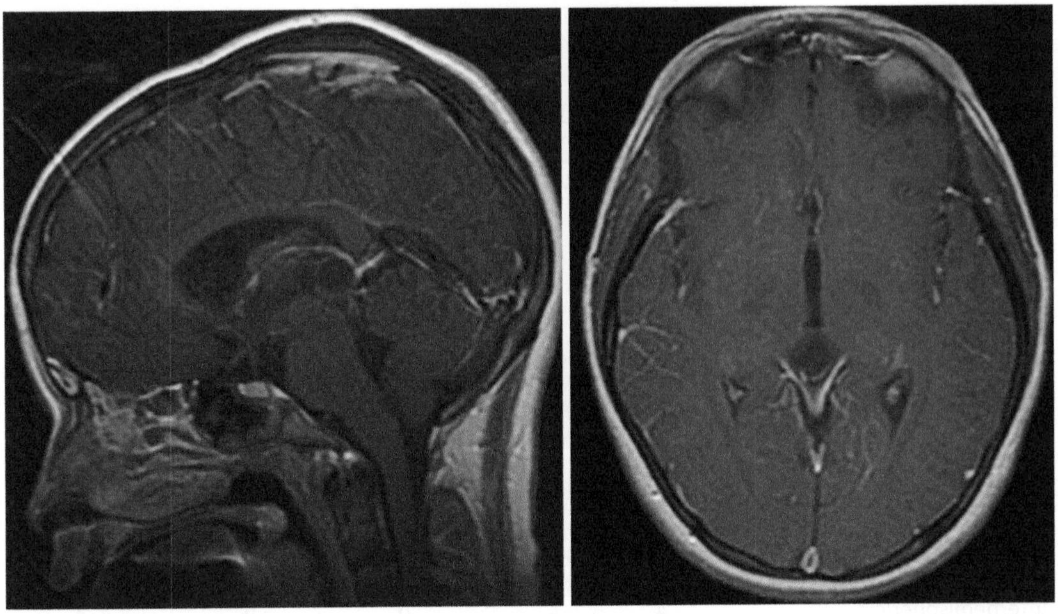

Fig. 2. Sagittal (*left*) and axial (*right*) T1-weighted MR images of asymptomatic pineal region cyst obtained after gadolinium administration. (*From* Al-Holou WN, Maher CO, Muraszko KM, et al. The natural history of pineal cysts in children and young adults. J Neurosurg Pediatr 2010;5:162–6; with permission.)

The clinical significance of these lesions was not well defined until recent analysis (**Table 3**). Several series found that the majority of patients with pineal cysts had no change in cyst size on follow-up imaging and clinical evaluation.[19,21,38–40] In one report of 32 patients with pineal cysts who underwent serial MR imaging, 75% of the cysts remained stable over time, 8% increased in size, and 16% regressed.[39] In another study of 26 children, all incidentally found pineal lesions were stable in size after a maximum of 8 years of follow-up. These findings were supported by a recent single-institution study of 106 patients that were followed over a mean 3-year interval.[38] In that report, 92% (98 of 106) of pineal cysts had no change in appearance on imaging (size or enhancement). Increased size at a mean patient age of 5.5 years was found in 6% (6 of 106), and 2% (2 of 106) had a change in imaging appearance without associated growth.[38] Initial cyst size and imaging characteristics were not predictive of interval growth or change in pineal cyst size, and cysts with atypical features were not significantly more likely to change in size over time.[38] Pineal cysts in younger patients were more likely to change than those found in older patients.

Pineal cysts almost never require surgical treatment. The indications for surgical intervention in

Table 3
Literature review of series reporting pineal cysts with MR imaging follow-up

			Results		
Authors and Year	**Follow-up Intervals**	**Number of Patients**	**Increase in Cyst Size**	**Stable**	**Decrease in Cyst Size**
Al-Holou et al,[38] 2010	Mean 3.0 y	106	6	99	1
Tamaki et al,[40] 1989	3 mo – 4 y	31	0	29	2
Golzarian et al,[19] 1993	>1 y	12	0	12	0
Sawamura et al,[21] 1995	Median 1.5 y	20	0	20	0
Barboriak et al,[39] 2001	Mean 3.7 y	32	3	24	5
Totals		201	9	184	8

Data from Al-Holou WN, Maher CO, Muraszko KM, et al. The natural history of pineal cysts in children and young adults. J Neurosurg Pediatr 2010;5:162–6.

several reported cases have included hydrocephalus, localizing neurologic symptoms, or the need to obtain a histologic confirmation for suspicious or rapidly expanding lesions. Management options for symptomatic pineal cysts have been a subject of debate over the past several years. Surgical options include open craniotomy for surgical excision followed by ventriculoperitoneal shunting for hydrocephalus, stereotactic cyst aspiration, and neuroendoscopy for lesion biopsy and endoscopic third ventriculostomy.[26,28,32,41–49] In most cases, the existing literature does not support surgical treatment for these lesions, except in extraordinary cases.

PEDIATRIC ARTERIOVENOUS MALFORMATIONS

Cerebral AVMs are abnormal connections between arteries and veins. Traditionally, AVMs have been considered congenital lesions, arising from a failure in embryogenesis of the cerebral vasculature.[50–54] Some have postulated that AVMs occur during the third week of embryogenesis, during the formation and absorption of surface veins.[54,55] Pediatric AVMs are thought to be dynamic in nature, constantly undergoing remodeling and angiogenesis.[54,56] The role of abnormal angiogenesis via vascular endothelial growth factor (VEGF) in the formation and progression of AVMs is unclear. Studies have noted increased VEGF levels in children who have recurrence of their lesion after an initial resection as well as increased local expression of VEGF in AVM tissue.[57,58] VEGF circulating in the plasma of patients with AVM has been found to be elevated compared with normal controls, with VEGF levels dropping soon after complete AVM resection.[57]

Although AVMs are most often discovered during the third through fifth decades of life, they remain a common cause of spontaneous intracerebral hemorrhage (ICH) in children.[52,59–65] Excluding hemorrhages of prematurity and early infancy, AVMs are the most frequently encountered structural cause of spontaneous ICH in childhood, and 80% to 85% of pediatric patients with AVM have intracranial hemorrhage as their presenting symptom.[51,60,61,66–69] Other presenting symptoms in children include seizures, visual disturbance, headaches, and progressive neurologic dysfunction.[70,71]

Three types of AVM have been identified. The most common type is high flow with a compact nidus, few arterial feeders, and draining veins. The diffuse variant with low flow and multiple arterial feeders and draining veins is less common.[54,72,73] Recently, the linear vein-based morphology with multiple arterial feeders draining into a single vein has been described (**Figs. 3** and **4**).[71] Linear vein-based AVMs may be more prevalent in children than in adults.[71]

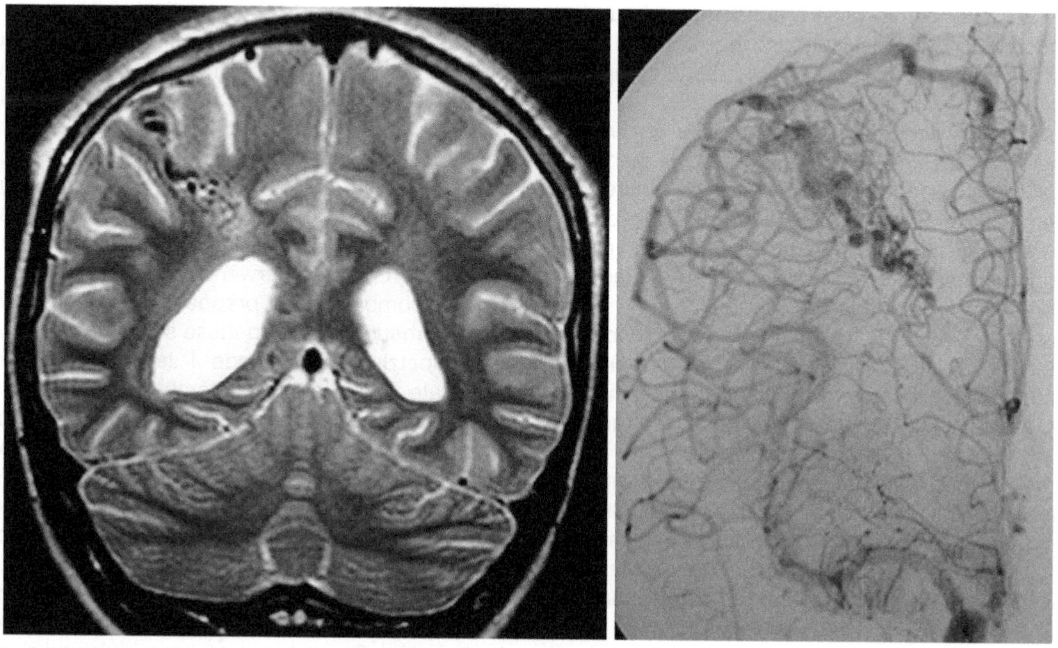

Fig. 3. Gradient echo coronal MR imaging study (*left*) and anteroposterior carotid injection angiogram (*right*) demonstrating the typical appearance of a linear vein-based AVM in a child. (*From* Maher CO, Scott RM. Linear vein-based arteriovenous malformations in children. J Neurosurg Pediatr 2009;4:12–6; with permission.)

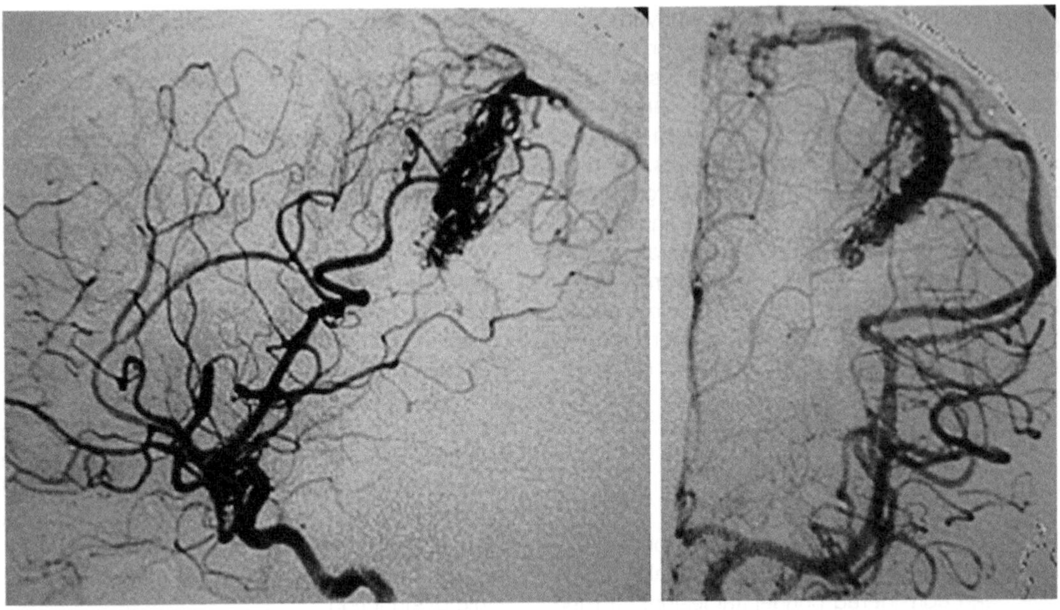

Fig. 4. Anterior circulation angiograms including lateral (*left*) and anteroposterior (*right*) views from another child with a typical linear vein-based AVM. (*From* Maher CO, Scott RM. Linear vein-based arteriovenous malformations in children. J Neurosurg Pediatr 2009;4:12–6; with permission.)

The natural history of pediatric AVMs is not well understood. The annual intracranial hemorrhage rate and mortality from AVM rupture in children is higher than that for adults. Hemorrhage is associated with 25% mortality in children compared with the 6% to 10% annual mortality rate in adult patients.[54,62,74] Factors that predict the bleeding risk of AVM hemorrhage are incompletely understood. Many reports suggest that children have a higher incidence of AVM hemorrhage compared with adults with an annual risk of 2%.[75–77] AVM association with intranidal or pedicle aneurysms increases the risk of AVM rupture in children.[78–80] Deep-venous drainage poses an increased hemorrhage risk.[77,78,81] Location and a previous hemorrhage appear to be quite important in predicting hemorrhage risk, because deep-seated and cerebellar AVMs pose a greater risk.[76–78,82–85] Size has been extensively studied with inconclusive results, because some find that smaller AVMs pose a greater risk of hemorrhage, whereas others suggest larger AVMs pose the greater hemorrhage risk.[76,77,81,85–87]

AVMs in children are generally treated with the goal of eliminating risk of rehemorrhage. Current treatment options include microsurgical resection, stereotactic radiosurgery, and endovascular surgery. Surgical resection remains the gold standard for pediatric AVMs in accessible areas of the brain. The choice of optimal treatment, however, depends on the location and size of the AVM, as well as the age of patients. AVMs in areas of eloquent brain may be considered for treatment with radiosurgery or endovascular therapy, given the higher risk of postoperative neurologic deficits with open microsurgery. Microsurgery should be considered the treatment of choice in children with Spetzler-Martin grade I to III AVMs.[52,54,88] The role of microsurgery in children with Spetzler-Martin grade IV and V AVMs is less clear. Ferch and Morgan[89] retrospectively reviewed 46 adults treated surgically with grade IV or grade V AVMs, noting a 44% morbidity in those with a deep, perforating arterial supply and 10% morbidity in those without a deep component.

Endovascular surgery has an important role in the treatment of pediatric vascular conditions, including AVMs. Several groups have reported on children who underwent treatment of AVMs using a combination of preoperative embolization and microsurgery.[60,66] In these series, all patients with Spetzler-Martin grade I to III AVMs had complete radiographic obliteration of their AVM with favorable clinical outcomes. The use of preoperative embolization has proven most beneficial in children with Spetzler-Martin grade II to V AVMs, thereby decreasing flow and size of the lesion, resulting in less blood loss during surgical resection.

Stereotactic radiosurgery has been used in children with AVMs in eloquent areas of the brain.[54,90,91] Several groups have reviewed their obliteration rates by AVM volume, showing higher obliteration rates with smaller AVMs (<10 mL).[90,92]

The long-term effects of ionizing radiation on the developing brain are incompletely understood. Although 32% of children will show radiation-induced changes on MR imaging after treatment, the short-term neurologic complications in published series are estimated at 5% and include ataxia and cerebral edema.[92–94]

CHIARI MALFORMATIONS

Chiari malformations represent a variety of congenital and acquired clinical syndromes involving structural defects in the cerebellum resulting in impaired CSF dynamics across the craniocervical junction. There are 4 distinct subtypes of Chiari malformations (Chiari I–IV), each representing some degree of hindbrain herniation or cerebellar hypoplasia, ranging from mild tonsillar ectopy to pronounced cerebellar and brainstem herniation through the foramen magnum.[95]

Chiari I malformation is characterized by the downward displacement of the cerebellar tonsils greater than 5 mm below the foramen magnum (as marked by McRae's line on radiograph imaging). Chiari type I is not typically associated with hydrocephalus and has no associated brainstem or supratentorial anomalies. Syringomyelia may be seen in association with Chiari I.

Chiari type II is characterized by herniation of the cerebellar vermis, brainstem, and fourth ventricle through the foramen magnum. Chiari II is typically associated with myelomeningocele and other congenital brain anomalies, as well as hydrocephalus and syringomyelia.

Chiari type III is characterized by an encephalocele at the foramen magnum containing elements of herniated cerebellar and brainstem tissue.

Chiari type IV is characterized by aplasia or hypoplasia of the cerebellum.

A comprehensive review of all subtypes of Chiari malformations is beyond the scope of this subsection; therefore, the authors focus on the clinical features, embryology, and neurosurgical management of Chiari I malformations, with some reference to Chiari II to IV when relevant.

Chiari I

Chiari I malformations are defined by a greater than 5-mm caudal tonsillar descent below the foramen magnum. Chiari I malformations may be congenital or acquired, and are associated with multiple other congenital syndromes.[96–107] Children may or may not be symptomatic from moderate tonsillar displacement; therefore, clinical correlation with radiological findings is essential. In several studies reviewing the position of normal cerebellar tonsils compared with those children who were symptomatic from Chiari I malformation, it has been suggested that tonsillar descent exceeding 5 mm below the foramen magnum was more likely to be pathologic.[108] Despite this commonly used criterion, it is clear that many asymptomatic individuals have greater than 5 mm of tonsillar descent below the foramen magnum. Age affects the normal position of cerebellar tonsils, leading some to define pathologic cerebellar herniation as a distance of greater than 2 standard deviations higher than the range of normal for the patients' age.[109]

Children with Chiari I malformations may present with a range of clinical symptoms. The most prevalent presenting symptom is occipital or cervical pain, seen in 70% of symptomatic children.[95,110–114] Characteristically, this pain is exacerbated by laughing, coughing, running, sneezing, or any other maneuvers resulting in bearing down against a closed airway (Valsalva maneuver). Although Valsalva maneuver-induced headaches associated with Chiari I malformations are often occipital, they may be retro-ocular or generalized in some cases.[114] Neurologic symptoms can be divided into 3 broad categories: cerebellar syndrome, spinal cord syndrome, and brainstem syndrome, representing 11%, 65%, and 22% of symptomatic patients, respectively.[95,113] Symptomatic younger children and infants tend to present with increased irritability, poor feeding, sleep apnea, failure to thrive, dysphagia, choking, and recurrent aspiration caused by lower cranial nerve dysfunction.[115,116] Spinal cord syndrome associated with Chiari I malformation may be the result of a syrinx. Syringomyelia is seen in as many as 70% of patients with Chiari I malformation in large surgical series.[117–119] The true association between Chiari and syrinx is almost certainly much lower, reflecting a bias for surgical treatment in those patients found to have a syrinx. Scoliosis is another common finding in Chiari I malformation, seen in 30% of patients with Chiari type 1 with an associated syringomyelia.[120,121] The mechanism by which a syrinx causes scoliosis is not well understood; however, some have postulated that the presence of a syrinx causes an asymmetry in strength of paravertebral spinal muscles.[119]

Although there are currently no randomized prospective studies, the benefit of surgery in patients with symptomatic Chiari I malformation has been characterized retrospectively.[117,122] In one large single-institution review, 85% of patients had improvement in presenting symptoms and the majority of cervical syringes resolved in size by 6 months after craniocervical decompression.[123,124] There are many differences in approach to treatment among neurosurgeons for patients with

Chiari I malformations; however, most practitioners agree that surgical consideration should be given to patients presenting with Chiari I malformation in the setting of progressive scoliosis or spinal cord syringes.[95,125,126] Furthermore, it is generally agreed that patients presenting with hydrocephalus and Chiari I malformation should receive treatment for their intracranial hypertension before considering suboccipital decompression.[127]

Chiari decompression is safe, with a low complication rate. The procedure typically involves a generous suboccipital decompression and removal of the posterior arch of the first cervical vertebra. The utility of opening the dura is still debated. Some surgeons open the dura and arachnoid completely, others split the outer leaf of dura, and still others leave the dura intact. Postoperative complications may include wound infection, CSF leak, or pseudomeningocele. Furthermore, craniectomies that are too large may lead to cerebellar slump, sometimes associated with chronic pain. Although differences in surgical technique exist, the majority of children report resolution of their preoperative symptoms after surgical decompression. Neurosurgeons and radiologists must continue to work together to develop better imaging modalities for these patients, because patient selection is paramount to the proper surgical treatment of this condition.

ENCEPHALOCELES

Encephaloceles represent a group of disorders in which a skull defect allows for extracranial herniation of leptomeninges, brain, and CSF. Primary encephaloceles are present at birth and secondary encephaloceles are acquired following trauma or surgery. This section focuses on primary (congenital) encephaloceles.

Although several classification systems have been proposed, classification based on anatomic location of the skull defect remains the most popular.[128] Primary encephaloceles can be divided into 3 major categories: fronto-ethmoidal (**Fig. 5**), cranial vault (**Fig. 6**), and basal. In North America and Western Europe, the overall incidence of encephaloceles is 1 to 3 per 10,000 live births and the most common location is occipital.[129,130] Seventy-five percent of children with occipital encephaloceles are girls, and 20% of these children have other neural tube defects.[131,132] Encephaloceles occur more frequently in Central America, Southeast Asia, Central Africa, and Russia. Encephaloceles are thought to result when surface ectoderm fails to separate from neuroectodermal elements during rostral nervous system development. The result is a skull defect, which allows neural elements, meninges, and CSF to migrate outside of the cranial vault. Although the diagnosis may be obvious at birth, encephaloceles can now be diagnosed prenatally in many cases with the use of prenatal ultrasonography.

The prognosis of children with encephaloceles is related to the degree of associated anomalies, the amount of neural tissue within the herniation sac, and the presence of hydrocephalus.[133] The occurrence of concurrent hydrocephalus varies between 16% and 65% in reported series.[134–137] Children with few CNS anomalies and a focal skull defect containing mostly CSF have an approximately 53% chance of being physically and

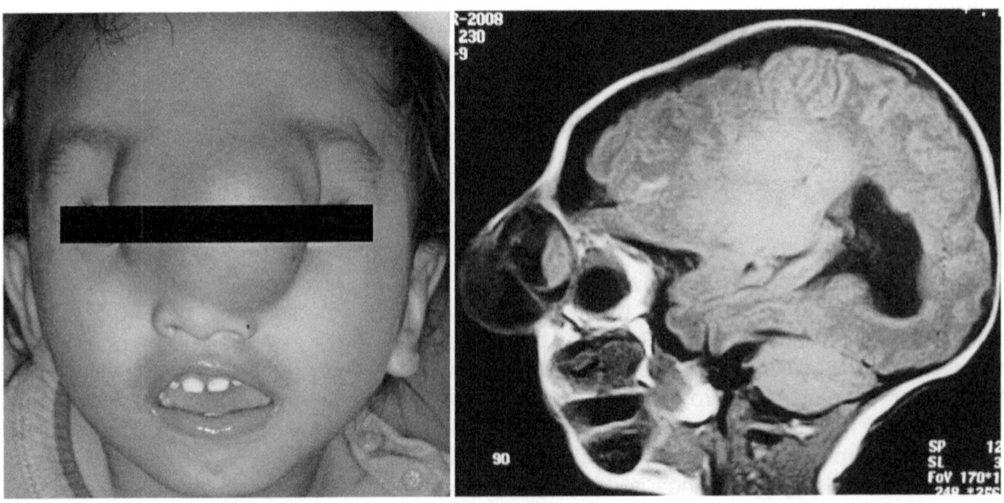

Fig. 5. Child with a frontoethmoidal encephalocele (*left*). Sagittal MR image (*right*) showing the encephalocele defect as well as the involved frontal lobe.

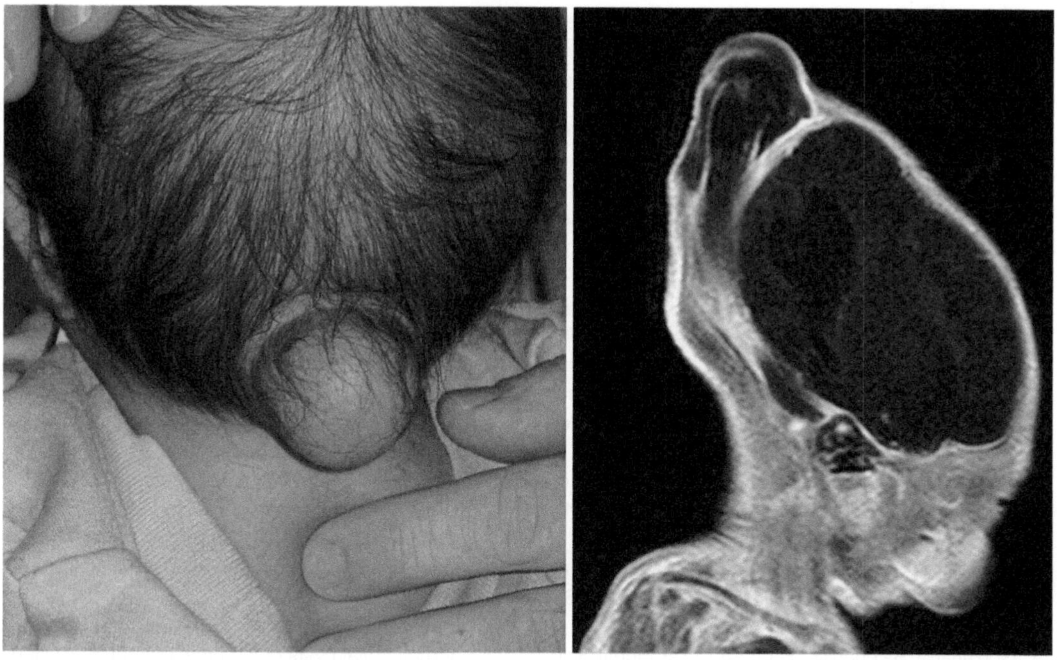

Fig. 6. A newborn with typical occipital encephalocele (*left*). Sagittal MR image (*right*) from a newborn baby with a slightly larger occipital encephalocele.

mentally normal. Mental disability is more likely in children with a larger encephalocele defect and a larger amount of neural tissue within the defect.[136]

Surgical repair of encephaloceles can be safely performed with the goals of providing a watertight dural closure and improving cosmesis. The choice of surgical approach varies greatly given the variability of this condition. A common surgical pitfall is inadequate dural closure resulting in postoperative CSF leakage or pseudomeningocele formation.

ACKNOWLEDGMENTS

We gratefully acknowledge the assistance of Holly Wagner in the preparation of this manuscript.

REFERENCES

1. Choi JU, Kim DS. Pathogenesis of arachnoid cyst: congenital or traumatic? Pediatr Neurosurg 1998; 29(5):260–6.
2. Gosalakkal JA. Intracranial arachnoid cysts in children: a review of pathogenesis, clinical features, and management. Pediatr Neurol 2002;26(2):93–8.
3. Al-Holou WN, Yew AY, Boomsaad ZE, et al. Prevalence and natural history of arachnoid cysts in children. J Neurosurg Pediatr 2010;5(6):578–85.
4. Catala M, Poirier J. [Arachnoid cysts: histologic, embryologic and physiopathologic review]. Rev Neurol (Paris) 1998;154(6–7):489–501 [in French].
5. Rengachary SS, Watanabe I. Ultrastructure and pathogenesis of intracranial arachnoid cysts. J Neuropathol Exp Neurol 1981;40(1):61–83.
6. Utsunomiya H, Yamashita S, Takano K, et al. Midline cystic malformations of the brain: imaging diagnosis and classification based on embryologic analysis. Radiat Med 2006;24(6):471–81.
7. Rao G, Anderson RC, Feldstein NA, et al. Expansion of arachnoid cysts in children: report of two cases and review of the literature. J Neurosurg 2005;102(Suppl 3):314–7.
8. Russo N, Domenicucci M, Beccaglia MR, et al. Spontaneous reduction of intracranial arachnoid cysts: a complete review. Br J Neurosurg 2008; 22(5):626–9.
9. Seizeur R, Forlodou P, Coustans M, et al. Spontaneous resolution of arachnoid cysts: review and features of an unusual case. Acta Neurochir (Wien) 2007;149(1):75–8.
10. Thomas BP, Pearson MM, Wushensky CA. Active spontaneous decompression of a suprasellar-prepontine arachnoid cyst detected with routine magnetic resonance imaging. Case report. J Neurosurg Pediatr 2009;3(1):70–2.
11. Weber R, Voit T, Lumenta C, et al. Spontaneous regression of a temporal arachnoid cyst. Childs Nerv Syst 1991;7(7):414–5.

12. Cagnoni G, Fonda C, Pancani S, et al. [Intracranial arachnoid cyst in pediatric age]. Pediatr Med Chir 1996;18(1):85–90 [in Italian].
13. Go KG, Houthoff HJ, Blaauw EH, et al. Arachnoid cysts of the sylvian fissure. Evidence of fluid secretion. J Neurosurg 1984;60(4):803–13.
14. Santamarta D, Aguas J, Ferrer E. The natural history of arachnoid cysts: endoscopic and cine-mode MRI evidence of a slit-valve mechanism. Minim Invasive Neurosurg 1995;38(4):133–7.
15. Schachenmayr W, Friede RL. Fine structure of arachnoid cysts. J Neuropathol Exp Neurol 1979; 38(4):434–46.
16. Di Costanzo A, Tedeschi G, Di Salle F, et al. Pineal cysts: an incidental MRI finding? J Neurol Neurosurg Psychiatry 1993;56(2):207–8.
17. Lee DH, Norman D, Newton TH. MR imaging of pineal cysts. J Comput Assist Tomogr 1987;11(4): 586–90.
18. Wisoff JH, Epstein F. Surgical management of symptomatic pineal cysts. J Neurosurg 1992;77(6): 896–900.
19. Golzarian J, Baleriaux D, Bank WO, et al. Pineal cyst: normal or pathological? Neuroradiology 1993;35(4): 251–3.
20. Mamourian AC, Towfighi J. Pineal cysts: MR imaging. AJNR Am J Neuroradiol 1986;7(6): 1081–6.
21. Sawamura Y, Ikeda J, Ozawa M, et al. Magnetic resonance images reveal a high incidence of asymptomatic pineal cysts in young women. Neurosurgery 1995;37(1):11–6.
22. Sener RN. The pineal gland: a comparative MR imaging study in children and adults with respect to normal anatomical variations and pineal cysts. Pediatr Radiol 1995;25(4):245–8.
23. Al-Holou WN, Garton HJ, Muraszko KM, et al. Prevalence of pineal cysts in children and young adults. Clinical article. J Neurosurg Pediatr 2009; 4(3):230–6.
24. Evans RW, Peres MF. Headaches and pineal cysts. Headache 2010;50(4):666–8.
25. Oi S, Matsumoto S. Controversy pertaining to therapeutic modalities for tumors of the pineal region: a worldwide survey of different patient populations. Childs Nerv Syst 1992;8(6):332–6.
26. Costa F, Fornari M, Valla P, et al. Symptomatic pineal cyst: case report and review of the literature. Minim Invasive Neurosurg 2008;51(4): 231–3.
27. Fain JS, Tomlinson FH, Scheithauer BW, et al. Symptomatic glial cysts of the pineal gland. J Neurosurg 1994;80(3):454–60.
28. Klein P, Rubinstein LJ. Benign symptomatic glial cysts of the pineal gland: a report of seven cases and review of the literature. J Neurol Neurosurg Psychiatry 1989;52(8):991–5.
29. Mandera M, Marcol W, Bierzynska-Macyszyn G, et al. Pineal cysts in childhood. Childs Nerv Syst 2003;19(10–11):750–5.
30. Maurer PK, Ecklund J, Parisi JE, et al. Symptomatic pineal cyst: case report. Neurosurgery 1990;27(3): 451–4.
31. Mena H, Armonda RA, Ribas JL, et al. Nonneoplastic pineal cysts: a clinicopathologic study of twenty-one cases. Ann Diagn Pathol 1997;1(1): 11–8.
32. Michielsen G, Benoit Y, Baert E, et al. Symptomatic pineal cysts: clinical manifestations and management. Acta Neurochir (Wien) 2002;144(3): 233–42.
33. Oeckler R, Feiden W. Benign symptomatic lesions of the pineal gland. Report of seven cases treated surgically. Acta Neurochir (Wien) 1991;108(1–2): 40–4.
34. Osborn RE, Deen HG, Kerber CW, et al. A case of hemorrhagic pineal cyst: MR/CT correlation. Neuroradiology 1989;31(2):187–9.
35. Vaquero J, Martinez R, Escandon J, et al. Symptomatic glial cysts of the pineal gland. Surg Neurol 1988;30(6):468–70.
36. Sumida M, Barkovich AJ, Newton TH. Development of the pineal gland: measurement with MR. AJNR Am J Neuroradiol 1996;17(2):233–6.
37. Pastel DA, Mamourian AC, Duhaime AC. Internal structure in pineal cysts on high-resolution magnetic resonance imaging: not a sign of malignancy. J Neurosurg Pediatr 2009;4(1):81–4.
38. Al-Holou WN, Maher CO, Muraszko KM, et al. The natural history of pineal cysts in children and young adults. J Neurosurg Pediatr 2010;5(2):162–6.
39. Barboriak DP, Lee L, Provenzale JM. Serial MR imaging of pineal cysts: implications for natural history and follow-up. AJR Am J Roentgenol 2001;176(3):737–43.
40. Tamaki N, Shirataki K, Lin TK, et al. Cysts of the pineal gland. A new clinical entity to be distinguished from tumors of the pineal region. Childs Nerv Syst 1989;5(3):172–6.
41. Gaab MR, Schroeder HW. Neuroendoscopic approach to intraventricular lesions. Neurosurg Focus 1999;6(4):e5.
42. Hellwig D, Bauer BL, List-Hellwig E. Stereotactic endoscopic interventions in cystic brain lesions. Acta Neurochir Suppl 1995;64:59–63.
43. Metellus P, Fuentes S, Levrier O, et al. Endoscopic treatment of a voluminous benign symptomatic cyst of the pineal region responsible for an obstructive hydrocephalus. Neurochirurgie 2005;51(3–4 Pt 1): 173–8 [in French].
44. Musolino A, Cambria S, Rizzo G, et al. Symptomatic cysts of the pineal gland: stereotactic diagnosis and treatment of two cases and review of the literature. Neurosurgery 1993;32(2):315–21.

45. Pople IK, Athanasiou TC, Sandeman DR, et al. The role of endoscopic biopsy and third ventriculostomy in the management of pineal region tumours. Br J Neurosurg 2001;15(4):305–11.
46. Sekiya T, Suzuki S, Iwabuchi T. [Pineal cyst: its diagnosis and treatment]. No Shinkei Geka 1994; 22(8):715–21 [in Japanese].
47. Stern JD, Ross DA. Stereotactic management of benign pineal region cysts: report of two cases. Neurosurgery 1993;32(2):310–4.
48. Tirakotai W, Schulte DM, Bauer BL, et al. Neuroendoscopic surgery of intracranial cysts in adults. Childs Nerv Syst 2004;20(11–12):842–51.
49. Turtz AR, Hughes WB, Goldman HW. Endoscopic treatment of a symptomatic pineal cyst: technical case report. Neurosurgery 1995;37(5):1013–5.
50. Akimoto H, Komatsu K, Kubota Y. Symptomatic de novo arteriovenous malformation appearing 17 years after the resection of two other arteriovenous malformations in childhood: case report. Neurosurgery 2003;52(1):228–32.
51. Di Rocco C, Tamburrini G, Rollo M. Cerebral arteriovenous malformations in children. Acta Neurochir (Wien) 2000;142(2):145–58.
52. Kiris T, Sencer A, Sahinbas M, et al. Surgical results in pediatric Spetzler-Martin grades I-III intracranial arteriovenous malformations. Childs Nerv Syst 2005;21(1):69–76.
53. Menovsky T, van Overbeeke JJ. Cerebral arteriovenous malformations in childhood: state of the art with special reference to treatment. Eur J Pediatr 1997;156(10):741–6.
54. Niazi TN, Klimo P Jr, Anderson RC, et al. Diagnosis and management of arteriovenous malformations in children. Neurosurg Clin N Am 2010;21(3): 443–56.
55. Mullan S, Mojtahedi S, Johnson DL, et al. Embryological basis of some aspects of cerebral vascular fistulas and malformations. J Neurosurg 1996; 85(1):1–8.
56. Shin M, Maruyama K, Kurita H, et al. Analysis of nidus obliteration rates after gamma knife surgery for arteriovenous malformations based on long-term follow-up data: the University of Tokyo experience. J Neurosurg 2004;101(1):18–24.
57. Kim GH, Hahn DK, Kellner CP, et al. Plasma levels of vascular endothelial growth factor after treatment for cerebral arteriovenous malformations. Stroke 2008;39(8):2274–9.
58. Sonstein WJ, Kader A, Michelsen WJ, et al. Expression of vascular endothelial growth factor in pediatric and adult cerebral arteriovenous malformations: an immunocytochemical study. J Neurosurg 1996; 85(5):838–45.
59. Forster DM, Steiner L, Hakanson S. Arteriovenous malformations of the brain. A long-term clinical study. J Neurosurg 1972;37(5):562–70.
60. Hoh BL, Ogilvy CS, Butler WE, et al. Multimodality treatment of nongalenic arteriovenous malformations in pediatric patients. Neurosurgery 2000; 47(2):346–58.
61. Humphreys RP, Hoffman HJ, Drake JM, et al. Choices in the 1990s for the management of pediatric cerebral arteriovenous malformations. Pediatr Neurosurg 1996;25(6):277–85.
62. Kondziolka D, Humphreys RP, Hoffman HJ, et al. Arteriovenous malformations of the brain in children: a forty year experience. Can J Neurol Sci 1992;19(1):40–5.
63. Perret G, Nishioka H. Report on the cooperative study of intracranial aneurysms and subarachnoid hemorrhage. Section VI. Arteriovenous malformations. An analysis of 545 cases of cranio-cerebral arteriovenous malformations and fistulae reported to the cooperative study. J Neurosurg 1966;25(4): 467–90.
64. Rodesch G, Malherbe V, Alvarez H, et al. Nongalenic cerebral arteriovenous malformations in neonates and infants. Review of 26 consecutive cases (1982–1992). Childs Nerv Syst 1995;11(4): 231–41.
65. Stein BM, Wolpert SM. Arteriovenous malformations of the brain. I: current concepts and treatment. Arch Neurol 1980;37(1):1–5.
66. Bristol RE, Albuquerque FC, Spetzler RF, et al. Surgical management of arteriovenous malformations in children. J Neurosurg 2006;105(Suppl 2): 88–93.
67. Matson DD. Neurosurgery of infancy and childhood. 2nd edition. Springfield (MA): Thomas; 1969. p. 749.
68. Millar C, Bissonnette B, Humphreys RP. Cerebral arteriovenous malformations in children. Can J Anaesth 1994;41(4):321–31.
69. Mori K, Murata T, Hashimoto N, et al. Clinical analysis of arteriovenous malformations in children. Childs Brain 1980;6(1):13–25.
70. Leblanc R, Feindel W, Ethier R. Epilepsy from cerebral arteriovenous malformations. Can J Neurol Sci 1983;10(2):91–5.
71. Maher CO, Scott RM. Linear vein-based arteriovenous malformations in children. J Neurosurg Pediatr 2009;4(1):12–6.
72. Chin LS, Raffel C, Gonzalez-Gomez I, et al. Diffuse arteriovenous malformations: a clinical, radiological, and pathological description. Neurosurgery 1992;31(5):863–9.
73. Klimo P Jr, Rao G, Brockmeyer D. Pediatric arteriovenous malformations: a 15-year experience with an emphasis on residual and recurrent lesions. Childs Nerv Syst 2007;23(1):31–7.
74. Celli P, Ferrante L, Palma L, et al. Cerebral arteriovenous malformations in children. Clinical features and outcome of treatment in children and in adults. Surg Neurol 1984;22(1):43–9.

75. Fullerton HJ, Achrol AS, Johnston SC, et al. Long-term hemorrhage risk in children versus adults with brain arteriovenous malformations. Stroke 2005;36(10):2099–104.
76. Hernesniemi JA, Dashti R, Juvela S, et al. Natural history of brain arteriovenous malformations: a long-term follow-up study of risk of hemorrhage in 238 patients. Neurosurgery 2008;63(5):823–31.
77. Stapf C, Mast H, Sciacca RR, et al. Predictors of hemorrhage in patients with untreated brain arteriovenous malformation. Neurology 2006;66(9): 1350–5.
78. Khaw AV, Mohr JP, Sciacca RR, et al. Association of infratentorial brain arteriovenous malformations with hemorrhage at initial presentation. Stroke 2004;35(3):660–3.
79. Meisel HJ, Mansmann U, Alvarez H, et al. Cerebral arteriovenous malformations and associated aneurysms: analysis of 305 cases from a series of 662 patients. Neurosurgery 2000;46(4):793–802.
80. Redekop G, TerBrugge K, Montanera W, et al. Arterial aneurysms associated with cerebral arteriovenous malformations: classification, incidence, and risk of hemorrhage. J Neurosurg 1998;89(4): 539–46.
81. Langer DJ, Lasner TM, Hurst RW, et al. Hypertension, small size, and deep venous drainage are associated with risk of hemorrhagic presentation of cerebral arteriovenous malformations. Neurosurgery 1998;42(3):481–9.
82. Arnaout OM, Gross BA, Eddleman CS, et al. Posterior fossa arteriovenous malformations. Neurosurg Focus 2009;26(5):E12.
83. da Costa L, Wallace MC, Ter Brugge KG, et al. The natural history and predictive features of hemorrhage from brain arteriovenous malformations. Stroke 2009;40(1):100–5.
84. Pollock BE, Flickinger JC, Lunsford LD, et al. Factors that predict the bleeding risk of cerebral arteriovenous malformations. Stroke 1996;27(1): 1–6.
85. Stefani MA, Porter PJ, terBrugge KG, et al. Large and deep brain arteriovenous malformations are associated with risk of future hemorrhage. Stroke 2002;33(5):1220–4.
86. Spetzler RF, Hargraves RW, McCormick PW, et al. Relationship of perfusion pressure and size to risk of hemorrhage from arteriovenous malformations. J Neurosurg 1992;76(6):918–23.
87. Waltimo O. The relationship of size, density and localization of intracranial arteriovenous malformations to the type of initial symptom. J Neurol Sci 1973;19(1):13–9.
88. Schaller C, Schramm J. Microsurgical results for small arteriovenous malformations accessible for radiosurgical or embolization treatment. Neurosurgery 1997;40(4):664–74.
89. Ferch RD, Morgan MK. High-grade arteriovenous malformations and their management. J Clin Neurosci 2002;9(1):37–40.
90. Pollock BE, Flickinger JC, Lunsford LD, et al. Factors associated with successful arteriovenous malformation radiosurgery. Neurosurgery 1998; 42(6):1239–47.
91. Pollock BE, Kondziolka D, Flickinger JC, et al. Magnetic resonance imaging: an accurate method to evaluate arteriovenous malformations after stereotactic radiosurgery. J Neurosurg 1996;85(6): 1044–9.
92. Levy EI, Niranjan A, Thompson TP, et al. Radiosurgery for childhood intracranial arteriovenous malformations. Neurosurgery 2000;47(4):834–42.
93. Buis DR, Dirven CM, Lagerwaard FJ, et al. Radiosurgery of brain arteriovenous malformations in children. J Neurol 2008;255(4):551–60.
94. Reyns N, Blond S, Gauvrit JY, et al. Role of radiosurgery in the management of cerebral arteriovenous malformations in the pediatric age group: data from a 100-patient series. Neurosurgery 2007; 60(2):268–76.
95. Tubbs RS, Lyerly MJ, Loukas M, et al. The pediatric Chiari I malformation: a review. Childs Nerv Syst 2007;23(11):1239–50.
96. Huang PP, Constantini S. "Acquired" Chiari I malformation. Case report. J Neurosurg 1994;80(6): 1099–102.
97. Lee J, Hida K, Seki T, et al. Pierre-Robin syndrome associated with Chiari type I malformation. Childs Nerv Syst 2003;19(5–6):380–3.
98. Mampalam TJ, Andrews BT, Gelb D, et al. Presentation of type I Chiari malformation after head trauma. Neurosurgery 1988;23(6):760–2.
99. Murphy RL, Tubbs RS, Grabb PA, et al. Chiari I malformation and idiopathic growth hormone deficiency in siblings. Childs Nerv Syst 2006;22(6): 632–4.
100. Tubbs RS, Oakes WJ. Pierre-Robin syndrome associated with Chiari I malformation. Childs Nerv Syst 2004;20(1):1–7.
101. Tubbs RS, Oakes WJ. Chiari I malformation, caudal regression syndrome, and Pierre Robin syndrome: a previously unreported combination. Childs Nerv Syst 2006;22(11):1507–8.
102. Tubbs RS, Rutledge SL, Kosentka A, et al. Chiari I malformation and neurofibromatosis type 1. Pediatr Neurol 2004;30(4):278–80.
103. Tubbs RS, Smyth MD, Oakes WJ. Chiari I malformation and cloacal exstrophy: report of a patient with both defects of blastogenesis. Am J Med Genet A 2003;119(2):231–3.
104. Tubbs RS, Smyth MD, Oakes WJ. Chiari I malformation and caudal regression syndrome: a previously unreported association. Clin Dysmorphol 2003;12(2):147–8.

105. Tubbs RS, Smyth MD, Wellons JC 3rd, et al. Hemihypertrophy and the Chiari I malformation. Pediatr Neurosurg 2003;38(5):258–61.
106. Tubbs RS, Wellons JC 3rd, Oakes WJ. Occipital encephalocele, lipomeningomyelocele, and Chiari I malformation: case report and review of the literature. Childs Nerv Syst 2003;19(1):50–3.
107. Welch K, Shillito J, Strand R, et al. Chiari I "malformations"–an acquired disorder? J Neurosurg 1981; 55(4):604–9.
108. Aboulezz AO, Sartor K, Geyer CA, et al. Position of cerebellar tonsils in the normal population and in patients with Chiari malformation: a quantitative approach with MR imaging. J Comput Assist Tomogr 1985;9(6):1033–6.
109. Mikulis DJ, Diaz O, Egglin TK, et al. Variance of the position of the cerebellar tonsils with age: preliminary report. Radiology 1992;183(3):725–8.
110. Levy WJ, Mason L, Hahn JF. Chiari malformation presenting in adults: a surgical experience in 127 cases. Neurosurgery 1983;12(4):377–90.
111. Nohria V, Oakes WJ. Chiari I malformation: a review of 43 patients. Pediatr Neurosurg 1990;16(4–5): 222–7.
112. Oakes WJ. Chiari malformations, hydromyelia, syringomyelia. In: Wilkins RH, Rengachary SS, editors. Neurosurgery. 2nd edition. New York: McGraw-Hill; 1996. p. 3593–616.
113. Paul KS, Lye RH, Strang FA, et al. Arnold-Chiari malformation. Review of 71 cases. J Neurosurg 1983;58(2):183–7.
114. Steinbok P. Clinical features of Chiari I malformations. Childs Nerv Syst 2004;20(5):329–31.
115. Greenlee JD, Donovan KA, Hasan DM, et al. Chiari I malformation in the very young child: the spectrum of presentations and experience in 31 children under age 6 years. Pediatrics 2002;110(6): 1212–9.
116. Nathadwarawala KM, Richards CA, Lawrie B, et al. Recurrent aspiration due to Arnold-Chiari type I malformation. BMJ 1992;304(6826):565–6.
117. Milhorat TH, Chou MW, Trinidad EM, et al. Chiari I malformation redefined: clinical and radiographic findings for 364 symptomatic patients. Neurosurgery 1999;44(5):1005–17.
118. Morioka T, Kurita-Tashima S, Fujii K, et al. Somatosensory and spinal evoked potentials in patients with cervical syringomyelia. Neurosurgery 1992; 30(2):218–22.
119. Oakes WJ. Chiari malformations and syringomyelia in children. In: Rengachary SS, Wilkins RH, editors. Neurosurgical operative atlas. Baltimore (MD): Williams & Wilkins; 1991. p. 59–65.
120. Isu T, Chono Y, Iwasaki Y, et al. Scoliosis associated with syringomyelia presenting in children. Childs Nerv Syst 1992;8(2):97–100.
121. Muhonen MG, Menezes AH, Sawin PD, et al. Scoliosis in pediatric Chiari malformations without myelodysplasia. J Neurosurg 1992;77(1):69–77.
122. Navarro R, Olavarria G, Seshadri R, et al. Surgical results of posterior fossa decompression for patients with Chiari I malformation. Childs Nerv Syst 2004;20(5):349–56.
123. Pillay PK, Awad IA, Little JR, et al. Symptomatic Chiari malformation in adults: a new classification based on magnetic resonance imaging with clinical and prognostic significance. Neurosurgery 1991;28(5):639–45.
124. Tubbs RS, McGirt MJ, Oakes WJ. Surgical experience in 130 pediatric patients with Chiari I malformations. J Neurosurg 2003;99(2):291–6.
125. Milhorat TH, Bolognese PA, Black KS, et al. Acute syringomyelia: case report. Neurosurgery 2003; 53(5):1220–2.
126. Schijman E, Steinbok P. International survey on the management of Chiari I malformation and syringomyelia. Childs Nerv Syst 2004;20(5):341–8.
127. Osuagwu FC, Lazareff JA, Rahman S, et al. Chiari I anatomy after ventriculoperitoneal shunting: posterior fossa volumetric evaluation with MRI. Childs Nerv Syst 2006;22(11):1451–6.
128. Suwanwela C, Suwanwela N. A morphological classification of sincipital encephalomeningoceles. J Neurosurg 1972;36(2):201–11.
129. Macfarlane R, Rutka JT, Armstrong D, et al. Encephaloceles of the anterior cranial fossa. Pediatr Neurosurg 1995;23(3):148–58.
130. Simpson DA, David DJ, White J. Cephaloceles: treatment, outcome, and antenatal diagnosis. Neurosurgery 1984;15(1):14–21.
131. Karch SB, Urich H. Occipital encephalocele: a morphological study. J Neurol Sci 1972;15(1): 89–112.
132. Naidich TP, Altman NR, Braffman BH, et al. Cephaloceles and related malformations. AJNR Am J Neuroradiol 1992;13(2):655–90.
133. Kiymaz N, Yilmaz N, Demir I, et al. Prognostic factors in patients with occipital encephalocele. Pediatr Neurosurg 2010;46(1):6–11.
134. Chapman PH, Swearingen B, Caviness VS. Subtorcular occipital encephaloceles. Anatomical considerations relevant to operative management. J Neurosurg 1989;71(3):375–81.
135. Lorber J, Schofield JK. The prognosis of occipital encephalocele. Z Kinderchir Grenzgeb 1979; 28(4):347–51.
136. Mealey J Jr, Dzenitis AJ, Hockey AA. The prognosis of encephaloceles. J Neurosurg 1970;32(2): 209–18.
137. Shokunbi T, Adeloye A, Olumide A. Occipital encephalocoeles in 57 Nigerian children: a retrospective analysis. Childs Nerv Syst 1990;6(2):99–102.

Neurosurgical Management of Congenital Malformations and Inherited Disease of the Spine

Shawn L. Hervey-Jumper, MD[a], Hugh J.L. Garton, MD[a], Nicholas M. Wetjen, MD[b], Cormac O. Maher, MD[c,*]

KEYWORDS

- Achondroplasia • Goldenhar syndrome
- Lipomyelomeningocele • Morquio syndrome
- Myelomeningocele • Osteogenesis imperfecta
- Spina bifida • Spondyloepiphyseal dysplasia

Congenital malformations encompass a diverse group of disorders present at birth, as result of genetic abnormalities, infection, errors of morphogenesis, or abnormalities in the intrauterine environment. Congenital disorders affecting the brain and spinal cord are now often diagnosed before delivery with the use of prenatal ultrasonography and maternal serum screening. Over the past several decades there have been major advances in the understanding and management of these conditions. This article focuses on the most common spinal congenital malformations, limiting the discussion to the neurosurgically relevant aspects of myelomeningocele, lipomyelomeningocele, and skeletal dysplasias, including achondroplasia, Goldenhar syndrome, Morquio syndrome, spondyloepiphyseal dysplasia (SED), osteogenesis imperfecta (OI), and Larsen syndrome.

Skeletal dysplasias are a heterogeneous group of more than 200 disorders in which there is abnormal formation, growth, or remodeling of cartilage and bone. This group of disorders affects 1 in 5000 live births, differing widely in natural history, inheritance, and etiology. Skeletal dysplasias may be classified as either osteochondral dysplasia (involving the whole skeleton) or dysostosis (involving a single group of bones). Craniocervical junction abnormalities, atlantoaxial subluxation, and kyphoscoliotic deformities are common spinal problems found in skeletal dysplasias. This discussion focuses on the key skeletal dysplasias and their neurosurgical implications in children.

ACHONDROPLASIA

Achondroplasia is the most common form of dwarfism and is the most common heritable skeletal dysplasia, characterized by a disproportionate shortening of the proximal limbs relative to the

Disclosure: The authors have nothing to disclose.

[a] Department of Neurosurgery, University of Michigan, 1500 East Medical Center Drive, Ann Arbor, MI 48109-5338, USA
[b] Department of Neurologic Surgery, Mayo Clinic, 200 First Street, Rochester, MN 55905, USA
[c] Department of Neurosurgery, University of Michigan, 1500 East Medical Center Drive, Room 3552 Taubman Center, Ann Arbor, MI 48109-5338, USA
* Corresponding author.
E-mail address: cmaher@med.umich.edu

Neuroimag Clin N Am 21 (2011) 719–731
doi:10.1016/j.nic.2011.05.009

trunk. This is sometimes referred to as rhizomelic dwarfism, describing the small forearms and thighs in relation to the entire limb and trunk. It occurs in 1 of every 28,000 live births.[1–3] Recognizable at birth, the characteristic morphology includes shortened limbs and long bones, macrocephaly, frontal bossing, genu varum abnormalities, and a low-set nasal bridge.[4] Achondroplasia follows an autosomal dominant inheritance pattern, although 80% of cases arise as a result of spontaneous mutations in the fibroblast growth factor receptor 3 (*FGFR3*) gene located on chromosome 4.[1,2,5] This gene mutation results in a decrease in the rate of endochondral bone formation with normal rates of membranous bone formation, calcification, and remodeling.[4,5]

Almost half of all children with achondroplasia have neurologic manifestations of their disease.[2] The neurologic manifestations of achondroplasia include ventriculomegaly, compressive spinal syndromes, and developmental delay.[6] Other than ventriculomegaly, foramen magnum stenosis resulting in cervicomedullary compression is the most frequent cause of neurosurgical consultation in infants. In older children and adults, multisegment spinal stenosis involving the subaxial cervical or thoracolumbar spine may also be present. Foramen magnum stenosis results from abnormal endochondral bone growth and fusion of posterior basal synchondroses.[3,7] The bones of the skull base, as well as bones of the neural arches, normally enlarge by endochondral ossification.[8,9] Because of defective endochondral bone formation at the cranial base and craniocervical junction, infants with achondroplasia may have a small foramen magnum, a short basicranium and clivus, a shallow posterior fossa with a horizontally oriented inferior occiput, an abnormal odontoid process, stenotic jugular foramina, and a narrow upper cervical canal.[1,3,8] Furthermore, premature fusion and abnormal development of the 2 posterior synchondroses contribute to thickening of the rim of the foramen magnum, which may project into the brainstem causing compression and severe angulations of the medulla and rostral cervical spinal cord.[1,8] The odontoid often projects superiorly and posteriorly into the small foramen magnum causing the anterior medulla to drape over the odontoid.[8,9] These changes lead to damage of the corticospinal tract and chronic ischemia to the medulla.[8]

Although foramen magnum stenosis is found in as many as 70% of achondroplasia patients, only between 10% and 35% of patients exhibit symptoms of cervicomedullary compression.[10,11] Cervicomedullary compression secondary to foramen magnum stenosis can present with dysfunction of the lower brainstem, high cervical spinal cord, and associated nerve roots in children with achondroplasia. Symptoms of cervicomedullary compression may include poor head control, excessive hypotonia, apnea, feeding difficulties, developmental delay, hydrocephalus, myelopathy, respiratory disorders, and sudden death due to respiratory arrest.[12] Less lethal respiratory disturbances in children with achondroplasia include central and obstructive sleep apnea.[13] Central sleep apnea in these children is thought to result from damage to the ventral medullary respiratory control centers from foramen magnum stenosis. Foramen magnum stenosis may also compress lower motor neurons leading to paralysis of the diaphragm and accessory muscles of respiration.[1] Apnea due to foramen magnum stenosis may improve dramatically after surgical decompression.[7,13–15] Hydrocephalus in children with achondroplasia is theorized to result from a combination of crowding of the foramen magnum, resulting in obstruction of cerebrospinal fluid (CSF) outflow, and jugular foramen stenosis, resulting in elevated venous sinus pressures.[9,13] In many instances, the ventriculomegaly found in children with achondroplasia arrests without treatment. Shunt placement can be considered for those who have failed conservative treatment.[1,13,14] Even without hydrocephalus, macrocephaly is extremely common in achondroplasia and relative head size should be assessed compared with disease-specific normative data.

The decision to recommend surgical decompression of foramen magnum and cervical stenosis in achondroplasia patients should be based on both clinical signs and symptoms and imaging data. The clinical signs and symptoms of most concern include lower cranial nerve palsies, apnea, hyperreflexia, clonus, and weakness. Concerning findings on magnetic resonance (MR) imaging include intramedullary T2-weighted changes, absence of CSF signal at the foramen magnum, and the presence of a syrinx. One prospective study of children with achondroplasia concluded that the signs and symptoms that best predicted the need for surgical decompression included central hypopnea, foramen magnum measurements below the mean for children with achondroplasia, lower-extremity hyperreflexia, and clonus.[10] Foramen magnum decompression via a suboccipital craniectomy with removal of the posterior arch of the atlas is performed in cases of proved symptomatic cervicomedullary compression. Even in apparently asymptomatic children, the presence of significant stenosis and T2 signal change in the spinal cord is strongly suggestive of the need for decompression or stabilization. The use of an intraoperative ultrasound to assess for adequate CSF pulsations around the brainstem may assist in determining the degree to which the dura mater should be opened. Marked improvement in neurologic function is often noted in symptomatic children after foramen magnum decompression. Bagley and colleagues[1] reported their single-institution series of 43 children with achondroplasia who underwent foramen magnum decompression. All patients in their series had complete or partial improvement in preoperative symptoms after surgery, in particular respiratory symptoms. Postoperative complications include re-stenosis at the level of the foramen magnum, particularly if the procedure is performed in infancy. If the procedure is performed with a durotomy, additional potential complications include CSF leaks and pseudomeningocele formation.[1,14]

Subaxial spinal stenosis in children with achondroplasia results from premature fusion of the ossification centers of the vertebral bodies and posterior neural arches. The vertebrae develop a characteristic morphology, including short and thick lamina, vertebral bodies with reduced height, and small neural foramina with a narrowed interpedicular distance.[8,16] Clinically the most commonly involved areas in order are thoracolumbar, pure lumbar, and cervical. A history of prior need for foramen magnum decompression has been associated with an increased likelihood of symptomatic spinal stenosis before adolescence.[17] Typically, however, stenosis becomes symptomatic in adolescence. Signs and symptoms depend on the level of spinal cord involvement and include ataxia, frequent falls, spasticity, bowel or bladder dysfunction, radiculopathy, temporary deterioration of spinal cord function after minor trauma, paraparesis, or quadriparesis. Surgical treatment usually involves posterior decompression with consideration given to spinal cord fusion if multiple-level laminectomies are required or preoperative spinal instability is present.

GOLDENHAR SYNDROME

Goldenhar syndrome, also known as oculoauriculovertebral dysplasia, is a clinically heterogeneous disorder occurring in 1 of every 3000 to 5000 live births in North America.[18] It is characterized by hemifacial microsomia, epibulbar dermoid appendages, and spinal defects. As many as 40% of patients with Goldenhar syndrome may have Klippel-Feil–type fusion anomalies of the spine.[19] Additionally, craniofacial, gastrointestinal, cardiac, renal, and ophthalmic anomalies may be seen.[20] Most cases occur sporadically due to a terminal deletion in the short arm of chromosome 5 and trisomy 7 and 9 mosaicism.[18,21–23] This is thought to lead to a disruption in development of the first and second branchial arches as well as in the intervening first pharyngeal pouch and branchial cleft within the first 6 weeks of intrauterine life.[18,20]

The spinal anomalies associated with Goldenhar syndrome include vertebral hypoplasia, segmentation failure, and failure of vertebral formation. Segmentation defects are more common in the cervical spine, whereas vertebral formation failure more often occurs in the thoracolumbar spine.[19,20] Unbalanced hemivertebrae and segmentation defects may result in scoliosis or thoracolumbar kyphosis, often requiring surgical treatment.[19,20] Gibson and colleagues[20] identified vertebral anomalies in 60% of children with Goldenhar syndrome. Among the spinal anomalies identified were block vertebrae (most often involving fusion of C3 and C4), unilateral hemivertebrae in the thoracolumbar spine, spina bifida occulta, butterfly vertebrae, and sacral agenesis.[20] In that series, all patients with scoliosis had an unbalanced hemivertebra.[20] Although several patients required surgical correction of their scoliosis, none of the children in that single-institution series demonstrated any neurologic dysfunction.[20]

Anomalies of the upper cervical spine, including platybasia, occipitalization of the atlas, and odontoid hypoplasia with atlantoaxial instability, have been identified in association with Goldenhar syndrome. One group reported a 12% incidence of platybasia and occipitalization of the atlas.[20] In a series of 8 children with Goldenhar syndrome reported by Healy and colleagues,[18] 3 patients had atlantoaxial subluxation with upward migration of the odontoid process. Two of the patients in that series had atlantoaxial subluxation greater than 7 mm and required occipitocervical fusion.[18] Although atlantoaxial instability may remain clinically silent in children who have not yet reached skeletal maturity, some surgeons advocate treatment in any child with greater than 6 mm of subluxation to reduce the possibility of catastrophic spinal cord impingement.[18] In cases of subluxation less than 6 mm, serial cervical flexion-extension films should be obtained at regular intervals.[18] In addition, due to the high frequency of upper cervical instability, preoperative flexion-extension imaging should be considered in all children with Goldenhar syndrome before undergoing elective endotracheal intubation.

SPONDYLOEPIPHYSEAL DYSPLASIA

SED encompasses several disorders characterized by flattened vertebral bodies and abnormal epiphyses.[24] Typically, children with SED have short-trunk dwarfism with shortened proximal and middle limbs but relatively normal-sized hands and feet. Epiphyseal abnormalities frequently result in precocious osteoarthritis by the third to fourth decade of life.[24] There are 2 major types of SED: SED congenita and SED tarda. SED congenita is the more severe form of the disorder with recognizable features present at birth. It is commonly associated with delayed ossification of vertebral bodies, coxa vara abnormalities of the hips, and retinal detachment.[25] Wynne-Davies and Hall[26] further classified SED congenita into mild or severe clinical subtypes, with the severe subtype marked by extremely short stature and severe coxa vara.

SED congenita is inherited in an autosomal dominant fashion, with most cases resulting from sporadic mutations in the collagen, type II, alpha 1 chain (*COL2A1*) gene on chromosome 12.[27] An X-linked recessive form of SED tarda has also been described with similar clinical manifestations.[28] Such mutations result in defective type II collagen, which is the major matrix protein in the nucleus pulposus, epiphyseal cartilage, and vitreous of the eye.[27]

The signs and symptoms of myelopathy due to SED may develop gradually, manifesting as delayed motor development, slowly progressive weakness, spasticity, or sleep apnea.[29] Atlantoaxial instability associated with odontoid hypoplasia or ligamentous laxity is the most common spinal manifestation of SED congenita in children. The incidence of cervical myelopathy due to atlantoaxial subluxation may be as high as 35% in children with SED congenita.[30] In a study of risk factors for myelopathy in patients with SED congenita, Nakamura and colleagues[29] found that atlantoaxial subluxation (defined as an atlantodental interval [ADI] of 5 mm or more in children) was present in most cases with myelopathy. Studies also suggest that atlantoaxial subluxation with increasing ADIs progress with age.[30] The sagittal axis diameter, measured between the posterior edge of the anterior arch of the atlas and the anterior edge of the posterior arch of the atlas, is small in most patients with SED congenita.[30] Those patients in whom sagittal cervical canal diameter at the level of the atlas is 10 mm or less are at increased risk of spinal cord compression, as are patients with the severe subtype of SED congenita.[29,30] Os odontoideum is frequently present in children with SED and is also associated with a narrowed sagittal axis diameter. In patients with a small sagittal axis diameter and atlantoaxial subluxation, reduction of the subluxation does not ensure an adequate sagittal canal diameter, even in extension.[30] In SED patients, stenosis at the C1 level may be multifactorial such that even with reduction of widened ADI, the canal diameter may still be unacceptably narrow from superimposed C1 stenosis. In these patients, removal of the posterior arch of the atlas in addition to a posterior occipitocervical fusion is recommended to reduce subluxation and to adequately decompress the spinal canal.[29] Preoperative reduction and immobilization in a halo vest may be helpful.[30] Depending on the extent of compression on preoperative imaging, additional procedures, such as a C2 laminoplasty and foramen magnum decompression, may also be required.[30] Perioperative airway management must be tailored to prevent spinal cord injury during induction of anesthesia.

MORQUIO SYNDROME

Morquio syndrome or mucopolysaccharidosis type IV (MPS IV) is an autosomal recessive lysosomal storage disease characterized by the inability to metabolize keratan sulfate, a glycosaminoglycan found predominantly in cartilage and in the cornea. There are 2 subtypes of MPS IV: MPS IV type A, which results from a deficiency in *N*-acetyl-galactosamine-6-sulfatase, and MPS IV type B, which results from a deficiency in β-galactosidase.[31,32] The clinical manifestations typically become apparent between ages 1 and 3 with marked abnormalities in the skeletal system. Individuals with MPS IV have short-trunk dwarfism with skeletal features that may include barrel chest with pectus carinatum, odontoid hypoplasia, thoracolumbar kyphosis, scoliosis, genus valgus, platyspondyly, flaring of the ribs, and joint hypermobility.[31] Corneal clouding is also common in patients with MPS IV. In contrast to patients with other mucopolysaccharidoses, patients with MPS IV have normal intelligence. Although skeletal abnormalities are present and radiologically evident within the first year of life, patients with MPS IV appear healthy at birth and often have normal growth and development for the first 2 years of life.[33] Clinical and phenotypical abnormalities progress rapidly between 2 and 6 years of age. MPS IV occurs in 1 in 40,000 live births, and although patients may survive to adulthood, many patients die in early adulthood, from either cardiopulmonary disease or neurologic complications of their disorder.[31,33]

As in SED congenita, a common and serious condition associated with MPS IV is atlantoaxial subluxation with spinal cord compression. Odontoid dysplasia—which can include hypoplasia, aplasia, or os odontoideum—is often present in MPS IV, as is ligament laxity.[34] Both are contributing factors for atlantoaxial subluxation in these patients.[33] In Stevens and colleagues'[33] series of patients with MPS IV and radiographic atlantoaxial subluxation, odontoid hypoplasia was present in every case. As in patients with SED, primary C1 sinal stenosis can coexist with odontoid and ligamentous abnormalities.[34]

Atlantoaxial subluxation has been identified in up to 42% to 90% of cases of MPS IV.[33,34] Not all patients with atlantoaxial subluxation have spinal cord compression or require surgery. Symptomatic patients or patients with a 50% reduction in spinal cord diameter, however, should be considered for posterior occipitocervical fusion.[33] The preferred time period for an elective operation is between 3 and 8 years of age, when skeletal anomalies are well developed.[33] Preoperative MR imaging is useful to assess extradural soft tissue elements and the degree of cord compression at the craniocervical junction. In patients who have undergone occipitocervical fusion, postoperative studies of the extradural compressive agents suggest a regression of the extradural soft tissue and ossification of previously unossified cartilage.[33]

OSTEOGENESIS IMPERFECTA

OI is an autosomal dominant congenital disorder characterized by osteopenia, fragile bones susceptible to fracture, variable degrees of short stature, and progressive skeletal deformities.[35] This disease results from mutations in 1 of 2 genes that code for the collagen, type I, alpha chains, *COLA1A1* and *COL1A2*, localized to chromosomes 17 and 7, respectively.[36] Type I collagen fibers are found in bone, organ capsules, fascia, cornea, sclera, tendon, meninges, and dermis.[36] There are several classification schemes for subtypes of OI; the most common of these categorizes OI into 4 subtypes. Type I is a mild form with no long bone deformities and a normal life expectancy; type II is lethal in the perinatal period with in utero fractures; type III is the most severe form in children who survive the perinatal period; and type IV is associated with moderate bone deformities and variable short stature with a near-normal life expectancy.[36–38]

Kyphosis and scoliosis are the most common spine manifestations of OI in children. The incidence of scoliosis in OI is reported to be age dependent but as high as 80% in some series.[39,40] Benson and colleagues[39] found that the incidence of scoliosis is 26% in children younger than 6 years of age and that the incidence of scoliosis rises significantly in children 6 years of age and older. There is a predictable, early progression of scoliotic curves in children with OI. The scoliotic curve in OI usually progresses despite bracing. Brace therapy in severe forms of OI is usually not indicated because of poor therapeutic results and a high complication rate. Furthermore, the ribs of affected patients with OI type III and type IV are too fragile to transmit corrective forces to the spine with bracing, and bracing often causes further deformities of the rib cage that can, in turn, compromise pulmonary function.[39–41] Early spinal fusion in children with curves less than 40° has been advocated by some to halt or slow progression of spinal deformity and cardiopulmonary dysfunction.[40] Kyphosis, like scoliosis, is often associated with more severe forms of OI.[35]

Patients with OI are at risk for compression fractures and vertebral body collapse.[39] The vertebrae assume a biconcave shape, and microfractures adjacent to vertebral growth plates can interfere with growth and cause deformity.[39] Ishikawa and colleagues[42] found that severe scoliosis (>50°) was likely to develop in prepubescent children with 6 or more biconcave vertebrae. Cyclic intravenous bisphosphonate pamidronate therapy given monthly was found to have beneficial effects on vertebral morphometry in children and adolescents with severe forms of OI.[43] With treatment, there is increased cortical long bone thickness and bone mineral density in the lumbar vertebral bodies, decreased fracture rates, and improved mobility.[38] Moreover, the effect is greatest in vertebral bodies that are more compressed.[38] Early treatment is advocated in children, and pretreatment may improve surgical outcomes for scoliosis.

A rare but potentially serious condition associated with OI is basilar impression due to repetitive microfractures of the base of the skull adjacent to the foramen magnum.[37] Janus and colleagues[37] report a series of 130 children with OI who were found to have basilar impression. None of these children displayed neurologic symptoms. The condition may progress slowly, and it is rare for children with OI to require surgical treatment. Surgery is indicated, however, if there is symptomatic compromise of the spinal cord. If there is significant anterior compression present, an anterior transoral approach for ventral clival-odontoid anterior atlas arch resection followed by posterior stabilization may be required.

LARSEN SYNDROME

Larsen syndrome is a rare congenital disorder of connective tissue characterized by cervical spine anomalies, anterior dislocation of the knees, dislocations of the hips and elbows, equinovarus deformities of the feet, supernumerary ossification of the hands and feet, long fingers with shortened metacarpals, dysmorphic facies with frontal bossing, hypertelorism, and a depressed nasal bridge.[44–49] The cervical spine is more often affected than the thoracic or lumbar spine, and typical vertebral anomalies include hypoplastic or flattened vertebral bodies, dysraphism, hemivertebrae, and wedged vertebrae.[44,45] Most cases occur sporadically, although autosomal recessive and dominant transmission have also been reported.[44,45]

Abnormal spinal curvatures are also common in Larsen syndrome, including cervical kyphosis, thoracic lordosis, lumbar kyphosis, scoliosis, and spondylolysis.[45] Midcervical kyphosis, seen most commonly at C4–C5, can lead to instability, myelopathy, weakness, and even sudden death in children with Larsen syndrome.[44,47,48,50] In Bowen and colleagues'[45] single-institution series, the incidence of cervical kyphosis was 12%. In another series of 38 children with Larsen syndrome, sudden death occurred in 37% of children with an average age at death of 1 year.[47] Micheli and colleagues[48] followed 3 children with Larsen syndrome and cervicothoracic segmental abnormalities, one of whom developed progressive instability and subluxation due to midcervical kyphosis and subsequently expired from sudden cardiorespiratory arrest. Subsequent postmortem studies of this patient revealed a C4–C5 subluxation in association with cervicomedullary compression and extensive gliosis and axonotmesis on histology studies.[48] Forese and colleagues[50] also reported 1 case of sudden death in a 6-month-old infant with Larsen syndrome and severe midcervical kyphosis.

Anteroposterior dissociation with cervical kyphosis due to absence of pedicles has been frequently reported in Larsen syndrome.[51,52] The result is near-complete separation of the laminae and vertebral bodies at multiple levels, making operative fusion difficult and requiring extension of the fusion for several levels beyond the affected segments.[52] Katz and colleagues[51] described 2 such patients with cervical kyphosis, anteroposterior dissociation, and quadriparesis in Larsen syndrome. One neonate was treated nonoperatively with early traction and cervicothoracolumbosacral orthosis and demonstrated clinical and radiographic improvement to at least 3 years of age.[51] Other practitioners have favored early treatment of cervical kyphosis by posterior fusion in patients with Larsen syndrome.[53,54]

Although the natural history and optimal treatment of cervical spine anomalies have not been clearly established via long-term studies, a common practice pattern is to radiographically evaluate patients with Larsen syndrome at baseline with radiographs, such as cervical plain films in neutral, flexion, and extension positions. These can be supplemented with CT and MR imaging. The value of routine (yearly) follow-up imaging is uncertain, but it is often done, even in the absence of neurologic deterioration.

SPINA BIFIDA

Spinal bifida is a birth defect resulting from incomplete closure of the neural tube during development. In the United States, neural tube defects affect 3000 pregnancies every year.[55] Included in this group of disorders are myelomeningocele, lipomeningocele, and several other forms of occult spinal dysraphism. A comprehensive review of spina bifida is beyond the scope of this article; therefore, this subsection focuses on neurosurgical considerations in diagnosis, workup, and treatment of myelomeningocele (MM) and lipomyelomeningocele.

Embryologically, the neural tube forms during primary neurulation, which occurs during days 17 to 27 of gestation. The ectoderm overlying the notochord proliferates and differentiates forming the neural plate. Midline cells overlying the notochord assume a wedge shape that, in cross section, creates a U shape from the original plate. The top edges of the U later fuse to form the neural tube. Neural tube closure begins by the twenty-first day of gestation and the posterior neuropore closes by the twenty-seventh day of gestation. Immediately after neurulation, the distal neural tube undergoes canalization. The distal neural tube develops into the conus medullaris, cauda equina, and filum terminale. Canalization ends by the forty-eighth day of gestation. Differential and simultaneous growth of the caudal spinal cord and vertebral bodies results in ascension of the conus and elongation of the filum terminale.

MYELOMENINGOCELE

MM is a congenital malformation arising from a local failure of primary neurulation (**Fig. 1**). MM results from a focal failure of dorsal fusion of the neural fold, leaving the vertebral arches open with the unfused spinal cord exposed. MM occurs in 0.41 to 1.43 per 1000 live births in North America.[56] MM is associated with many neurologic abnormalities, including hydrocephalus, Chiari type II malformation, syringomyelia, and tethered cord syndrome. Most children with MM have some degree of lower-extremity weakness. Muscle imbalance resulting from denervation

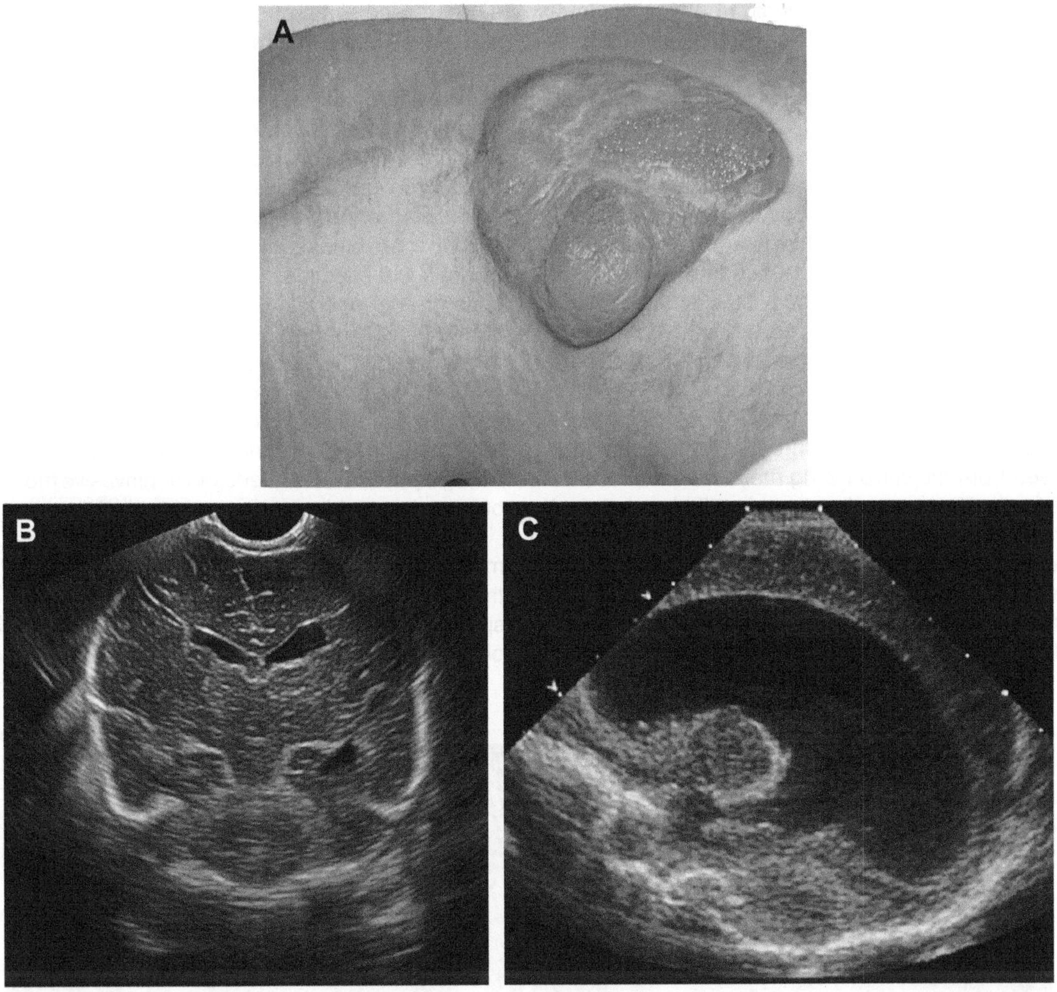

Fig. 1. (*A*) Typical appearance of a newborn baby with myelomeningocele. (*B*) Cranial ultrasound initially demonstrated only mild ventriculomegaly. Given this finding and a reassuring physical examination, the decision was made to postpone shunt placement. (*C*) Four days later, the anterior fontanelle was full and a repeat cranial ultrasound confirmed worsening ventriculomegaly. A ventriculoperitoneal shunt was placed.

may cause orthopedic abnormalities of the hip, knee, or feet. Compromise of nerves supplying the bladder results in bladder dysfunction. Proper management of these associated conditions may significantly improve patient outcomes. In developed nations, due to early primary surgical repair and close follow-up by a multidisciplinary team of physicians, a large percentage of patients with MM can be expected to reach adulthood, with 82% of survivors achieving independence in their activities of daily living.[56]

The prenatal diagnosis of MM relies on maternal serum α-fetoprotein, fetal ultrasonography, and amniocentesis. Elevated maternal serum α-fetoprotein levels measured at 16 to 18 weeks gestation are 75% sensitive for detecting open neural tube defects.[57] Prenatal counseling for parents of children with MM may help clear up confusion, relieve fears, and allow practitioners to present an accurate picture of MM and the expected clinical course.

The initial neurosurgical treatment of children with MM involves closure of the MM and treatment of hydrocephalus. Before MM closure, the placode should be covered with a moist dressing. It is generally accepted that emergent operative intervention is not necessary and repair may be safely performed within 48 hours after delivery.[58] A thorough examination of the newborn should be performed, with focus on lower-extremity sensorimotor function. Physical examination should include assessment for signs of hydrocephalus, including split cranial sutures, a bulging or tense anterior fontanelle, or paresis of upgaze. Cranial and spinal ultrasound, including both the cranio-cervical junction as well as the remainder of the spine, may help a surgeon assess for hydrocephalus, the extent of Chiari type II malformation, and any other associated abnormalities.

A meticulous initial repair of MM may reduce the incidence of secondary lesions, such as dermoid cysts later in life. The exposed neural placode is dissected beginning at the lateral aspect at the junction of the zona epitheliosa and the edge of the zona cutanea. The edges of the neural placode should be inspected to ensure that no dermal elements are included in the placode. Nerve roots can be seen passing from the placode down to the spinal canal. The floor of the sac under the placode is formed by the underlying dura, which must be freed from the surrounding mesodermal elements laterally. The dural edges are identified and closed in a watertight manner. The lumbodorsal fascia and overlying defect skin should then be closed, excluding any compromised areas of skin. Recent studies suggest a benefit to local or myofascial flap closure in MM. Long-term results suggest a decreased rate of postoperative CSF leaks and infection in children following a myofascial closure.[59]

Associated hydrocephalus occurs in approximately 75% of children with MM.[60] In children who present with obvious clinical signs and symptoms of hydrocephalus, CSF shunting may be considered concurrently with MM repair. Several retrospective studies suggest there is no increased risk of shunt infection or closure-related complications if the operations are performed concurrently.[61,62] Although shunt placement is required for patients with obvious signs of hydrocephalus, patients with asymptomatic, mild ventricular enlargement may be followed with frequent clinical examinations and imaging follow-up. Cranial ultrasonography is a convenient and noninvasive means of following ventricular size in these patients.

Tethered cord syndrome (TCS) occurs in as many as 32% of patients with MM (**Fig. 2**). It is theorized that this is a result of stretching of the spinal cord from a combination of scarring of the placode to the surrounding structures and

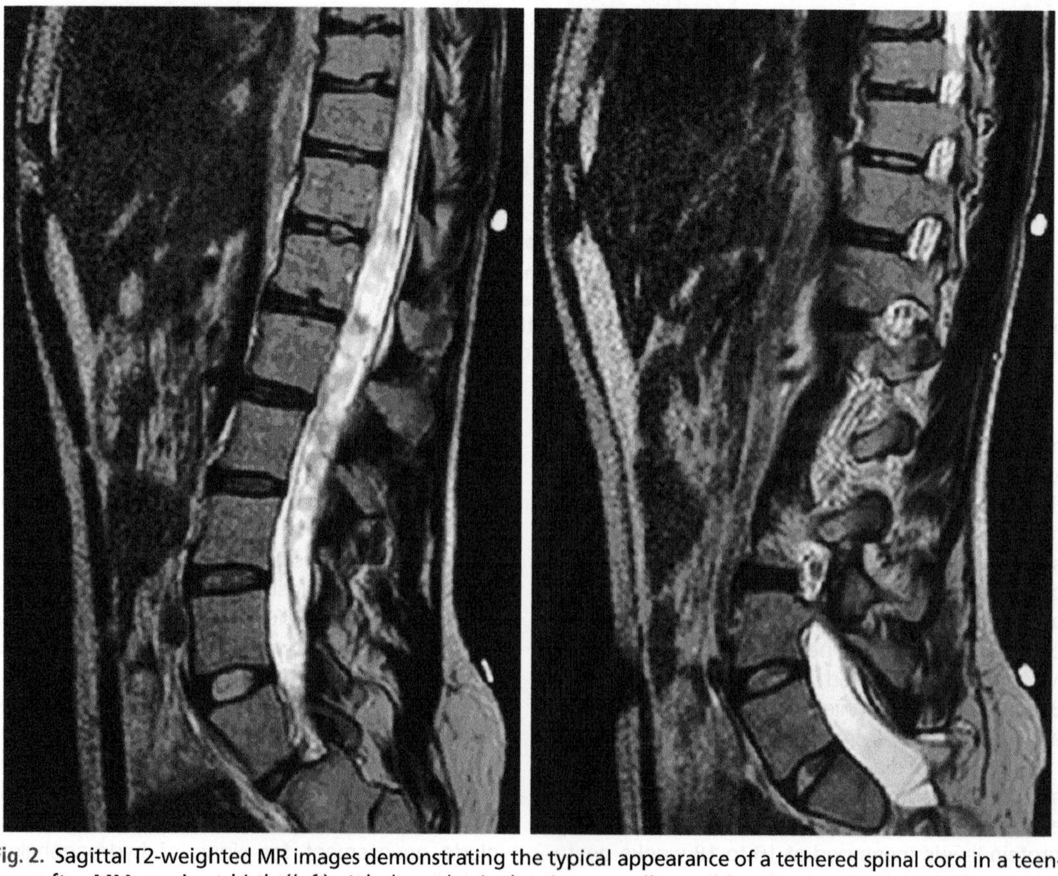

Fig. 2. Sagittal T2-weighted MR images demonstrating the typical appearance of a tethered spinal cord in a teenager after MM repair at birth (*left*). A holocord spinal syrinx as well as mild scoliosis may also be appreciated (*right*).

vertebral column lengthening during growth.[63–67] Symptoms typically present between ages 6 and 13 years but can occur at any age.[68,69] As the length of the spinal canal changes during normal movements, such as flexion and extension, the length of the spinal cord must also change with the spinal canal. The spinal cord is normally attached caudally to the filum terminale, which is a thin band of connective tissue that extends from the caudal end of the spinal cord to the inferior termination of the spinal canal. This attachment of the spinal cord to the filum terminale does not normally apply significant traction to the cord itself during normal movements. Similarly, although nerve roots leave the cord at each functional spinal level, they do not normally tether the cord in an anatomic position. Therefore, the spinal cord is not normally physiologically tethered by its attachments within the caudal dural sac. In contrast, in cases of TCS there is an abnormal

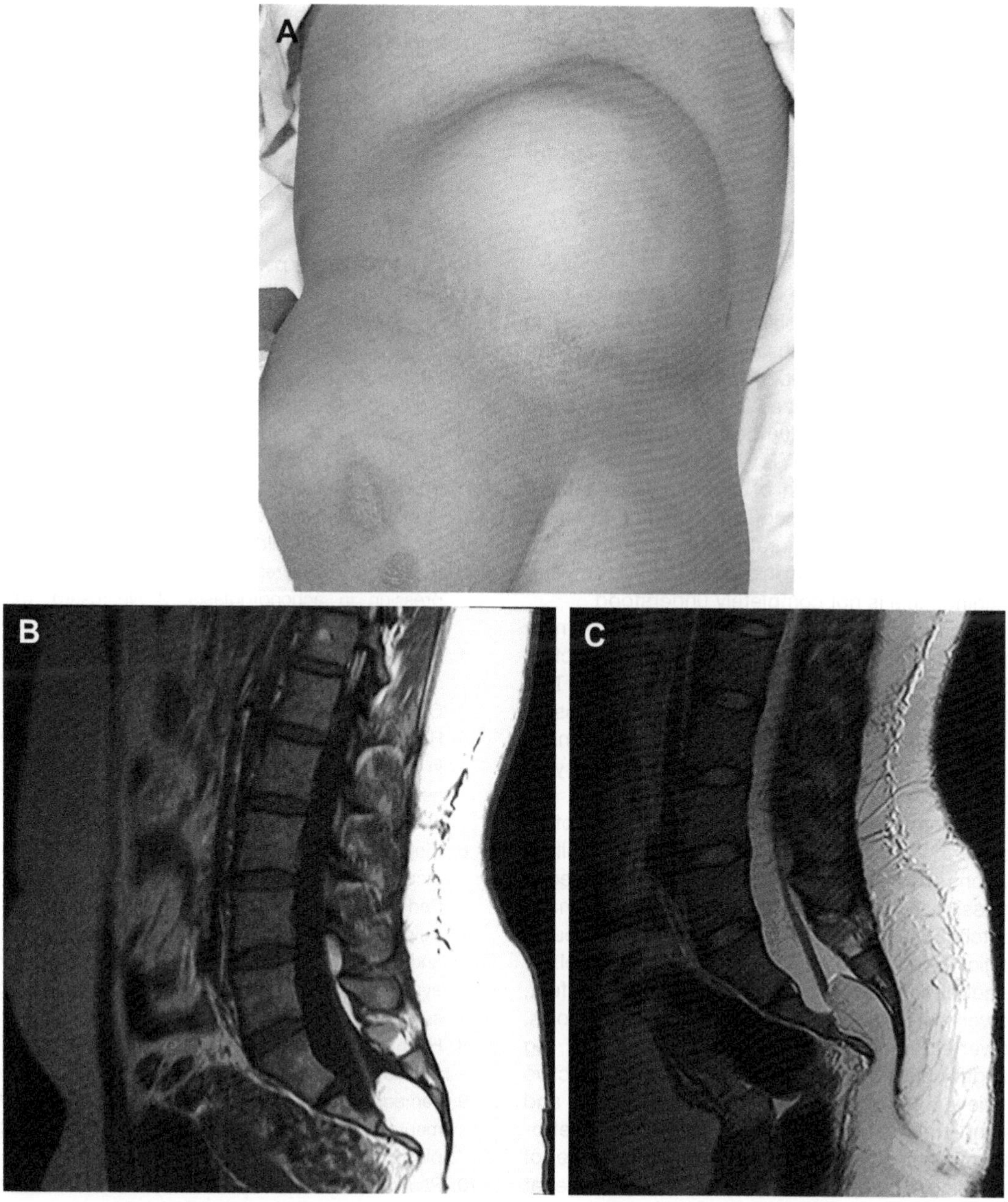

Fig. 3. (*A*) Typical appearance of a newborn baby with a lipomyelomeningocele. Sagittal T1-weighted (*B*) and T2-weighted (*C*) MR images from a teenager demonstrate the typical imaging appearance of a terminal lipomyelocele with a tethered spinal cord.

attachment of the cord, most often caudally, to surrounding structures. These abnormal attachments limit movement of the cord.[68,70,71] Tethering and subsequent traction of the spinal cord during motion of the spinal canal have been shown to cause derangements in blood flow and oxidative metabolism, ultimately leading to cord ischemia and worsening neurologic function.[72,73]

Although anatomic tethering of the spinal cord is a nearly universal finding on MR imaging after MM repair, only those patients with progressive symptoms due to spinal tethering are considered to have TCS. Symptoms of TCS can include back pain, progressive leg weakness or ambulation difficulties, leg numbness, or a progressive decline in bladder function.[69] Patients with severe or progressive symptoms should be considered for secondary untethering surgery.[69]

LIPOMYELOMENINGOCELE

Lipomyelomeningocele is the most common form of occult spinal dysraphism (**Fig. 3**). It occurs in 16 of 100,000 live births in North America, with a slightly increased incidence in girls.[74] The condition is typically recognized in children with a cutaneous lipoma in the lumbosacral region of the spine. The condition is characterized by an abnormal accumulation of subcutaneous fat extending to the conus medullaris, leading to spinal cord tethering. The natural history and pattern of neurologic deterioration in children with lipomyelomeningocele is not completely understood.

Lipomyelomeningoceles are disorders of primary neurulation, resulting from a focal nondisjunction of cutaneous ectoderm from neuroectoderm. This allows mesenchymal derivatives (adipose tissue) to enter the neural tube. Histologically, the mass is composed of clusters of mature adipocytes with intervening bands of collagen.[75]

Children with lipomyelomeningocele often present with both clinical and neurologic manifestations of the disease. In addition to a subcutaneous mass, many have depigmented areas of skin, hairy patches, hemangiomas, or skin tags.[76,77] Neurologic symptoms include neurogenic bowel or bladder, an arched instep in one or both feet, lower-extremity weakness, progressive scoliosis, lower-extremity spasticity, back pain, and leg length discrepancy.[77,78] In one retrospective review, 52% of patients presented with signs and symptoms of neurologic deterioration.[76] Retrospective analysis suggests that the degree of neurologic symptoms relates to patient age at time of diagnosis. Hoffman and colleagues[76] showed that 62.5% of patients who presented at less than 6 months of age were asymptomatic, whereas only 29% of children older than 6 months were asymptomatic at diagnosis. Other studies found no asymptomatic children older then 5 years of age at diagnosis.[79] Studies reviewing long-term follow-up over 20 years after untethering of children with lipomyelomeningocele suggest that although bowel and bladder function often do not improve, lower-extremity sensorimotor function often shows some recovery.[76,77,79] Because the deterioration pattern in many series seemed unpredictable and many of the neurologic symptoms (in particular those involving bowel and bladder function) are incompletely reversed after untethering, many surgeons recommend untethering at the time of diagnosis, regardless of neurologic function or patient age.[80]

ACKNOWLEDGMENTS

We gratefully acknowledge the assistance of Holly Wagner in the preparation of this manuscript.

REFERENCES

1. Bagley CA, Pindrik JA, Bookland MJ, et al. Cervicomedullary decompression for foramen magnum stenosis in achondroplasia. J Neurosurg 2006;104(Suppl 3):166–72.
2. Ruiz-Garcia M, Tovar-Baudin A, Del Castillo-Ruiz V, et al. Early detection of neurological manifestations in achondroplasia. Childs Nerv Syst 1997;13(4):208–13.
3. Ryken TC, Menezes AH. Cervicomedullary compression in achondroplasia. J Neurosurg 1994;81(1):43–8.
4. Frigon VA, Castro FP, Whitecloud TS, et al. Isolated subaxial cervical spine stenosis in achondroplasia. Curr Surg 2000;57(4):354–6.
5. Rimoin DL. Cervicomedullary junction compression in infants with achondroplasia: when to perform neurosurgical decompression. Am J Hum Genet 1995;56(4):824–7.
6. King JA, Vachhrajani S, Drake JM, et al. Neurosurgical implications of achondroplasia. J Neurosurg Pediatr 2009;4(4):297–306.
7. Keiper GL Jr, Koch B, Crone KR. Achondroplasia and cervicomedullary compression: prospective evaluation and surgical treatment. Pediatr Neurosurg 1999;31(2):78–83.
8. Hecht JT, Butler IJ. Neurologic morbidity associated with achondroplasia. J Child Neurol 1990;5(2):84–97.
9. Yamada Y, Ito H, Otsubo Y, et al. Surgical management of cervicomedullary compression in achondroplasia. Childs Nerv Syst 1996;12(12):737–41.
10. Pauli RM, Horton VK, Glinski LP, et al. Prospective assessment of risks for cervicomedullary-junction compression in infants with achondroplasia. Am J Hum Genet 1995;56(3):732–44.

11. Reid CS, Pyeritz RE, Kopits SE, et al. Cervicomedullary compression in young patients with achondroplasia: value of comprehensive neurologic and respiratory evaluation. J Pediatr 1987;110(4):522–30.
12. Hecht JT, Francomano CA, Horton WA, et al. Mortality in achondroplasia. Am J Hum Genet 1987;41(3):454–64.
13. Kao SC, Waziri MH, Smith WL, et al. MR imaging of the craniovertebral junction, cranium, and brain in children with achondroplasia. AJR Am J Roentgenol 1989;153(3):565–9.
14. Aryanpur J, Hurko O, Francomano C, et al. Craniocervical decompression for cervicomedullary compression in pediatric patients with achondroplasia. J Neurosurg 1990;73(3):375–82.
15. Morgan DF, Young RF. Spinal neurological complications of achondroplasia. Results of surgical treatment. J Neurosurg 1980;52(4):463–72.
16. Fortuna A, Ferrante L, Acqui M, et al. Narrowing of thoraco-lumbar spinal canal in achondroplasia. J Neurosurg Sci 1989;33(2):185–96.
17. Sciubba DM, Noggle JC, Marupudi NI, et al. Spinal stenosis surgery in pediatric patients with achondroplasia. J Neurosurg 2007;106(5 Suppl):372–8.
18. Healey D, Letts M, Jarvis JG. Cervical spine instability in children with Goldenhar's syndrome. Can J Surg 2002;45(5):341–4.
19. Tsirikos AI, McMaster MJ. Goldenhar-associated conditions (hemifacial microsomia) and congenital deformities of the spine. Spine (Phila Pa 1976) 2006;31(13):E400–7.
20. Gibson JN, Sillence DO, Taylor TK. Abnormalities of the spine in Goldenhar's syndrome. J Pediatr Orthop 1996;16(3):344–9.
21. Choong YF, Watts P, Little E, et al. Goldenhar and cri-du-chat syndromes: a contiguous gene deletion syndrome? J Aapos 2003;7(3):226–7.
22. Hodes ME, Gleiser S, DeRosa GP, et al. Trisomy 7 mosaicism and manifestations of Goldenhar syndrome with unilateral radial hypoplasia. J Craniofac Genet Dev Biol 1981;1(1):49–55.
23. Wilson GN, Barr M Jr. Trisomy 9 mosaicism: another etiology for the manifestations of Goldenhar syndrome. J Craniofac Genet Dev Biol 1983;3(4):313–6.
24. Williams CJ, Considine EL, Knowlton RG, et al. Spondyloepiphyseal dysplasia and precocious osteoarthritis in a family with an Arg75–>Cys mutation in the procollagen type II gene (COL2A1). Hum Genet 1993;92(5):499–505.
25. Bethem D, Winter RB, Lutter L, et al. Spinal disorders of dwarfism. Review of the literature and report of eighty cases. J Bone Joint Surg Am 1981;63(9):1412–25.
26. Wynne-Davies R, Hall C. Two clinical variants of spondylo-epiphysial dysplasia congenita. J Bone Joint Surg Br 1982;64(4):435–41.
27. Anderson IJ, Goldberg RB, Marion RW, et al. Spondyloepiphyseal dysplasia congenita: genetic linkage to type II collagen (COL2AI). Am J Hum Genet 1990;46(5):896–901.
28. Whyte MP, Gottesman GS, Eddy MC, et al. X-linked recessive spondyloepiphyseal dysplasia tarda. Clinical and radiographic evolution in a 6-generation kindred and review of the literature. Medicine (Baltimore) 1999;78(1):9–25.
29. Nakamura K, Miyoshi K, Haga N, et al. Risk factors of myelopathy at the atlantoaxial level in spondyloepiphyseal dysplasia congenita. Arch Orthop Trauma Surg 1998;117(8):468–70.
30. Miyoshi K, Nakamura K, Haga N, et al. Surgical treatment for atlantoaxial subluxation with myelopathy in spondyloepiphyseal dysplasia congenita. Spine (Phila Pa 1976) 2004;29(21):E488–91.
31. Northover H, Cowie RA, Wraith JE. Mucopolysaccharidosis type IVA (Morquio syndrome): a clinical review. J Inherit Metab Dis 1996;19(3):357–65.
32. Piccirilli CB, Chadduck WM. Cervical kyphotic myelopathy in a child with Morquio syndrome. Childs Nerv Syst 1996;12(2):114–6.
33. Stevens JM, Kendall BE, Crockard HA, et al. The odontoid process in Morquio-Brailsford's disease. The effects of occipitocervical fusion. J Bone Joint Surg Br 1991;73(5):851–8.
34. Takeda E, Hashimoto T, Tayama M, et al. Diagnosis of atlantoaxial subluxation in Morquio's syndrome and spondyloepiphyseal dysplasia congenita. Acta Paediatr Jpn 1991;33(5):633–8.
35. Engelbert RH, Gerver WJ, Breslau-Siderius LJ, et al. Spinal complications in osteogenesis imperfecta: 47 patients 1-16 years of age. Acta Orthop Scand 1998;69(3):283–6.
36. Rauch F, Glorieux FH. Osteogenesis imperfecta. Lancet 2004;363(9418):1377–85.
37. Janus GJ, Engelbert RH, Beek E, et al. Osteogenesis imperfecta in childhood: MR imaging of basilar impression. Eur J Radiol 2003;47(1):19–24.
38. Land C, Rauch F, Munns CF, et al. Vertebral morphometry in children and adolescents with osteogenesis imperfecta: effect of intravenous pamidronate treatment. Bone 2006;39(4):901–6.
39. Benson DR, Donaldson DH, Millar EA. The spine in osteogenesis imperfecta. J Bone Joint Surg Am 1978;60(7):925–9.
40. Widmann RF, Bitan FD, Laplaza FJ, et al. Spinal deformity, pulmonary compromise, and quality of life in osteogenesis imperfecta. Spine (Phila Pa 1976) 1999;24(16):1673–8.
41. Hanscom DA, Winter RB, Lutter L, et al. Osteogenesis imperfecta. Radiographic classification, natural history, and treatment of spinal deformities. J Bone Joint Surg Am 1992;74(4):598–616.
42. Ishikawa S, Kumar SJ, Takahashi HE, et al. Vertebral body shape as a predictor of spinal deformity in

osteogenesis imperfecta. J Bone Joint Surg Am 1996;78(2):212–9.
43. Astrom E, Soderhall S. Beneficial effect of long term intravenous bisphosphonate treatment of osteogenesis imperfecta. Arch Dis Child 2002;86(5): 356–64.
44. Banks JT, Wellons JC 3rd, Tubbs RS, et al. Cervical spine involvement in Larsen's syndrome: a case illustration. Pediatrics 2003;111(1):199–201.
45. Bowen JR, Ortega K, Ray S, et al. Spinal deformities in Larsen's syndrome. Clin Orthop Relat Res 1985; 197:159–63.
46. Larsen LJ, Schottstaedt ER, Bost FC. Multiple congenital dislocations associated with characteristic facial abnormality. J Pediatr 1950;37(4):574–81.
47. Laville JM, Lakermance P, Limouzy F. Larsen's syndrome: review of the literature and analysis of thirty-eight cases. J Pediatr Orthop 1994;14(1): 63–73.
48. Micheli LJ, Hall JE, Watts HG. Spinal instability in Larsen's syndrome: report of three cases. J Bone Joint Surg Am 1976;58(4):562–5.
49. Weisenbach J, Melegh B. Vertebral anomalies in Larsen's syndrome. Pediatr Radiol 1996;26(9):682–3.
50. Forese LL, Berdon WE, Harcke HT, et al. Severe mid-cervical kyphosis with cord compression in Larsen's syndrome and diastrophic dysplasia: unrelated syndromes with similar radiologic findings and neurosurgical implications. Pediatr Radiol 1995; 25(2):136–9.
51. Katz DA, Hall JE, Emans JB. Cervical kyphosis associated with anteroposterior dissociation and quadriparesis in Larsen's syndrome. J Pediatr Orthop 2005;25(4):429–33.
52. Luk KD, Yip DK. Congenital anteroposterior spinal dissociation in Larsen's Syndrome: report on two operated cases with long-term follow-up. Spine (Phila Pa 1976) 2002;27(12):E296–300.
53. Francis WR Jr, Noble DP. Treatment of cervical kyphosis in children. Spine (Phila Pa 1976) 1988; 13(8):883–7.
54. Johnston CE 2nd, Birch JG, Daniels JL. Cervical kyphosis in patients who have Larsen syndrome. J Bone Joint Surg Am 1996;78(4):538–45.
55. Au KS, Ashley-Koch A, Northrup H. Epidemiologic and genetic aspects of spina bifida and other neural tube defects. Dev Disabil Res Rev 2010;16(1):6–15.
56. Dias MS. Neurosurgical management of myelomeningocele (spina bifida). Pediatr Rev 2005;26(2):50–60.
57. Cuckle HS. Screening for neural tube defects. In: Bock G, Marsh J, editors. Neural tube defects. CIBA foundation symposium 181. West Sussex (England): John Wiley & Sons Ltd; 1994. p. 253–69.
58. Charney EB, Weller SC, Sutton LN, et al. Management of the newborn with myelomeningocele: time for a decision-making process. Pediatrics 1985; 75(1):58–64.
59. Lien SC, Maher CO, Garton HJ, et al. Local and regional flap closure in myelomeningocele repair: a 15-year review. Childs Nerv Syst 2010;26(8):1091–5.
60. Swank M, Dias L. Myelomeningocele: a review of the orthopaedic aspects of 206 patients treated from birth with no selection criteria. Dev Med Child Neurol 1992;34(12):1047–52.
61. Epstein NE, Rosenthal AD, Zito J, et al. Shunt placement and myelomeningocele repair: simultaneous vs sequential shunting. Review of 12 cases. Childs Nerv Syst 1985;1(3):145–7.
62. Parent AD, McMillan T. Contemporaneous shunting with repair of myelomeningocele. Pediatr Neurosurg 1995;22(3):132–6.
63. Bowman RM, McLone DG, Grant JA, et al. Spina bifida outcome: a 25-year prospective. Pediatr Neurosurg 2001;34(3):114–20.
64. Phuong LK, Schoeberl KA, Raffel C. Natural history of tethered cord in patients with meningomyelocele. Neurosurgery 2002;50(5):989–93 [discussion: 993–5].
65. Selber P, Dias L. Sacral-level myelomeningocele: long-term outcome in adults. J Pediatr Orthop 1998;18(4):423–7.
66. Shurtleff DB, Duguay S, Duguay G, et al. Epidemiology of tethered cord with meningomyelocele. Eur J Pediatr Surg 1997;7(Suppl 1):7–11.
67. Tamaki N, Shirataki K, Kojima N, et al. Tethered cord syndrome of delayed onset following repair of myelomeningocele. J Neurosurg 1988;69(3):393–8.
68. Herman JM, McLone DG, Storrs BB, et al. Analysis of 153 patients with myelomeningocele or spinal lipoma reoperated upon for a tethered cord. Presentation, management and outcome. Pediatr Neurosurg 1993;19(5):243–9.
69. Maher CO, Goumnerova L, Madsen JR, et al. Outcome following multiple repeated spinal cord untethering operations. J Neurosurg 2007;106(Suppl 6):434–8.
70. McLone DG, La Marca F. The tethered spinal cord: diagnosis, significance, and management. Semin Pediatr Neurol 1997;4(3):192–208.
71. Schoenmakers MA, Gooskens RH, Gulmans VA, et al. Long-term outcome of neurosurgical untethering on neurosegmental motor and ambulation levels. Dev Med Child Neurol 2003;45(8):551–5.
72. Tani S, Yamada S, Knighton RS. Extensibility of the lumbar and sacral cord. Pathophysiology of the tethered spinal cord in cats. J Neurosurg 1987;66(1):116–23.
73. Yamada S, Zinke DE, Sanders D. Pathophysiology of "tethered cord syndrome". J Neurosurg 1981;54(4): 494–503.
74. McNeely PD, Howes WJ. Ineffectiveness of dietary folic acid supplementation on the incidence of lipomyelomeningocele: pathogenetic implications. J Neurosurg 2004;100(Suppl Pediatrics 2):98–100.
75. Naidich TP, McLone DG, Mutluer S. A new understanding of dorsal dysraphism with lipoma (lipomyeloschisis): radiologic evaluation and surgical

correction. AJR Am J Roentgenol 1983;140(6):1065–78.

76. Hoffman HJ, Taecholarn C, Hendrick EB, et al. Management of lipomyelomeningoceles. Experience at the Hospital for Sick Children, Toronto. J Neurosurg 1985;62(1):1–8.
77. Kanev PM, Lemire RJ, Loeser JD, et al. Management and long-term follow-up review of children with lipomyelomeningocele, 1952-1987. J Neurosurg 1990;73(1):48–52.
78. Kanev PM, Bierbrauer KS. Reflections on the natural history of lipomyelomeningocele. Pediatr Neurosurg 1995;22(3):137–40.
79. Koyanagi I, Iwasaki Y, Hida K, et al. Surgical treatment supposed natural history of the tethered cord with occult spinal dysraphism. Childs Nerv Syst 1997;13(5):268–74.
80. Cochrane DD. Cord untethering for lipomyelomeningocele: expectation after surgery. Neurosurg Focus 2007;23(2):1–7.

Index

Note: Page numbers of article titles are in **boldface** type.

Neuroimag Clin N Am 21 (2011) 733–736
doi:10.1016/S1052-5149(11)00100-6
1052-5149/11/$ – see front matter

FPO

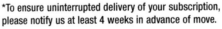

Printed and bound by CPI Group (UK) Ltd, Croydon, CR0 4YY
03/10/2024
01040348-0014